ICD10 & CPT/HCPCS COMPREHENSIVE PHYSICIAN MEDICAL CODING WITH TEST PREPARATION (CPC & CCS-P)

By Dr. Lyn Olsen
RHIT, CCS, CPC-H, CCS-P, CPC

This book is dedicated to the children who teach us the most valuable lessons in life, especially how to love another with our whole hearts as my daughters and grandchildren have done for me… you are my miracles from God.

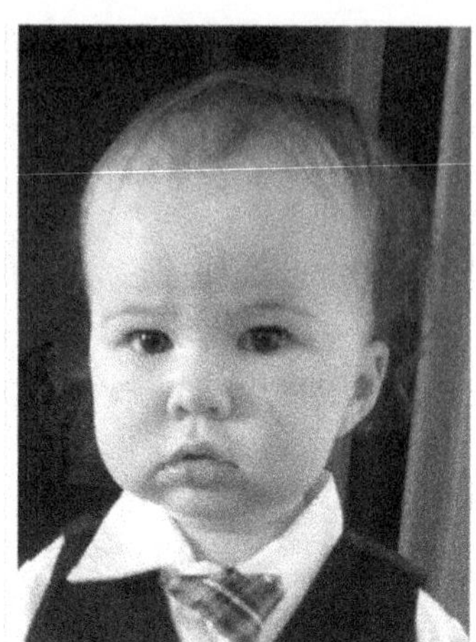

TABLE OF CONTENTS

CHAPTER 1

MEDICAL CODING CAREER

You will learn the following objectives in this chapter:

A. Importance of Coders
B. Responsibilities of Coders
C. Career Ladder for Coders
D. Future for Coders
E. Education

Section 1.1: IMPORTANCE OF CODERS IN HEALTHCARE ADMINISTRATION

Times have changed, and nowhere is this more evident that in the field of healthcare administration which has become highly complex and regulated. The essential ingredient in all of these changes and in the vitality of healthcare institutions is the critical role of medical coders because they ensure the successful continuance of physician practices and hospitals and proper provision of healthcare to patients. The reasons for the critical role of medical coders will be discussed thoroughly in this book as well as the importance for quality in instruction of medical coding so that medical coders can, not only be nationally certified, but also perform all levels of job responsibilities.

Despite the increased central role of medical coding in the proper functioning and continuance of healthcare, too often physicians and healthcare administrators fail to recognize the importance of highly qualified medical coders, and all too often they suffer the consequences of not hiring and maintaining qualified medical coders. An important lesson to be learned is that medical coding is not data entry, and the adoption of this attitude can, and has, produced devastating consequences.

To be a highly qualified medical coder, it is best for the coder to have certain qualities and knowledge including, not only the specifics of medical coding, but also of reimbursement, regulations, medical terminology, anatomy and physiology, fraud and abuse, compliance, confidentiality, and auditing plus more which should be achieved through the process of critical thinking. Critical thinking is vital because medical coding is a highly professional and complex profession requiring extensive education and experience and failure to perform these duties properly today will definitely result in increased regulation and severe penalties executed by government agencies. Medical coders are, therefore, at the center of the practice of healthcare today.

While there are time and money constraints within a healthcare practice, it must be recognized that a qualified coder is a necessary expense because, not only do they capture all proper reimbursement for services provided by a healthcare provider within the proper time frame, but they also can recapture lost reimbursement from previous improper billing and reduce or eliminate regulatory penalties Never should the importance of these responsibilities be underestimated and relegated to data entry positions.

Coding responsibilities may be concentrated in a few selected employees or may be diluted throughout a healthcare practice amongst a myriad of employees whose duties can vary. In larger healthcare practices, there may be several coders whose specific duties are solely associated with responsibilities relating to coding and related training. It is the expectations of payers, particularly, the government, that healthcare practices have adopted proper administrative and reimbursement procedures and policies that ensure proper reimbursement. It is essential that there are well-qualified coders assigned to develop, implement and monitor related policies and procedures to ensure proper coding and reimbursement.

Section 1.2: RESPONSIBILITIES OF CODERS

Duties of a coder are, therefore, vast and highly valuable to the well-being of the healthcare practice. These duties can include:

(1) Proper coding of all types of medical records including office and hospital visits, surgical procedures, anesthesia services, radiology and laboratory services, medicine services and many other services utilizing proper and updated coding manuals.
(2) Determine performance of quality and quantity of other employees' work performed through regular audits.
(3) Providing teaching to staff and physicians determined by audits.
(4) Abstract proper codes and information from medical records.
(5) Ensure optimal and proper reimbursement.
(6) Ensure compliance with government regulations and rules.
(7) Development of compliance plan.
(8) Ensure confidentiality by the exercise of proper security and implementation of privacy rules and policies.
(9) Maintain high levels of standards and knowledge by maintaining certification by engaging in learning activities, such as seminars and courses.
(10) Ensure maintenance of proper medical record formatting and data collection through chart reviews.
(11) Participate in accreditation processes such as the Joint Commission on Accreditation of Health Organizations (JCAHO).

The nationally recognized organizations (which will be discussed later) which certify medical coders also have their Code of Ethics which are a listing of professional and ethical qualifications and responsibilities required of their certified coders. This is particularly important with regards to proper reimbursement and confidentiality practices which include security and privacy concerns. These Code of Ethics are as follows:

American Health Information Management Associations (AHIMA)'s code of ethics are:

I. Advocate, uphold and defend the individual's right to privacy and the doctrine of confidentiality in the use and disclosure of information.

II. Put service and the health and welfare of persons before self-interest and conduct themselves in the practice of the profession so as to bring honor to themselves, their peers, and to the health information management profession.
III. Preserve, protect, and secure personal health information in any form or medium and hold in the highest regard the contents of the records and other information of a confidential nature, taking into account the applicable statutes and regulations.
IV. Refuse to participate in or conceal unethical practices or procedures.
V. Advance health information management knowledge and practice through continuing education, research, publications, and presentations.
VI. Recruit and mentor students, peers and colleagues to develop and strengthen professional workforce.
VII. Represent the profession accurately to the public.
VIII. Perform honorably health information management association responsibilities, either appointed or elected, and preserve the confidentiality of any privileged information made known in any official capacity.
IX. State truthfully and accurately their credentials, professional education, and experiences.
X. Facilitate interdisciplinary collaboration in situations supporting health information practice.
XI. Respect the inherent dignity and worth of every person.

American Academy of Professional Coders (AAPC)'s code of ethics are:

(1) Members of the American Academy of Professional Coders shall be dedicated to providing the highest standard of professional coding and billing services to employers, clients and patients. Professional and personal behavior of AAPC members must be exemplary.
(2) AAPC members shall maintain the highest standard of personal and professional conduct.
(3) Members shall respect the rights of patients, clients, employers and all other colleagues.
(4) Members shall use only legal and ethical means in all professional dealings and shall refuse to cooperate with, or condone by silence, the actions of those who engage in fraudulent, deceptive or illegal acts.
(5) Members shall respect and adhere to the laws and regulations of the land and uphold the mission statement of the AAPC.
(6) Members shall pursue excellence through continuing education in all areas applicable to their profession.
(7) Members shall strive to maintain and enhance the dignity, status, competence and standards of coding for professional services.
(8) Members shall not exploit professional relationships with patients, employees, clients or employers for personal gain.
(9) Above all else we will commit to recognizing the intrinsic worth of each member.

Section 1.3: CAREER LADDER FOR CODERS

Medical coding provides an excellent career path, even for those who do not have extensive experience or education, but it does require a great deal of motivation and hard work because the field demands excellence, integrity, and a great depth of knowledge. Medical coding provides a great opportunity for those who may not even have worked within the healthcare field or who are in beginning level positions within a healthcare practice. With medical coding, as well as with various other career opportunities in healthcare administration, no matter what the current career field in which a person may be, they can advance into a career with great variety and opportunities for advancement. The healthcare administration career field is vast with a great variety of jobs and high growth in the number of jobs. The great variety of jobs is highly advantageous because no matter what your preference may be with employment, you can find a job that will suit your needs. There are jobs that require a lot of patient contact to jobs that require little, from a variety of duties to more singular duties, from small practices to large hospital departments, and from large practices to small practices.

There are a wide variety of employment opportunities for certified coders in a rapidly growing and well-paying field of medicine. The medical field has been rated as one of the fastest growing occupations in the country. Certified coders make average salaries of $50,000 annually. These figures are dependent on where in the country the coder is employed, their educational level, and in what employment capacity. Coding consultants, auditors, analysts, and specialist can earn up to $70,000 to $80,000 per year. Career opportunities will depend on your ambition, which can be enhanced by additional education. Do not limit yourself unnecessarily. Earning national certification in coding is a great accomplishment and only an indication of what else you can achieve. *Check out*: www.bls.gov and www.advanceweb.com.

Do not despair if you are not successful in getting a job that involves only coding. Get experience in billing, medical records, and/or medical office management. Many duties in the medical field are not limited to strictly coding but will include other tasks, such as billing or medical records. Oftentimes, you may have to take a job that is beginning level despite your certification because it is easier to get into an organization at the beginning levels where many jobs are. Your additional knowledge and education will only help you gain promotions quicker and easier, so the extra knowledge is definitely to your advantage.

Additional opportunities for coders include positions such as inpatient and outpatient hospital billers, clinic coders, claim reviewers, supervisors, compliance specialists, billers, analysts, auditors, consultants, educators, case managers, medical record technicians, and medical office specialists. There are a wide variety of employers for whom a coder can work, for example, private or governmental, hospitals or agencies, schools, insurance companies, physician offices, or clinics. Some positions may involve a great deal of patient contact, some may involve contact with physicians and insurance companies, and some may involve little contact with anyone. Some positions may combine both the billing and coding into office duties, even including patient checkout. There is a great diversity on how medical practices divide the responsibilities among employees, but learning the most will always be to your benefit, so do not confine yourself to strictly coding. Other than in hospitals, most positions will include other duties, which may be due in part to the smaller structure of the medical practice. Often within a medical practice, a position may be exclusive to one particular area or may be generalized. If a coding position is specialized, it may include strictly coding from a cover sheet, whereas some may involve the abstracting of codes from actual files. Specialization may be confined to coding and billing for a particular insurance company or Medicare. Keep the door of possibilities open in your search for employment, and remember that you have many skills by which you can mold your job.

When a person becomes certified as a coder, many opportunities open up for advancement including positions that are strictly involved with coding and management positions. Usually a person begins as a physician-based coder within a clinic, doctor's office, or outpatient hospital. While many coders choose to remain practicing at the physician level, some will opt to advance to inpatient coding which is generally the highest paying type of coding position. A coder can also become certified and/or experienced in specialty areas of coding, such as radiology, cardiovascular, or orthopedic. From there, a coder may advance into higher-level positions such as analysts or auditors. Since the introduction of the electronic health record, many coders are able to go home to work but this usually is obtained by gaining several years experience in coding.

Another career opportunity derived from the coding field is that a person may enter the field as a biller or clerk, or even a coder, and then continue their education for a position as a nurse, radiologist, doctor, or laboratory technician. This career opportunity is advantageous because many healthcare organizations will pay for further education if the person stays with the organization for a certain time period afterwards.

Perhaps the best incentive of the healthcare field as a career is that it does provide security, good environments, professionalism, respect and good pay as compared to some other fields. As a person advances within the healthcare field, they can make up to $100,000 a year, particularly if they advance into management which may be furthered by obtaining national certification as a Registered Health Information Technician (RHIT which requires completion of an associate's degree by an AHIMA-accredited college) or Registered Health Information Administrator (RHIA which requires completion of a bachelor's degree by an AHIMA-accredited university or college).

Section 1.4: FUTURE FOR CODERS

The future for medical coders is very bright indeed as the need for them only continues to intensify. The need for qualified coders is enhanced by the increase in government regulations and oversight of healthcare. In addition, the complexity of new services and discoveries require greater knowledge and expertise to accurately portray healthcare service provided and to ensure full and proper payments for physicians and healthcare practices. But the bottom line is proper coding ensures that patients do receive the healthcare they need, especially without overly burdensome costs which could otherwise devastate patients.

The challenge also grows from the financial and physical limitations within the healthcare field in the effort to provide quality healthcare to a highly diverse world population. For these reasons, the value of a qualified coder has grown significantly within the past ten years and will continue to grow. In addition, labor reports indicate that healthcare administration will continue to be one of the career fields with the fastest job growth, so coding and the career ladder opportunities it provides will continue to be a highly professional, well-respected, interesting, and good-paying occupations of the future.

Section 1.5: EDUCATION

Perhaps the most secure and practical way to advance from a lower level position in healthcare is to participate in an educational program, such as in a certificate or a college degree program. Many educational programs have developed over the past ten years to accommodate the increasing need for knowledgeable healthcare administrative staff; however, schools and training programs differ greatly so it is wise to thoroughly investigate the schools. Remember that short cuts are usually just that and unable to provide in-depth training and education – in healthcare administration it is always best to get as much education and training as you can because it is a highly responsible and complex career field.

Your education can also include earning other certifications within the medical field. Within the coding field, there is certification as a hospital coder. AAPC provides certification for outpatient hospital known as Certified Outpatient Coder for the hospital (COC), Certified Inpatient Coder for the hospital (CIC). AHIMA provides certification for inpatient hospital based coding known as Certified Coding Specialist (CCS). In addition, AHIMA offers certification known as Certified in Healthcare Privacy (CHP); Certified in Healthcare Security (CHS), sponsored by HIMSS, administered by AHIMA; Certified in Healthcare Privacy and Security (CHPS), co-sponsored with HIMSS; Registered Health Information Administrator (RHIA); and Registered Health Information Technician (RHIT). There are other organizations that offer other certifications, but check the legitimacy of the organization and its national recognition.

Your endeavors can project even further, onto associate, bachelor, and master degrees, maybe even a doctorate. Your knowledge is something no one can ever take away from you and builds a solid future for you and is a great boost to your self-esteem.

Do not forget additional future opportunities that your experience and education can provide you. Beginning with your success as a coder, you need to make education a part of your career goals. *Don't limit yourself.* In obtaining your national coding certification, you certainly have demonstrated that you have the potential to be your best.

CHAPTER 2
INTRODUCTION TO MEDICAL CODING

You will learn the following objectives in this chapter:

F. Knowledge of the beginning and development of the health administration field.
G. Definition and history of a hierarchial system.
H. Knowledge of the history and development of ICD-10-CM.
I. Define terminology used for understanding ICD-10-CM.
J. Current role and application of coding within health administration.

Section 2.1: HISTORY OF MEDICAL CODING

One of the primary systems used in medical coding is the International Classification of Diseases (ICD). The origin of this concept dates back to the ancient civilizations for the purpose of tracking and classifying diseases and causes of illnesses and death which have always intrigued mankind, but also has the purpose of promoting better health and eliminating causes of death. Today, ICD is the world's most widely used classification system.

More recently, in the 17th century, the English statistician, John Graunt, developed the London Bills of Mortality which identified the number of children who died before reaching age 6 and mimicked the same basis of earlier disease and death classification systems. Later in 1838, William Farr, registrar general of England, developed a system to classify deaths.

It was the Bertillon Classification of Causes of Death, however, that was developed in 1893 that became the precursor for the ICD system. This was developed by a French physician, Jacques Bertillon at the International Statistical Institute in Chicago. Subsequently, in 1898 the American Public Health Association (APHA) recommended the adoption of the Bertillon System with revisions every ten years. In 1900 the first international conference was convened to revise what now is known as the International Classification of Causes of Death.

The Mixed Commission, a group composed of representatives from the International Statistical Institute and the Health Organization of the League of Nations, was responsible for the early revisions. Early revisions contained minor changes, but there were major changes in the sixth revision when it changed from one book to two books (known as tabular and alphabetical volumes) as well as changing of the title to Manual of International Statistical Classification of Diseases, Injuries and Causes of Death (ICD). Ever since there have been numerous revisions which are a reflection of the changes in healthcare, diseases, and knowledge within the health field.

Section 2.2: DEVELOPMENT OF ICD

It was in 1948 that the World Health Organization (WHO), headquartered in Geneva, Switzerland, assumed responsibility for the revisions of the ICD with the production of the 7th

version in 1957 and the eighth revision in 1968. WHO designed ICD for classification of morbidity and mortality information for statistical purposes and for indexing medical records by disease and operations.

It was in 1968 that the Eighth Revision of International Classification of Diseases (ICD) was published in the United States and served as the basis for coding diagnostic data for official morbidity and mortality statistics in the U.S. When revised by United States, ICD was modified and utilized for purposes of billing, thus this version became known as the Clinical Modification (CM); therefore, this revision became known as ICD-8-CM.

The current version, the tenth, is known as ICD-10-CM and has been in use since October 2015. The purpose of the book has remained to encompass the great variety and complexity, as well as technological advances in healthcare, in the diagnosis and treatment of diseases and other conditions that influence a person's well-being. It was able to emphasize what was happening clinically; namely, to serve as a useful tool in the area of classification of morbidity data for identification of diagnoses, demonstrating medical necessity, indexing of medical records, medical review, ambulatory and other medical care programs, as well as for basic health statistics.

Section 2.3: UPDATES TO ICD

Regardless of the version of the ICD, there are updates added October 1st of every year with clarifications and explanations provided routinely which can be accessed through the government's Federal Register. Updates are issued periodically by what is now known as the Centers for Medicare and Medicaid Services (CMS) or formerly known as the Health Care Financing Administration (HCFA). CMS is a part of the United States Federal Government's Health and Human Services Department.

Section 2.4: NATIONAL CODING ORGANIZATIONS

There are two national organizations recognized for national certification of medical coders which is the American Health Information Management Association (AHIMA) and American Academic of Professional Coders (AAPC).

AMERICAN HEALTH INFORMATION MANAGEMENT ASSOCIATION (AHIMA): AHIMA is a well known health administration national organization that has been in existence for over 75 years. It was formed in 1928 by the Association of Record Librarians to standardize and professionalize the health care administration field. Currently there are over 70,000 registered members and many more professionals who have been certified through the various certifications offered by AHIMA. AHIMA is headquartered in Chicago, Illinois. The organization provides a wide variety of other services besides certification which includes development of standards and government regulations, seminars, training, accreditation, publications, and continuing education.

While a person may gain certification, they do not necessarily have to be members although additional benefits are provided to members such as lower costs for tests, publications, and conferences in addition to access to information and publications. Membership costs are reduced for students who are attending an accredited AHIMA school. AHIMA offers an immense variety of publications, including textbooks and sample certification tests.

Various certifications through AHIMA include Registered Health Information Technicians (RHITs) and Registered Health Information Administrators (RHIAs). These national certifications are often required for various administrative positions within hospitals or large clinics. In addition, AHIMA now offers certifications for management of privacy and security programs within medical practices. These certifications are known as Certified in Healthcare Privacy (CHP) and Certified in Healthcare Security (CHS); a combined certification, can be obtained.

AHIMA provides coding certification for both physician (Certified Coding -Specialist–Physician Based, CCS-P) and hospital (Certified Coding Specialist, CCS for inpatient and outpatient hospital coding). In addition, there is certification for entry-level coders (Certified Coding Associate, CCA). It is also recommended that you have several years' experience within the coding and billing fields before taking the CCS-P and CCS exams.

AHIMA can be contacted at their website (www.ahima.org), where applications, forms, and information are provided. In addition, this website provides sample tests, description of available references, listing of AHIMA-certified educational resources, correspondence material, and various other coding-related information. Materials can be purchased for a home study course in coding, but not for RHIT or RHIA which requires an associates or bachelor's degree from an AHIMA accredited school.

AMERICAN ACADEMY OF PROFESSIONAL CODERS (AAPC): The American Academy of Professional Coders (AAPC) was formed in 1988 and provides national coding certification for both physician (Certified -Professional Coder, CPC) and hospital (Certified Outpatient Coder, COC and Certified Inpatient Coder, CIC). They also offer certification in auditing, management, and compliance. AAPC is composed of a national advisory board with members selected from state organizations. AAPC is supported by a national physician advisory board. There are now more than 150,000 members throughout 250 local chapters. There are state and local groups that provide educational opportunities and meetings for its members.

AAPC can be contacted at their website (www.aapc.com), where form, dates, application, and information are provided. In addition, this website provides sample tests, description of available references, listing of AAPC-certified educational resources, correspondence material, and various other coding-related information. Coursework can be purchased for a home study course. Dates are also available in AAPC's publication, "The Coding Edge," or by calling the national office. Locations and dates of exams are determined by local AAPC chapters.

CHAPTER 3
TEST PREPARATION

You will learn the following objectives in this chapter:

A. AHIMA certifications.
B. AHIMA test structures and rules.
C. AAPC certifications.
D. AAPC test structures and rules.

Section 3.1: AHIMA TESTS

AHIMA offers a number of national certifications which can be accessed by visiting their website at http://ahima.org. The handbook for testing should also be downloaded as it is very important that you know the content of this handbook as it will prepare you well for the exam. Test applications can be completed at this website.

AHIMA offers the CCS and CCS-P coding certifications. The CCS (Certified Coding Specialist) signifies that a person is qualified to perform inpatient and outpatient hospital coding. This is the most advanced national coding certification in that it requires extensive experience and knowledge and is also the most difficult certification exam. CCS-P (Certified Coding Specialist – Physician) signifies that a person is qualified to perform physician billing and oftentimes these certified individuals are also recruited for outpatient hospital coding. The career path is fairly clear in that a person should seek physician certification first and gain experience as a coder before proceeding onto the hospital certification due in large part to the fact that employers do not wish to hire inpatient hospital coders who are not certified and do not have experience. In fact, before proceeding into hospital coding and certification, a person should evaluate if this is the right career choice for them as many coders do not proceed into hospital coding. Many physician certified coders are very successful and productive as physician coders within offices and clinics.

The CCS hospital certification is difficult as it pertains to both inpatient and outpatient coding and, therefore, has many differences as compared to physician coding. Such differences include the use of groupers (DRGs and APCs), coding of symptoms and principal diagnosis, and use of Volume 3 of the ICD-10 book. A word of advice is to obtain your physician certification (CCS-P) and gain experience before proceeding onto hospital coding because the differences in the coding rules and practices can be confusing when taking the national exams.

AHIMA also offers the CCA (Certified Coding Associate) which is an apprentice-type certification which is an introductory step to being a fully certified coder. This certification allows people to enter the coding field who may not yet have the experience or knowledge to pass the national exams.

CCS-P: Applications can be accessed online at www.ahima.org. Once a person has submitted their application for the test, they are sent an Authorization to Test letter and then they are allowed four months to schedule and take the test at a Pearson Vue Center which are located in most cities throughout the United States. Because of the use of the testing centers and computerized tests, candidates are allowed to select the date and time that works best for them and they can reschedule if adequate notice is provided. This is highly advantageous over the previous system in which tests were administered once or twice a year at specified locations throughout the country. You can reschedule with a fee if necessary but there must be adequate notice.

Requirements to be eligible to take the CCS or CCS-P test are that the candidate must meet one of the following eligibility requirements:

By Credential: RHIA, RHIT, or CCS/CCS-P;
OR
By Education: Completion of a coding training program that includes anatomy and physiology, pathophysiology, pharmacology, medical terminology, reimbursement methodology, intermediate/advanced ICD diagnostic/procedural and CPT coding;
OR
By Experience: Minimum of two (2) years of related coding experience directly applying codes;
OR
By Credential with Experience: CCA plus one (1) year of coding experience directly applying codes;
OR
Other: Coding credential from other certifying organization plus one (1) year coding experience directly applying codes.

The CCS-P exam consists of:
88 Multiple Select (18 unscored/pretest)
8 Multiple Select (2 unscored/pretest)
13 medical record cases

Exam Time: 4 hours

The areas (domains) of the test are:
DOMAIN I: Health Information Documentation (8-12%)
DOMAIN II: Diagnosis and Procedure Coding (60-64%)
DOMAIN III: Regulatory Guidelines & Reporting Requirements for Outpatient Services (8-12%)
DOMAIN IV: Data Quality & Management (5-7%)
DOMAIN V: Information & Communication Technologies (2-4%)
DOMAIN VI: Privacy, Confidentiality, Legal & Ethical Issue (4-6%)
DOMAIN VII: Compliance (3-5%)

ICD-10-CM CPT, and HCPCS are allowed for use during the exam as well as a medical dictionary. It is strongly suggested that you use a professional edition of the CPT book because

The coding abstracts may contain a single report, such as a progress note, or may contain various reports, such as operative, discharges, history and physicals, and lab/pathology. From these reports, you must then determine the proper codes after going through all of the reports. Sequencing is not considered in scoring, so you do not have to worry about this on the exam.

It is important to emphasize at this time that the handbook for the tests must be downloaded from AHIMA's website and should be thoroughly read and understood as specific rules are provided. It is also important to stress that the notes within the coding books, medical terminology, reimbursement, and regulatory information are critical to successfully passing the exam.

In the CCS-P exam, information is provided concerning the levels of each element used to determine the evaluation and management codes. The test now indicates how many ICD-10 and CPT/HCPCS codes are needed to answer the coding abstracts.

Tests results may or may not be given immediately because sometimes AHIMA collects a group of tests to evaluate the reliability and validity of the tests. If this occurs, results are usually provided within a month.

CCS: Number of Questions on Exam:
97 multiple-choice questions (79 scored/18 pretest)
8 medical scenarios (6 scored/2 pretest)
Exam Time: 4 hours

The areas (domains) of the test are:
DOMAIN I: Health Information Documentation (8-10%)
DOMAIN II: Diagnosis and Procedure Coding (64-68%)
DOMAIN III: Regulatory Guidelines and Reporting Requirements for Acute Care (Inpatient) Service (6-8%)

For more specifics regarding what is contained in each domain, view the candidate's handbook.

CCA: For the CCA exam, you must have two forms of identification. One must be a picture ID, and one must have your signature. A Social Security card is not acceptable. No paper, dictionaries, or other reference materials are allowed. The CCA exam is offered online at Pearson Vue and can be arranged at a time convenient for you within the allotted time frame. An application must be submitted and confirmed. There is a sample test -on-line at AHIMA's website.

There are 100 questions with two hours allowed for testing. Content of the exam includes rules and regulations for health data, coding classification and reimbursement procedures, and delivery and technology of health information. At the end of the exam, you will have the opportunity to provide comments and feedback to AHIMA via the computer. You will be notified at the conclusion of the exam by the test proctor if you passed or failed the exam.

Section 3.2: AAPC EXAMS

AAPC offers coding certification for both physician (Certified Professional Coder, CPC), outpatient hospital (Certified Outpatient Hospital Coder COC), and Certified Inpatient Hospital Coder (CIC). It also offers certification for coders who work with reimbursement (Certified Professional Coder – Payer). Therefore, the CPC is similar to AHIMA's CCS-P. Both the CIC and CCS do include outpatient hospital coding. Applications can be completed on the website (aapc.com). Be sure to download the handbook for testing as the information is important to be prepared for the exam and will direct your studies.

Coding tests are paper and pen at this time. The tests can be scheduled by visiting the website (aapc.com) and selecting the state where you want to take the exam. The location and date can then be selected. The certification examinations are administered through the AAPC's local chapters and Professional Medical Coding Curriculum (PMCC) sites. These examinations are proctored by AAPC's approved local chapter officers and/or PMCC instructors.

Qualifications to take the exam include at "least two recommendation letters verifying 2 years of on the job experience using the CPT®, ICD-10, or HCPCS code sets. At least one letter must be from a supervisor outlining your coding experience and amount of time in that capacity OR a minimum 80 hour coding course AND one letter verifying one year of on the job coding experience from a supervisor. Proof of education may be sent in the form of a letter from the instructor stating the amount of contact hours or a completion of certificate" (aapc.com) describing the number of hours. If you do not meet these qualifications, you may still take the exam, and if you are successful in passing it then you will be awarded the status of apprentice until these qualifications have been met.

Current editions of the ICD-10, CPT, and HCPCS books must be brought to the exam. Other version of the books other than the standardized versions (which includes the professional edition of the CPT book which is highly recommended) are not allowed, such as the Expert or Plus versions. No other books or materials are allowed to be brought in. Officially published errata update sheets can also be brought to the exam. "Tabs may be inserted, taped, pasted, glued, or stapled in the manuals so long as the obvious intent of the tab is to earmark a page with words or numbers, not supplement information in the book. No materials may be inserted, taped, glued, or stapled in the books. Writing is allowed in the manuals" (aapc.com).

The test is 150 multiple choice questions and five hours and 40 minutes are allowed to complete the exam. There are three sections to the exam:

You can obtain an application online or by ordering one from AAPC. It must be mailed and received four weeks before the exam date. The cost of the exam is approximately $300 (you have to be a member in order to take the exam, which costs $120 per year). It is recommended that you have several years' experience within the coding and billing fields before taking the exam.

"A CPC® must have at least two years medical coding experience (member's with an apprentice designation are not required to have two years medical coding experience.) Membership is required to be renewed annually and 36 Continuing Education Units (CEU's) must be submitted every two years for verification and authentication of expertise" (AAPC.com). If designated as an apprentice, then two letters on letterhead need to be sent indicating that the apprentice has gained two years' experience on the job or else attended an 80-hour course in addition to one letter confirming at least one-year experience on the job.

For the COC exam, the sections are: Section 1: Clinical Knowledge, Medical Terminology (20), Anatomy (20); Section 2: Reimbursement Concepts & Terminology, General Insurance (6), Payment Systems (5), HIPAA (3), Payment Impacts (5), Inpatient (8); Section 3: Applied Coding Concepts & Rules, ICD-10-CM Coding Rules (12), HCPCS (4), CPT® Rules (13), CPT® Sections/Applied Coding (13), Hospital Coding/Applied Coding (6), ICD-10-CM Sections (21), HCPCS Level II (7), Modifiers (7). The order of these sections may vary over the years.

You must pass all three sections to earn certification. If you do not pass the first time, you are allowed to take the exam one more time at no charge.

Section 3.3: TEST PREPARATION:

The CPC and CCS-P exams are based on the services provided by physicians and as coded by experienced coders. Therefore, you must evaluate your combination of education and experience to determine whether you are prepared to take the exam or whether you need to study or work more. ICD-9-CM, CPT-4, and HCPCS Level II codes are included on the exam. V codes are used. Each section of the CPT-4 coding book is included on the exam; therefore, if you have worked in a specialty area for many years, you will need to study all of the other areas of the CPT-4 book.

BOOKS: Choose your books wisely. Stay current with AHIMA's and AAPC's policies because they can change in any year. Although the time frame can vary, you may be allowed to use the current year CPT-4, ICD-10-CM, and HCPCS books for the exam up through spring of the following year. Be aware that some versions of (e.g., CPT Expert) or changes to (e.g., taping or copying of information) in these books may not be allowed in the exams. In addition, AHIMA allows the use of a medical dictionary. There is a wide range of books from the basic to professional.

Features vary from book to book, such as indentations for indexes, extra information, drawings, and descriptions, so check the book carefully because all information is valuable when taking the exam. For example, some ICD-9-CM books have notations for fourth and fifth digits which is very helpful. Some CPT-4 books will list the three main criteria, history, exam, and medical decision-making levels for you under the E/M codes, which is also very helpful. Some coding books may change the order of the volumes, such as placing volume 1 first or second in the ICD-9-CM book. Books can be purchased as spiral bound, regular binding, or in a notebook. Much of this is simply preference, but you should be familiar and comfortable with your code book. As you study, you can mark in your books, but remember that only coding-pertinent information is allowable and not excessive information, such as medical terminology and definitions. It is advisable that you have a medical dictionary; don't limit yourself to a small one because it is cute and handy.

BEWARE OF SHORTCUTS: There are no shortcuts in preparing for the national exams. Whether you study by yourself or with an established program for 40 hours, then you have only studied for 40 hours. The tests are designed for those who have worked for many years within the field of coding which means that they probably have many more hours of learning than you do if your only source of knowledge is what you are studying.

MEDICAL TERMINOLOGY: Medical terminology is crucial and is not limited to a few specialties, so you must know your terminology, including combining forms (roots, suffixes, and prefixes). It is very important that you have recently taken a comprehensive medical terminology course including anatomy and physiology, unless your medical terminology background is all encompassing and in depth already. Abbreviations should be included in your study of medical terminology. Although not every question will involve abbreviations, there will be some on the national exams. Not only may there be particular medical terminology questions and abbreviations on the national exams, but the medical terminology and abbreviations will be used extensively in the descriptions of coding scenarios.

PRACTICE: There is nothing that can substitute for practice. Practice both short descriptions and long reports in which more abstracting will be required. The most valuable attribute of practice is that it makes you feel more confident. You must also practice pacing yourself—take timed tests with short answers, but also with long abstracting scenarios. Also, practice taking long exams so that you can endure both the fast pace and long hours that are required for the national exams.

STUDY SCHEDULE: *Do not procrastinate!* About four months before the exam, you should be studying seriously. You need to set this as your top priority and put other things aside to be completed or done after your test. You should commit at least one hour per day every day of the week to studying study guides and textbooks and practicing coding. At two weeks before, start studying 2 to 3 hours per day and also check with the testing center to be confirm dates, times, and place. In the last week, studying the notes and guidelines should be your final focus.

STUDY TECHNIQUES: Study groups are highly recommended, as are traditional coding courses. Ask questions! Study groups help you learn to argue with yourself in a practiced setting with input from others, instead of just by yourself. This will help immensely on the exam; it is better to have practiced it and refined it so you can argue sensibly with yourself about your coding choices.

There are various coding publications and courses available in various formats including online and lecture. Check them out. They are not all the same: some are hands-on, while others are lecture; some are 40 hours long and others may be more than 100. Ask questions and check with local employers, coders working in the field, and national or state associations and chapters.

When reading the coding books, make notes and highlight important information, which will then be readily visible during the exam and can prompt your memory. Studies have found that a good night's sleep actually does help you retain more after each time you study prior to the exam. For these exams, you need to understand and think critically, not memorize, how coding is done. You will be a little unsure during the test itself because it is not like traditional tests; these tests focus on your ability to apply your knowledge, interpret information, and think. Surround yourself with people who can help you remain positive and study effectively because success feeds off of positive thinking.

Section 3.4: TAKING THE TEST

EXAM DAY: Arrive half an hour or an hour early. Bring your admission paperwork and two forms of ID including picture ID. Bring your books: ICD-10-CM, CPT, and HCPCS. With AHIMA a medical dictionary is allowed. You may want to bring a watch and ruler. You should also bring several #2 pencils.

There are limitations on what can be written in them, such as no extensive medical terminology with definitions. The concept is that additional information that would be used on the job is allowed within the coding book. No stapled or taped pages are allowed.

DETAILS: Coding is all about details. Find out *who* you are coding for, whether it is the surgeon, anesthesiologist, or whomever. Keep this frame of reference—who are you billing for and what services did he or she provide?

Find out *where* the patient is, whether it is in the office or hospital, emergency room, urgent care, or wherever. Codes used for locations are listed at the front of the CPT book.

Find out whether they are a *new or established* patient. If a patient has not seen the physician/practice in over three years, then he or she is considered a new patient for billing and coding purposes. Look for words that indicate an established patient, such as "he returns again," or "he is here for follow-up."

Details include reference to notes, guidelines, and information in the ICD-10 and CPT books. *Take your time to check things out.*

It is critical when coding that you take the extra time to read the notes and other notations in the ICD10 and CPT books including the coding guidelines in the front of the ICD-10 and the notes throughout the CPT books.

In addition, it is advisable that you take a few extra moments to scan before (above) and after (below) a selected code. One code may seem correct, but if you examine other surrounding codes, you may find another code that more specifically describes the service. This is also true of the alphabetic index. If you find several codes listed in the alphabetic index, you may want to check them out, even if one appears correct. Take the few extra moments to read notes and check other codes.

It is also important to take your time and check the documentation in the patient's file. Starting with a final diagnosis on whatever document it may appear (e.g., progress note or discharge summary), proceed onto other parts of the report and other documentation. When you find anything that can be coded, such as diagnoses, symptoms, procedures, and services, write those codes above the description. By looking up the codes at this stage and writing them down, you will know what you need to look for in the reports and you will not have to look them up again if you need to come back to the scenario later. This will alleviate confusion because you know what you are looking for and don't have to reread all of the reports.

ANSWERS: Very importantly, answer first what is easiest. This will probably be the sections in the following order: medical terms and A&P, HCPCS, billing, general healthcare information, anesthesia, radiology, pathology/lab, medicine, E/M and finally surgery. Remember that if you do the easier sections first and you finish half the test in half the time, then you will have done a better job to that point and now all you will need is to get about half of the remainder of the test correct to pass. Do not get obsessed with a question and spend too much time on it – if you start to overthink a question and are taking too much time, then you need to leave that question until later.

Psychologically, it is critical for you to answer a couple of questions right in the beginning so that your brain will unlock. This will give you confidence. Do not confuse yourself or discourage yourself within the first few minutes of the exam by spending too much time on hard questions. (Be sure to mark in the column with star or check any questions that you did not answer, did not complete, or for which you need to recheck your answer because you were uncertain about the answer you selected.) Do this for several reasons. You do not want to waste precious time on a difficult question. It is better to answer 10 questions, rather than just one. After you have answered a few easy question, your brain will unlock and so it will get easier. When you return to an unfinished question later, it may make more sense, especially after you have gained confidence and answered other questions. It is much easier to tackle the harder questions when you have already answered three fourths of the questions.

Answer what you do know. If you are fairly sure of your answer, mark it. You can return to the question later and review it to ensure that your answer was correct or make another selection if you decide otherwise. Don't waste any of your thought processes, so mark an answer if you are fairly confident it is correct because you will have to make many educated guesses. If the answer requires several answers, mark what you know and return to the question later to finish marking the other answers. If a question becomes very confusing, just put down what you can or leave it until later to answer. You will not be getting a 100% on the exam, so you can miss a few.

Be careful of skimming and making **ass**umptions. Although you cannot conceivably read everything, particularly when abstracting, and you certainly cannot read and reread everything on these tests, the detail is critical. If you skim or assume, you can miss the detail, such as which physician you are coding for or whether the patient is new or established. *Take time to read the details.*

This exam is tough for everyone, so you are not the exception if you find it difficult. Many who take the exam have thought they failed, when in truth they find they actually passed.

Failure does not define you, life is a learning process that can help you become better. The only failure is to not try. With all of the emphasis on coding certification, it is sometimes forgotten that being able to do the coding job well is more important. Fear of failure keeps us from being our best. You can take the exam again and you can still have a great career without the certification, so be kind to yourself.

When it is the day of the exam, if you have studied and worked hard, then you have done your best. There is nothing more to be done at this time. Take the exam to the best of your ability and realize that you cannot anticipate everything or know everything.

CODING: Every scenario must have an ICD-10-CM code and a CPT code on the AHIMA's coding scenarios, just as in the real world. However, on AAPC tests there are questions that may only have ICD codes or CPT codes.

Read directions. Read the testing handbook before you come to the test so you do not have to waste time reading it during testing time. Make sure that you read the instructions well. Although you must be concerned with time, especially on the AAPC exam, if you fail to read the directions or questions carefully, you can easily miss points.

Make sure that you read all of the possible answers, particularly with multiple choice. Do not read one and assume that it is right without reading the rest of the choices.

If you finish early, go back and check your answers. Use all of your time if you can. Remember, your first answer has a greater chance of being right. If you decide to change your first answer, make sure that you have good justification. Sometimes the first choice represents your unconscious thought which may recall something that your conscious does not.

Remember also to check before codes to determine if there are any other criteria that apply to this code, such as "code also" or fifth digits.

Be sure to put your answers in the right place on the answer sheet. This is particularly important with test forms that require bubbles to be filled in with a pencil such as the AAPC exam. It is easy to get off by just one line when marking your answer which could result in many more answers being answered in the wrong answer line. Use a piece of paper or other straight edge to mark where your answers go to ensure that you are marking the answer in the right line.

DOCUMENTATION: Documentation is the basis of coding. "Not documented, not done" is the motto of coders. Although this concept is frustrating to some who like to overanalyze, it is critical to remember for the exam, as in all coding, that if it is not documented, then it never happened. Do not diagnose the patient. Only the physician can do this. You can only code from the documentation. If there are inadequacies in the documentation, these can be addressed in the future through education of the physicians and staff.

SKIPPING: If you skip a question, only partially complete it, or if you are unsure of your answer, mark it in the outside column with perhaps a star so that you can find it easily when you recheck the exam. If you do not mark these questions, odds are that you will miss finding one when you recheck to see what you have not completed. Maybe even worse, you may spend too much time looking for what questions you did not finish. Marking them makes everything easier and more certain.

NOTES: You cannot write on the answer key. If you can, in the test booklet circle and underline any valuable information so that you do not have to constantly reread everything. When you find a code, mark it next to the description in the test booklet. This saves time and diminishes confusion because you will not have to constantly refind the codes.

MULTIPLE CHOICE: When you are completing a multiple-choice section, through the **process of elimination,** cross off answers when you have determined that they are wrong. The wrong answers will tell you what is right, as much as the right answer will. Therefore, you do not have just one way to find the right answer, but many. You can determine that codes are wrong in a multiple choice sometimes by examining just a few codes. Begin by selecting a code that that varies slightly in several answers and compare the differences. Check them and see if they are valid. If you find that they are not valid, such as the patient is insulin-dependent but the code does not signify this, then cross off all answers that indicate non-insulin dependence. You can then continue onto another code that occurs in several answers and cross off what you know to be definitely wrong until you have found the right answer. Usually within one code or another, you can find that you are fairly definite about your answer obtained through this process of elimination.

For example, in selecting the proper codes for the following scenario:

A 63-year-old diabetic male has returned to his physician for treatment of diabetic cataract and problems with peripheral angiopathy of his feet due to Type 1 diabetes, which patient has had problems controlling. The patient is insulin dependent.

A E10.3, E10.51
B E11.51, E10.3
C E10.3, E11.36
D E10.3, E10.51, H25.011

Let us find the right answer by a process of elimination. It is Type 1 diabetes so B and C are not the correct answers since E11.51 and E11.36 are for Type 2 diabetes. D is not right because H25.011 is for cataract but this is a diabetic cataract which is already included in the E10.3 code. So, A is the correct answer.

Make **educated guesses.** The purpose of exams is to test your ability to abstract knowledge from your previous experience and education and apply it to new situations as given in the exam. The national coding exams are not a test of memorization but of thinking skills with the application and interpretation of that knowledge to coding scenarios. Since you are relying upon educated guesses, stick with your first answer. Often when we are thinking hard, our brain remembers something that we cannot consciously perceive at the time, particularly under stress; so, our first guess often reflects this unconscious knowledge of a fact. Your first guess is frequently the right guess! Therefore, if you start constantly second-guessing yourself, you will be wrong more than you will be right. It is good to review your test once you have finished, but you must hesitate in changing an answer—remember, there is a strength of knowledge in your first answer. You must have some solid information before you change your first educated guess. *Be careful.*

Get as close as you can. Sometimes, particularly when using the alphabetic index, you will not find the exact description of a diagnosis or procedure. Get as close as you can then. Find some terminology that is related. Keep trying several different terms. Even when you sometimes think you may have found something, take the time to look a little further. This is particularly true when there are several codes listed as possibilities under a term. For example, transfer of a shoulder muscle lists several codes in the alphabetical index, that is, 23395–23397, 24301, 24320. Briefly examine each to determine which is correct. You may still find more information and important differences. Although you are on a time frame, taking a few extra seconds to explore may help you not make mistakes. Sometimes, a code listing in either Volume 1 or Volume 2 may contain references to the use of other codes that would be more appropriate. Essentially all of the answers when coding from abstracts are in front of you because they are contained within your coding books—they are in the details. These tests are not about memorization but about knowing how to research and think. *Be sure to read the notes.*

The details are also important in the alphabetical -index. When the alphabetical index directs you somewhere specifically, then you must do so. This is particularly true with the **ICD-10-CM** coding book.

Section 3.5: POST TEST

AAPC exam results are mailed to you within four to six weeks after the exam although they are usually much faster; however, you can usually access it online through your account within a few days. You must pass all three parts of the exam to become certified. AHIMA exam results are provided at the time of completion of the computerized test; however, on some occasions these results will not be given immediately but will be mailed to you because AHIMA periodically evaluates the test to be sure it is valid. Passing scores for the AHIMA exam are not necessarily a set score but can range around the 70th percentile for both parts of the exams due to their evaluation of testing throughout the nation. You must pass all parts of the exam. Since the exams vary from year to year, the difficulty of the exams may fluctuate. To level the playing field for all candidates, the testing agency uses a statistical equating process to determine the passing exam scores for a given year. The AHIMA website explains this as a process that provides adjustment for the "fluctuations in difficulty across examination forms. After individual examinations are scored, an item analysis is performed and reviewed with members of the Examination Construction Committee before final scoring. Because of the use of this statistical equating process and a post-examination item analysis to ensure that the examination is psychometrically sound and valid, a passing score cannot be established prior to examination administration."

CERTIFICATION: Every successful applicant who passes the certification exam will receive a certificate identifying their credentials. AAPC examinees will receive the distinction of Certified Professional Coder (CPC) and AHIMA examinees will receive the distinction of Certified Coding Specialist–Physician Based (CCS-P) or Certified Coding Associate (CCA). AAPC apprentices will receive certification as CPC-Apprentice.

COMPLAINTS/APPEALS: Although comments are allowed on the exams during examination time and can also be given on the evaluation form at the end of the testing period regarding concerns about the test, there is also an appeals process. It is important that you take this seriously because the national organizations do consider these complaints/appeals. If you can prove the validity of your complaints, these national organizations may make accommodations.

For AHIMA, the complaint/appeal must be submitted within 30 days after the completion of the exam and must be written. Addresses for mailing of complaints/appeals are listed in the application handbook.

TESTING AGAIN: With AHIMA, you can take the CCS-P exam again but will have to pay for it again. With AAPC, you can take the examination again, one more time, at no extra charge but no sooner than 30 days after taking the first exam and not more than one year later. You must resubmit your request to take the exam again.

Section 3.6: RENEWING CERTIFICATION

AAPC and AHIMA will send you information regarding recertification and how to earn continuing education units (CEUs). You can also access this information on the Internet at their websites. With AAPC, in your certification process you become a member. For AHIMA, membership is a separate process from certification.

AHIMA CEUS: AHIMA certification must be renewed every two years. With AHIMA, you must renew your certification every two years by earning 20 CEUS or 30 CEUs if dual certified as CCS and CCS-P. As a part of this, a self-assessment exam must be completed each year, which counts for 5 CEUs for a total of 10 CEUs for the two-year renewal period. The self-assessment costs members $25 each year and nonmembers $50 each. The self-assessment is mailed to the certified coder and is self-administered, then mailed back to AHIMA when completed. The self-assessment is composed of short-answer and multiple-choice questions with some medical scenarios. The self-assessments are not graded, but rather the experience of taking it should provide an educational opportunity. Additional CEUs can be earned by attending preapproved CEUs, including seminars, workshops, -web-based training, audio conferences, subscriptions, local meetings, teaching, and more. Programs not on the preapproved list include many of the same listings for preapproved, such as seminars. These do not need to be necessarily preapproved by AHIMA before attending them.

AAPC CEUS: AAPC certification must be renewed every two years. With AAPC, you must be earning CEUs throughout the year by attending coding seminars and preparing coding materials in order to meet renewal deadlines. For the CPC, COC, or CIC, you must demonstrate that you have earned 36 CEUs within two years. With AAPC, if you have dual certification in, then you must submit documentation for 48 CEUs for every two years. To earn CEUs, you should be attending seminars, workshops, and presentations throughout the year(s) that are approved for CEUs through AHIMA or AAPC. In addition, CEUs can be obtained through instruction of coding courses, attending local organizational meetings, publication or presentation of coding materials, development of coding scenarios, and more.

Certified apprentices with AAPC must complete their coding experience and submit proper documentation that demonstrates the completion of the one or two years of medical coding experience, as well as maintaining CEUs yearly, to become a fully certified coder, and no longer an apprentice.

ACTIVITIES THAT QUALIFY FOR CEU CREDIT: The national organization will assess what activities you have presented as qualifying for satisfying the requirements for CEUs and how many CEUs are awarded per activity. AHIMA and AAPC do differ some on what they will accept and for how many CEUs. The organization will send you information prior to the recertification time that will provide the application and qualifying activities for CEUs. Some activities do require prior approval by the national organization. These include participation in related educational programs; attendance at AHIMA meetings; national convention; state, local, or regional meetings; vendors; seminars; publication or presentation of coding seminars or materials; speaker or panel participant at a related event; approved quizzes; and study from related publications.

NATIONAL RECOGNITION: National certification as a coder does provide a unique recognition anywhere in the country. Some states and organizations actually do require that coders are certified to obtain employment. Its well-recognized status provides many new career opportunities and professional status that earns respect from administrators and coworkers within governmental agencies, hospitals, regulatory agencies, and physician offices. This professionalism can be magnified through attendance and networking at seminars, at national and state organizational meetings, and in educational institutions. Networking is an important factor in furthering your career opportunities and in creating a source of information and feedback for coding issues. The certification is certainly earned through hard work and should be valued by you as well.

CHAPTER 4
REGULATIONS AND COMPLIANCE

You will learn the following objectives in this chapter:

A. Definitions of fraud and abuse.
B. Legislation pertinent to fraud and abuse.
C. Agencies involved in fraud and abuse prosecution.
D. Elements of a compliance program.
E. OIG Workplan
F. Auditing

Section 4.1: TYPES OF OFFENSES

There are three levels at which healthcare offenses can occur. Fraud is the most severe offense as it is considered the purposeful intent to gain funds from the rendering of healthcare in an illegal manner. Abuse is based on the failure to perform fair and reasonable billing and coding practices as illustrated by the standardized practices throughout other healthcare providers. The least offensive are acts of omission and mistakes since they are supposed to not contain any purposefully intent to defraud. The classification of these errors are evaluated based on the practices of the healthcare provider, so if a provider is attempting in good faith to comply with the rules and regulations and has instituted standard practices and procedures, then errors would most likely be considered to be actions of omissions and mistakes.

The importance of fraud and abuse concepts within a healthcare practice are critical and fearsome to healthcare providers. The government estimates that billions of dollars are lost every year to healthcare fraud and abuse. Providers who act properly should not have to worry, however, as qualified personnel who are knowledgeable and up-to-date on rules and regulations can ensure that proper procedures are instituted to protect the practice and to ensure proper reimbursement. One important aspect of a certified coder or health administration would be the institution of a compliance program to ensure proper controls and procedures are instituted to assure compliance with federal rules and regulations, as well as state and local.

While computerized programs are utilized to create profiles of healthcare practices, these are used to determine inconsistencies or poor practices and which may trigger federal audits. Examples of fraud or abuse can include:

(1) Upcoding means the selection of codes at a higher level than as justified by the documentation within the patient's record.
(2) Downcoding means the selection of codes at a lower level than as justified by the documentation with the patient's record.
(3) Billing for noncovered services using codes for covered services.
(4) Billing for services provided that were not medically necessary.
(5) Misuse of modifiers.
(6) Misuse of place of service on the billing form.
(7) Using ICD-10 codes to justify billing when the patient does not have the

diagnosis.

(8) Altering claims fraudulently after they have already been submitted in order to increase payment.
(9) Billings for services not rendered.
(10) Billing for office visits when only surgical procedures were performed.
(11) Unbundling of global services.
(12) Overutilization and billing of laboratory or radiological services.
(13) Billing for consultations when an office visit was provided.
(14) Improper billing for physician services when services are provided by other staff who are not qualified to provide the service for billing purposes.
(15) Billing for services by two physicians for a surgical procedure that is not billable as a team procedure.
(16) Changing of dates of service to ensure additional payments.
(17) Duplicate billing.
(18) Billing and/or performing a more costly procedure, lab, or test when not justified as medically necessary.
(19) Misidentifying the person receiving the services for billing purposes.
(20) Kickbacks, bribes, rebates or other remuneration in exchange for services and referrals.
(21) Routine waivers of copays and deductibles which can be construed to be an inducement to gain referrals and patients.

Section 4.2: LEGISLATION

There are many pieces of legislation that affect healthcare reimbursement and practice, as well as there are many governmental agencies that monitor, deny reimbursement, and prosecute false or inaccurate claims. If a claim is successfully prosecuted, the monies can amount fast due to various aspects of legislation. Fines can include $10,000 per incident in addition to three times the amount of the fraud. Although this may not sound ominous at first, it must be recognized that such an event of fraud and abuse may be found to have occurred in 5% of the files over a number of years, so the fine is computed based on each incident and can easily amount to millions of dollars. Penalties can also include prison time and loss of privileges to serve government patients, such as Medicare patients who may constitute the larger portion of a healthcare practice's business and, therefore, put them out of business. In addition, the government will issue a corporate integrity agreement (CIA) which lists the specifics of the operations of the practice to ensure proper compliance and correction of abuse procedures. To view examples, the government's website can be accessed at www.oig.hhs.gov.

Legislation to combat fraud and abuse include the False Claims Act, Stark Laws, anti-kickback laws, Qui Tam actions, Health Insurance Portability and Accountability Act (HIPAA), and the deficit reduction act.

The False Claims Act was designed during the Civil War to address false claims by military contractors but is still actively used today. It prohibits the submission of false claims to the government.

The anti-kickback laws are to prevent fraud and abuse by ensuring that providers do not recommend that their patients receive services from an organization or provider who is affiliated with the initial provider. This includes companies owned by the referring provider or their families or associates or with whom the provider or their family or associates are partners which, therefore results in the referring provider receiving benefits, including monetary or otherwise. These types of kickbacks are addressed under the Stark laws. This also includes the referring of patients by a provider to someone he may not know professionally or personally, but who are giving the provider benefits for the referral. In other words, the provider cannot refer a patient to any entity from which he or she will benefit either monetarily or in any other manner. Kickbacks have occurred with pharmaceutical companies, durable medical equipment companies, and laboratories.

Qui tam means that a private plaintiff files a lawsuit in place of the government.

In the Deficit Reduction Act, it became mandatory for some healthcare providers to comply, required education of staff regarding fraud and abuse laws, provided penalties for failure to comply, and provided incentives to state to adopt similar anti-fraud laws.

HIPAA provided more means for prosecution of fraud and abuse and increased penalties in addition to coordination of law enforcement at all levels and establishment of standardized practices. It provided greater means for enforcement, just as the Deficit Reduction Act did. HIPAA's goals include providing insurance portability, promote the use of medical savings account, decrease the costs of health care administration by simplifying insurance processes, and combating waste, fraud and abuse. HIPAA allows the government to mandate the use of standards for electronic exchange of health information and is known as Electronic Transactions and Code Sets Rule. Under HIPAA, a covered entity includes physicians, other healthcare providers, health plans, and healthcare clearinghouses who process claims. Business associates are those who do business with a covered entity. Both the covered entity and business associates must comply with HIPAA. There are two parts to HIPAA for security: the Privacy Rule and the Security Rule. The Privacy Rule refers to the concept of protected health information and its transmission and use. With the Privacy Rule only the minimal amount of patient information should be shared as required by law and no further information should be shared. The Security Rule refers to the concept of establishing protection for purposes of confidentiality and integrity of data.

Most investigations for fraud and abuse are initiated by complaints from current or former company employees who are then known as whistle-blowers. If a lawsuit develops from this it is known as qui tam action meaning that a private person stands in place of the government for the filing of charges. If the suit initiated by a whistle-blower is successfully prosecuted, that person will receive approximately 10% of the final award which could be considerable when awards are in the millions of dollars. Although there are laws that protect whistleblowers from retaliation, this is not always enforced.

Patient Protection and Affordable Care Act (PPACA) is the new healthcare reform legislation signed into law on March 30, 2010. It expands Medicaid eligibility, provides subsidies for insurance premiums for eligible persons and requires others to purchase their own health insurance if they have none, prohibits denial of healthcare coverage due to pre-existing conditions, and provides for intensified audits, investigations, penalties and limitations on payments to healthcare providers.

In 1996 the Health Care Financing Administration (HFCA), now known as the Center for Medicare and Medicaid Service (CMS) instituted the National **Correct Coding Initiative** (NNCCI) to assist in proper coding and billing of health care services, including issues regarding bundling. The CCI establishes rules for the determination of the correct methods to combine codes. CCI edits will inform the coder when combinations are not acceptable, such as the coding for an episiotomy when charging for vaginal delivery, which would be included in the cost of the vaginal delivery (global). Because of the National Correct Coding Initiative, you must be knowledgeable and be current in the field of coding and its applications through such things as study programs, seminars, research materials, and publications. CCI are published on a quarterly basis (Jan. 1–March 31; April 1–June 30; July 1–Sept. 30; Oct. 1–Dec. 31).

An additional piece of legislation is the Balanced Budget Act (BBA) of 1997 which requires the implementation of performance measures within the reimbursement/coding process. This type of legislation is important because of the effort to standardize the health record and the provision of health services through the development of performance measures and data sets. A performance measure inventory can be found at http://www.qualitymeasures.ahrq.gov/browse/browseorgsbyLtr.aspx?Letter=*Dozens.

Section 4.3: REGULATORY/GOVERNMENTAL AGENCIES

Many federal agencies are involved in the investigation and prosecution of fraud and abuse cases. Primary amongst these is the Office of Inspector General (OIG). In addition, the Department of Health and Human Services (HHS) is involved, as well as the Federal Bureau of Investigation (FBI), Department of Justice, Internal Revenue Service (IRS), Defense Criminal Investigative Services (DCIS), Drug Enforcement Agency (DEA), and the Post Office.

There are several additional agencies and programs which are used to audit and collect inappropriate and improper payments by governmental agencies to healthcare providers within OIG/CMS which are described below.

RECOVERY AUDIT CONTRACTORS (RACs): RACs are a recent creation of CMS which focus on recovery of improper payments based primarily on coding errors. RACs are entitled to 20% of the amount recovered. RACs were formed as part of Section 306 of the Medicare Prescription Drug, Improvement, and Modernization Act of 2003 (MMA) and was made permanent by Section 302 of the Tax Relief and Health Care Act of 2006 (TRHCA). In its initial 3-year trial, over $1 billion were collected due to improper payments by Medicare. There are two types of RAC reviews: the Automated (no medical record needed – just claims such as for double billing) and the Complex (medical record required). Reasons for recovery of funds by RACs included services that:

1. were found to be medically unnecessary

2. were incorrectly coded
3. had insufficient documentation in the record to support the treatment and services billed
4. contained other inconsistencies in the record and quality of care processes suggestive of billing that led to overpayment.

RACS will first send a demand letter containing some of the following: (1) Provider's identity, (2) Reason for the review, (3) List of claims, with findings, reasons for any denials, and amount of the overpayment for each claim, (4) Explanation of Medicare's right to charge interest on unpaid debts, (5) Instructions on paying the overpayments, (6) Explanation of the provider's right to submit a rebuttal statement and/or an appeal, (7) Description of the overpayment situation, including the reasons for the overpayment and suggested corrective actions, (8) Other demand letter requirements for written notifications, including the citation of the specific coverage, coding, or payment policies that the organization may have violated leading to the overpayment.

Following the initial demand letter, an appeal consists of the following: (1) Rebuttal, (2) redetermination, (3) reconsideration, (4) administrative law judge, (5) medicare appeal council, (6) US District Court.

Medicaid Integrity Program (MIPs) was created by the Deficit Reduction Act of 2005 to audit and collect Medicaid overpayments to healthcare providers with enforcement by Medicaid Integrity Contractors (MICs). Their role is to review provider actions, audit claims, identify overpayments; and educate providers, managed care entities, beneficiaries and others with respect to payment integrity and quality of care. The MIC mails a notification letter to the provider giving at least two weeks' notice before the audit is to begin.

Section 4.4: ELEMENTS OF A COMPLIANCE PROGRAM

A proper compliance program is the best insurance to proper reimbursement and office management practices. A proper compliance program should include

1. The development and institution of written standards for all aspects of the office management, including reimbursement and coding,
2. The selection of a compliance and security officer within the practice to develop and ensure institution and compliance with the written compliance program.
3. Provision of proper training to all staff and healthcare providers.
4. Established complaint process.
5. Enforcement policies for violations.
6. Audits and other evaluation techniques.
7. Investigation and remediation of violations and problems.

Section 4.5: OIG WORKPLAN

Each year, the Office of Inspector General publishes its work plan which highlights what coding areas will be focused on during that year for investigation. This is a valuable resource in that it can provide guidance as to proper coding so that proper measures and study can be taken by a healthcare provider to ensure that they are in compliance with those issues which may help thwart an audit or noncompliance (http://oig.hhs.gov/reports-and-publications/workplan/index.asp)

Section 4.6: AUDITING

Audits are reviews of practices and procedures to establish baselines and determine deviations, otherwise known as fraud, abuse, and/or omissions and mistakes. They can be initiated by external, internal, governmental or regulatory agencies with respect to possible fraud, abuse, or omissions/mistakes. The purpose of the auditing is to ensure proper compliance with rules and regulations with the ultimate purpose being the provision of quality healthcare. Auditing can involve coding as well as issues concerning reimbursement, privacy, legal, reimbursement, management, and compliance with regulatory requirements. Audits also ensure accuracy, consistency, timeliness and completeness.

Audits should be conducted on a regular basis which can be based on a certain percentage of charts reviewed or focused such as on certain specialties or doctors. Audits can be either retrospective or prospective. A retrospective audit is done after a claim has been submitted; Prospective audits are done before the claim is submitted.

Audits should include auditing of the superbill on a regular basis to ensure that: (1) the codes are updated and current; (2) applicable and highly used codes are included on the superbill; (3) physicians and staff are selecting proper codes that are justified as medically necessary by the documentation in the patient's record.

Other reasons that may evoke the need to conduct an audit include rejected claims, OIG work plan, suspected problems due to staff comments, physician or administrative requests, and other changes in the reimbursement or coding processes.

REASONS FOR AUDITS: Reasons in the past for audits include:

1. Up-coding
2. Using a code that does not properly define the services provided.
3. Not documented not done services as reported.
4. Billing for services not performed.
5. Unnecessary treatment, not medically necessary which is not justified by diagnoses.
6. Too many codes of the same type
7. Performing disallowed procedures and billing them as allowed ones
8. Unbundling
9. Billing for procedures that are already covered under other global time periods.
10. Improper use of "multiple procedure codes."

PRE-AUDIT: Once the audit is approved and has full support of administration, requests must be made for the proper records and information. Charts and actual reports should be used for the audit. All staff, including physicians, should be notified to ensure their full cooperation.

It can be helpful to query staff and physicians about possible problem areas or issues to help guide the audit to determine if there are any particular areas of concern that should be focused on. This is particularly true of the billing and medical records department since employees may know of current issues that should be investigated. EOBs (explanation of benefits) can also be reviewed to investigate why claims were denied.

AUDIT: To conduct the audit full clinical records (either paper or electronic) need to be available. Forms can be developed to assist with collection of consistent and focused data from various people, including staff, physicians, and external agencies. The audit can be used to compare ICD-10 and CPT/HCPCS codes to ensure proper coding from the documentation, claim and EOBs completion and processing, determination of discrepancies, and to provide feedback to administration, staff and physicians through training, meetings and workshops.

POST AUDIT: The final report should contain the following:

1. Review of the purpose, objectives and methodology of the audit.
2. Report major coding deficiencies including coding errors and sources of errors.
3. The report containing the findings including areas of good practice, analysis of errors and recommendations.

DENIALS/APPEALS: Appeals are becoming a critical element in the reimbursement process since there are many external agencies which conduct audits and assess denials and penalties on healthcare providers. Because a healthcare provider may receive a notice of denial of payment or findings from an audit does not mean that they were not in compliance, so it is important that the staff/coder understand the process and are highly knowledgeable so that they can file proper appeals and ensure proper reimbursement and compliance for their healthcare providers.

CMS requires that RACs operate web-based systems so that providers who are involved in an audit will have secure online access to information that explains the status of their claims. CMS oversight will ensure that providers are not unduly burdened or second-guessed by the RACs. CMS will also require the RACs to identify and publish vulnerability analyses so that the provider community can better understand where mistakes are being made and have the opportunity to correct.

DOS AND DONTS FOR AUDITS:

1. Don't procrastinate by doing your response on the last day.
2. Don't expect to answer all of your audit complaints, but make an attempt to do each one.
3. Separate out each complaint into the "type of classification" usually by error type, diagnoses or procedure.
4. Don't throw away the demand letter or their audit report.
5. Less said the better. Responses should be written and carefully thought out.
6. Include documents that support your position.

REGULATIONS QUIZ 1

1. What does OIG stand for?
2. What does HIPAA stand for?
3. Explain the Stark Laws.
4. What are the fines for healthcare fraud?
5. What other prosecutory actions are levied besides fines for healthcare fraud?
6. What is the three areas of healthcare offenses and describe them.
7. Where can you find what areas OIG will be focusing on for fraud and abuse for that year?
8. Describe the components of a good compliance program.
9. What does Qui Tam mean?
10. Who is responsible for development of the ICD codes?

CHAPTER 5
MEDICAL REPORTS AND FORMATS

You will learn the following objectives in this chapter:

A. The health record in coding
B. Health record factors.
C. Types of report formats.
D. Types of Reports

Section 5.1: THE ESSENTIAL ROLE OF HEALTH RECORDS IN CODING

The health record provides the heart of coding because only descriptions and services contained in a legitimate health record can be coded; it is essential to remember the coder's motto "not documented, not done." This motto stresses that if the physician does not provide proper and adequate documentation of the patient's status, health condition, prior history, and services rendered, then proper reimbursement and, therefore, proper medical care may be jeopardized. In addition, the health record must be properly completed and signed at which time it becomes a legal record; otherwise, there are serious repercussions that can result, including not only federal government sanctions and fines, but also legal ramifications if the records were involved in a lawsuit.

Perhaps one of the most important functions of a proper medical record is that it provides the supporting documentation that verifies medical necessity. Medical necessity has become a cornerstone in proper coding and reimbursement because if a record cannot validate the need for services provided then the issues of fraud and abuse can arise. From the medical report, the coder then selects proper ICD-10 codes which are listed on the CMS-1500 billing form and linked to the CPT/HCPCS codes for services. This linkage is what proves medical necessity and so it is critical that a qualified coder understands how codes are assigned and linked on the CMS-1500 billing form . The importance of the health record has become critical in proper reimbursement and operations of a healthcare practice because it illustrates medical necessity and stands as a legal document to protect the practices of a healthcare provider with the courts.

For these reasons, a well prepared health record with a good format ensures easy and proper coding and billing as all relevant information is provided and easy to find and read as will be discussed more thoroughly later.

Section 5.2: HEALTH RECORD DATA STANDARDIZATION

There are a number of important policies/procedures and data that must be followed and provided to ensure standardization on the medical record to reduce any misinterpretations since records may be shared amongst different medical specialties and across the country or nations.

As part of the effort to standardize health record data, the Uniform Hospital and Discharge Data Set (UHDDS) was established. UHDDS required that certain information be included in all medical records across the country which includes: patient full name, patient identifier number, address, date of birth, gender, marital status, race or ethnic group, social security number, primary and secondary insurance companies and information, guarantor for patient's account, employer's name and address, parent information for minor child, occupation, emergency contact information, primary care physician contact information and referring physician. This ensures that if a patient moves to another part of the country they can still receive optimal healthcare in that it is not jeopardized by a lack of communication or information.

Other data sets collect similar data as well as additional data relative to the type of care. These include the Minimum Data Set for Long-Term Care (MDS) used for nursing home patients, the Uniform Ambulatory Care Data Set (UACDS) for ambulatory patients, the Outcomes and Assessment Information Set (OASIS) for home health patients, Data Elements for Emergency Department Systems (DEEDS) for emergency room patients, and Health Plan Employer Data and Information Set (HEDIS) for healthcare purchasers and patients.

To ensure proper completion of health records, other practices and procedures that should be followed include:

1. Only black ink can be used for handwritten entries.
2. Handwriting must be legible. If it is not legible, then it is considered to not exist.
3. Entries within the health record must be made in a timely fashion.
4. All entries must have a date and time with initials of who made the entries.
5. All entries and records must have proper healthcare provider signatures.
6. To make changes in a health record, a line should be drawn through the error, followed by a date and initials of who made the change and when.
7. An option to making changes in a health record is to add an addendum with a reference to the addendum within the health record with date and time and signature provided.

Section 5.3: TYPES OF HEALTH RECORD FORMATS

There are three main types of health record formats: source oriented, integrated, and problem oriented.

A source-oriented health record is based on what department, specialty, or other group is involved in the patient's care. This type of report makes it easy to find and follow specific treatment of a patient. For instance, all of the x-rays for a patient diagnosed with cancer would be located together and it would be easy to follow the progression of the disease. The problem, though, is that it can result in fragmentation of the history of care as other specialties may provide services pertinent to other services which results in a less congruent time frame of care. It is also dependent on the knowledge of what kind of records and care is being sought before reports can be located which may result in some information being overlooked.

An integrated health record is where all reports are strictly situated within the record chronologically. Although this may provide a more congruent time line for the patient's care, this can be highly cumbersome, particularly for lengthy files in which there may be many reports. In this type of format, each report would be viewed in order to progress to the next one until the desired report is found.

A problem-oriented health record is based on the diagnosis or problem for which the patient is being treated. This type of format is also known as POMR (problem oriented medical record). This format presents the difficulty of comprehending the patient's record of care if a patient has numerous problems and many services are provided.

An alternative to these three types of health record formats include a format which combines various aspects of each format which can be selected and implemented according to the needs of the healthcare practice.

Progress notes are used often by healthcare providers and may be presented in several formats. The SOAP is the most common format consisting of four categories. This consists of the description of each category sometimes contained within a couple of sentences in the order of SOAP. The S stands for subjective which is the symptoms and history as stated by the patient and usually obtained from the health history record completed by the patient prior to services being provided. The O stands for objective which is the findings of the healthcare provider. A stands for Assessment which is the evaluation and determination by the healthcare provider of the patient's condition. The P stand for plan which is the healthcare provider's decision regarding what type of care will be provided to the patient. This format is enhanced in the SNOCAMP format. The additional elements are N which means nature of presenting problem, C which means counseling and/or coordination of care, and M which means medical decision making.

Section 5.4: TYPES OF REPORTS

There are numerous reports that can be found within a medical record. The main ones for hospitalization include History and Physical, Operative, Consultations, Pathology, Radiology, and Discharge Summary. Offices frequently use progress notes as previously described, but the other report types will be described here.

It is important to understand medical record formats as a coder because documentation is where the codes are derived from during abstracting. Abstracting is the higher level process in which coders take the entire medical record with all reports and research through them to find the ICD-10 diagnostic codes and CPT/HCPCS codes in physician billing. With hospital coding, Volume 3 ICD-10 procedural codes would be used instead of CPT codes. As a coder, you will have to read and review the many reports found within the record and, therefore, the more familiar you are with the record format and what is contained within the reports, the easier it will be to find the right information to ensure proper coding.

The best reports have clearly defined headings which include patient information at the beginning followed by specific headings relative to the report which will be discussed for each report. As a coder, you will use these headings to help you scan a record and know where important information is located and where your analysis as a coder should begin and what it should include. When you first begin abstracting from reports you will find it cumbersome and slow but as you progress you will learn where crucial information is located and, therefore, will became faster.

As with all reports, the History and Physical report begins with demographics, such as the patient's name, patient number, physician's name, etc. There is usually an ADMITTING DIAGNOSIS listed. This heading section is then followed by paragraphs. These paragraphs usually begin with a HISTORY OF PRESENT ILLNESS, followed by PAST FAMILY SOCIAL HISTORY, ALLERGIES, and REVIEW OF SYSTEMS. You will learn more about the value of these sections in determining the level of evaluation and management codes with CPT coding later. The paragraphs then progress onto the EXAM, and an IMPRESSION. When these reports are properly done, the REVIEW OF SYSTEMS and EXAM sections will contain subsections highlighted by the different systems of the body, such as HEENT, CARDIOVASCULAR, RESPIRATORY, INTEGUMENTARY, DIGESTIVE, etc.

The Operative Report consists of the regular headings as previously mentioned including a listing of the diagnoses and the operative procedure. It is this brief description of the procedure in this heading that is a critical beginning point for determining what services were provided for CPT coding purposes. The report then proceeds into the paragraph sections which consists primarily of a description of the procedure. Remember as you gain experience you will get faster with abstracting information from the reports.

Pathology reports usually consist of the standard headings in addition to the postoperative diagnoses, specimens, gross description, and microscopic description. Radiology consists of the standard headings in addition to the type of test and the findings.

The last report is typically the Discharge Summary which also contains the standard headings but includes a DISCHARGE DIAGNOSES. It is this heading that is the most important within all of the reports because it is the most definitive diagnoses and is where you should start when you are abstracting. You should use other diagnostic listings and descriptions to verify this or add to it, in addition to various paragraphs throughout the patient's chart. There is usually a description of the hospital stay, a brief description of the procedure, and then a discharge plan.

See Appendix B for samples of these types of reports.

Section 5.5: PATIENT RECORDS

A personal health record (PHR) contains personal health information (PHI) which if stored electronically is known as electronic health record (EHR).

Minimum required information in the data set for the these can include demographic information, medical information, allergies, conditions, hospitalizations, surgeries, medications, immunizations, provider information, health status, medical, personal and family history, insurances, and payments.

It must be remembered that the PHI is owned by the patient, the PRH is controlled by the patient, but the EHR are property of the healthcare provider. The PHR differs from the EHR in that the patient controls the information in the PHR and maintains it.

There are various methods used with the EHR. This includes voice recognition, bar code readers, computer templates, computerized data entry systems, document imaging, computerized physician order entry (CPOE), and optical character readers.

With an electronic system, there must be a process in which signatures can be authenticated. This means that the computer system can provide electronic signatures by various means which are used to indicate that the person entering the information entered into the electronic record is the authorized person and not somebody else. This can be achieved by the use of passwords, user ID, and other means of identification. It is critical that the person who is authorized with that signature is the one entering the information and that nobody else ever enters information on another person's electronic signature.

Release of information (ROI) is as form that allows the release of patient information to another agency or party. The information provided should follow the minimum necessary standards in which health information should be limited to the minimum amount that will achieve the purpose of the request. Per HIPAA, the information on the ROI should include

- The patient's name and date of birth
- Doctor's full name
- What is being requested and who is requesting
- Expiration date or event that relates to the individual or the purpose of the use or disclosure
- Revocable clause
- AIDS confidentiality clause
- Signed recently
- A statement regarding the potential for redisclosure of information

Section 5.6: HEALTHCARE QUALITY

Healthcare quality is overseen by Centers for Medicare and Medicaid Services (CMS) as well as Agency for Healthcare Research and Quality (AHRQ) which is also part of HSS. The National Committee for Quality Assurance (NCQA) also works with promoting quality healthcare. They are responsible for developing the Health Plan Employer Data and Information Set (HEDIS) and are involved in accreditation and certification with the purpose that employers are able to select healthcare plans. The American National Standards Institute (ANSI) provides accreditation to organizations to ensure utilization of proper standards. The American Society for Testing and Materials (ASTM) establishes standards for materials and products.

REPORT FORMAT QUIZ 2

1. Name and describe the three types of health record formats.
2. Describe the advantages and disadvantages of each type of health record format.
3. Describe the two types of progress notes.
4. What are five types of medical reports?
5. Describe the content of the history and physical report.
6. What are the two most important parts of medical reports for coding purposes?
7. Describe abstracting.
8. Describe two ways in which changes can be made to a medical report.
9. Describe four criterion for proper completion of medical records.
10. What is the coder's motto concerning medical records?

CHAPTER 6
ICD-10 STRUCTURE

You will learn the following objectives in this chapter:

You will learn the following objectives in this chapter:

1. History of ICD-10
2. Reasons for Change
3. Structure of ICD-10-CM Book
4. Differences between ICD-10 Books
5. ICD-10 Description
6. ICD-10 Classification

K. Characters of the codes
   1. Character Notations3

L. Description of Volume 2

M. Selection of Codes from Volume 2
   1. Main terms and subterms

N. Z Codes

O. S, T, V and Y Codes

Section 6.1: HISTORY OF ICD-10

ICD-10 was endorsed by the Forty-third World Health Assembly in May 1990 and was in application in 1994 throughout most of the world, except for United States although it is used for mortality purposes.

The first edition of ICD was known as the International List of Causes of Death originating in 1850. In 1948 WHO took over the responsibility for the ICD for the purposes of compilation of national mortality and morbidity statistics and subsequent classification of this data for the purposes of statistics, world-wide health management, research, records, storage of information, and compilation of national mortality and morbidity statistics throughout the world.

ICD has been regularly updated and changed to meet the greatly changing times within the healthcare field by WHO. Currently, the United States has been utilizing the 9th revision, while rest of the world has been using the ICD-10. One of the main reasons that United States has not adopted ICD-10 is because the revision needed to be altered for reimbursement and implementation purposes within United States, so the version ICD-10-CM needed to be developed.

The ICD is the largest classification system based on a hierarchial system. It classifies a wide variety of healthcare data with one of its main purposes being to provide statistics for healthcare research. In its purest form, ICD translates healthcare into numbers so that it can be processed in a meaningful way for reports and narratives.

Most importantly, the use of ICD codes was widely promoted by Medicare's requirement in the

1980's that they be used for all reporting and billing. Without the use of proper ICD codes, a healthcare provider would not be paid because the codes justify medical necessity of services provided.

Section 6.2: REASONS FOR CHANGE

With the ICD-10, countries are more able to track and respond to public health emergencies and utilize electronic records and SNOMED-CT more effectively. ICD-9 was no longer able to accomplish these goals because it lacked the ability to be more specific and detailed because it was running out of capacity and structure of numbers which, therefore, could not accommodate the vast advances and reimbursement issues in the healthcare field, specifically technology and quality, the continuous changes within diseases, and the ever-changing regulations and structure of healthcare practices, most specifically the electronic medical record. As a reflection of our times, ICD-10 is also better able to document and track terroristic attacks, biochemical attacks, and new and changing diseases through its alphanumeric format which allows for considerably more space for future revision without disruption of the numbering system.

ICD-10 provides greater compatibility and usability with SNOMED-CT. SNOMED-CT is the Systematized Nomenclature of Medicine -- Clinical Terms which is a computerized set of medical terminology covering diseases, findings, procedures, organisms, etc which, therefore, promotes the ability to electronically index, store, retrieve, and aggregate medical data from many healthcare sources which is contained within the electronic medical record (EMR) and is utilized with computer-assisted coding (CAC).

ICD-10 provides the ability of the United States to compare and share data about diseases with other countries who are utilizing ICD-10 now which promotes better public health surveillance and research. It also provides better measures of patient care quality since it is more attune to new technologies and procedures since it adds more detail and expands codes for medical complications and safety issues, particularly for the top causes of mortality and diseases, even those related to terroristic attacks. This also promotes greater response to reimbursement issues, such as medical necessity, and less errors; therefore, promoting better management and institutional performance.

ICD-10 provides the ability to rate the severity of diseases which is critically important in the outcomes of the patient's care and assessment of institutional and practice practices.

External cause of injury codes detailing external factors that produced the injury are also much more detailed in ICD-10-CM which help in ensuring injury prevention and developing safety programs, including in the workplace and for violent crimes.

ICD-10-CM index, tabular, guidelines, and general equivalence mapping files on the National Center for Health Statistics Web site at: www.cdc.gov/nchs/about/otheract/icd9/icd10cm.htm.

General Equivalence Mappings (GEMs) are provided from various sources which help with crosswalking from ICD-9 codes to ICD-10 codes although it must be strongly noted that, like with any type of translation, the codes are not equivalent as there are many differences and additions/deletions which compromise the accuracy of crosswalking.

Section 6.3: ICD-10 DESCRIPTION

ICD-10-CM is an acronym which stands for "International Classification of Diseases, 9th Revision, Clinical Modification." ICD-10-CM is a clinical modification (CM) of the World Health Organization's ICD-10 for use within the United States in the same fashion as the ICD-9-CM and is maintained by the U.S. National Center for Health Statistics. ICD-10-PCS is developed by the Center for Medicare and Medicaid Services (CMS) and is used by hospitals to code for procedures and services that are performed as inpatient. CMS also provides regular updates and information which can be found through the Correct Coding Initiative and Federal Register, as well as many other sources such as insurance companies, state health departments, and organizations.

With ICD-10-CM, there are two sections, ICD-10 and ICD-10-PCS. ICD-10 is reminiscent of the traditional Volumes 1 and 2 from ICD-9 and ICD-10-PCS is reminiscent of Volume 3 which provided codes for in-hospital procedures. ICD-10-PCS codes are alphanumeric codes comprised of 7 characters.

There are more than 68,000 codes in the ICD-10-CM compared to the approximately 13,000 ICD-9-CM diagnosis codes. There are more than 87,000 procedure codes in the ICD-10-PCS. Both of these numbers demonstrate that clearly there is greater specificity in the ICD-10-CM and PCS.

The structure of the ICD-10 is similar to ICD-9 in that there are three volumes with chapters and categories. There are 21 chapters in ICD-10 whereas there were only 17 in ICD-9. There are two new chapters, Chapter VII "Diseases of the eyelid and adnexa" and Chapter VIII "Diseases of the ear and mastoid process". Other chapters have new and expanded names. Some chapters, such as "symptoms, signs and ill-defined conditions" have increased by more than 300%.

The ICD-10-CM book is divided into three volumes:

Volume 1: Tabular List of Diseases and Injuries
Volume 2: Alphabetic Index to Diseases
Volume 3: Tabular List of and Alphabetic Index to Procedures

These will be described later in this module and throughout all of the modules.

First, although there are three volumes in ICD-10-CM books, for physician coding only the first two volumes are used. The third volume is for coding of procedures in the hospital. Many ICD-10-CM books do not contain a third volume because this is used strictly for inpatient hospital coding and is not used for physician coding. Therefore, there is no reason for a person to pay additional monies for a book with three volumes if they are not going to be coding for inpatient hospital procedures. For this course which focuses on coding for the physician offices, we are only interested in the first two volumes. It is advised that you do not study for the inpatient hospital coding unless you are going to be doing inpatient hospital coding because it does differ from physician coding. Studying for inpatient hospital coding can be confusing when preparing to take the test for physician coding and may result in lost points and possible test failure.

Section 6.4: DIFFERENCES BETWEEN ICD-10-CM BOOKS

There are many versions of the ICD-10-CM book published by various companies with many differences. It is recommended when you take the national coding exams that you use a regular book and not any described as expert or otherwise. In fact, alternative versions may not be allowed on exams so do not jeopardize your chances of passing your national exam by using an alternative book. The reason for this is that some of those differences could affect the outcome of your test because you may not have access to some important information. During this course, you will learn about what are the most helpful and important attributes to look for in an ICD-10-CM book.

Also, there are different publishers and different features to each type of book. One of these differences is that some publishers will put the alphabetic index first and the tabular index second. Note, at the beginning of this section, however, that Volume 1 is known as the Tabular List and Volume 2 is known as the Alphabetic Index. Even though these volumes may be switched in the order of their presentation, it still remains that Volume 1 is the Tabular List and Volume 2 is the Alphabetic Index. It is important to emphasize that, because of this, you should become familiar with the use of your book, particularly before testing, so that you can easily and quickly find your way through the book without confusion as it could result in errors and lost time which are not desirable during a national test.

Section 6.5: DIFFERENCES BETWEEN ICD-9 AND ICD-10 BOOKS

Although the differences between the ICD-9 and ICD-10 codes will be discussed and illustrated throughout this entire book, a general presentation is provided now.

- There are 21 chapters in ICD-10 but in ICD-9 there were only 17.
- ICD-10 codes are alphanumeric rather than the ICD-9 where most codes were only numeric.
- There are additional characters possible for codes in ICD-10, up to seven, whereas the most characters possible in ICD-9 were five.
- Codes in ICD-10 now specify laterality which was not available ICD-9 codes.
- There is the use of a placeholder denoted by X which is used when a space is not filled in with other characters but rather the X is used to hold the place for future use when additional expansion may be needed for codes.
- There are full code descriptions in ICD-10 rather than the breakdown of common fourth and fifth characters into one box which were then applied to numerous codes as seen in ICD-9.
- There are now combination codes for poisonings and their causes in ICD-10 rather than the additional E codes for causes that were used in ICD-9.
- There is greater specification within codes such as pregnancy codes further distinguished by trimesters for ICD-10.
- V and E codes of the ICD-9 are now incorporated into the main code classification

in ICD-10.

- ICD-10 does classify some codes by anatomic site such as injuries which are first coded by site and then by injury; ICD-9 classified by injury.
- There are new separate chapters in ICD-10 for eye and ear conditions which did not exist in ICD-9.
- Changes in time frames in ICD-10 for some codes such as MI which are now 4 weeks instead of 8 weeks.
- There are many reclassifications of diseases and conditions to other chapters in ICD-10 which differ from where the codes were placed in ICD-9 including more use of combination codes.
- Postoperative complications are now included in each chapter by procedure-body system in ICD-10 rather than in their own section at the end of Volume 1 as they were in ICD-9.
- In ICD-10 there are now two types of exclude notes. Exclude 1 indicates "not coded here" in which the excluded code cannot be listed with the condition described in the original code. Exclude 2 indicates "not included here" as it is not part of the condition described in the code.

Section 6.6: DESCRIPTION OF VOLUMES

ICD-10-CM has an alphabetical index and tabular list similar to those of ICD-9-CM including indentations and use of sections, categories, and subcategories which creates the familiar hierarchical system. The main terms are in bold.

There are two parts to the ICD-10-CM alphabetical index which are the index to diseases and injury and index to external causes of injury. As with the ICD-9 the table of drugs and chemicals and the neoplasm table are contained with the alphabetical index. There no longer is a table for hypertension.

Volume 1 is known as the Tabular List of Diseases and Injuries. This is where the codes are located. Again, it does not matter where the book organizes the volumes, Volume 1 remains as the Tabular List and lists the actual codes. The Alphabetic Index is Volume 2 and contains alphabetical listing of conditions as well as the Neoplasm Table and, Index for External Causes of Injury, and Table of Drugs and Chemicals.

HIERARCHIAL SYSTEM: The Tabular List is organized in a hierarchical classification system. Understanding and properly using the hierarchical system is critical to proper coding, so be sure to understand this system of indentations, highlighting, and other notations that will be discussed as the means to classifying diseases and injuries.

The hierarchical systems are categorized by alphanumeric characters. Codes can vary from three to seven characters. The various characters can symbolize details of diseases, injuries, and conditions which prompt the need for medical care. These will be discussed within each section where it is applicable.

RULE: A critical rule involving the use of the hierarchical system in ICD-10-CM coding is **CODE TO THE HIGHEST LEVEL OF SPECIFICITY,** which will be discussed below.

Section 6.7: CLASSIFICATIONS

The hierarchical system is based on classifications (or subdivisions). Again, it is not as important to remember the exact definition of what each level signify but rather to understand the application. The change to a different level of classification is indicated by indentations within the Tabular List.

The first subdivision is by **CHAPTER.**

Volume 1 consists of 21 chapters, rather than the 17 of ICD-9. Chapters are based on body system or condition. The first character is alphabetical but the remaining characters may be either alphabetical or numeric.

These chapters are:

1.	Infectious and Parasitic Diseases	A00-B99
2.	Neoplasms	C00-D49
3.	Diseases of the Blood and Blood-Forming Organs	D50-D89
4.	Endocrine, Nutritional, and Metabolic Diseases, and Immunity Disorders	E00-E89
5.	Mental & Behavioral Disorders	F01-F99
6.	Diseases of the Nervous System And Sense Organs	G00-G99
7.	Disease of Eye & Adnexa	H00-H59
8.	Diseases of Ear & Mastoid Process	H60-H59
9.	Diseases of the Circulatory System	I00-I99
10.	Diseases of the Respiratory System	J00-J99
11.	Diseases of the Digestive System	K00-K95
12.	Diseases of the Skin and Subcutaneous Tissue	L00-L99
13.	Diseases of the Musculoskeletal System & Connective Tissue	M00-M99
14.	Diseases of the Genitourinary System	N00-N99
15.	Complications of the Pregnancy, Childbirth, and Puerperium	O00-O9A
16.	Certain Conditions Originating in the Perinatal Period	P00-P96
17.	Congenital Malformations, Deformations & Chromosomal Abnormalities	Q00-Q99
18.	Symptoms, Signs, and Abnormal Clinical & Laboratory Findings, Not elsewhere classified	R00-R99
19.	Injury, Poisoning & Certain Other Consequences of External Causes	S00-T88

20.	External Causes of Morbidity	V01-Y99
21.	Factors Influencing Health Status & Contact With Health Services	Z00-Z99

Codes are further broken down by categories, subcategories and valid codes. SUBCATEGORIES are indicated by either four or five characters. It is important to remember to code to **THE HIGHEST LEVEL OF SPECIFICITY RULE** by putting the correct number of characters required for a code. There are notes and indications at the bottom of each page to denote when an additional character is required.

X is used as a placeholder in some codes which allows for future expansion of codes.

Section 6.8: CHARACTERS

ICD-10 has a new name, "International Statistical Classification of Diseases and Related Health Problems".

The first most important concept is that almost all of the codes were only numeric in ICD-9-CM but are alphanumeric in ICD-10-CM and structured on a hierarchical system. It is very important that the correct number of characters are applied or payment will be denied and the coding will be wrong.

The importance of learning this hierarchical system can be seen in the selection of a wrong code by not following the hierarchical system which results in serious errors which will be seen repeatedly throughout the modules as we go more in depth. In other words, if the condition requires the use of four characters as directed by the ICD-10-CM book, then four characters must be coded. The same for five characters and so forth for all characters.

DETERMING CHARACTER NOTATIONS: The first character for ICD-10 codes is always alphabetical. All letters of the alphabet are used with the exception of U which has been reserved by WHO for assignment of new diseases of uncertain etiology and for drug-resistant bacteria.

The remaining characters can be either alphabetical or numeric with the exception of the second character which is always numeric. Seventh characters are used to denote encounters or sequelae for injuries and external causes.

As with ICD-9, the period is placed after the first three characters.

Do not neglect to include the proper number of characters when coding because it is wrong as previously noted. For example, do not use only four characters when five characters are required.

First, there are notations in the tabular list which indicate the proper number of characters, as well as sometime an indication of which specific character should be used, which will be discussed further in later chapters. These notations can include a notation by the side of various codes that indicate the need for a fourth or fifth character.

Second, most additional characters are indicated with full descriptions following the initial code. For example, Multiple myeloma (C90.0) has further specification such as C90.00 for multiple myeloma not having achieved remission, C90.01 in remission and C90.02 in relapse.

Third, in the alphabetical index, a hyphen (-) is listed after some codes to indicate that additional characters are required.

> **IMPORTANT! When it is noted that a character needs to be added, be sure to add the character in its proper place.**

In other words, a notation will indicate if a fourth or fifth character needs to be listed so be sure that your code has the proper number of characters. The first character is the third character to the left of the period. The second character is the second character to the left of the period. The third character is the first character to the left of the period. The fourth character is the first character to the right of the period. The fifth character is the second character to the right of the period and so on. If a character is required in a specific location, but there are there no values associated with a previous character space assigned yet, then "x" is used as a placeholder. For example, T38.4X1. The X does not represent any value yet but a seventh character is required so the "X" holds the space to ensure proper use of character spacing.

BE CAREFUL! Do not transpose characters. Again, using the example above, do not enter T37.4X5 when the code is T37.5X4. It in these transpositions that many coding errors are made.

An additional source of common errors in coding is selecting the code from the wrong line. This is a significant problem and be sure you are overly cautious concerning this selection from the wrong line as it is extremely easy to do. This error occurs due to the complex and extensive hierarchical system of coding as previously explained and will be discussed further in discussion about the alphabetical index. In other words, be sure that you did not go into another section of classification and indentation. This is particularly a problem when you change to another column or page. The alphabetical index for ICD-10 has tried to eliminate this problem by adding grey bars along the side of the pages which indicate when categories begin and when another code is listed under that code or has its own subcategory.

Section 6.9: DESCRIPTION OF VOLUME 2

Volume 2 is known as the Alphabetical Index. Again, this may be listed second in the ICD-10-CM book which is why it is known as Volume 2; however, some books are printed with the Volume 2 listed first.

Volume 2 is divided into:

1. Alphabetical Index listing diseases and injuries.
2. Table of Drugs and Chemicals.
3. Alphabetic Index to External Causes of Injury and Poisoning (E codes).

There are some basic critical rules to remember about utilizing Volume 2.

RULE: NEVER CODE DIRECTLY FROM VOLUME 2!

If there are discrepancies or debate regarding selection of the proper code, the ICD-10-CM book is used as the final authority, the basis for all coding decisions, and the tabular index is the final authority. The ICD-10-CM book is very clear and precise. Therefore, if either the Tabular List or the Alphabetical Index provides direction on selecting the proper code, then you must follow these directions. When coding, always remember – YOU MUST USE THE ICD-10-CM CODING BOOK TO JUSTIFY YOUR SELECTIONS, so if someone came two years later questioning why you selected certain codes, then you would need to demonstrate a rationale from the ICD-10-CM code book for why you chose the code you did.

It is important to remember this because oftentimes the Alphabetical Index will provide instructions on selecting on the proper code. If the Index tells you to do so, then do so. Do not interpret (misinterpret) the codes because of information you may think you know that contradicts the information in the ICD-10-CM book. If you have a disagreement with codes as they are, the proper place to ask those question is not when you are coding to bill, but by addressing the questions to CMS.

Section 6.10: SELECTION OF CODES FROM VOLUME 2

MAIN TERMS: Of course, the alphabetical index is set up alphabetically; however, there are some idiosyncrasies that can complicate finding the correct code. Basically, the index is set up in a hierarchical system beginning with main terms which can be based on anatomical site, diseases, eponyms, conditions, general nouns and adjectives. These terms are bolded. An eponym is a term named after a person which is common in the medical field, such as Parkinson's disease and Lou Gehrig's Disease. The main terms are also listed at the top of each page, much as it would be found in a dictionary. It is important to acknowledge general terms because many codes are listed here and not elsewhere. Examples of general terms include "failure", "disease", "examination", "disturbance", "disorder", "dependence, "problem", etc.

IMPORTANT! In the alphabetical index for ICD-10-CM, if there is a hyphen (-) listed at the end of a code entry, this indicates that additional characters are needed.

SUBTERMS: Below the main terms there is usually a listing of subterms which are further elaborations (modifications) of the main term. Under subterms, you will find more subterms (carryovers) which are further elaborations (modifications) of the subterms, which forms the hierarchical system of the ICD-10-CM codes. To create the hierarchical system, these subterms are indented under the term that it is connected to. For example, if you locate contusion in the alphabetical index, you will see there are many subterms, but that the indentation of the terms varies. The subterms, "with", "abdomen", "adnexa", are the first set of subterms and are indented but are the farthest indentation to the left under the main term, "contusion." Notice under "with" that there subterms which are further indented, which include "crush injury", "dislocation", etc. This means that these terms are all a subterm of "contusion". Now notice that under "contusion, with, internal injury", there are more subterms which are further indented, such as "heart", "kidney," and "liver". These are subterms of "contusion", but only of "contusion, with, internal injury". They are not subterms of "abdomen" or "adnexa" under "contusion".

Due to this hierarchical system, you will find that the terms are categorized in several ways. First, the subterms are categorized alphabetically. Most of the subterms can be found this way. But this becomes complicated because there are subterms under subterms which disrupts the alphabetical nature of this index.

Second, subterms under other subterms will be listed alphabetically, but this disrupts the original alphabetical indexing for the first subterm. In other words, you will have multiple alphabetical indices, so there are alphabetical indices contained within other alphabetical indices which, again, form the hierarchical nature of ICD-10-CM coding. Let's examine our example again of "contusion." Locate "arm" under "contusion". You will find that it has a couple of subterms further indented under it. This means that "lower" and "upper" are referring to a contusion on the arm and not any other term, such as abdomen or adnexa. This process of indentations is very important to understand and to use properly; otherwise, you may be selecting your codes from the wrong terms.

Third, as noted above, there are other subterms that disrupt the alphabetical indexing. These oftentimes are connecting terms or nouns other than diseases, conditions, or anatomic sites. There are a variety of these terms that occur commonly throughout the alphabetical index and they do disrupt the alphabetical listing but they are oftentimes very important in helping to find the correct code. In fact, if you cannot find your term alphabetically, you may find it under one of these terms. These general terms that are used throughout the alphabetical index include "with", "due to", "during", "following", "involving", "in", "secondary to", "with mention of", "complicated by", "management affected by", "administration of", "adjustment," etc. Therefore, you must be check in several places for a term: (1) traditional alphabetical ordering, (2) subterms under terms, (3) and general terms.

Therefore, when a term is indented under another term, it means that it is a subdivision or modifier of the term under which it is indented. This can vary from a few subterms to a lot. This is where the use of the alphabetical index becomes tricky, mainly because there are so many subterms and indentations that it becomes difficult to know if you are under the right term. For this reason, it becomes important that you take time to search through the main terms and subterms to be sure that you have found the right code and did not miss it somewhere.

Therefore, when you are looking for a code in the alphabetical index, you may have to look in several places and you must be sure that you do not get into the wrong main term or subterms. To achieve this, you must keep track of indentations and the alphabetical indexing, so if you are looking under terms that go from A to C to F, etc., and then you notice that the next term is B, then you know that you are no longer under the term you were originally looking under. For example, if you are looking for "pregnancy, complicated by", and you are then looking under "hemorrhage, threatened abortion" but you notice that you are looking at "h's" again, under hepatitis and hypertension, then you know that you have gone out of the subterms you wanted because "h" does not come before "t" in the alphabet.

Section 6.11: Z CODES

Z codes are what used to be Y codes. They are a supplementary classification system located at the end of the Tabular List in Volume. They are a listing of "Factors Influencing Health Status and Contact with Health Services." They contain a large variety of codes which are applied to services which do not meet the typical description of diseases and conditions as listed in the Tabular Index itself. These codes can be found in the Alphabetical Index for the tabular codes. These will be discussed later in their own packet. Oftentimes in ICD-10-CM codes the factors influencing health status and contact are included in the core code rather than having a separate code.

Section 6.12: S, T, V AND Y CODES

S, T, V, and Y codes are what used to be E codes. They are a supplementary classification system that is now before the Z codes in Volume 1. They are the supplementary classification of External Causes of Injury and Poisoning. Oftentimes in ICD-10-CM codes the external causes of injury and poisoning are included in the core code rather than having a separate code.

CHAPTER 7
ICD-10 CODING CONVENTIONS

You will learn the following objectives in this chapter:

A. Guidelines
    1. Placeholder
    2. Combination Codes
    3. Laterality
    4. New Codes
B. Late Effects
C. Medical Care Complications
    1. Postsurgical Complications
    2. Prosthetics/Grafts
    3. Infections
    4. Transplants
    5. Other
D. Code First
E. Cross-Referencing
F. Inclusion Notes/Nonessential Modifiers
G. Exclusion notes
H. Punctuation
    1. Parentheses
    2. Colon
    3. Square Brackets
    4. Slanted Brackets
I. Abbreviations
    1. NEC
    2. NOS

Section 7.1: GUIDELINES

PLACEHOLDERS: New to ICD-10-CM is the use of placeholders. X is always used as the placeholder in that it holds the place of that position for future use so that the structure of the code is not distorted, because if a character is required in the seventh position then it must be in the seventh position and not moved to fifth or sixth just because there are no values yet for those positions.

COMBINATION CODES: There are now more combination codes in the ICD-10 in which the cause and condition are coded together.

Combination Codes for Conditions and Common Symptoms:

- I25.110, Arteriosclerotic heart disease of native coronary artery with unstable angina pectoris

- K50.013, Crohn's disease of small intestine with fistula
- K71.51, Toxic liver disease with chronic active hepatitis with ascites

Combination Codes for Poisonings and the External Cause

- T39.011, Poisoning by aspirin, accidental (unintentional)
- T39.012, Poisoning by aspirin, intentional self harm
- T39.013, Poisoning by aspirin, assault
- T39.014, Poisoning by aspirin, undetermined

LATERALITY: ICD-10 codes are now more specific about the area of the body involved including right or left, such as left lower eyelid.

- C50.212, Malignant neoplasm of upper-inner quadrant of left female breast
- H02.835, Dermatochalasis of left lower eyelid
- I80.01, Phlebitis and thrombophlebitis of superficial vessels of right lower extremity
- L89.213, Pressure ulcer of right hip, stage III

NEW CODES: There are many new codes for conditions that did not have a specific code in ICD-9, e.g., Chronic fatigue syndrome (G93.3), chronic intractable pain (R52.1) and stress NOS (Z73.3.).

In addition to new codes, some codes have been moved to other chapters, e.g., transient cerebral ischemic attacks and related syndromes are now in the chapter for "Diseases of the Nervous System," rather than the circulatory chapter of the ICD-9.

Section 7.2: LATE EFFECTS: Late effects are now coded in the chapter to which they apply anatomically e,g, sequelae of injury of nerve of lower limb (T93.4). A late effect is a residual or sequelae that has continued after the treatment for the causal or etiological condition has concluded. Residuals and sequelae are conditions caused by another condition (etiology).

Late effects may be temporary or permanent. There is no time limit to determine a late effect; it will depend upon the condition and the patient.

Late effects in the alphabetical index of the ICD-10 book instruct to look under "sequelae". You can also find late effects listed under specific conditions, e.g., under hemiplegia there is a listing for "late effects or residual".

Section 7.3: MEDICAL CARE COMPLICATIONS

POSTSURGICAL COMPLICATIONS: Many postsurgical complications are now coded at the end of the chapter to which they are associated anatomically instead of in the last chapter of the coding book, e.g., vomiting following gastrointestinal surgery (K91.0) or infection due to foreign object left during a procedure (T81.6). However, some non-specific disorders are still coded in the last chapter, such as shock and air embolism.

Medical care complications are conditions and complications that result from medical care and are known as misadventures. Codes for complications of medical care are only used for unanticipated/undesirable conditions that result from the medical care itself; not for common and anticipated conditions of medical care. In other words, swelling is a common aftercare condition of a surgery, so it would not be coded as a complication of medical care. On the other hand, if a patient has an indwelling catheter and develops an infection, this would be considered a complication of the medical care and would be coded because, although infections do occur, it is not an acceptable outcome of medical care. There is no time limit on when conditions and complications of medical care can develop.

Medical care complications can be found in the alphabetical index under a variety of terms, including the complication itself, postsurgical, complications, medical care, and surgical procedures.

PROSTHETICS/GRAFTS: A common category that can produce postsurgical complications involve prosthetics and grafts. Prosthetics include a wide variety of devices and implants, such as heart valves, pacemaker, catheters, shunts, electrodes, contraceptive device, colostomy, screws, nails, and plates, . Medical care complications can include breakdown, displacement, perforation, protrusion, leakage, or obstruction by the devices. Although these conditions do occur, it is not an acceptable outcome of the surgery. These are coded as complications, prosthesis and under the specific prosthesis such as graft. Usually T codes are used to code for these.

INFECTION: Although infections also do occur from medical care, again they are not acceptable outcomes. They can be coded with T codes also such as T81.4.

TRANSPLANTS: Transplants oftentimes result in medical care complications and are coded by anatomic site; however, complications are only coded if they impair the functioning of the transplant. T86 codes are used to code for these complications.

OTHER: Other medical care complication codes include postoperative shock, hemorrhage, puncture or laceration, disruption of wound, foreign body left in the operation site, emphysema, non-healing surgical wound, air embolism, and infusion reactions.

Section 7.4: CODE FIRST/USE ADDITIONAL CODE

There is the use of "code also" and "use additional code if desired" in ICD-10 as there was in ICD-9. The use of the terms "due to" and "resulting in" do indicate causal relationship, but the use of terms "with", "with mention of", "associated with", and "in" do not necessarily indicate a causal relationship. The use of term "and" means they are not connected.

Section 7.5: CROSS REFERENCES

Under main terms and subterms, there are many cross-references in the alphabetical index which are extremely helpful. Cross references may be denoted by the terms, "see also," "see condition," etc. followed by the term of where to check or there may be a reference or duplication of terms. For example:

1. You can find references to pregnancy conditions under pregnancy, labor and delivery, postpartum, antepartum, etc.
2. You can find references to a condition under its own name, anatomical site, modifier, or condition, such as cortical blindness which can be found under cortical or blindness. If you look in the alphabetical index under cortical, you will see a note that says "see also condition." This means to check under "blindness."

When the alphabetical index makes a cross-reference, be sure to use the exact term. For instance, when a cross reference says, "see condition," it does not mean to look up the word "condition," but to look for the condition, such as "failure" for heart failure.

When the index makes references or notations, you must follow the directions completely. Do not alter or re-interpret what the alphabetical index or even the tabular list tells you to do. Follow it precisely. This point will be emphasized repeatedly throughout the packets.

Section 7.6: INCLUSION NOTES/NONESSENTIAL MODIFIERS

You will also find terms in the alphabetical index in parenthesis. These are known as nonessential modifiers because they do not need to be described in the patient's chart to allow for the use of this code. They are simply providing extra information to assist in more accurate coding.

Inclusion notes are similar to nonessential modifiers in that they do not exclude the use of codes to conditions not listed, but rather are simply providing more information. In other words, if a condition is not listed in the include notes of a code, the code may still be the correct code. The inclusions notes simply provide additional information to assist in the selection of the proper code, but again, do not preclude the use of the code for a condition that is not listed in the inclusion notes.

Again, if you have determined that this is the correct code from the use of the diagnostic statements provided by the physician and the use of the alphabetical index and tabular index but it is not described in these terms, you will still use these codes. Remember, inclusion notes do not exclude the use of the code for other descriptive diagnostic statements.

Section 7.7: EXCLUSIONS NOTES

There are two new exclude notes definitions.

Excludes 1 note means "not coded here" which means the excluded code is never used with the original code, they are exclusive of each other, i.e. they cannot exist together at the same time.

Excludes 2 note means "not included here" which means the excluded condition is not coded as part of the original code; therefore, if the patient does have both conditions they can both be coded but they are not coded as part of each other.

Exclusion notes are critical! They must be read in detail and followed precisely. The term

EXCLUDE is bolded in the ICD-10-CM book. Again, details are critical in coding and this is one detail that is! The exclusion note will apply to all codes within that main code.

Section 7.8: PUNCTUATION

PARENTHESIS: As discussed earlier, there are nonessential modifiers (supplementary words) which are additional information provided by the ICD-10-CM book to assist in proper coding which are included in parenthesis. Remember those that these do not exclude the use of this code for other diagnostic descriptions that are not included in the parenthesis.

COLON: A colon indicates additional modifiers of a term and these modifiers are indented below the term they modify.

SQUARE BRACKETS: Square brackets in the tabular list enclose alternate wording for a diagnostic description, including synonyms, abbreviations and phrases. In the alphabetical index, brackets are used to identify manifestation codes such as nephrosis in amyloidosis E85.4 [N08].

Section 7.9: ABBREVIATIONS

NEC: Not elsewhere classified. This category of codes is used when other information is provided about a code, but there is no specific code for it. This is usually indicated by the use of an "8" in the fourth position. It is also known as "other specified". For example, notice in code E22.8, it states "other". Again, this indicates that the specific site was not listed by itself and so this code contains a number of groups or sites. While this is the common practice of using 8 to signify "other", it does not mean that the description of the codes always follow this protocol, so always be sure to read the descriptions carefully. "8" can be used for other factors such as anatomic site.

NOS: Not otherwise specified. This category of codes is used when no other information is available and is usually indicated by the use of a "9". Notice also that the code's description may also say "unspecified", which means the same thing in referring to there being no further information provided. For example, see code D27.9 or D26.9 where the term "unspecified" is used. While this is the common practice, it does not mean that the description of the codes always follow this protocol of assigning "9" to NOS, so always be sure to read the descriptions carefully. "9" can be used for other factors such as anatomic site. Sometimes the NOS description is used in the beginning of a subcategory but only because the entire category is the last category.

CHAPTER 8
ICD-10 BASIC CODING GUIDELINES

You will learn the following in this chapter:

A. Basic coding guidelines and rules
    1. Medical Necessity
    2. Not documented, not done
B. Proper Coding with ICD-10
C. Multiple Codes
    1. Etiology/Manifestation
    2. Additional Codec/Code Also
    3. Code First
D. Combination Codes
E. Sequencing
F. Comorbidities and complications
G. Symptoms
H. Rule outs

Section 8.1: BASIC CODING GUIDELINES AND RULES

MEDICAL NECESSITY: The ICD-10-CM codes are used to prove medical necessity….this is a critical term on which all payment is based which is why providing the proper ICD-10-CM code is important. Services provided will not be paid if the ICD-10-CM code does not prove that the service was necessary. For example, if a patient is seen for a fractured leg and receives a stress test for a heart problem, then this service will be denied because it was not related to the care of the fracture. This is a huge problem nowadays as there are practices that will charge for services, such as tests, which they either do not provide or which should not have been provided because the patient's condition did not require it.

NOT DOCUMENTED, NOT DONE: This means that you can only code what the physician or healthcare provider has stated in the reports and notes within the patient's file. You cannot re-interpret, change, or ignore what is written in the patient's record. So, you cannot code more than or less than what the physician or healthcare provider has written.

If you find when you are attempting to code a report you cannot make a coding choice because the information is not clear, you can make queries of the physician at that time for the purpose of clarification. For example, if a report states that a patient is on insulin but the physician does not classify it as Type I, you may want to inquire of the physician if the patient is Type I diabetic.

Remember – **NOT DOCUMENTED, NOT DONE.** You can only code what the physician has reported and you cannot make your own interpretations. If a physician tells you he meant to put certain information in the report but failed to do so, then explain to him that in the future he must be sure to include it but you cannot code it unless it was in the signed final report.

When you are coding for a physician, you should derive your codes from the physician's statements as he determines the diagnosis, not you. This is a part of the "not documented, not done" concept because the physician must provide the information and make the diagnosis.

So, **NEVER** give a patient a diagnosis they do not have, and you can ensure that by never coding a diagnosis unless the physician has stated it which is a basic rule of coding, **NOT DOCUMENTED, NOT DONE.** This is one area of coding that causes enormous problems for nurses as they are accustomed to always trying to figure out what is wrong with the patient, but coders cannot do that – two completely different scenarios. So, nurses in particular, but others as well, may try to determine diagnosis, but remember that only the physician can do this, so avoid the urge (despite any available information or verbal directives) to select a code based on your making a diagnosis and not the physician's written statements.

This also applies to the physician making a report, signing a report, and then the physician wishing to later verbally add to the report after the bill has been sent so that a higher code can be billed. If the physician did not put the information in the report, it cannot be billed. This is poor practice and is a red flag for auditors and government agencies.

What can be done for situations where physicians are not reporting proper information to ensure correct billing and coding is that the coder should be involved in the education and training of the physician (and all office and healthcare staff) with regards to report formats and what they need to include in their reports to receive proper reimbursement. This education and training will then ensure that the proper procedures will be followed in the future and prevent future failures to receive full reimbursement.

Section 8.2: PROPER CODING WITH ICD-10-CM

There are many ways that the ICD-10-CM book provides valuable information in the selection of the codes. For this reason, you must follow the book's direction closely. Do not re-interpret what it tells you to do, nor disregard any information it provides.

How informative the ICD-10-CM book is will depend on the book you are using. Some books provide not only inclusion and exclusion notes, but also coding guideline notes, definitions, and references. Some provide additional table formatting. It is for this reason you should become familiar with the structure of your coding books before the national exam to ensure that you can quickly and easily find the correct codes and utilize all of the advantages that a book may offer.

IMPORTANT! At the front of the book are coding guidelines which are very helpful in further explaining the proper use of codes and are very helpful, especially during testing.

The process of selecting the right code begins with locating it in the alphabetical index. However, remember that you never select a code from the alphabetical index. This is because there are many notes, as are being described in this packet and others, which are listed in the tabular list and which are critical to the selection of the correct code.

Therefore, begin by searching for what you believe is the main term from the diagnostic statement (located on superbills or ideally in charts or reports). If you cannot find your code under this term, then pick the next best term to describe the condition. If that does not work, continue through the terms you have until you find the correct code. If you still cannot find the correct code, then you should think of terms that are similar to the terms describing the patient's condition.

Remember in our description of the structure of the book and conventions that you need to look for other terms as well, such as "with", "due to", "disease," etc. You may also need to follow instructions within the ICD-10-CM book, such as "see" and "see also."

Remember, follow the instructions within the alphabetical index and tabular list precisely. Correct coding depends heavily on the following of details precisely from the ICD-10-CM book.

If codes are listed in the alphabetical index in parenthesis, do not use them as the selected code. These signify other information about the code which varies by the codes, but is never the actual code to be selected.

Section 8.3: MULTIPLE CODES

Several diagnostic statements may be present in a report and linked to each other (such as etiology and manifestation) as per the physician's statement, so they will either be coded together as one code or as multiple codes. You can find referrals to code additional diagnostic statements with another code in either the Tabular List or Alphabetical Index.

Multiple coding means that more than one code is required to code for a condition:

(1) ETIOLOGY/MANIFESTATION: There may be an etiology code and a manifestation code which would both need to be coded. Etiology is the cause and manifestation is the condition that results from the etiology. Usually the etiology will be listed first in reporting the codes and the manifestation second.

(2) ADDITIONAL CODE/CODE ALSO: There may be a notation in the ICD-10-CM book that states "use additional code, if desired" or "code also." Ignore the "desired" term; you must code the additional code. You must be careful to ensure that you find any of these notations, even if you have to search back to the beginning of the section because the additional code must be coded, if known. For example, J13 instructs to code also associated lung abscess. Most use additional code listings include a category now for tobacco use (Z72.0) such as J37, Chronic laryngitis.

(3) CODE FIRST: Another notation in the ICD-10-CM book is "code first underlying disease." You must be careful to ensure that you find any of these notations, even if you have to search back to the beginning of the section because the additional code must be coded, if known. This notation is particularly important in that it is providing you information about the order of the codes. For example, J12 instructs to code first associated influenza.

On occasion with multiple coding, information may not be provided in the report which allows for coding the second code. Under these circumstances, you cannot code the extra code. If the second code cannot be coded, however, this may result in denial of payment since the medical necessity of the services provided may not be justified, so it is important that physicians provide all the necessary information so that the correct code can be selected.

Section 8.4: COMBINATION CODES

Combination codes are comprised of one code that contains more than one diagnostic statement and does not require coding of any additional codes.

In contrast to ICD-9, in ICD-10-CM there are more combination codes which then do not require the coding of additional codes, such as diabetes codes, e.g. E10.21 for type diabetes mellitus with diabetic nephropathy. This also applies to poisonings, such as T41.291 for accidental poisoning by general anesthetic which also includes the mode of poisoning.

Be careful when selecting either combination or multiple codes because you do not code them as related unless the doctor makes a statement that they are related. This is because a patient may have a condition that can be coded as associated or due to another condition, but may in their case not be related. For example, a patient may be seen for treatment of cataracts and the patient has diabetes, but the two are not related and the cataracts are not caused by the diabetes. Therefore, the healthcare provider must clearly state that they are connected; otherwise, you would code them separately as having no relationship to each other.

Section 8.5: SEQUENCING

The linking of ICD-10-CM codes to CPT and HCPCS code is critical in physician coding. This will be discussed further in the CPT section. Sequencing is based on several formats:

First, sequencing is required when the ICD-10-CM book directs you to code a certain code first. Information regarding sequencing can be found in the coding guidelines in the front of the book which are very helpful when coding either on the job or during a test.

Sequencing can also be determined by determining which condition is the etiology and which is the manifestation. A manifestation is a condition that results from another condition known as the etiology. The etiology is the original condition that caused the manifestation. In these scenarios, the etiology is usually listed first. Oftentimes this will be denoted by explanatory notes within the codes, such as "code first" which is usually listed in the etiology code descriptions. For manifestation codes, there is usually a description of "code also" meaning that the etiology code should also be listed. In the alphabetical index this sequencing is denoted by the etiology code listed first and the manifestation code listed after in square brackets.

Second, the concept of sequencing is that the code for the main reason the patient received services is usually listed first.

Section 8.6: COMORBIDITIES/COMPLICATIONS

Comorbidities are conditions that are oftentimes associated with another condition and complications are conditions that can result from a condition. Although we do not always code conditions that exist at the time healthcare is provided for another condition, we do code them if they either receive treatment themselves or if they may influence the patient's care or the outcome and, therefore, MAY result in additional care and/or extended hospital stay which many comorbidities and complications do, such as diabetes or COPD.

With this definition, there are some comorbidities and complications that are typically coded in addition to the primary diagnosis for which the patient received care. These comorbidities and complications are coded also because either they require care for themselves or they are known to pose a great probability of affecting the outcome of the patient's care.

Probably the most familiar are diabetes and AIDS. These two conditions complicate most all other healthcare. For example, if a patient receives sutures for a minor wound, the diabetes may complicate things and result in longer healing and/or infection. Other conditions that are oftentimes coded in addition to the primary code are hypertension, heart problems, COPD and other breathing problems, and renal failure.

Section 8.7: SYMPTOMS

For physician coding, do not code symptoms if you have a diagnostic statement. Code only the diagnostic statement then such as diabetes, not the symptoms associated with it. Typically, with physician coding, you code the diagnostic statement and nothing else.

However, there are several scenarios in which you would code symptoms. First, this includes when no diagnostic statement is given or possible. This can occur because the symptoms are transient and were, therefore, not diagnosable. It can also occur if the tests are negative or abnormal but no definitive diagnosis is determined from it. If a physician is not able to conduct enough tests at the time of the visit, then he may not be able to determine the diagnosis. Cases may also be referred to another practice or hospital for determination of the diagnosis. You must code something and since you don't have a diagnostic statement, you will code the symptoms.

You would also code symptoms even if they are contained within the diagnosis code if they are being treated, such as a headache, fever, or dehydration.

Common symptoms may include fever, dehydration, headache, syncope, convulsions, dizziness, weakness, stomach ache, nausea, vomiting, diarrhea, urination problems, skin problems, palpitations, and breathing problems.

Section 8.8: RULE OUTS

Physician coding and hospital inpatient coding vary in many ways. One of the most prominent differences is that we never code diagnostic statements that contain "rule out," "possible," "probable", or any other term that is not a definite diagnosis for physician coding. This is because healthcare providers may not always have the time or ability to fully test and determine the cause of symptoms (the diagnosis), so we do not know if the "rule out" statement by a healthcare provider is true or not as opposed to the testing in the hospital which can be much longer and more intensive, therefore more defining and certain.

Remember, if a physician provides symptoms, and even if he uses a "rule out" diagnostic statement, we can only code the symptoms because **WE NEVER MAKE A DIAGNOSIS, so NOT DOCUMENTED, NOT DONE.** If you remember this critical coding rule, it will simplify your coding responsibilities and ensure correct coding. It is vital that you remember this because you can get into trouble if you start diagnosing the patient and use these codes to bill. It is a very serious situation in which a patient is given a diagnosis they do not have – this can have huge implication in many ways on their future care and may impact their lives in a myriad of ways. This serious situation is also complicated because once a patient is given a wrong diagnosis, that diagnosis becomes disseminated throughout a wide network of providers and organizations which makes it more difficult to remove and/or correct. In addition, the process to remove an incorrect diagnosis is extremely difficult and frustrating.
So, never code any diagnostic statement that does not clearly posit a diagnosis. Instead, you will have to code the symptoms.

If a condition is described as "borderline," code it as definitive unless there is a code that describes the condition as borderline in which case you would use that code.

Section 8.9: ACUTE/CHRONIC

Acute and chronic are definitions that come up repeatedly throughout the ICD-10 codes and will be discussed throughout the remainder of the packets in this course.

Acute means the condition has developed recently and is being treated at the present time. Chronic means that the condition has been ongoing in treatment over time. It is very important to distinguish between chronic and acute when coding because it makes a difference in several ways. The physician must describe it as chronic in order to be coded as chronic.

First, some codes do not distinguish between acute and chronic codes. If this is the case, the one code would be used for either one. If a condition is reported as both acute and chronic, but the code does not distinguish, you still only need to use the one code to describe both.

Second, some codes distinguish between acute and chronic codes. If this is the case, then you must select which code is accurate, either acute or chronic.

Third, some conditions may be both acute and chronic. A person may have a chronic condition which is present at the same time as the acute condition. In this case, you would have to code both acute and chronic, which again is reflected in the previously mentioned scenarios that you will use either one code that includes both acute and chronic or two separate codes, one for acute and one for chronic.

STRUCTURE QUIZ 3

1. What number most often represents an unspecified code?

2. What is the code for encephalopathy that is not specified?

3. Derangement of a previous ligament of the right knee is what code?

4. What are the codes for a perforation of the esophagus that was traumatic?

5. What number most often represents a code in which more information is provided but there is no specific code for the condition?

6. What is the code for spina bifida occulta?

7. What are the codes for otitis due to impetigo?

8. What are the codes for excessive vomiting in a pregnant woman?

9. What does NEC stand for?

10. What is the code for postviral encephalitis?

11. What is the code for a patient who is seen today for crushing chest injury?

12. A patient is seen today for a headache and polyneuropathy due to Type 1 diabetes. What are the codes?

13. A patient is seen today to rule out a hernia due to abdominal pain. What are the codes?

14. A patient is seen today for arthropathy due to TB of the hip. What are the codes?

15. A patient is seen today for a stomach ache and headache and was found to be due to botulism. What are the codes?

CHAPTER 9
ICD-10 INFECTIOUS DISEASES

You will learn the following objectives in this chapter:

A. Coding for Organisms
B. Infections
    1. Intestinal
    2. Tuberculosis
    3. Other
C. Sepsis
D. Sexually Transmitted
E. Viral
    1. Hepatitis
F. HIV/AIDS
G. Mycosis/Others
H. Sequelae

Section 9.1: CODING FOR ORGANISM

Chapter 1 is described as "Certain Infectious and Parasitic Diseases" and is coded as A00-B99. The term "certain' indicates that some related codes may be found in other sections, such as respiratory if related to colds or pneumonia. For example, tetanus during pregnancy may be found under code A34. HIV may be found under B20.

As with most of the codes in ICD-10, there is a much greater specificity and many conditions are now combined with the organism as one code, such as typhoid.

When coding for infectious and parasitic diseases be sure to use an additional code to identify the organism's resistance to antimicrobial drugs (Z16).

Remember, as with ICD-9, some conditions caused by an organism are included in the code for the organism. When coding for conditions caused by organisms, there are several coding scenarios that you may encounter so you must determine correct codes including those that involve multiple and combination coding.

When coding for conditions caused by an organism, you want to code the condition and the organism. If the organism is known and not included in a selected code, then a code from the section for infectious diseases needs to be coded also for the organism, such as B96.

One possible scenario in coding infectious diseases is combination coding scenarios in which one code can be found in the ICD-10 book which includes in its description both the condition and the organism.

If an organism is drug-resistant, this must also be coded such as with Z16, resistance to antimicrobial drugs as well as the combination code for the condition and the organism, such as MRSA, e.g. J15.212, if available. If there is not a combination code, then code the condition and organism separately. Sometimes a patient may be carrying a drug-resistant organism but display no symptoms. This is known as colonization and can be coded with Z22.322. If the patient is determined to be both carrying it and does have symptoms, then code both.

Organisms should always be coded, if known whether in a combination code or as an additional code to the condition. If not known, A41.9 could be used associated with sepsis.

INTESTINAL: Intestinal infectious diseases are coded as A00-A09. This includes typhoid, salmonella, shigellosis, and many others including food poisoning and dysentery.

Typhoid Fever (A01.0) and Amebic infections (A06.8) have a fifth character added which indicates site or type. Many other codes have been expanded to include manifestations such as Listeriosis (A32) and Whooping cough (A37).

TUBERCULOSIS: Tuberculosis is coded as A15-A19. While most TB codes are included in these codes, some are not, such as congenital TB which is coded as P37.0 which is in the congenital section of codes.

Tuberculosis can occur in various parts of the body such as nervous system, eyes, spine, intestines, and organs other than just the lungs. There are various related conditions that are now included in some TB codes such as arthritis.

A positive TB test but no symptoms is coded as R76.11 as noted under the exclude notes as well as other excluded conditions.

OTHER BACTERIAL INFECTIONS: A wide variety of bacterial conditions are coded from A20 to A38 such as the plague, anthrax, cat-scratch fever, meningitis, tetanus, staph, strep, whooping cough, and scarlet fever.

Leprosy (A30) has been expanded with regards to type, e.g. Tuberculoid leprosy (A30.1) or lepromatous leprosy (A30.4).

Section 9.2: SEPSIS

There are various names used to refer to an infection caused by an organism within the human body. If allowed to grow, this infection can progress throughout the body and result in death. Although some of the terms used to denote this condition may be used interchangeably by healthcare providers, there are distinct differences within the terms and may involve the progression and severity of the infection within the body. If the infectious organism is not known, this is known as cryptogenic.

The progression of the infection is bacteremia to septicemia which is now known as sepsis to severe sepsis to severe sepsis with septic shock to multiple organ dysfunction to death. Sepsis is an infection. Urosepsis is a nonspecific term and should not be used. If used, the doctor should be queried as to whether this is sepsis or not. Puerperal sepsis refers to sepsis following childbirth. Cellulitis is infection of the skin. Lymphangitis is infection of the lymph glands.

Septicemia is when an organism has invaded the blood and is systemic. Forms of septicemia include bacteremia and sapremia. Bacteremia is when a bacteria has caused the infection and is further defined by the organism. Sapremia is when a toxin has caused the infection. Sepsis is coded from the other bacterial infection section and is specified by streptococcal (A40) and other (A41). Related septicemia and bacteremia are coded as R78.81.

There are several "code first" notes in this section for sepsis related to pregnancy, abortions, postprocedural, immunizations and infusions. There are also many "exclude" notes when sepsis is associated with specific organisms.

As sepsis continues, it can result in SIRS (systemic inflammatory response syndrome) which refers to an overwhelming septic infection and is coded with R65.1. Sometimes in the latter stages of infection, a physician may refer to the condition as severe sepsis which is coded as R65.2- with additional conditions listed after the code which denote what conditions make the sepsis qualify as severe. This includes shock and organ failure which would also be coded in addition to the sepsis code. The severe sepsis codes are now differentiated by the absence or presence of septic shock with R65.20 without and R65.21 with shock. Postprocedural septic shock is coded as T81.12.

Regarding sequencing, the underlying infection should be coded first and then the R65 codes for the sepsis. If the sepsis is due to a noninfectious process such as trauma, then code the trauma first.

Section 9.3: SEXUALLY TRANSMITTED

Codes A50-A64 include sexually transmitted diseases (STDs) other than AIDS which are highly differentiated such as whether they are congenital, late, early, secondary, symptomatic or asymptomatic and include related conditions such as endocarditis. This includes syphilis, gonococcal, chlamydia, and herpes, trichomoniasis.

OTHER: Other diseases include yaws, fevers, and lyme disease. There are also codes for rickettsiosis (A75-A79) which includes tick borne illnesses.

Section 9.4: VIRAL

Viral infections (A80-A89) include poliomyelitis, Creutzfeldt-Jakob disease, rabies, and mosquito-borne encephalitis. It also includes arthropod-borne viral diseases such as dengue fever, west nile, and yellow fever. Viral infections of the skin include herpes, chickenpox (varicella), smallpox, measles, rubella and viral warts.

HEPATITIS: Hepatitis is inflammation of the liver and can be viral or nonviral. Hepatitis codes are coded as being acute or chronic and if the delta-agent (Hepatitis D) is present with relationship to Hepatitis B.

There are several types of hepatitis.

Type A (B15) is highly contagious and usually transmitted fecally or orally. It was formerly known as infectious hepatitis and is the least serious form. Contaminated food is oftentimes the source and is typically spread under unsanitary conditions.

Type B (B16) is transmitted by contaminated blood, feces, and other human secretions. It was formerly known as serum hepatitis and is also known as chronic hepatitis. It can result in death from cirrhosis. It is transmitted by donated blood or serum transfusions, as well as sexually, which also includes dirty needles from drug use. The codes are differentiated by whether Hepatitis D and a coma are present.

Type C is usually transmitted by blood transfusions and use of dirty needles and sexual contact. C is the leading viral cause of chronic liver disease and can result in end-stage renal disease; however, some Type C hepatitis can be fulminating in that there is rapid onset.

Type D (also known as delta) is seen only in patients with Type B hepatitis because it cannot reproduce if the cell is not infected with Type B. Note that the fifth character also defines if Type D (delta) is mentioned.

Type E is transmitted enterally. Although not common in United States, it is common throughout the rest of the world due to infected water sources and causes epidemics.

These hepatitis codes also are further defined by whether there is a coma and if they are acute or chronic.

Other hepatitis include alcoholic, chemical, amebic, dirty-needle, cholestatic, giant cell, interstitial, peliosis, posttransfusion, serum, syphillic, toxic, tuberculous, etc.

OTHER VIRAL: Other viral include CMV (B25), mumps (B26), infectious mononucleosis (B27) further specified by the type and the manifestation, conjunctivitis (B30) and numerous others.

Section 9.5: HIV/AIDS

There are some special coding circumstances surrounding the coding of HIV and AIDS. It is transmitted by sexual contact, body fluids, and dirty needles. There have been many misconceptions and limited information about HIV. There are two types of HIV: HIV-1 and HIV-2. It is HIV-1 that is known to cause AIDS

HIV (human immunodeficiency virus) means that the person has tested positive for the organism (a retrovirus) but may not have experienced any symptoms yet, so they are not considered to have the disease, AIDS (acquired immunodeficiency syndrome). AIDS is now pandemic in that it is an epidemic that has spread throughout various parts of the world. Most cases are in Africa.

HIV is coded as B20. If a patient has demonstrated symptoms due to HIV, then they are coded as having AIDS or symptomatic HIV disease using the code B20.

The manifestations should also be coded, that is what condition or symptoms the patient is experiencing that has resulted from the HIV virus. For example, if a patient has Kaposi's sarcoma due to HIV, then the person has the disease, AIDS, which would be listed first and the sarcoma second. HIV disease resulting in multiple infections in addition to the other conditions, B37.0 Candidal stomatitis, B37.1 Pulmonary candidiasis, and J99 respiratory disorders in other diseases specified elsewhere.

The B20 code should always be coded first, and any related conditions second. However, if a patient is seen for a condition, such as a fractured leg that is unrelated to the AIDS/HIV, then the condition would be listed first, and the AIDS/HIV second.

If the patient has tested positive for HIV, but has demonstrated no symptoms, then the correct code for their condition is Z21, asymptomatic HIV. If a patient is admitted for AIDS testing but there is no definitive positive diagnosis of HIV or AIDS, then code Z11.4.

If the patient is pregnant and is admitted for AIDS related condition, then code O98.7- followed by B20 as well as the related condition. If the HIV is asymptomatic in a pregnant patient, then code as O98.7- and Z21.

Once a patient is coded as B20 due to having manifestations of AIDS at some time, then they are always coded as B20 and never again as Z21.

If a patient's test has been inconclusive for HIV, then the correct code would be R75. If the results were negative, code Z71.7.

Section 9.6: MYCOSIS

Mycosis are fungal infections and can occur in various tissues such as different parts of the skin on different parts of the body (e.g. tinea pedis of the feet B35.3), candidiasis of various anatomic sites (B37), coccidiodomycosis (B38), histoplasmosis (B39), aspergillosis (B44), and cryptococcosis (B45).

OTHERS: Protozoal diseases (B50-B64) include malaria further specified by type and complications, e.g. plasmodium vivax malaria with rupture of spleen (B51.0). It also includes Chagas disease (B57), leishmaniasis (B55) and toxoplasmosis (B58). Helminthiasis (B65-B83) include schistosomiasis, flukes, taeniasis, filiariasis, hookworm, and enterobiasis. Pediculosis, acariasis, and other infestations are coded as B85-B89. Scabies is a parasitic infection of the skin characterized by pruritus. Tinea (ringworm) is a fungal infection of the skin, such as tinea corporis (ringworm) and tinea pedis (athlete's foot).

Section 9.7: SEQUELAE: Codes for sequelae of infections and parasitic disease are found at the end of the Chapter for infectious diseases (B90-B94).

INFECTIOUS DISEASES QUIZ 4

1. Is AIDS pandemic or epidemic?
2. What are the codes for septicemia due to anthrax?
3. What are the codes for a patient seen today for septic urinary tract infection due to E. coli?
4. What are the codes for a patient seen with hepatitis D associated with Hepatitis B?
5. What are the codes for a patient with uveitis due to syphilis?
6. What are the codes for a patient who has H. influenza due to meningitis?
7. What are the codes for a patient who has infection of the colon due to Clostridium difficile?
8. What are the codes for a patient seen today for HIV and related Kaposi's sarcoma of the lymph nodes?
9. What are the codes for a patient seen today with HIV?
10. What are the codes for chronic spondylitis?
11. What are the codes for a patient seen today for bacteremia with septic shock?
12. What are the codes for a patient with acute bronchitis due to Pseudomonas?
13. What are the codes for a patient with pernicious complications of malaria with nephropathy?
14. What are the codes for a patient seen today for SIRS with septic shock?
15. What are the codes for a 23-year-old patient who is seen today for MRSA?

CHAPTER 10
ICD-10 NEOPLASMS

You will learn the following in this chapter:

A. Types of Neoplasms
    1. Benign neoplasm
    2. Uncertain behavior
    3. Unspecified behavior
    4. Malignant neoplasm
        a. In situ
        b. Primary/Secondary
B. Grading and staging systems
    1. Grades
    2. TNM
C. Location
D. Alphabetical Index
E. Sites
    1. Overlapping
    2. Multiple
    3. No Specification
F. Chemotherapy/Follow-Up
G. Neoplasm Table
H. Complications
I. Excision/History

Section 10.1: TYPES OF NEOPLASMS

A neoplasm is a growth (tumor) and can be benign, malignant, in situ, unspecified, or unknown as listed in the table. They are located in the second chapter of the Tabular Index with codes ranging from C00-D49. If your book is designed as such, please note that the indentation or color coding of the outer edges of the book designate the neoplasm section.

BENIGN NEOPLASM: A benign neoplasm is not cancerous (or bad) or spreading. The suffix, -oma, refers to benign neoplasms. For example, an osteoma is a benign neoplasm of the bone. This includes moles, polyps, lipoma (fatty tumor), adenomas (tumor of a gland), myoma (tumor of the muscle), angiomas (blood or lymph tissue tumors), papilloma (papillary tumor), meningiomas (brain tumors), cyst, and fibroids.

Although benign neoplasms are not associated with the dangers of a malignant (or cancerous) tumor, they can still pose health problems due to the pressure or complicating conditions they may cause on vital organs or structures.

Some benign neoplasms can progress to malignancy which is why they are observed and tested over time.

UNCERTAIN BEHAVIOR: Neoplasm of uncertain behavior means that it could not be determined from the tests if the neoplasm was malignant or benign.

UNSPECIFIED BEHAVIOR: Neoplasms that are unspecified means that no information was provided in the report to determine if the neoplasm was benign or malignant.

MALIGNANT NEOPLASM: A malignant neoplasm is cancerous and the term, malignancy, refers to bad. There are many terms used to indicate malignancy which are oftentimes designated by the location of the cancer. Cancer can occur in several places at the same anatomic site, for example, cancer could be in the bone, tissue, or skin on the leg.

Sarcomas are malignant neoplasms of the connective tissue, such as bone, fat, muscle, and cartilage, plus others. Melanomas are cancer of the pigment producing cells called melanoctyes which appear on the skin. PSA (prostate specific antigen) is a tumor market measured in the blood which is elevated in men with prostate cancer.

Malignant neoplasms are further described as in situ, primary, or secondary.

IN SITU: If it is contained and not spreading, the malignant neoplasm is known as "in situ". This classification, "in situ" can only be used if the physician states the neoplasm is in situ. Additional terms that indicate "in situ" include non-infiltrating, non-invasive, intraepithelial, and pre-invasive carcinoma.

PRIMARY/SECONDARY: Primary or secondary cancerous neoplasm are indicated by terms such as infiltrating and invasive which indicate the cancer is spreading.

Primary malignant neoplasms are the originating site for the cancer. Secondary malignant neoplasms are the sites where the cancer spread to (or metastasized).

Sometimes physicians may use terms other than "metastasis" to denote the spreading of the primary neoplasm to other sites. When you are not certain of the use of the term metastatic, substitute "spread" and you will be able to understand the term better. These terms include "spreading to/from" or "invasion to/from". Note the difference in the use of "to" or "from" and its relationship to either primary or secondary as the type of cancer. For example, if the physician states the liver cancer was metastatic or spreading from the breast, then it means the primary site was the breast and the liver cancer was the secondary site. If the physician states the colon cancer was metastatic or spreading to the bone, then the colon cancer was the primary site and the bone cancer was the secondary site.

There are some areas that are considered to be secondary if the morphology is not stated as to whether it is primary or secondary. These include:

Bone
Brain
Heart
Diaphragm

Liver
Lymph nodes
Mediastinum
Meninges
Peritoneum
Pleura
Retroperitoneum
Spinal Cord

Section 10.2: GRADE/STAGING

Grades are the degree of maturity or differentiation of the malignancy and are oftentimes used in assessing the prognosis for cancers, for example with PAP tests. There are four grades. Grade I are well differentiated tumors so they resemble their parent cell closely. This differentiation continues to decline as you progress through the other grades, from II to III and then finally to IV which carries the poorest prognosis.

TNM: TNM is the system used for staging. Staging is the extent of the malignancy's metastasis within the body. T refers to the size and degree of the malignancy; N refers to the number of regional lymph nodes involved, and M refers to metastasis. The numbers range from 0 to 4 with 0 being the least (undetectable) and 4 being the most advanced. T stages range from 1 to 4; N stages range from 0 to 3; and M stages range from 0 to 1. Therefore, a malignancy might be coded as T1, N2, M1 which indicates the tumor is less than 3 cm in diameter (T1), metastasis to the lymph nodes in the trachea area (N3), and distant metastasis present (M1).

Section 10.3: LOCATION

Codes are differentiated initially by anatomic site. It is important to note that a neoplasm can occur in several areas of the same location on the body, so you must be careful that you code it correctly. For example, a neoplasm can occur in the skin, muscle, organ, bone, or other structure at the same anatomical site, such as the knee. Sometimes the neoplastic terms will indicate the specific location, such as sarcoma which indicates cancer of the skin or osteosarcoma which is cancer of the bone.

Section 10.4: ALPHABETICAL INDEX

If you are feeling confused by all of the various names for the many types of cancer and are wondering how you can embrace all of this, the alphabetical index is very helpful. If you do not know what the terms mean that a physician uses to describe a neoplasm, you can simply look it up in the alphabetical index, and it will tell you what the neoplasm is, whether it is benign or malignant and what type it is with reference to its location. If the index lists it as being one or the other because some tumors can occur as malignant or benign, then you know what type of code to select. However, if the index lists the neoplasm as being either, then you must search the medical report to find out if it is malignant or benign.

Second, when the alphabetical index provides specific codes for a site under the tumor's name, such as leiomyoma of the uterus, you can simply use that code.

Third, if the alphabetical index does not provide a specific code under the term, then you must reference the neoplasm table as indicated in the alphabetical index.

Section 10.5: SITES

OVERLAPPING SITES:

The character 8 is oftentimes used in the fourth character to indicate that the neoplasm has spread to other contiguous or overlapping sites, e.g. C15.8 says "overlapping lesion of esophagus". If the site of origin is not known and the neoplasm is overlapping, there are also codes used to indicate this, e.g. C26.9 overlapping lesion of digestive system.

NO SPECIFICATION OF SITE: If no site is specified for the malignant neoplasm, then code C80, "Malignant neoplasm without specification of site", should be listed which can be used for primary or secondary sites.

Section 10.6: CHEMOTHERAPY/FOLLOW-UP

Remember in the ICD-9 book the V codes have codes for chemotherapy and follow-up exams. In ICD-10, those codes change to Z08.0 for follow-up exam (remember, a follow-up exam can only be coded as follow-up if treatment for the original condition has been completed as determined by the physician). Code Z51.1 is for chemotherapy and should be coded first if this is the reason the patient is seen. Personal history code for neoplasms are coded as Z85 codes.

If there is organ removal for prophylactic treatment of cancer, it would be coded as Z40.0. Z12 is for visits in which there is screening for cancer.

OTHER: The codes for malignant neoplasm of the esophagus (C15) has been changed from the ICD-9 in that reference to cervical, thoracic and abdominal has been eliminated. For other neoplasms, there has been an expansion of the codes by site, such as carcinoma in situ of skin, e.g. carcinoma in situ of skin or right eyelid, including canthus (D04.11).

There are new notes that direct the additional coding of factors that may have influenced the condition, such as tobacco dependence (F17) and exposure to tobacco smoke in the perinatal period (P96.81).

Hodgkin's Disease (C81) has been expanded to include types and lymph node involvement.

Section 10.7: NEOPLASM TABLE

When you know what terms you are looking for in the Neoplasm Table, then you can go to the Table and find the correct code. The Neoplasm Table lists the codes according to the specific location. For example, if you are coding osteosarcoma of the elbow, when you look under sarcoma in the alphabetical index, it directs you to check in the neoplasm table under bone and malignant. Remember to follow the directions of the alphabetical index precisely! Be sure to look under bone first, and not elbow. Once you have found bone in the neoplasm table, then you will look for elbow which has a code of C40.0.

VERY IMPORTANT! WHEN CODING FROM THE NEOPLASM TABLE AND ALPHABETICAL INDEX......BE SURE TO PICK THE CODE FROM THE CORRECT LINE

Section 10.8: COMPLICATIONS

Complications should always be coded in addition to the neoplasm codes. Complications are sequences first if their treatment is the primary reason for the visit. Anemia is an exception in which the malignancy code would be listed first.

Section 10.9: EXCISIONS/HISTORY

If a malignancy has been removed, then it no longer exists. As long as the patient is treated for this malignancy, despite its removal, you will code the malignancy as existing. For example, if a patient has breast cancer and it is removed but the patient remains under chemotherapy for it and the physician does not describe the treatment as completed for the malignancy, then the code for breast cancer continues to be used. However, once the physician completes the treatment, then the breast cancer would be coded as a personal history of breast.

If a primary malignant neoplasm was removed but reoccurs at the same site then this should be coded as primary again.

NEOPLASMS QUIZ 5

1. What are the codes for intramural leiomyoma of the uterus?
2. What are the codes for a patient who is seen today for nausea and vomiting due to chemotherapy two days ago for metastatic brain cancer?
3. What are the codes for traumatic asphyxiation?
4. What are the codes for benign leiomyoma of the abdomen?
5. What are the codes for a patient who has metastatic brain cancer?
6. What are the codes for Paget's disease of the extramammary skin?
7. What are the codes for a patient with carcinoma of the body of the uterus and contiguous sites?
8. What are the codes for carcinoma of the rectum and colon metastatic from the anterior wall of the bladder?
9. What are the codes for adenoma of the chief cell?
10. What are the codes for a patient who is seen today for prophylactic chemotherapy a year after having a mastectomy due to breast cancer with treatment completed three months ago?
11. What are the codes for a patient who has Hodgkin's lymphoma of the lymph nodes of the neck and axilla and the spleen?
12. What are the codes for patient with malignant schwannoma of the abdomen?
13. What are the codes for leiomyoblastoma (include the M code) of the chest?
14. What are the codes for osteochondroma of the coccyx?
15. What are the codes for patient with UTI due to E. coli?

CHAPTER 11
ICD-10 BLOOD DISORDERS

You will learn the following objectives in this chapter:

A. Types of Blood Cells
B. Types of Blood Groups
C. RH Factor
D. Types of Blood Disorders
    1. Anemias
    2. Coagulation Defects
    3. Purpura/Hemorrhage
    4. White Blood Cell Disorders
    5. Other Diseases
E. Operative/Post Procedural
F. Immune Disorders
G. Leukemia
H. Multiple Myeloma

Chapter 3 is described as "Diseases of the Blood and Blood-forming Organs and Certain Disorders Involving the Immune Mechanism" and range from D50-D89. Some blood conditions are not coded in this chapter because other chapters have precedence over this chapter and so the blood condition may be coded in another chapter, such as neoplasms, pregnancy, perinatal, and organisms have a greater priority than the chapter for blood disorders for where conditions are coded, e.g. leukemia (cancer of the blood) are coded in Chapter 2, Neoplasms.

Section 11.1: TYPES OF BLOOD CELLS

Blood is composed of different types of cells. Erythrocytes are red blood cells. Leukocytes are white blood cells. There are five types of leukocytes: lymphocytes, basophils, eosinophils, neutrophils, and monocytes. Also known as thrombocytes, platelets are blood cells which are important in the process of blood clotting.

Section 11.2: TYPE OF BLOOD GROUPS

Blood groups are distinguished by the type of antigens and antibodies are present. The four blood types are:

Type A contains A antigen and anti-B antibodies
Type B contains B antigen and anti-A antibodies.
Type AB contains both A and B antigens and no anti-A or anti-B antibodies.
Type O contains no A or B antigens and both anti-A and anti-B antibodies.

The problem with donating blood is that if someone is Type B and they are given Type A, their anti-A antibodies will attack the blood which will result in hemolysis (breakdown of the blood) which can have serious consequences.

People with Type O blood are known as the universal donor because they have no A or B antigens so their blood can be accepted by anyone as there are no antigens to cause an attack by the antibodies. However, because Type O contains both types of antibodies, they cannot accept blood from anyone else except another Type O person.

Section 11.3: RH FACTOR

Rh factor is also an important issue with blood type, particularly with pregnancies. If a fetus is Rh+ (they have the Rh antigen), then their blood will incite the mother's blood to create antibodies to the Rh, so the first pregnancy does not pose any problems. The problem occurs when this mother gets pregnant again with another fetus that is Rh+ because now the mother's antibodies will attack the fetus' blood and destroy the Rh+ red blood cells. This condition is also known as erythroblastosis fetalis.

Section 11.4: ANEMIAS

Anemia is a deficiency in hemoglobin (a protein found inside red blood cells), either qualitative or quantitative. Hypoxia (lack of oxygen) occurs in anemia because sufficient blood with oxygen does not get to the cells. Anemia can result from several conditions, including hemorrhaging, iron deficiency, B12 deficiency (pernicious anemia), folic acid deficiency, hemolysis (red blood cell death), genetic (sickle cell anemia and thalassemia), nutritional deficiencies, and diseases.

The codes for anemia (D50-D64) have been expanded greatly to include more information about the type, e.g. thalassemia, beta type (D56.1). Secondary anemias are coded from D63 codes which are anemias due to other illness which will also need to be coded. If the anemia is drug-induced, there are coding notes that instruct the coding of E codes to identify the drug responsible. If caused by a poisoning, then the coding instruct that the substance should be coded first from T codes.

Nutritional anemias, such as iron deficiency anemia, are coded from D50-D53. Sickle cell anemia is coded as D57 and is subdivided by whether it is with or without crisis.

Sickle cell anemia is a genetic defect in which red blood cells exhibit a sickle shape resulting in severe hemolysis and pain, oftentimes resulting in death. With sickle cell anemia, there is a code for a person who has the genetic disease, but there is also a code for someone who is a carrier of the gene but does not have the symptoms. This is known as sickle cell trait (D57.3).

Hemolytic anemia (D59) is when the red blood cells are destroyed prematurely. It can be genetic or acquired (that is due to condition that occurs during a person's life). Acquired hemolytic anemia is broken into autoimmune and non-autoimmune. Non-autoimmune can be due to drugs, toxins, trauma, infections, liver disease, or septicemia. Autoimmune means the body is attacking the cells.

Aplastic anemia (D60) occurs when the bone marrow does not produce enough red blood cells. Included under this category of codes is pancytopenia which means deficiency in numbers of all cells, including red blood cells, white blood cells, and platelets.

Section 11.5: COAGULATION DEFECTS

Coagulation defects, purpura and other hemorrhagic conditions are coded as D65-D69. Other diseases are coded as D65-D69. Disorders involving the immune system are coded from D80-D89, such as sarcoidosis of lymph nodes (D86.1).

Coagulation is also known as blood clotting or the forming of a thrombus. Coagulation defects can occur due to genetic defects in clotting factors in the blood, synthesis problems, or breakdown of clotting factors. Vitamin K deficiency is one disorder that can result in coagulation defects. Hemophilia (D66) is a sex linked genetic recessive disorder in which a person bleeds easily and experiences difficulties in stopping the flow of blood due to the inability of the blood to clot. Bleeding can occur internally as well as externally. Von Willebrand disease (D68.0) is a genetic bleeding disorder in which a person bruises easily, has frequent nosebleeds, and has difficulty in profuse bleeding when cut, such as with surgeries.

Section 11.6: PURPURA/HEMORRHAGE

Hemorrhage is excessive bleeding. Purpura is red or purple colored discolorations of the skin caused by hemorrhaging. If the discolorations are smaller, they are known as petechiae and when they are larger they are known as ecchymoses. These conditions are frequently seen in thrombocytopenia (D69) which occurs when there is a low number of platelets in the blood.

Section 11.7: WHITE BLOOD CELL DISORDERS

Neutropenia (D70) is a reduction in circulating neutrophils which increases the risk of bacterial and fungal infections since the body does not have the means to fight the infections. Neutropenia occurs frequently in people receiving chemotherapy or other medications that suppress the immune system (D70.2). There are also codes for decreased or increased white blood cell count (D72).

Section 11.8: OTHER DISEASES

Other blood diseases include polycythemia (D75.1). This is an increase in the mass of the red blood cells or decrease in the volume of plasma and is measured in a lab as the hematocrit. Primary polycythemia can be caused by an abnormality of the bone marrow. Secondary polycythemia can be caused by heart or lung disease, smoking, renal or liver tumors, and endocrine abnormalities.

Section 11.9: OPERATIVE/POST PROCEDURAL

Hemorrhage and hematomas resulting from procedures are coded as D78. Codes for the spleen have been expanded to include intraoperative and postprocedural complications (D78), e.g. accidental puncture or laceration during a procedure on the spleen (D78.1).

Section 11.10: IMMUNE DISORDERS

Immunodeficiencies other than AIDS are coded with D80-D89 codes. This includes hereditary, nonfamilial, antibody, selective, combined, variable and those with other major defects such as SCID (severe combined immunodeficiency), sarcoidosis, and graft-versus-host disease wherein the body reacts against grafts.

Section 11.11: LEUKEMIA

Leukemia is an increase in the cancerous white blood cells, but it is not coded from this section of the codes, but rather from the neoplasm chapter. Oftentimes treatment consist of chemotherapy and/or bone marrow transplants.

Section 11.12: MULTIPLE MYELOMA

Multiple myeloma is cancer of the bone marrow and is also coded in the neoplasm codes.

BLOOD DISORDERS QUIZ 6

1. What are the codes for a patient with senile dementia?
2. What are the codes for a patient experiencing septic shock due to UTI?
3. What are the codes for a patient suffering from dipsomania?
4. What are the codes for a patient with goat's milk anemia?
5. What are the codes for a patient who metastatic cancer of the uterus?
6. What are the codes for an anemic patient due to hemorrhaging of a lower leg wound caused by a car accident?
7. What are the codes for a patient who has sickle cell anemia Hb-SS with acute chest syndrome?
8. What are the codes for a patient who has vegan anemia?
9. What are the codes for a patient who has malignant schwannoma of the hip?
10. What are the codes for a patient experiencing a crisis with sickle cell anemia?
11. What are the codes for a patient who is diagnosed with anemia due to a chronic gastric ulcer?
12. What are the codes for a patient with Hodgkins lymphoma of the spleen and axillary and neck lymph nodes who has neutropenia due to chemotherapy?
13. What are the codes for a patient with traumatic asphyxiation?
14. What are the codes for a patient with a coagulation defect due to Vitamin K deficiency?
15. What are the codes for a patient who Pelger-Huet anomaly?

CHAPTER 12
ICD-10 ENDOCRINE

You will learn the following objectives in this chapter:

A. Endocrine System
B. Endocrine Glands
C. Diabetes
    1. Diabetes Mellitus
    2. Other
D. Operative Complications
E. Nutritional/Metabolic

Chapter 4 is described as "Endocrine, Nutritional and Metabolic Diseases" and range from E00-E89. There are many new subchapters in this Chapter including diabetes and malnutrition.

Section 12.1: ENDOCRINE SYSTEM

The endocrine system involves various glands within the body which secrete a large variety of hormones into the blood that control in many ways the vital functions of our body. In contrast, the exocrine system secrete their chemical substances into ducts and out of the body which include sweat, mammary, salivary, lacrimal (tear), and mucous glands.

Major endocrine glands include the hypothalamus, pituitary gland, pineal, thymus, parathyroids, pancreatic islets of Langerhans, thyroid, adrenals, ovaries, and testicles. The pituitary gland is known as the master gland as it controls most of the glandular activities. The endocrine section of the codes also includes nutritional, metabolic, and immunity disorders and diseases.

The pituitary gland is located in the brain and is also known as the hypophysis. It secretes a wide variety of hormones including the thyroid stimulating hormone and various growth hormones. Inadequate secretion of the growth hormones may result in hypopituitarism and dwarfism.

The thyroid glands secrete thyroxine (T4) and tri-iodothyronine (T3) which influences metabolism and control of the body temperature. A goiter of the thyroid may result which is enlargement of the thyroid gland due to hypoactivity or hyperactivity of the thyroid or a deficiency in iodine. Graves' disease may occur in hyperthyroidism. Hypothyroidism is known as myxedema and may result in mental retardation and dwarfism.

There are four parathyroid glands are located on the posterior sides of the thyroid glands. These glands regulate the calcium and phosphate in the body.

Adrenal glands are located above the kidneys. They secrete steroids which regulate salt balance, metabolism, and sex development (androgens and estrogen) as well as epinephrine, norepinephrine, cortisone and cortisol. Hyperadrenalism can result in Cushing's Syndrome or Addison's disease.

In the medical field, this is probably the most neglected field with large cities oftentimes only have a couple of physicians who specialize in this area; yet, this area of medicine is probably one of the most critical to our general health and is found to contribute significantly to many symptoms and conditions as evidenced by the rapid growth in autoimmune diseases and diabetes.

Various deficiencies can result from the failure of these glands which are aggravated by poor nutrition and exposure to toxins and can be due to trauma, tumors, surgery, radiation, or genetic defects. Deficiencies can result in the over or under production of hormones.

Section 12.2: ENDOCRINE GLANDS

Disorders of the thyroid gland are coded as E00-E07 including goiters, iodine-deficiency, thyrotoxicosis and thyroiditis. Disorders of other endocrine glands are coded as E20-E35, such as hypoparathyroidism, hypopituitarism, Cushing's syndrome, hyperaldosteronism, ovarian and testicular dysfunction.

Section 12.3: DIABETES

There are two types of diabetes: mellitus and insipidus. There are significant differences between the two types. Symptoms for both diabetes include polydipsia (excessive thirst) and polyuria (excessive urination), but there is also hyperglycemia (excessive sugar) and glycosuria (sugar in the urine) in diabetes mellitus. The presence of ketones and rapid weight loss may also indicate diabetes mellitus.

DIABETES MELLITUS: The most common type is diabetes mellitus which is caused by the improper secretion and utilization of insulin which is produced by the pancreas and, therefore, the body is not able to properly utilize sugar and instead excretes it in the urine. Diabetes mellitus can be controlled or uncontrolled.

There are two types of diabetes mellitus: Type I and Type II. Type II is the most common type and does not require insulin therapy; however, there may be times when this type of diabetes is treated with insulin; therefore, a person being on insulin does not necessarily mean they are Type I so the physician must describe if the diabetes is Type I or Type II. If not known, then it would be coded as Type II/unspecified.

Type I is known as juvenile type or insulin-dependent diabetes mellitus (IDDM) because it develops most often in childhood. In Type I there is a complete lack of insulin so Type I is treated with insulin through injections or orally with daily blood monitoring and diet.

The two major changes to the diabetes codes are there are now five categories for diabetes and manifestations and complications are now indicated by the fourth or fifth character so there is no need for additional codes for them.

Diabetes is coded in three levels as Type I insulin-dependent/juvenile (E10), Type II non-insulin-dependent (E11), and other specified (E13). If the type of diabetes is not specified, then it should be coded as Type II, even if they are given insulin. Type I or juvenile just be specified in order to code Type I.

There are also codes for secondary diabetes mellitus due to underlying conditions (E08) and due to drugs or chemicals (E09) in which the underlying condition should be coded first as directed by the coding notes.

There are then fourth character classifications by complications which are much more extensive than they were in the ICD-9 codes. A fourth character of 6 indicates that the complication is not listed in the previous classifications, so this is an "other" code. A fourth character of 7 indicates that there are multiple complications. A fourth character of 8 indicates complications were mentioned but not identified. A fourth character of 9 indicates there are no identified complications. Remember, if the complication is known, then it should also be coded, e.g. diabetic cataracts would be coded as E13.36 and then H28 for the diabetic cataracts whose positioning as second denoted by an asterisk. Be careful to assure that the physician has diagnosed the complication as being related to the diabetes in order to code them together. If the condition is not due to the diabetes, then do not code the complication as being due to the diabetes.

There are new codes for diabetes mellitus caused by drugs or chemicals (E09), e.g. drug or chemical induced diabetes mellitus with renal complications (E09.2).

There is also a note in these codes that directs the coding of long-term insulin use (Z79.4).

If there are complications due to an insulin pump, this should be coded as T85.614.

OTHER: Hypoglycemia is coded with E15 and E16 codes with many differentiations of codes based on related conditions.

Diabetes insipidus is caused by the body's failure to adequately utilize antidiuretic hormone (ADH) which results in the kidneys not being able to properly reabsorb water into the bloodstream. Because the water is not reabsorbed, it is excreted in urine which is why urine in diabetes insipidus is watery and tasteless. In contrast, urine in diabetes mellitus is sweet due to the presence of excessive amounts of sugar which was not properly used by the body and, therefore, excreted in the urine. Diabetes insipidus can be treated by the administration of ADH either by injection or orally. Diabetes insipidus is coded with E23.2.

Gestational diabetes can occur when a woman is pregnant and is due to increased metabolic demands during this time, so a woman may be diagnosed with gestational diabetes who is not diabetic when not pregnant, but she does have the potential to become diabetic in the future if not treated. This is not coded in this section but is listed in the pregnancy chapter.

Section 12.4: OPERATIVE COMPLICATIONS:

Intraoperative or postprocedural complications are coded as E36 for complications of the endocrine system developed from a procedure, e.g. postprocedural hemorrhage of an endocrine organ following an endocrine procedure (E36.01). Postprocedural complications for endocrine and metabolic are coded as E89.

Section 12.5: NUTRITIONAL/METABOLIC

Malnutrition is coded with codes E40-E46. Other nutritional deficiencies (E50-E64) include deficiencies of various vitamins such as B12, thiamine, D, E, and K as well as nutrients such as copper, magnesium and iron.

Weight codes (E66-E68) include overweight, obesity, and hyperalimentation.

Metabolic disorders (E70-E88) include albinism, PKT, maple-syrup-urine disease, fatty acid metabolism, carnitine, glycoprotein, lipid storage, lactose intolerance, X-linked disorders, fructose intolerance, Cori disease, Niemann-Pick disease (Type A, B, C or D), uricemia, bilirubin, minerals, volume depletion, hyperkalemia, and fluid overload. Cystic fibrosis is coded as E84. Hypercholesterolemia and hyperlipidemia are coded as E78 codes. Dehydration is coded as E86.0.

ENDOCRINE QUIZ 7

1. What are the codes for a patient with drug-induced Cushing's syndrome?
2. What are the codes for a patient with H. influenza with meningitis?
3. What are the codes for a patient with anemia and ALS?
4. What are the codes for a patient with polyuria due to possible diabetes mellitus?
5. What are the codes for a Type I diabetic patient with cataracts?
6. What are the codes for a patient with arthritis due to chronic gout?
7. What are the codes for a patient with Hodgkins lymphoma of the spleen and axillary and neck lymph nodes?
8. What are the codes for a patient treated with insulin in the emergency room due to severe ketoacidosis due to their diabetes mellitus?
9. What are the codes for a patient who experienced hypovolemic shock due to trauma?
10. What are the codes for a patient with goiter related to hyperthyroidism with storm?
11. What are the codes for a patient with diabetic retinal microangiopathy with edema?
12. What are the codes for a patient with a headache and possible concussion?
13. What are the codes for hypopituitarism due to the administration of radiotherapy?
14. What are the codes for a patient experiencing a thyrotoxic crisis due to Graves' Disease?
15. What are the codes for a patient who has amputation of two toes on the right foot due to gangrene related to Type 2 diabetic peripheral vascular disease?

CHAPTER 13
ICD-10 MENTAL

You will learn the following objectives in this chapter:

A. DSM-IV-TR
B. Mental Disorders due to Physiological Conditions
C. Psychoactive Substances
D. Psychosis
E. Neurosis
F. Behavioral Syndromes
G. Disorders of Adult Personality
H. Intellectual Disabilities
I. Developmental Disorders
J. Childhood Disorders

Chapter 5 is described as "Mental and Behavioral Disorders" and range from F01-F99.

Section 13.1: DSM-IV-TR

Another form of coding used with mental disorders is the DSM-IV (Diagnostic and Statistical Manual of Mental Disorders, Fourth Edition, Text Revision) published by the American Psychiatric Association. It is composed of Axis I, Axis II, Axis III, Axis IV, and Axis V. Axis I is for Clinical Disorders and Other Conditions including all psychiatric disorders which are now described by the use of ICD-10 codes. Axis II contains the personality disorder and mental retardation classifications. Axis II contains the medical conditions. Axis IV contains psychological and environmental conditions that influence the care. Axis V contains the psychological, social,

Section 13.2: MENTAL DISORDERS DUE TO PHYSIOLOGICAL CONDITIONS

Mental disorders due to physiological conditions (F01-F09) (formerly described as organic) include mental conditions and disorders that developed due to an actual physical condition such as dementia, amnesia, delirium, hallucinations, catatonic, mood, personality, and behavioral which may be caused by conditions such as epilepsy, concussions, and Alzheimer's. Dementia is the loss or impairment of thinking and distinguished as senile or presenile with other conditions such as delirium, delusions, and depression. Senile dementia is dementia occurring in people over the age of 65. Presenile dementia is dementia occurring in people younger than 65 years of age. The same codes are now used for both senile and presenile (F03). Delirium is acute temporary disturbance of consciousness in which a patient may be incoherent and disoriented.

Mental conditions due to alcohol or drugs are excluded from this section and are coded with F10-F19.

Section 13.3: PSYCHOACTIVE SUBSTANCES

Disorders due to psychoactive substances, such as alcohol, opioids, cocaine, and tobacco are coded with codes F10-F19. The fourth character specifies the clinical state as .0 acute intoxication; .1 harmful use; .2 dependence syndrome; .3 withdrawal state; .4 withdrawal state with delirium; .5 psychotic disorder; .6 amnesiac disorder; .7 residual and late-onset psychotic disorder; .8 other; and .9 unspecified. Fifth and sixth characters provide greater specificity about complications, such as sleep disturbance or delusions.

There are notes indicating that an additional code needs to be listed for blood alcohol level (Y90).

There is greater emphasis on nicotine use which is coded with F17 codes.

Alcoholism denotes an ongoing long-term abuse of alcohol in which a person mentally and physically has become dependent on alcohol as defined by the doctor, therefore it is described as a dependence. Continuous refers to regular ingestion of large amounts of alcohol, usually daily or weekly. Episodic refers to alcoholic binges which can last weeks or months which can be followed by periods of sobriety. In remission means that the patient is no longer consuming alcoholism or is in the process of significant reduction in their consumptions. However, once a person is diagnosed with dependence, they are treated as having dependence for life although it may be in remission because any encounter with alcohol can result in the return of their mental and physical dependencies. With alcoholism there may be other conditions that also need to be coded such as cirrhosis or hepatitis since alcoholism damages the health of a patient in many ways. Acute alcohol abuse refers to a one time abuse of alcohol which may occur in someone who is either dependent or not dependent on alcohol.

Section 13.4: PSYCHOSIS

Codes F20-F29 describe more serious psychosis including schizophrenia, bipolar disorder, and manic depressive disorder.

Schizophrenia (F20) is characterized by disturbances in thinking, mood and behavior with an altered concept of reality with possible hallucinations and delusions. Schizophrenia is classified by type: simple, disorganized, catatonic, paranoid, schizophreniform, latent, residual, schizoaffective, other, and unspecified. In catatonic schizophrenia, the patient is unresponsive and characterized by rigid positioning. Disorganized schizophrenia includes a lack of ability to associate with rapid shifting between thoughts so that the patient appears incoherent. In paranoid schizophrenia, the person imagines feelings of grandeur or persecution. Schizoaffective disorder (F25) is schizophrenia combined with affective mood disorders.

Affective mood disorders (F30-F39) are characterized by mood disturbances, such as manic, depressive, and bipolar. Mood disorder codes have been expanded to further describe the severity of bipolar disease (manic episode), e.g. manic episode without psychotic symptoms, mild (F30.11). Other nonpsychotic disorders have also been expanded through the use of fourth, fifth and sixth characters, e.g. blood, injection, injury type phobia, fear of other medical care

(F40.232).

Bipolar disorder (F31) is a mood disorder in which a person experiences rapid mood swings from manic levels of high to lows, known as mania and depression. Bipolar I are manic episodes with some depressive episodes, while Bipolar II is primarily depressive episodes marked by some periods of high manic behavior. Cyclothymia is a milder form of bipolar disorder. Major depression (F32) can be mild, moderate or severe with or without psychotic features and as a single episode or recurrent.

Depression can be major involving long continuous periods of depression marked by the patient's belief that the depression will not end. Dysthymia (F34.1) is a less severe form of depression that does not typically last as long and does not involved psychotic features such as hallucinations and paranoia.

Section 13.5: NEUROSIS

These codes (F40-F48) describe less severe mental conditions known as neurosis or personality disorders, in other words "nonpsychotic". This includes anxiety disorders, panic disorder, hysteria, phobias, histrionic and schizoid personality disorders, gender disorders, eating disorders, adjustment reaction, autism, sleep disorders, depression, speech and language disorders, conduct disorders, hyperactivity, and drug problems. Histrionic is when a patient is emotional and attention-seeking characterized by outbursts and tantrums. Schizoid is when the patient is cold and indifferent to other's emotions.

Anxiety disorders are coded with F40 codes, such as phobias like agoraphobia. Phobias are when a person has a great fear of something to the point of irrationality and debilitation. Phobias include agoraphobia which is a fear of being out in public. Social anxiety disorder is a phobia of social interaction. Claustrophobia is a fear of closed-in areas. Acrophobia is a fear of heights.

Other anxiety disorders include panic attacks (F41.0). Obsessive-compulsive disorder is coded as F42. Obsessive-compulsive disorders are when a person experiences recurrent thoughts and experience a dominant need to perform repeated acts. Obsessive-compulsive disorder is not coded the same as obsessive-compulsive personality disorder (F60.5) because it is not a personality disorder.

Dissociative disorders are when a patient has impairment of perception and consciousness and can include split personalities which can be a means of compensation for trauma or conflicts.

Another condition that develops from the attempt to compensate for past trauma is post traumatic stress disorder. Reaction to severe stress is coded as F43 such as post traumatic stress disorder (PTSD) which is coded as F43.1.

Adjustment disorders are coded as F43.2. Dissociative and conversion disorders are coded as F44 which include fugues, stupors, seizures, convulsions and motor symptoms related to the disorder.

Somatoform disorders (F45) are disorders which are evidenced in physical symptoms. This includes hypochondriasis which is an abnormal preoccupation with illnesses and physical problems. In a conversion disorder the patient experiences loss of physical functions based on their fear.

Section 13.6: BEHAVIORAL SYNDROMES ASSOCIATED WITH PHYSIOLOGICAL DISTURBANCES

There are several behavioral syndromes with physiological disturbances (F50-F59) that can occur. Eating Disorders (F50) include bulima nervosa, anorexia nervosa, pica, and rumination. Bulima is binge eating followed by self-induced vomiting. Anorexia nervosa is the failure to eat sufficient food to sustain life as evidenced by severe weight loss and a development of many other life-threatening conditions. Pica is the eating of inedible substances. Rumination is the regurgitation and re-swallowing of food, which is typically described as occurring in cows but is performed by some people.

Sleep disturbances (F51) include insomnia, hypersomnia, sleepwalking, nightmares, and sleep terrors.

Sexual dysfunctions (F52) include hypoactive sexual desire, sexual aversion, and sexual arousal disorders as well as orgasmic disorders. Postpartum depression is coded as F53.

Abuse of non-psychotic substances (F55) include abuse of antacids, laxatives, steroids, and vitamins.

Section 13.7: DISORDERS OF ADULT PERSONALITY

Disorders of adult personality and behavior (F60-F69) include paranoid, antisocial, borderline, histrionic, obsessive-compulsive, avoidant, and dependent. Impulse disorders (F63) include pathological gambling, pyromania, kleptomania, and trichotillomania (hair plucking). Gender identity disorders are coded as F64. Various paraphilias (F65) include fetishism, pedophilia, sadomasochism, necrophilia, and voyeurism.

Section 13.8: INTELLECTUAL DISABILITIES

Intellectual disabilities (F70-F79) include mental retardation which is coded as mild (F70), moderate (F71), severe (F72), profound (F73), other (F78) and unspecified (F79). Impairment of behavior is coded in the fourth character as .0 for no or minimal impairment of behavior, .1 for significant impairment, .8 for other impairments, and .9 for no mention of impairment. Notice that .0 is for when there is a statement that there is no or minimal impairment, but .9 is when there is no mention.

Section 13.9: DEVELOPMENTAL DISORDERS

Pervasive and specific developmental disorders (F80-F89) include disorders with language, speech, scholastic (reading and math), writing, learning disabilities, and clumsy child. Autism (F84.0) is also included as well as Rett's syndrome and Asperger's syndrome.

Section 13.10: BEHAVIORAL AND EMOTIONAL DISORDERS IN CHILDHOOD

Behavioral and emotional disorders with onset usually occurring in childhood and adolescence (F90-F98) may be used regardless of the patient's age as long as the disorder developing during childhood or adolescence. These codes include attention deficit hyperactivity disorder, conduct disorders, separation anxiety, selective mutism, reactive attachment disorder, tic disorders (Tourette's and motor), enuresis, encopresis, feeding disorders, pica, thumb-sucking, and nail-biting.

MENTAL QUIZ 8

1. What are the codes for a patient with carcinoma of the lower outer quadrant of the breast metastatic to the left lung?
2. What are the codes for patient experiencing panic attack with agoraphobia?
3. What are the codes for a patient who is experiencing combat fatigue?
4. What are the codes for a patient who has chronic alcoholism with cirrhosis?
5. What are the codes for a patient with anorexia?
6. What are the codes for a patient suffering from depression due to the death of her husband?
7. What are the codes for a teenager who has been experiencing problems with significant school truancy?
8. What are the codes for a patient with subacute borderline schizophrenia?
9. What are the codes for a patient with a long history of alcoholism who was binge drinking over the superbowl weekend and seen for drunkenness?
10. What are the codes for a patient with dementia due to alcohol intoxication?
11. What are the codes for a 62-year-old patient with paranoid senile dementia?
12. What are the codes for a patient with bulima nervosa?
13. What are the codes for a patient with chronic PTSD?
14. What are the codes for a patient who has an IQ of 65?
15. What are the codes for a patient with acute exacerbation of chronic myeloid leukemia?

CHAPTER 14
ICD-10 NERVOUS SYSTEM

You will learn the following in this chapter:

A. Nervous System
   1. Central Nervous System
   2. Peripheral Nervous System
B. Inflammatory Conditions
   1. Meningitis
   2. Encephalitis
   3. Myelitis
C. Movement Disorders
   1. Systemic Atrophies
   2. Extrapyramidal
   3. Degenerative
D. Epilepsy
E. Migraines/Headaches
F. Nerve Disorders
G. Cerebral Palsy/Paralytic Syndromes
H. Other Disorders
I. Procedural Complications

Chapter 6 is described as "Diseases of the Nervous System" and range from G00-G99. Most of these codes are secondary codes because many of these conditions are listed in other chapters, such as perinatal, pregnancy, neoplasms, and injuries.

Section 14.1: NERVOUS SYSTEM

The codes relating to the nervous system include the central nervous system and the peripheral nervous system. Remember, these codes refer to the nervous system and not the bones of the spinal cord which are included in the musculoskeletal section of the codes.

The central nervous system (CNS) includes the brain and the spinal cord. The brain is surrounded by three layers of connective tissue known as the meninges. The outermost layer is known as dura mater, the second layer is known as arachnoid membrane, and the third layer is pia mater. Between the first and second layer is the subdural space and between the second and third there is a space called subarachnoid space.

The peripheral nervous system (PNS) consists of 11 pairs of cranial nerves (cranial nerve II is not included in the PNS) outside of the brain and spinal cord. They carry impulses throughout the rest of the body. Peripheral nerves carry impulses from the CNS to nerves that function involuntarily or voluntarily. The autonomic nervous system (ANS) is a part of the PNS which can be enteric, sympathethic or parasympathetic. The sympathetic and parasympathetic react in opposite ways to each other to either increase or decrease body functions such as fight or flight response which increases blood pressure from the sympathetic opposite to the parasympathetic response of reducing blood pressure. The enteric influences the GI tract. There is a fluid that circulates throughout the brain and spinal cord which provides a cushion to prevent shock and is known as cerebrospinal fluid (CSF).

Section 14.2: INFLAMMATORY CONDITIONS

Meningitis is coded as G00-G04. Meningitis is the inflammation of the meninges that surround the brain and is caused by microorganisms. The organism is now included in the meningitis code such as bacterial or other.

Encephalitis (G04) is the inflammation of the brain, which derives from the term encephalo. Myelitis is the inflammation of the spinal cord. Encephalomyelitis is inflammation of the brain and spinal cord. Intracranial and intraspinal abscess and granulomas are coded as G06 or as in other diseases (G07). Intracranial and intraspinal phlebitis and thrombophlebitis is coded as G08.

Sequelae of inflammatory disease of the CNS are coded as G09.

Section 14.3: MOVEMENT DISORDERS

SYSTEMIC ATROPHIES: Systemic atrophies primarily affecting the central nervous system (CNS) (G10-G14) include Huntington disease coded as G10. These codes also include hereditary ataxia such as cerebellar, spinal muscular atrophy, and atrophies affecting the CNS in other diseases. Postpolio syndrome (G14) is also included.

EXTRAPYRAMIDAL AND MOVEMENT DISORDERS: Extrapyramidal and movement disorders (G20-G26) include Parkinson's disease coded as G20-G26 and has been expanded to include type. Parkinson's disease due to other conditions is coded as G21. Other disorders include dystonia which can be drug induced, genetic torsion, tremors, myoclonus, chorea, tics restless leg syndrome, and stiff-man syndrome with many differentiated by whether they are drug induced or not.

OTHER DEGENERATIVE DISEASES: Alzheimer's disease is coded as G30 which is further specified by age at onset, either early or late. Other degenerative disorders include Pick's disease and degeneration with separate codes for drug induced.

DEMYELINATING DISEASES: Demyelinating diseases of the CNS (G35-G37) include multiple sclerosis. Other diseases include demyelinations such as of the central pontine or myelitis.

Section 14.4: EPILEPSY

Grand mal seizures, also known as generalized tonic-clonic seizures, are characterized by involvement of the entire body including muscle rigidity, muscle contractions, and loss of consciousness. In the tonic phase, the muscles tighten up and in the clonic phase the muscles experience spasms. Petit mal seizures, also known as absence seizures, are characterized by a very short loss of consciousness and functions demonstrated by an absent look with or without twitching movements of muscles. Idiopathic epilepsy means the cause is not known.

Epilepsy is coded as G40 and is further specified by the type of seizure and epilepsy (localized, idiopathic, generalized, petit mal and grand mal) as well as types of seizures, if intractable and with or without status epilepticus. Epilepsy is a paroxysmal disorder characterized by recurrent seizures. The codes are differentiated by the terms generalized, complete partial, or simple partial. In a partial seizure, the disturbance is limited to a specific area of the brain as opposed to generalized which is not specific in area. Generalized codes are further classified by intractable or not intractable (intractable means not responding to treatment), and with or without status epilepticus. There are codes for drug-induced epilepsy (G40.5). There are also codes for absence epileptic syndrome (G40.A) and Juvenile (G40.B). Other epileptic codes include Lennox-gastaut syndrome (G40.81) and spasms (G40.82).

Grand mal and petite male seizures are no longer differentiated and are coded as G40.4, generalized epilepsy NEC.

Section 14.5: MIGRAINES/HEADACHES

Migraines are coded as G43 and have been expanded to fifth characters to indicate the presence of status migrainosus. If drugs are involved, then the drug needs to be identified using T codes. Migraines are differentiated as with or without auras and intractable or not intractable. Other types of migraines include hemiplegic, persistent with or without cerebral infarction, chronic (G43.7), cyclical vomiting, ophthalmoplegic, periodic, abdominal, and menstrual.

General description of headache is coded as R51. However, this section of the codes include some types of headaches (G44) which include cluster headaches, vascular, tension, post-traumatic, and drug-induced.

Sleep disorders (G47) include insomnia other than due to alcohol or drugs as well as other exclusions as noted in the chapter on mental disorders. Hypersomnia, circadian rhythm sleep disorders, apnea, narcolepsy, cataplexy, parasomnia, and bruxism are included in this section too.

Section 14.6: NERVE DISORDERS

Nerve, nerve root and plexus disorders (G50-G59) include disorders of the various nerves such as the trigeminal, facial, cranial, and brachial plexus. Bell's palsy is coded as G51.0. Phantom limb (G54.6) syndrome is now differentiated as to whether pain is present or not.

Mononeuropathies (G56) include carpal tunnel syndrome and other lesions/causalgias of various nerves of the limbs, both arms and legs.

Polyneuropathies are coded as G60-G65 and can be hereditary, idiopathic, inflammatory, drug-induced, radiation-induced, or due to diseases. Sequelae of polyneuropathies are coded as G65.

Myoneural disease (G70-G73) include myasthenia gravis, muscular dystrophy (G71.0), myotonic disorders, and congenital myopathies. Myopathies (G72) can also be drug-induced, alcoholic, inflammatory, critical illness, or due to toxic agents.

Section 14.7: CEREBRAL PALSY & PARALYTIC SYNDROMES

Cerebral palsy and other paralytic syndromes are coded as G80-G83. Cerebral palsy (G80) can be spastic, quadriplegic, diplegic, hemiplegic, ataxis, or athetoid. Spastic includes congenital that develops when a child is young and is a result of brain damage from birth trauma or intrauterine pathology. Cerebral palsy refers to various disorders within the development of muscles and their coordination so it affects body movement, posture, and balance. Paralysis, such as quadriplegia and hemiplegia, are common as well as muscle stiffness and poor tone, uncontrolled movements, mental retardation, skeletal deformities, problems with speech and swallowing, and many more.

Hemiplegia and hemiparesis (G81) both mean paralysis of one side of the body but hemiparesis is less severe as it is weakness rather than complete paralysis. These codes are differentiated as to whether they are flaccid, spastic, other, or unspecified. Flaccid is loss of muscle tone. Spastic means rigidity of paralysis in combination with muscular contractions or spasms. The fifth character specifies if the paralysis is affecting the dominant or nondominant side of the body. Dominant side means if they are right-handed, the right side is dominant and the left side is non-dominant. If they are left-handed, the left side is dominant and the right side is non-dominant. Remember from anatomy and physiology that there is a cross-over between the brain and the body, so if the right side of the brain was damaged, then the left side of the body is affected and vice versa for damage to the left side of the brain. Remember though, the physician needs to document this. If none of this information is provided, then you must use the unspecified code.

Other kinds of plegia (G82) include quadriplegia which means complete paralysis of the body from the neck down and is also known as tetraplegia. Paraplegia refers to complete paralysis from the waist down. For quadriplegia the exact cervical location of the damage to the spine must be specified. These are further defined as complete or incomplete. While complete refers to complete loss of sensory or motor function below where the spinal cord injury occurred, incomplete indicates that there is some sensory or motor function below the injury site.

Monoplegia (G83) are described as to location, such as limbs and dominant or non-dominant side.

Section 14.8: OTHER DISORDERS

Other disorders of the nervous system (G89-G99) include pain which has many exclude notes. It can be differentiated as to acute or chronic and due to trauma or post-procedural. Chronic pain syndrome is coded as G89.4.

Other disorders include autonomic dysreflexia, complex regional pain syndrome (CRPS), hydrocephalus, encephalopathy, cerebral cysts, anoxic brain damage excluding that due to anesthesia or neonatal, compression of brain, brain death, cord compression, and cerebrospinal fluid leak.

Section 14.9: PROCEDURAL COMPLICATIONS
Intraoperative and postprocedural complications of the nervous system are coded as G97 including hypotension, puncture, laceration, hemorrhage and hematoma.

NERVOUS QUIZ 9

1. What are the codes for a patient with a classic migraine with aura?
2. What are the codes for a patient with an IQ of 45 who has ringworm?
3. What are the codes for a patient who has MS?
4. What are the codes for a patient who has pars planitis?
5. What are the codes for a patient who has double vision?
6. What are the codes for a patient who has pigmentary open-angle glaucoma?
7. What are the codes for a patient who has Fusarium keratitis?
8. What are the codes for a patient who has tonic-clonic epilepsy?
9. What are the codes for a patient who has restless leg syndrome?
10. What are the codes for a patient who presents today because she has not been taking her insulin as prescribed for her for the past four years and she is now experiencing polyneuropathy due to Type 2 diabetes?
11. What are the codes for a patient who has presenile cortical cataract of the left eye and is Type I diabetic?
12. What are the codes for a patient who has epilepsy marked by grand mal seizures which is not responding to treatment?
13. What are the codes for a patient who has tic douloureux?
14. What are the codes for a patient who has pseudocyesis?
15. What are the codes for a patient who has Huntington's dementia?

TEST 1
ICD-10 CHAPTERS 1 - 14

1. What is the code for a patient who is seen today for chest pains due to possible MI?

2. What is the code for a patient who is seen today for crushing chest injury?

3. What are the codes for a patient who has metastatic brain cancer?

4. What are the codes for a patient seen today for chemotherapy for ongoing treatment of breast cancer which was excised two months ago?

5. An 8-year-old patient is seen today for enteritis due to Clostridium difficile. What are the codes?

6. What does HIPAA stand for?

7. What other prosecutory actions are levied besides fines for healthcare fraud?

8. What number most often represents an unspecified code?

9. What is Volume 2 of the ICD book known as?

10. Derangement of a previous ligament of the knee is what code?

11. What are the codes for a perforation of the esophagus that was traumatic?

12. What is the code for postviral encephalitis?

13. /3 indicates what in M codes?

14. What are the two supplementary classifications in Volume 1?

15. Name and describe the three types of health record formats.

16. Describe the two types of progress notes.

17. What does CPC mean?

18. What types of coding does a CPC perform?

19. What types of coding does a CCS perform?
20. Explain the Stark Laws.
21. What are the codes for traumatic asphyxiation?
22. What are the codes for benign leiomyoma of the abdomen?
23. What are the codes for a patient who was binge drinking over the weekend and was seen in the emergency room who experienced alcoholic stupor?
24. A patient is seen today for arthropathy due to TB. What are the codes?
25. ICD-10-CM stands for what?
26. What federal department is CMS a part of?
27. How many volumes are there in the ICD today?
28. What are the codes for a patient seen today for septic urinary tract infection due to E. coli?
29. What are the codes for a patient seen with hepatitis D associated with inactive Hepatitis B?
30. What are the codes for a patient with uveitis due to syphilis?
31. What is the code for a patient with acute bronchitis due to Pseudomonas
32. What are the codes for malaria with pernicious complications with hepatitis?
33. What are the codes for a 23-year-old patient who is seen today for MRSA?
34. What are the codes for leiomyoma of the uterus?
35. What are the codes for a patient who is seen today for nausea and vomiting due to chemotherapy?
36. What are the codes for a patient with carcinoma of the breast metastatic to the left lung?

37. AHIMA stands for what?

38. What does CCS-P mean?

39. What are the codes for patient experiencing panic attack with agoraphobia?

40. What are the codes for a patient who has MS?

41. What are the codes for a patient who has pars planitis?

42. What are the codes for a patient who is experiencing combat fatigue?

43. A patient is seen today for a stomach ache and headache and was found to be due to E. coli food poisoning. What are the codes?

44. Define presenile dementia.

45. What are the codes for a patient with anorexia?

46. What are the codes for a patient suffering from depression due to the death of her husband?

47. Describe the CNS.

48. What are the codes for a patient with a classic migraine with aura?

49. What are the codes for a patient who has meningitis due to Aerobacter aerogenes?

50. What are the codes for a patient who has double vision?

51. What is the difference between hemiplegia and hemiparesis?

52. Infantile cerebral palsy occurs when?

53. What are the codes for a patient who has Fusarium keratitis?

54. What are the codes for a patient who has osteitis with chronic mastoiditis due to TB?

55. What does idiopathic mean?

56. When two major changes were added in the ninth revision?

57. What are the codes for septicemia due to anthrax?

58. What are the codes for a patient who has Huntington's dementia?

59. What is the difference between a TIA and a CVA?

60. What are the fines for healthcare fraud?

CHAPTER 15
ICD-10 EYE

You will learn the following in this chapter:

A. Injuries
J. Inflammation
K. Foreign Body
L. Cataracts
M. Glaucoma
N. Other Disorders
O. Visual
P. Procedural Complications

Chapter 7 is described as "Diseases of the Eye and Adnexa" and range from H00-H59. These codes have been expanded greatly with fourth, fifth and sixth characters that further describe the site and laterality. If the cause of the eye condition is known then it should be coded with the external codes.

Section 15.1: INJURIES

Many eye conditions are excluded due to other conditions as indicated by the exclude notes. Superficial injury and open wounds of the eye are coded with S00-S01 codes.

Section 15.2: INFLAMMATION

Various inflammations of the eyes are coded with H01 codes including blepharitis (ulcerative or squamous), dermatoses/dermatitis, and xeroderma which are also differentiated by laterality and upper or lower eyelid.

Conjunctivitis (H10) includes conjunctivitis that is mucopurulent, acute, atopic, toxic, serous, chronic, simple, follicular and vernal. Conjunctivitis can also include the eyelid which is known as blepharoconjunctivitis.

Iridocyclitis (H20) due to disease are not coded in this section as described in the exclude notes. Various types of iridocyclitis include primary, recurrent, hypopyon, chronic lens-induced, and other syndromes.

Section 15.3: FOREIGN BODY

Retained foreign body in the eyelid is coded as H02.81 with the use of Z codes to indicate the type of foreign body. Also contained in the H02.8 codes are cysts, dermatochalasis, edema, elephantiasis, hypertrichosis and vascular anomalies. Foreign body in the orbit is coded as H05.5. Foreign bodies in these sites (H44.6) are differentiated by if the foreign body was magnetic or not or unspecified.

Section 15.4: CATARACTS

Disorders of the lens (H25-H28) include cataracts which are now described as age-related cataract instead of senile. Cataracts are the clouding or opacification of the lens of the eye or its capsule and can result in loss of vision. Senile cataracts occur in old age when there are characteristics of impaired memory or the inability to perform certain mental tasks. Presenile cataracts occur before the period of senility which is typically 65 years of age.

Fourth characters classify conditions by type of cataract. All other types of cataracts are coded as H26 such as infantile/juvenile, traumatic, complicated, and flecks. H28 codes are for cataracts that are due to another condition.

Section 15.5: GLAUCOMA

Glaucoma contains a group of diseases of the optic nerve which is characterized by intraocular pressure and resulting in visual impairment. Glaucoma (H40) is differentiated as suspect, open-angle, primary angle-closure, secondary to trauma or inflammation, or drugs. There are boxes for seventh characters in this section for stages. Open angle occurs from an increase in the fluid pressure in the eye due to a blockage of the ocular fluid. This type of glaucoma is also described as chronic and develops slowly. Closed angle is described as acute with rapid onset due to blockage of the chamber angle where the iris and cornea meet and, therefore, the aqueous fluid cannot drain.

Section 15.6: OTHER DISORDERS

Styes (hordeolums) are coded as H00 on either the external or internal portion of the upper or lower eyelid on either the right or left side. Abscess of the eyelid and chalazion are also coded in this section.

Other disorders of the eyelid are coded as H02 such as entropion, trichiasis, ectropion, lagophthalmos, blepharochalasis, ptosis (drooping), innervation syndrome, retraction, xanethelasma, cholasma, madarosis and vitiligo.

Disorders of the lacrimal system (H04) include dacryoadenitis either acute or chronic, dacryops, dry eye syndrome, cysts, atrophy, dislocation, epiphora, inflammation, stenosis, insufficiency of lacrimal passages, fistula, and granuloma.

Disorders of the eye orbit (H05) include inflammation, displacement, edema, hemorrhage, exophthalmos, deformity due to many conditions such as disease, trauma or surgery, atrophy, enlargement, exostosis, and enophthalmos.

Other conditions of the conjunctiva (H11) includes a benign growth on it known as pterygium with specification as to exact location. Also included are codes for degeneration, deposits, concretions, xerosis, pigmentation, scars, granuloma, hemorrhage, vascular abnormalities, edema, hyperemia, cysts and conjunctivochalasis

Disorders of the sclera (H15) include scleritis and staphyloma. Disorders of the sclera (H16) include many types of keratitis, ulcers, keratoconjunctivitis, and neovascularization. Corneal scars and opacities are coded as H17.

Other disorders of the cornea (H18) include pigmentations, deposits, keratopathy, edema, changes of the membranes, degeneration, keratomalacia, arcus senilis, hereditary dystrophies, keratoconus, ectasia, staphyloma, anesthesia, hypoesthesia, disorders due to contact lens, and erosion.

Other disorders of the iris and ciliary body (H21) include hyphema, degeneration, iridoschisis, cysts, pupillary membranes, adhesions, and floppy iris syndrome.

Other disorders of the lens (H27) include aphakia which is absence of the lens and dislocation.

Disorders of the choroid and retina (H30-H36) include inflammation, cyclitis, Harada's disease, scars, retinopathy, degeneration, atrophy, hemorrhage, rupture, cysts, retinoschisis, occlusions, changes in appearance, aneurysms, vasculitis, hemorrhages, separation, and detachment. Retinal detachment is coded as H33 which include single or multiple breaks. Retinopathy in premature babies is coded as H35.1 and is differentiated by stages. Proliferative retinopathy not due to diabetes is coded as H35.2. Macular degeneration, (loss of central vision) is coded as H35.3. Peripheral retinal degeneration is coded as H35.4. H40 is highly specific for glaucoma differentiated by stages, tension, and laterality.

Disorders of the vitreous body and globe (H43-H44) include prolapse, hemorrhage, crystalline deposits, opacities, adhesions, degeneration, endophthalmitis, and hypotony.

Disorders of the optic nerve and visual pathways (H46-H47) include neuritis, neuropathy, hypoplasia, hemorrhage, papilledema, atrophy, coloboma, inflammation, cortical blindness, or due to neoplasm.

Other disorders of the eyes (H55-H57) include nystagmus, anomalies such as mydriasis, and pain.

Section 15.7: VISUAL

Disorders of ocular muscles, binocular movement, accommodation and refraction (H49-H52) include strabismus. Strabismus is the inability of the both eyes to look in the same direction due to muscle weakness of one eye. Strabismus is coded as paralytic, esotropia either alternating or monocular, exotropia, vertical, intermittent heterotropia heterophoria, and mechanical.

Other disorders include binocular movement, refraction, accommodation, myopia (nearsightedness), astigmatism (defective curvature of the cornea or lens), hyperopia (farsightedness), and presbyopia (impairment of vision due to old age).

Visual disturbances (H53-H54) include amblyopia, discomfort, sudden visual loss, transient vision loss, day blindness, diplopia, scotoma, defects, contraction of visual field, color vision deficiencies, and night blindness.

Also coded in this section is blindness and low vision (H54) with fourth characters classifying which eyes are involved and if there is blindness or low vision, e.g. blindness in both eyes are coded as H54.0 and blindness in one eye and low vision in the other is coded as H54.1. If a cause is known for the blindness, the code instructs the additional coding of the underlying cause. Legal blindness is coded as H54.8. Visual impairment is differentiated as 1, 2, 3, 4, 5 or 9 depending on visual acuity with 5 indicating no light perception and 9 undetermined or unspecified.

Section 15.8: PROCEDURAL COMPLICATIONS

Complications and disorders to the eyes due to a procedure either during the procedure or after are coded as H59 which include keratopathy, fragments in the eyes, edema, hemorrhage, hematoma, accidental puncture or laceration, inflammation, and scars.

CHAPTER 16
ICD-10 EAR

You will learn the following in this chapter:

B. Otitis
   1. Suppurative
   2. Serous
   3. Otitis Media
   4. Otitis Externa
Q. Diseases
   5. Inner Ear
   6. External Ear
   7. Middle Ear
R. Other Disorders
S. Procedural Complications

Chapter 8 is described as "Diseases of the Ear and Mastoid Process" and range from H60-H95. These codes are broken into five blocks: external ear, middle ear and mastoid, inner ear, other disorders, and intraoperative and postprocedural complications.

Section 16.1: OTITIS

There are various disorders of the ear which include tinnitus (ringing sensation in the ears), vertigo, deafness, and otitis media. Otitis media is inflammation of the ear. There are two types of otitis media: suppurative is characterized by the accumulation of pus due to an infection and serous is characterized by an accumulation of serous fluid. It is important that otitis media is treated immediately as it can result in hearing impairment or loss. There is also otitis externa which is inflammation of the outer ear and is also known as swimmer's ear. Diseases of the middle ear are coded as H65-H75 such as suppurative otitis media (H66.0) and chronic serous otitis media (H65.2).

There is much greater specificity as to site and laterality through the use of fourth, fifth, and sixth characters for these codes, acute and subacute allergic otitis media (mucoid) (sanguinous) (serous), right ear (H65.111). There are also many more "code first underlying disease" notes.

Section 16.2: DISEASES

Diseases of the inner ear are coded as H80-H83. Other disorders are coded as H90-H94.

Diseases of the external ear (H60-H62) include otitis externa which can involve abscesses, cellulitis, hemorrhagic, swimmer's ear, cholesteatoma, noninfective (from chemicals, actinic, contact, eczematoid, etc), chronditis, hematomas, acquired deformities, impacted cerumen, stenosis and due to other diseases.

Diseases of the middle ear and mastoid (H65-H75) include nonsuppurative otitis media (serous and mucoid), suppurative (producing pus), in diseases classified elsewhere, salpingitis or obstruction in Eustachian tube, myringitis, atrophic flaccid or nonflaccid tympanic membrane, sclerosis, adhesive disease, discontinuity, dislocation, ankylosis or loss of ear ossicles, polyp, mastoiditis, and cholesteatoma. If the tympanic membrane has been perforated, code H72 should be used in addition to instructions to code first any associated otitis media.

Diseases of the inner ear (H80-H83) include otosclerosis, Meniere's Disease, vertigo, neuronitis, other diseases of the inner ear, and noise effect conditions.

Section 16.3: OTHER DISORDERS

Other disorders of the ear (H90-H94) include hearing losses (conductive, sensorineural, mixed, ototoxic, and presbycusis) otalgia, effusion (otorrhea), otorrhagia, degeneration, deafness, tinnitus, hyperacusis, in other diseases, and temporary loss of hearing.

Section 16.4: PROCEDURAL COMPLICATIONS

Codes for intraoperative or postprocedural complications are coded as H95.

CHAPTER 17
ICD-10 CIRCULATORY SYSTEM

You will learn the following objectives in this chapter:

A. Circulatory System
B. Rheumatic Fever/Heart Disease
C. Hypertension
D. Ischemic Heart Disease
E. Diseases of Pulmonary Circulation
F. Other Forms of Heart Disease
    1. Pericarditis/Endocarditis/Myocarditis
    2. Conduction Disorders
    3. Dysrhythmias
    4. Heart Failure
    5. Cerebrovascular Diseases
G. Diseases of the Arteries
H. Diseases of the Veins
I. Other
J. Operative Complications

CIRCULATORY SYSTEM: Chapter 9 is described as "Diseases of the Circulatory System" and range from I00-I99. Remember, these are I's, not the number one.

Section 17.1: CIRCULATORY SYSTEM

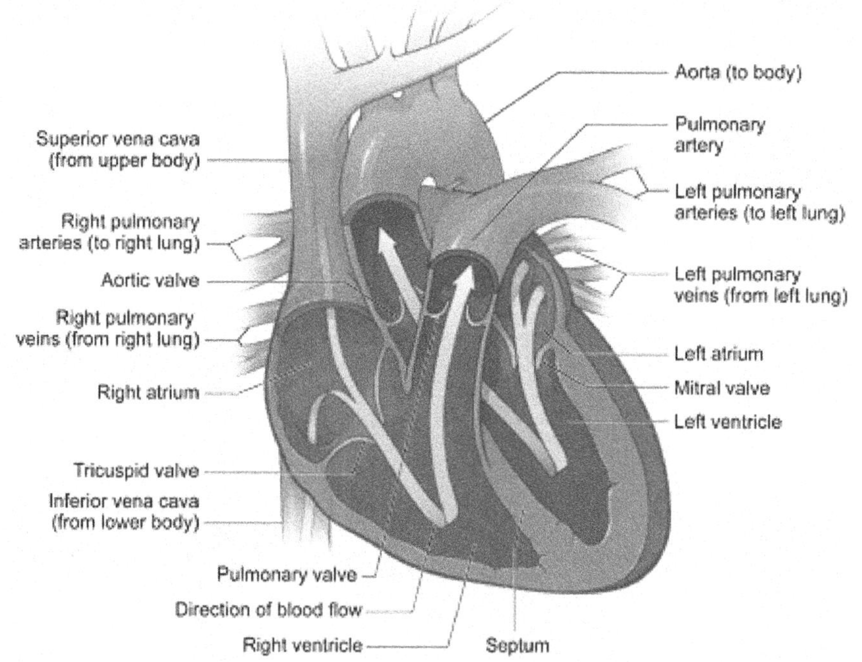

nih.gov

The circulatory system is extensive and so is the complexity of the coding that accompanies it. In fact, some of the most proficient coders are cardiovascular coders. This complexity is due to the vast vascular system of which knowing the anatomy and physiology is a great challenge, in addition to multitude, severity, and prominence of related diseases and conditions and the complexity and rapid advancements in procedures.

The cardiovascular system is comprised of the heart and the vascular system. The cardiovascular system is the means by which all nutrients, water, and oxygen are distributed to the rest of our body.

The vascular system is comprised of a hierarchial system of blood vessels. Arteries are the larger blood vessels that carry oxygen-rich blood away from the heart and is the color red. Once the blood has been depleted of oxygen, nutrients, and water, the blood returns to the heart through the veins.

It is important to understand the flow of the blood, not only through the arteries and veins, but also through the heart and will continue to be very critical in the selection of CPT codes. Blood flow begins when the blood enters the right atrium of the heart:

(1) Blood enters the right atrium (upper) of the heart through the superior vena cava from the upper portions of the body and through the inferior vena cava from the lower portions of the body.
(2) Blood then passes through the tricuspid valve into the right ventricle of the heart.
(3) Blood then passes through the pulmonary valve into the pulmonary artery and into the lungs where it is enriched with oxygen. This is the only artery of the body that contains oxygen-poor blood which is blue.
(4) The blood then returns from the lungs now rich with oxygen through the pulmonary vein and into the left atrium. This is the only vein of the body that contains oxygen-rich blood and is red.
(5) The blood then passes through the mitral valve into the left ventricle.
(6) The blood then passes out of the left ventricle through the aortic valve and into the aorta, then into the rest of the body through the arterial system.

LAYERS OF HEART: There are three layers to the heart, the endocardium which lines the interior of the heart, the myocardium which is the thick muscular middle portion of the heart, and the pericardium which surrounds the heart.

PHASES: There are two phases to a heartbeat: diastole and systole. Diastole is the phase when the ventricles are relaxing and the heart is filling with blood. Systole is when the ventricles are contracting and pushing blood into the pulmonary artery and aorta. The phases are indicated by the blood pressure reading in which the systole number is on top and the diastole number is on the bottom as a fraction. For example, blood pressure of 120/80 means the systole is 120 and the diastole is 80. Blood pressure in which the systole rate is sustained at above 140 and/or a diastole rate is sustained above 90 is considered hypertension and constitutes a health risk. An abnormal heart rate is known as a murmur.

CONDUCTION: The heartbeat is initiated by an electrical impulse from the sinoatrial node (SA node) located in the right atrium. It is also known as pacemaker, albeit the natural one and not an implanted pacemaker. This electrical impulse causes the atrium to contract and push blood into the ventricle; thereby, starting the flow of the blood through the heart and the continuing ripple of the electricity throughout the heart. This electrical impulse then passes to the atrioventricular node (AV node), to the AV bundle (bundle of His), which then divides into the right and left bundle branches. These terms are important when coding as blockages of these areas can result in serious health issues.

Section 17.2: RHEUMATIC FEVER/HEART DISEASE

Rheumatic fever is a sequela of a streptococcal infection, group A, and can result in serious damage to the heart, known as rheumatic heart disease. It occurs most often in younger people.

Rheumatic fever can be coded alone if it the heart is not involved, as described by the physician. The codes are also distinguished by which layer of the heart is involved: pericarditis is inflammation of the outer layer; endocarditis is inflammation of the inner layer; and myocarditis which is inflammation of the middle layer.

These conditions can be acute or chronic. The physician must describe it as chronic to be listed as chronic; otherwise, it would be coded as acute which means the condition is currently occurring.

The inflammation from the infection and fever can result in damage to the valves, including stenosis, which can be heard as a murmur during a cardiac examination. Most oftentimes it is the mitral valve that is damaged. The codes are distinguished by which valve is damaged.

Acute rheumatic heart disease or rheumatic chorea are coded as I00-I09 and are further specified as to with or without heart involvement. Chronic rheumatic heart disease is coded as I05-I09. Other rheumatic heart disease include myocarditis, pericarditis and heart failure. There are notes indicating the need to code additional codes for type of condition such as heart failure.

Rheumatic valvular disease is coded as I05-I09 for the mitral valve, arotic valve, and tricuspid which can involve multiple valves together. Rheumatic valvular disease can include stenosis or insufficiency. ICD-10 assumes that valvular disease was caused by rheumatic heart fever caused by streptococci unless it is described as non-rheumatic (I34). Only aortic valvular disease is assumed to be non-rheumatic unless otherwise stated.

Section 17.3: HYPERTENSION

Hypertension is the elevation of the blood pressure, either or both the systole and diastole pressures. Hypertension is considered a major factor in atherosclerosis, cardiovascular disease, heart failure, coronary artery disease, and stroke. Hypertension is certainly a condition that complicates the care of the patient, so if a patient is described as having hypertension by the physician, then it is usually coded even if the hypertension is not the main reason for the visit nor does the patient receive any care for it.

Hypertension is coded as I10-I15. It is specified as it was previously in ICD-9, i.e. primary or secondary and with or without heart or renal involvement. However, there is no specification of type of hypertension (malignant, benign, or unspecified). Fourth characters further classify the hypertension codes as to presence of congestive heart failure and renal failure. When a patient has only high blood pressure with no diagnosis of hypertension (also known as transient hypertension) it is coded as R03.0.

The great majority of hypertension is primary (essential) and its cause is not known. The remainder is secondary to renal disease which is due to the physiological relatedness of the renal system and blood pressure. The condition causing the hypertension should also be coded (multiple coding).

There is no longer a table in the alphabetical index for hypertension.

Additional codes should be listed for exposure to tobacco smoke.

There are separate codes for a hypertensive condition in a pregnant mother (O10-O11) which is known as transient. A hypertensive condition in the baby is coded as P92.2. This is an important distinction because a mother may develop hypertension while pregnant but it is only transient due to the pregnancy and should cease once she is no longer pregnant.

There are several scenarios for coding hypertension codes when heart or kidney conditions are occurring at the same time. First, the term hypertension may be described as a diagnosis in addition to a heart condition, but they are not described as related. If the physician does not link these two conditions with statements such as "hypertensive heart disease" or "heart disease complicated by hypertension", etc, then you must code the heart condition and the hypertension separately. However, if the physician does describe the hypertension and heart condition as being related, such as "hypertensive heart disease" or "due to", then I11 should be used. The code directs the additional coding of the heart problem. Hypertension can affect the heart because it causes the heart to work harder which results in thickening of the left ventricle and can result in heart failure.

WARNING: The use of conjunctions may be confusing so beware! If a physician describes a condition as "heart problem with hypertension," the "with" may not necessarily mean that the two conditions are related to each other although the hypertension codes do use the "with" to denote a relationship. Therefore, you should check with a physician or check the report for further information to be sure if the heart condition and hypertension should be coded with one code if they are related.

The term hypertension may be described as a diagnosis in addition to a renal (kidney) condition. If the renal condition is described as acute and the physician does not describe the renal condition being related to the hypertension, then the two conditions are coded separately (as we did with the heart condition).

However, if the renal condition is chronic, then hypertension and the renal condition are coded as related. Chronic renal conditions are considered related to hypertension because the hypertension causes damage to the kidneys. This is also known as hypertensive nephropathy, hypertensive nephrosclerosis, hypertensive renal disease, chronic renal disease (CRD), or chronic kidney disease (CKD). If the renal condition is chronic, then the hypertension and renal disease are related and code them together in one code (I13) even if the doctor does not define them as being related, such as if he said hypertension and chronic renal disease. In addition, another code is needed for the renal disease and its stage as denoted in the hypertension notes in the coding book. Renal diseases codes are differentiated by stages with stage V being end stage renal disease (ESRD).

A physician may describe both a heart and renal condition as being related to hypertension, and this is also coded with I13 codes. This is also known as cardiorenal hypertension.

Secondary hypertension is coded as I15.

Section 17.4: ISCHEMIC HEART DISEASE

Ischemic heart disease is caused by arteriosclerotic heart disease (ASHD) (I70) in that the arteries of the heart are hardened and narrowed, resulting in coronary ischemia and coronary artery disease (CAD). This occurs when atherosclerosis causes a lack of blood flow (ischemia) and, therefore, a lack of oxygen which can result in impaired functions, infarctions, or necrosis (death). The area of dead tissue is known as an infarction (not infraction). Chest pain is known as angina pectoris.

Heart problems may be indicated by Mobitz II heart block, ventricular fibrillation and angina pectoris (chest pain, I20) which can be unstable or with spasms.

If this infarction is of the heart, it is known as a myocardial infarction (MI) and is also known as a heart attack or cardiac arrest. MIs are coded with I22 codes if the duration is less than four weeks. The codes are based on where the ST elevation (STEMI) is in the heart or if there is non-ST elevation (NSTEMI). Additional codes are also required for tobacco exposure and if status post administration of tPA within last 24 hours at another facility.

Cardiac arrest (I46) occurs when the heart stops. Heart attack refers to a blockage in a coronary artery resulting in heart muscle damage and is commonly known as a myocardial infarction (MI) (I21). It is important to understand the differences between heart attack, cardiac arrest, and heart failure.

If a subsequent MI occurs within four weeks after a previous MI, then the correct codes would be I22. Certain complications to the MI should be coded additionally with I23 codes such as atrial septal defect, rupture of cardiac wall, and thrombosis of atrium.

If ischemic heart disease does not result in an MI, then codes I24 should be used, such as a thrombosis or postmyocardial infarction syndrome.

If the patient is diagnosed as having an old or healed MI or if an MI was diagnosed on an EKG (ECG) but is not presenting any problems at this time, it should be coded with I25.2.

Chronic ischemic heart disease (I25) includes atherosclerosis. Atherosclerosis precedes arteriosclerosis in that atherosclerosis is the accumulation of fatty deposits in the arterial system. This then results in arteriosclerosis, which is hardening of the arteries due to the development of plaque from the fatty deposits. With these deposits of plaque, a clot can form which is known as a thrombosis. If this thrombosis dislodges and is released into the rest of the arterial system it is known as an embolus and can be deadly.

Within the codes, atherosclerosis can be defined with angina pectoris or spasms and occurring in a native artery or area with a bypass graft or of a transplanted heart. Chronic total occlusion of a coronary artery is coded as I25.82 which can be coded in addition to atherosclerosis.

Aneurysms (I25.3) are weakened areas of the vascular walls which can result in rupture.
NOTE that although hyperlipidemia (elevation of fats in the blood) and hypercholesterolemia (high levels of cholesterol in the blood) are major factors in the development of arteriosclerosis and hypertension, they are coded from endocrine/metabolic codes.

Section 17.5: DISEASES OF PULMONARY CIRCULATION

Diseases of the pulmonary circulation (I26-I28) refer to conditions related to the pulmonary vein or artery, such as arteriosclerosis, hypertension, aneurysm, infarction, and embolism. Remember that iatrogenic means the condition resulted from medical care.

Pulmonary embolisms are coded as I26 if it not related to surgery or is a complication of pregnancy.

There are references in some descriptions of the codes to septic involvement which needs to also be coded, as described in an earlier packet and as noted in the ICD-10 book.

An arteriovenous fistula (I28.0) is an abnormal connection or passageway between an artery and a vein. Aneurysm of the pulmonary artery is coded as I28.1.

Section 17.6: PERICARDITIS/ENDOCARDITIS/MYOCARDITIS

Pericarditis (I30) is inflammation of the sac surrounding the heart; endocarditis (I33) is inflammation of the interior tissue of the heart; and myocarditis (I40) is inflammation of the heart muscle. Inflammation can be due to an infectious organism or idiopathic which means the cause is unknown. Remember, you must code the organism also, if known. Many of these codes include acute and subacute. Subacute refers to a condition being less severe or having less duration than an acute condition and not long enough to be considered chronic.

Disorders of valves include insufficiency, incompetence, regurgitation, and endocarditis of the mitral valve (I34), the aortic valve (I35), the tricuspid valve (I36), and the pulmonary valve (I37). Incompetence can result from stenosis, which is narrowing of the valves and the failure of the valve to operate properly. Insufficiency and regurgitation occurs when the valve allows backward flow of blood.

Cardiomyopathy is disease involving the heart (I42). Cardiomyopathy may be due to many factors, such as diseases, arteriosclerosis, alcohol abuse, nutritional deficiencies, and diseases.

Section 17.7: CONDUCTION DISORDERS

Conduction codes (I44) include such terms as left bundle branch block and atrioventricular (AV) blocks. The bundle of His branches into three bundle branches, the right, left anterior and left posterior bundle branches which can experience blockage causing a defect in the electrical system of the heart. RBBB is a right bundle branch block and LBBB is a left bundle branch block. AV blocks involve impairment of the conduction from the atrium to the ventricular Bundle of His. There are three types of AV blocks: in the first degree AV block there is a slowing of the conduction as noted on an EKG as a prolonged PR interval; a second degree AV block, also known as Mobitz I or II, or Wenckebach, involves a greater slowing of the conduction and some missed beats; third degree AV block, also known as a complete heart block, occurs when there is complete blockage of the conduction from the atria to the ventricle. Usually this requires the implantation of a pacemaker.

Peripheral vascular disease (PVD) is included in this section (I44). PVD is any disease caused by obstruction of the arteries in the legs and arms. It is also known as peripheral artery disease (PAD) or peripheral artery occlusive disease (PAOD).

Section 17.8: DYSRHYTHMIAS

Cardiac dysrhythmias (I48-I49) are abnormal electrical currents in the heart which can result in irregular, slowed, or fast heart beats. These codes are differentiated by being supraventricular or ventricular. Supraventricular are those arrhythmias generated within the SA node, atria, and AV node. Ventricular are those arrhythmias generated in the ventricular conduction system. The result of dysrhythmias can include tachycardia (fast heartbeat), bradycardia (slow heart beat), and fibrillation/flutter (disorganized current flow).

Section 17.9: HEART FAILURE

Heart failure (I50) is the insufficiency of the heart to pump adequate amounts of blood. Differentiation of codes is based on congestive heart failure which includes right heart failure due to left heart failure since heart failure usually begins in the left heart and then progresses to the right. Because the failure can begin in the left, there is a code for left heart failure only (I50.1). The codes are also differentiated based on systolic or diastolic heart failure. There are many notes about coding first for a variety of reasons including following surgery or hypertension.

Section 17.10: CEREBROVASCULAR DISEASES

Cerebrovascular diseases (I60-I69) refer to conditions pertaining to the blood vessels or blood flow to the brain through the vascular system. These include hemorrhages (bleeding), occlusion (closure due to blockage), stenosis (narrowing), and ischemia (restriction in blood flow). These codes are usually referenced by the artery involved.

There are many additional codes that need to be coded if present which includes alcohol abuse, exposure to tobacco, and hypertension.

Nontraumatic subarachnoid hemorrhages are further specified by site, e.g. nontraumatic subarachnoid hemorrhage from carotid siphon and bifurcation, I60.0.

Embolism and thrombus are listed under occlusion because they cause an occlusion, thus resulting in a cerebral infarction (I63). These occlusions, stenosis, or hemorrhaging (known as aneurysms) can result in a cerebrovascular accident (CVA), better known as a stroke. CVA is a lack of blood to the brain which can result in the loss of brain functions and related activities, such as speech, motor ability and vision.

Transient cerebral ischemia (TIA) (G45.9) is a temporary loss of blood to the brain, as transient means temporary, and is not coded from this section.

Stroke is coded as I63.9. Sequelae from a CVA are coded as I69 plus a code for the specific condition. Late effects of cerebrovascular diseases (I69) have been expanded to include laterality, trauma, site, dominance, and deficits, e.g. monoplegia of upper limb following nontraumatic subarachnoid hemorrhage affecting right dominant side, I69.031. A late effect is a sequela or residual that is caused by an acute condition but which remains after the treatment of the acute condition is completed.

Section 17.11: DISEASES OF THE ARTERIES

These codes (I70-I79) include conditions involving the arteries, arterioles and capillaries, such as atherosclerosis, aneurysm, embolism, thrombus, polyarteritis, and fistulas.

These codes are further classified by additional complications, such as claudication (cramps in the legs caused by poor circulation within the arteries), rest pain, ulceration, and gangrene.

Section 17.12: DISEASES OF VEINS AND OTHERS

These codes, I80-I89, include some of the conditions previously described in the arterial system, such as embolism for veins, lymphatic vessels, and lymph nodes, but does contain other categories.

Phlebitis and thrombophlebitis (I80.0) are inflammation of veins and creation of thrombus and are classified by the veins involved.

Varicose veins (I83) of the lower extremities are veins that have become enlarged and tortuous because the valves that prevent the backward flow of blood no longer functioning properly and so a leakage of blood occurs. Not only can this cause unsightly veins which become enlarged, but it can result in ulceration which is a disruption in the layers of the skin so that a sore appears. The codes are differentiated by the presence of ulcers, inflammation or other complications. There are separate codes for varicose veins of other anatomic sites, such as gastric (I86.4) which can be deadly.

Hemorrhoids (K64) are contained in the digestive system chapter. They are dilated, swollen, painful veins in the anus or rectum. These can be complicated by thrombosis, bleeding, strangulation, ulceration, and prolapse (falling down or slipping out of place). They are classified as internal or external. External hemorrhoids protrude from the rectum through the anus.

Section 17.13: OTHER

Lymphadenitis (I88) has been moved to this section of codes. Gangrene has also been moved to this section (I96). Hypotension (I95.9) is an abnormally low blood pressure which can be caused by various conditions such as hemodialysis, drugs, idiopathic (origin not known) or postprocedural.

Section 17.14: OPERATIVE COMPLICATIONS

Intraoperative and postprocedural complications are coded as I97 and include hemorrhage, hematoma, puncture, laceration, cardiac insufficiency, cardiac arrest, heart failure, and cerebrovascular infarction.

CIRCULATORY QUIZ 10

1. What are the codes for a patient with congestive heart failure and hypertension?
2. What are the codes for a patient with elevated blood pressure?
3. What are the codes for a patient with malignant hypertensive stage IV CKD?
4. What are the codes for a patient with benign CKD stage 4 and ASCVD due to hypertension?
5. What are the codes for a patient with acute and chronic pericarditis?
6. What are the codes for a patient who has a complete AV heart block?
7. What are the codes for a patient who has strangulated internal hemorrhoids with bleeding?
8. What are the codes for a patient who has hemiplegia after experiencing a CVA 6 months ago?
9. What are the codes for a patient who was diagnosed nine weeks ago with chronic coronary insufficiency?
10. What are the codes for a patient who had an appendectomy due to appendicitis who has postoperative hypertension?
11. What are the codes for a patient who is not presenting with any symptoms but was diagnosed as having MI on an EKG reading?
12. What are the codes for a patient diagnosed with intermediate coronary syndrome?
13. What are the codes for a patient with chest pain due to acute MI of the inferoposterior wall as part of initial care?
14. What are the codes for a patient with RBBB?
15. What are the codes for a patient who has aplastic anemia due to radiation therapy?

CHAPTER 18
ICD-10 RESPIRATORY SYSTEM

You will learn the following objectives in this chapter:

A. Respiratory System
B. Acute Respiratory Infections
C. Upper Respiratory Tract Conditions
D. Pneumonia/Influenza
E. Acute Lower Respiratory Infections
F. Other Upper Respiratory Infections
G. Chronic Lower Respiratory Infections
H. Chronic Obstructive Pulmonary Disease
I. Other Lung Diseases Due to External Agents
J. Other Respiratory Diseases
K. Suppurative and Necrotic Conditions
L. Procedural Complications

Chapter 10 is described as "Diseases of the Respiratory System" and range from J00-J99.

Section 18.1: RESPIRATORY SYSTEM
The respiratory system includes airways, lungs, and the respiratory muscles and the process of allowing gas exchange (respiration), primarily of oxygen and carbon dioxide. Respiration consists of internal and external respiration. External respiration involves the lungs and the air sacs of the lung. Internal respiration involves the exchange of gases at the cellular level in which oxygen passes into the cells and carbon dioxide passes out so that it can be exhaled from the body through the lungs.

Air enters through the nose and proceeds through the pharynx (throat). The nose area contains the sinuses, which include the maxillary, frontal, ethmoidal, and sphenoidal. The pharynx is comprised of the nasopharynx where the tonsils and adenoids are located, then into the oropharynx, and lastly the laryngopharynx. The laryngopharynx divides into two branches, the larynx (voice box) and the esophagus. While the esophagus leads into the stomach, the larynx leads into the lungs. The epiglottis is a flap that controls the opening of the laryngopharynx so that either the larynx or the esophagus branch is open.

PARANASAL SINUSES: The paranasal sinuses are the frontal, maxillary, ethmoid and sphenoid.

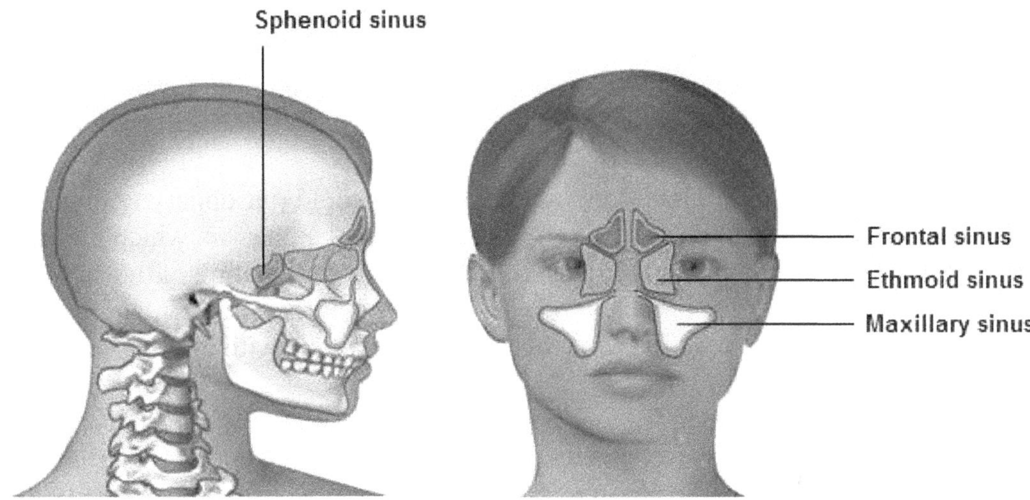

National Pain Foundation

The larynx then opens into the trachea (windpipe) which branches into the bronchial tubes (bronchi) thus leading into the right and left lungs. These then branch into bronchioles which end in clusters of air sacs called alveoli. It is here that the exchange of gases occur with the capillaries so that oxygen can pass into the blood and be dispersed to the cells. (American Lung Association)

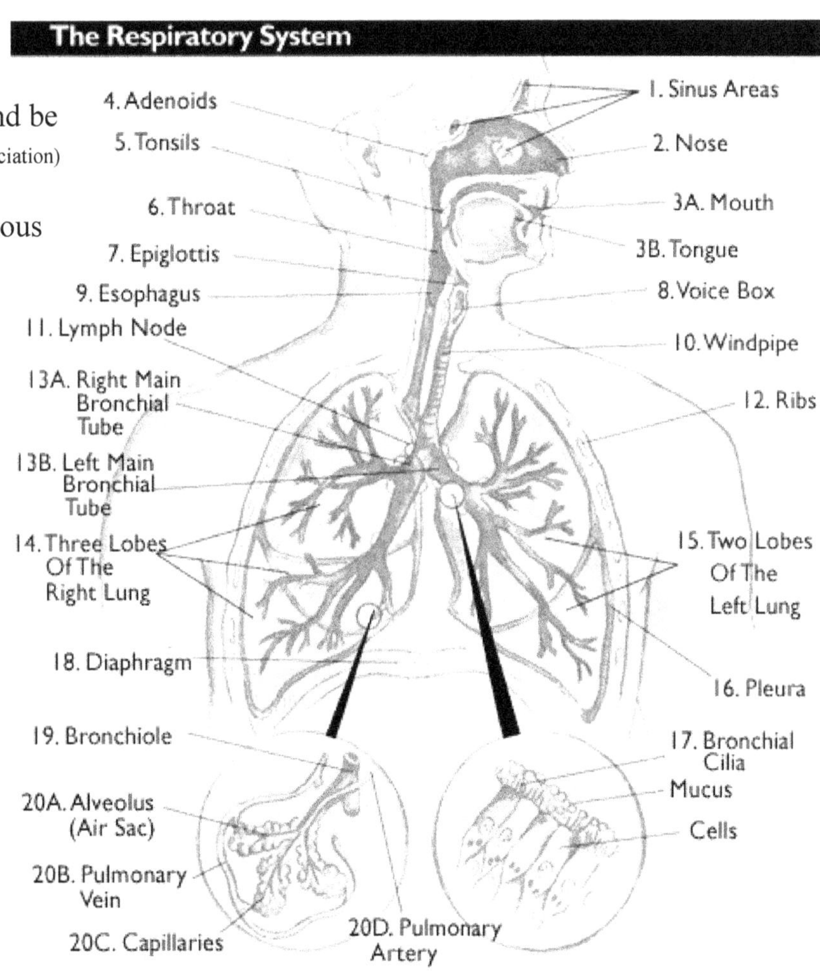

Each lung is covered by the membranous pleura. The outer layer is called the parietal pleura and the inner layer is called the visceral pleura (surrounding an organ).

The diaphragm is a muscle that separates the thoracic cavity from the abdominal cavity. It is involved in the inhalation and exhalation of the lungs through contractions.

The right lung is divided into three lobes and the left lung has two lobes, so they are not mirror images of each other and cannot be coded as bilateral if a procedure is done on both sides.

Section 18.2: ACUTE RESPIRATORY INFECTIONS

For all codes in this chapter, when a respiratory condition occurs in more than one site, if there is not a code specifying these multiple sites, then the lowest anatomic site location should be used to select the code as noted in the book.

Acute respiratory infections (J00-J06) include the common cold (nasopharyngitis) (J00), sinusitis (inflammation of the sinuses), pharyngitis (inflammation of the pharynx which includes sore throat), tonsillitis (inflammation of the tonsils), laryngitis (inflammation of the larynx), bronchitis (inflammation of the bronchial tubes), and bronchiolitis (inflammation of the bronchioles). Croup is coded as J05, acute obstructive laryngitis with or without obstruction.

Tonsillitis codes have been expanded to include organisms with the fourth character and the level (acuity or recurrent) with the fifth character, e.g. acute tonsillitis due to other specified organisms (J03.80). Pharyngitis similarly has been expanded in the fourth character to specify the organism, e.g. acute pharyngitis due to strep (J02.0). Remember, the organism should also be coded, in addition.

Section 18.3: UPPER RESPIRATORY TRACT CONDITIONS

Acute upper respiratory infections (URI) of multiple or unspecified sites are coded as J06. Acute (LRI) is coded as J22. Chronic lower respiratory infection is coded as chronic bronchitis.

Section 18.4: PNEUMONIA/INFLUENZA

Influenza and pneumonia are coded as J09-J18. Fourth characters provide classification based on presence of pneumonia and manifestations, such as myocarditis.

Influenza is coded according to what type of virus is involved and some manifestations such as gastrointestinal or respiratory. There are notes to code the virus for some of the codes as well as to additionally code pleural effusion or sinusitis.

Pneumonia is inflammation of the lung that produces exudates. These codes are differentiated as viral (J12), Strep (J13), other bacterial (J15), Hemophilus (J14), staph (J15.2) as well as others. Notice that pneumonia due to MRSA is coded as J15.212. Pneumonia due to other diseases classified elsewhere is coded as J17 such as Q fever and rheumatic fever with a note to code the disease first.

Other types of pneumonia include bronchopneumonia (J18.0), lobar (J18.1) and hypostatic (J18.2) (hypostasis is pooling of the blood in the area of the body closest to the ground). J69 describes pneumonitis due to solids and liquids.

Section 18.5: ACUTE LOWER RESPIRATORY INFECTIONS

Acute lower respiratory infections (J20-J22) include acute and subacute bronchitis and bronchiolitis which can be differentiated by organism.

Section 18.6: OTHER UPPER RESPIRATORY TRACT DISEASES

These codes contain many of the chronic conditions, as well as conditions such as polyps (nonmalignant growth or tumor), deviation, hypertrophy (overgrowth), abscesses (collection of pus due to the body's reaction to an infection), allergic responses, paralysis, edema (swelling), stenosis, and cellulitis.

Allergic rhinitis is coded as J30 differentiated by what the cause is, such as food, animals, or pollen. Chronic rhinitis (J31) include pharyngitis and nasopharyngitis which requires the use of additional codes for any exposure to tobacco.

Chronic sinusitis (J32) is differentiated by which part of the sinus is involved such as frontal, maxillary, ethmoidal, or sphenoidal. If all sinuses are involved, then it is coded as pansinusitis, but if only some of the sinuses are involved, this would be coded as other (J32.8).

Nasal polyps are coded as J33 and other disorders of the nose and nasal sinuses (J34) include abscess, furuncle, carbuncle, cyst or deviated nasal septum.

Chronic diseases of the tonsils and adenoids (J35) include tonsillitis, adenoiditis, and hypertrophy which can be coded singly or together. Chronic laryngitis/laryngotracheitis is coded as J37.

Disease of the vocal cords and larynx (J38) include paralysis, polyp, nodules, abscess, cellulitis, leukoplakia, edema, spasm, or stenosis.

Section 18.7: CHRONIC LOWER RESPIRATORY INFECTIONS

Chronic lower respiratory infections (J40-J47) begin with bronchitis (J40) specified as neither chronic nor acute, chronic bronchitis (J41-J42) described as simple, mucopurulent or mixed simple and emphysema (J43) (chronic respiratory condition characterized by loss of elasticity of lung tissue which results in the collapse of the airways).

Chronic obstructive pulmonary disease (COPD) codes have changed in that the term COPD is now included with the chronic condition. COPD is a general term which has been used to indicate any disorder that persistently obstructs bronchial airflow. COPD is coded as J44 which includes chronic bronchitis, emphysema, and chronic asthma. You can now code COPD in addition to other chronic pulmonary diseases as indicated in the notes; some will require that you code the other condition as well such as emphysema.

Asthma (J45) includes many types including atopic, extrinsic, and idiosyncratic and can include bronchitis and rhinitis. Asthma is a chronic respiratory condition characterized by inflammation, airflow obstruction, and bronchospasm, also known as reactive airway disease (RAD). Extrinsic asthma is caused by factors outside of the body such as food allergies, while intrinsic asthma is caused by internal factors. Asthma can also be induced by exercising or coughing.

Code J45, asthma, has a fourth character for degree of persistence such as mild, moderate or persistent and either persistent or intermittent. It also has a fifth character classification that is uncomplicated, exacerbated or with status asthmaticus which is an acute attack in which the asthma is not relieved by usual treatments. Status asthmaticus is also known as intractable, refractory, and severe prolonged. There is no longer specification in the asthma codes to specify extrinsic, intrinsic, chronic obstructive and unspecified (J45).

Bronchiectasis (J47) can be coded as with acute lower respiratory infection, exacerbated, or uncomplicated

Section 18.8: LUNG DISEASES DUE TO EXTERNAL AGENTS

Various lung diseases that can be caused by external agents (J60-J70) include coalworker's pneumoconiosis, black lung disease, anthracosis, pneumoconiosis due to asbestos, silica, inorganic dusts, or tuberculosis.

Specific codes are provided for diseases or hypersensitivity (allergy) caused by organic dust (J66-J67) such as flax-dresser's disease, farmer's lung, bird fancier's lung, maple-bark-stripper's lung, air conditioner lung, or cheese-washer's lung.

Inhalation of chemicals, gases, fumes and vapors can cause various respiratory conditions (J68) including bronchitis, pneumonitis, and URI. The cause should be coded first with T51-T65 codes. Any associated respiratory conditions should also be coded such as respiratory failure (J96).

Pneumonia can be caused by the inhalation of solids and liquids into the lungs (J69) which can include food, vomit, oils and essences.

Other external agents that can cause respiratory conditions (J70) include radiation, drugs, and smoke inhalation.

Section 18.9: OTHER RESPIRATORY DISEASES

Other respiratory diseases principally affecting the interstitium (J80-J84) include acute respiratory distress syndrome, pulmonary edema, eosinophilia, fibrosis, idiopathic pneumonia, and hyperplasia. Acute Respiratory Distress Syndrome (ARDS) is coded as J80. ARDS is a serious reaction to injuries of the lung and result in inflammation, hypoxemia and can result in multiple organ failure.Empyema is coded as J86.9 and involves infection with pus in the lungs and is not the same as emphysema. Pleurisy is inflammation of the pleura.

Section 18.10: SUPPPURATIVE AND NECROTIC CONDITIONS OF LOWER RESPIRATORY TRACT

Other conditions of the lower respiratory tract that are suppurative or necrotic (J85-J86) include abscess with gangrene or necrosis and pyothorax.

There are several types of pleural effusion (J90-J91) including malignancy or heart failure but some of these require the use of other codes so be sure to check the exclude notes. Pleural effusion is the inflammation of the pleural cavity.

Pneumothorax and air leak (J93) is when air or gas is present in the pleural cavity oftentimes due to trauma. It can be spontaneous, primary, or secondary. In secondary pneumothorax, the underlying condition needs to be coded first. There are numerous types of pneumothorax that are excluded such as traumatic (S27.0), iatrogenic (J95) as caused by medical treatment. Spontaneous means the air is able to enter the pleural space but not leave it.

Section 18.11: INTRAOPERATIVE/POSTPROCEDURAL Respiratory conditions that develop during or after a procedure has been performed are coded as J95 which can include tracheostomy complications, pulmonary insufficiency, chemical pneumonitis due to anesthesia, hemorrhage, hematoma, puncture, laceration, air leak, and complications from the use of a ventilator (respirator) for breathing.

Respiratory failure and insufficiency (J96) is the inability of the respiratory system to provide adequate levels of oxygen and to adequately remove carbon dioxide.

RESPIRATORY QUIZ 11

1. What are the codes for a patient with lower respiratory infection?
2. What are the codes for an asthmatic patient with status asthmaticus and COPD?
3. What are the codes for a patient with COPD and emphysema?
4. What are the codes for a patient with chronic respiratory failure and chronic edema?
5. What are the codes for a patient with ARDS?
6. What are the codes for a patient who is dehydrated and has pneumonia of the right lobe?
7. What are the codes for a patient with pleurisy due to TB?
8. What are the codes for a collapsed lung?
9. What are the codes for a patient with a sore throat?
10. What are the codes for a patient with tonsillitis and adenoiditis?
11. What are the codes for a patient who is seen today for a high fever and chest congestion due to the common cold?
12. What are the codes for a patient with COPD with pneumonia?
13. What are the codes for a patient with acute and chronic bronchitis and COPD?
14. What are the codes for a patient with chronic bronchitis and emphysema?
15. What are the codes for a patient with asthma that was precipitated by exercise?

CHAPTER 19
ICD-10 DIGESTIVE SYSTEM

You will learn the following objectives in this chapter:

A. Digestive System
B. Diseases of the Mouth
C. Diseases of Esophagus and Stomach
D. Diseases of the Appendix
E. Hernias
F. Enteritis/Colitis
G. Other Diseases of the Intestines
H. Diseases of the Peritoneum
I. Liver Diseases
J. Disorders of Gallbladder and Pancreas
K. Other Diseases of the Digestive System
L. Procedural Complications

Chapter 11 is described as "Diseases of the Digestive System" and ranges from K00-K95. There are two new sections for liver diseases (K70-K77) and disorders of gallbladder, biliary tract and pancreas (K80-K87).

Section 19.1: THE DIGESTIVE SYSTEM

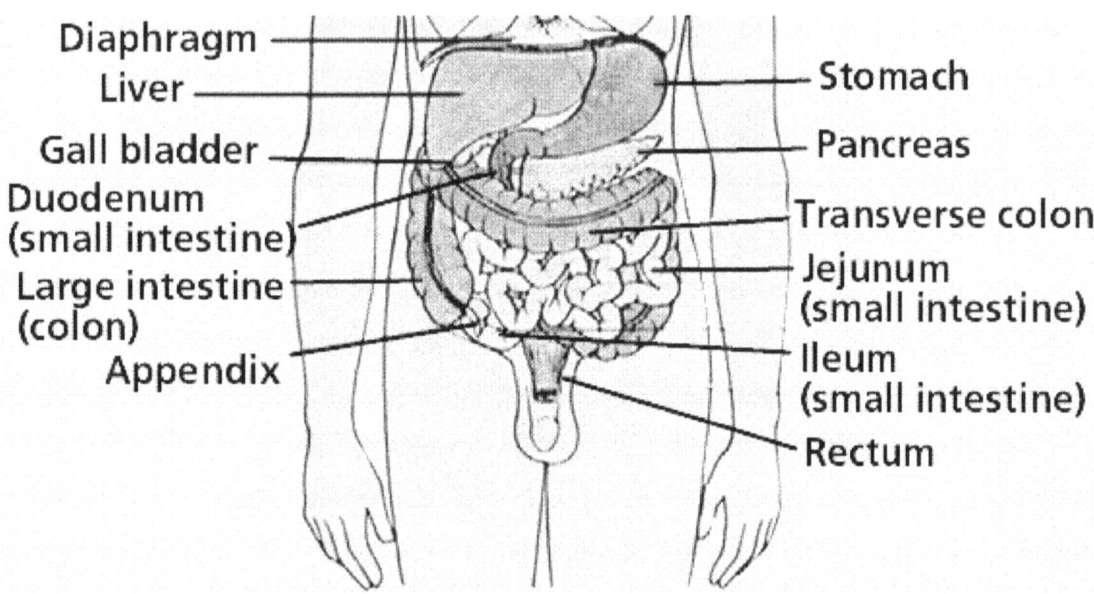

http://www.niddk.nih.gov/digesyst/digesyst.html.

The digestive system (also known as the gastrointestinal tract) includes from the top (mouth) to the bottom (anus).

The pharynx (throat), as discussed in the respiratory packet, extends from the mouth downwards where it separates into the trachea (windpipe) and the esophagus which is controlled by the epiglottis. It is through the esophagus that food travels into the stomach through contractions of muscles known as peristalsis.

The pyloric sphincter separates the stomach from the duodenum, which is the first part of the small intestine (small bowel). The next part of the small intestine is the jejunum, and then last is the ileum. Please note the spelling, ileum is part of the small intestine and should not be confused with the ilium.

From the ileum, the digestive system continues with the large intestine (large bowel) composed of the cecum, the colon (ascending colon, transverse colon, descending colon), then the sigmoid colon, and the rectum which terminates in the anus. The appendix hangs from the cecum.

Section 19.2: DISEASES OF THE MOUTH

This chapter contains many new notes that direct the coding of external causes, underlying conditions, and additional factors influencing the patient's condition, e.g. tobacco dependence (F17) and alcohol abuse and dependence (F10).

Alcohol and tobacco abuse are most oftentimes coded additionally as indicated in the notes for diseases in this chapter.

This section of codes begin with dental conditions and progress through the oral cavity and salivary glands (K00-K14). These include anodontia (K00.0) (absence of teeth), supernumerary teeth, disturbances in tooth formation and eruption, and teething (K00.4) in children.

The codes then continue into diseases of the hard tissues in the mouth (K02-K03) which includes caries, excessive wearing away of the teeth, abrasions and erosions. Conditions of the pulp and gum follow (K04-K08). This includes gingivitis which is a bacterial inflammation of the gums. Periodontitis is rapid onset of inflammation of the gums (gingiva) or peridontium (tissue supporting the teeth). Abnormalities of the dentofacial structures (including the jaw and bones follow next and include malocclusion (improper alignment of teeth and/or arches). Lastly, there are codes for other or unspecified conditions such as loss of teeth.

The codes then proceed into codes for diseases of the salivary glands (K11) including atrophy and sialoadenitis. Diseases of the mouth (K12-K13) include lips and oral mucosa such as abscess, cheilosis, cheek biting, leukoplakia, and fibrosis. The final section is diseases of the tongue (K14) which includes glossitis, hypertrophy, geographic tongue, plicated tongue, and glossodynia.

Section 19.3: DISEASES OF ESOPHAGUS, STOMACH & DUODENUM

Diseases of the esophagus and stomach (K20-K31) begin with disease of the esophagus and include esophagitis, ulcers, stricture, diverticulum, and laceration.

Reflux esophagitis (K21) is a similar condition to gastric esophageal reflux diseases (GERD), but it does not include the stomach. GERD is coded as K21 and includes the esophagus and stomach. It is caused by reflux of acidic stomach fluids up through the esophagus which can result in erosion of the esophagus.

Ulcers are lesions that form necrotic tissue due to inflammation which leaves a hole. Ulcers, again, are coded by what anatomic sites are involved, so the codes vary by anatomic site. Esophageal ulcers (lesion) are coded as K22.1 and are differentiated with or without bleeding. If drugs or poisonings are involved with the ulcer, then these should be coded also with T36-T65.

Gastric ulcers (K25) are also known as peptic ulcers that include the stomach and pylorus.

Duodenal ulcers (K26) are ulcers of the duodenum which is part of the small intestine. This is coded similar to gastric ulcers. Previously peptic ulcers were listed under gastric ulcers although they are of the stomach so they are known as gastroduodenal ulcers.

Gastrojejunal ulcer (K28) occurs in both the stomach and jejunum but excludes primary ulcer of the small intestine as directed in the ICD-10 book.

For all of the ulcers, fourth characters further classify codes by being acute or chronic and with hemorrhage or perforation, e.g. chronic gastric ulcer with hemorrhage and perforation is coded as K25.6, but they are not classified as bleeding. Bleeding is only used to refer to gastritis, dudodenitis, diverticulosis and diverticulitis. The reference to obstruction has been eliminated.

Gastritis and duodenitis (K29) include acute, alcoholic, chronic as either superficial or atrophic, and unspecified as specified by the fourth digits. The fifth digits indicate if there is bleeding or not.

Other disease of the stomach and duodenum (K31) include dilatation of stomach, hypertrophic pyloric stenosis, hourglass stricture and stenosis of stomach, pylorospasm, fistula, and gastroparesis.

Diverticulum is a pouch or sac that can be acquired or genetic. Acquired means that the diverticulum was a result of an occurrence and that the person was not born with it (genetic). This can occur in various locations of the digestive tract, i.e. esophagus (K22.5), appendix (K38.2), and stomach (K31.4); these codes do not provide a description of inflammation (diverticulitis) or the abnormal condition of having diverticulum (diverticulosis) which are coded with K57 codes.

Section 19.4: DISEASES OF THE APPENDIX

Diseases of the appendix (K35-K38) include appendicitis which is inflammation of the appendix. This code is differentiated as including generalized or localized peritonitis (inflammation of the peritoneum). The peritonitis code includes appendicitis that also includes perforation or rupture. Other diseases of the appendix include hyperplasia, concretions, and fistula.

Section 19.5: HERNIAS

Hernias (K40-K46) are protrusions of any part of tissues and organs through an abnormal break in the muscular wall. A hiatal hernia is a hernia of the digestive system, specifically a protrusion of the stomach into the hernia. Inguinal hernia is a hernia of the groin area. An incisional hernia are hernias located at an incompletely-healed surgical wound. If the incisional hernia is in the stomach area, these are known as ventral hernias.

Both acquired and congenital hernias are coded from codes K40-K46 except for congenital diaphragmatic hernia (Q79.0) and congenital hiatus hernia (Q40.1). Like the ICD-9 codes, the hernias are coded as to site, e.g. inguinal, and are further specified in the fourth character as to the presence of obstruction and/or gangrene. Laterality and recurrence are also coded.

Obstructive hernias include hernias that are strangulated and incarcerated. A hernia is considered strangulated when the blood supply is compromised due to a constriction. A hernia is considered incarcerated when the bowels are completely obstructed.

Irreducible hernia is a hernia that cannot be returned to its original place.

An incomplete hernia has not completely gone through the break but in a complete hernia the protrusion has gone entirely through the opening.

Section 19.6: ENTERITIS & COLITIS

Noninfective enteritis and colitis (K50-K52) include Crohn's disease of the small or large intestines. Fifth characters indicate bleeding, obstruction, fistula or abscess. Manifestations should also be coded additionally.

Ulcerative colitis (K51) includes inflammation of the ileum (ileitis), rectosigmoid, and rectum (proctitis). It also includes inflammation of polyps in the colon. The fifth digit indicates bleeding, obstruction, fistula, abscess or other.

Other noninfective gastroenteritis and colitis (K52) can be due to radiation, allergy, dietary, or toxic adverse effects.

Section 19.7: OTHER DISEASES OF THE INTESTINES

Vascular disorders of the intestines (K55) include various types of colitis, infarction, ischemia, thrombosis, and angiodysplasia of the colon. Paralytic ileus and intestinal obstructions without hernia are coded as K56 which includes the bowel, colon and intestine. These codes include intussusception, volvulus, gallstones in the ileus, fecal impaction, and intestinal adhesions. Intussusception occurs when one section of the intestine collapses within another section. A volvulus is when the intestine twists upon itself.

Diverticular disease of intestines (K57) include diverticulitis and diverticular disease but diverticulum alone was previously coded in other sections. These codes are differentiated with the fourth digit as to location and with or without perforation and abscess. The fifth digit indicates with or without bleeding.

Irritable bowel syndrome is coded as K58 with or without diarrhea.

Other intestinal disorders and diseases (K59-K63) include constipation, diarrhea, neurogenic bowel, anal spasm, megacolon, fissures, fistulas, abscess, polyp, stenosis, hemorrhage, ulcer and proctitis due to radiation. Anal fissures are cuts or tears in the tissue of the anus and anal fistulas are abnormal connections between the anus or rectum and the skin.

Hemorrhoids (K64) are dilated, swollen, painful veins in the anus or rectum. These can be complicated by thrombosis, bleeding, strangulation, ulceration, and prolapse (falling down or slipping out of place). They are classified by grades/stages from I to IV based on various factors such as bleeding, prolapse, and manual replacement. There are also hemorrhoidal skin tags and perianal venous thrombosis coded in this section.

Section 19.8: DISEASES OF PERITONEUM AND RETROPERITONEUM

Peritonitis (K65) is inflammation of the peritoneum. There are many excludes to these codes such as for various infections, foreign substances and neonatal. If peritonitis is coded from K65 then the infectious agent should also be coded, as would be with any infection. These peritonitis codes include generalize, spontaneous bacterial, abscess, sclerosing mesenteritis, and others.

Other disorders of the peritoneum (K66-K67) include for diseases classified elsewhere, adhesions and hemoperitoneum (traumatic coded as S36.8 instead).

Disorders of retroperitoneum (K68) include abscess including postprocedural.

Section 19.9: LIVER DISEASES

Diseases of the liver (K70-K77) are differentiated by cause such as alcohol or toxic substance. Fifth digits refer to the presence of various conditions such as ascites, sclerosis, fibrosis, hepatitis, cirrhosis, failure, cholestasis, and necrosis across the various causes.

Hepatitis can be persistent, lobular, active or other. Necrosis is death of the liver. Liver failure is differentiated as to with or without coma and as either acute, subacute or chronic.

Chronic liver disease leads to damage to the liver with cirrhosis and hepatitis. Cirrhosis is the destruction of liver cells and replacement of normal liver tissue with fatty tissue and can be caused by alcohol, malnutrition, or other conditions.

Other diseases that involve the liver (K76-K77) include fatty liver, congestion, hemorrhagic necrosis, infarction, occlusive disease, hepatorenal syndrome, and in diseases classified elsewhere.

Section 19.10: DISORDERS OF GALLBLADDER, BILIARY TRACT & PANCREAS

Cholecystitis and cholelithiasis are coded as K80 and now specify presence of cholangitis, e.g. calculus of bile duct with cholangitis (K80.3). Cholelithiasis (K80) is formation of calculus in the gallbladder and/or bile ducts, more commonly known as stones. These codes are differentiated as to whether acute or chronic cholecystitis is present or not. Cholecystitis is inflammation of the gallbladder and/or bile ducts and can be coded singly as K81.

Choledocholithiasis (K80.6) is obstruction of the common bile duct by calculus. Calculus of the bile ducts with cholangitis is coded as K80.3 and is differentiated as to being with or without obstruction and acute or chronic.

Other disease of the gallbladder (K82) include obstruction, hydrops, perforation, fistula, and cholesterolosis. Other diseases of the biliary tract (K83) include cholangitis, obstruction, perforation, fistula, cyst and spasm of sphincter of Oddi (SOD).

Acute pancreatitis and other diseases of the pancreas (K85-K86) can be idiopathic, biliary, alcohol or drug induced. Other diseases of the pancreas include alcohol-induced chronic pancreatitis or other cause, cyst, pseudocyst, and other such as necrosis and cirrhosis.

Section 19.11: OTHER DISEASES OF DIGESTIVE SYSTEM

Oftentimes, a person may be ingesting sufficient food but the body is not able to process the food which is known as malabsorption. Other diseases of the digestive system (K90-K95) include various diseases that affect the digestive process such as celiac disease, tropical sprue, blind loop syndrome, steatorrhea, malabsorption due to intolerance, and Whipple's disease. Celiac disease occurs when the stomach is coated by the gluten from grain products which then prevents the stomach from absorbing and distributing the food that is processed in the stomach. Steatorrhea occurs when there is the presence of excess fats in the stool due to the processing and malabsorption of fats.

GI hemorrhaging includes hematemesis (K92.0) which is spitting up blood and melena/hematochezia (K92.1) which is black tarry stools due to the presence of digested blood. Hematochezia is bright red blood in the stools. Vomiting blood and spitting blood are not the same diagnosis. Spitting blood is known as hemoptysis (R04.2).

Other diseases include ulcerative gastrointestinal mucositis (K92.8) with the need to code also if therapy such as for cancer was administered (T45.1X).

Section 19.12: INTRAOPERATIVE AND POSTPROCEDURAL

Complications and disorders associated with the digestive system due to medical procedures (intraoperative and postprocedural) (K91) include vomiting, dumping syndrome, postgastrectomy syndrome, malabsorption, obstruction, postcholecystectomy syndrome, hemorrhages, hematoma, puncture, laceration, hepatic failure, and pouchitis.

Complications from an artificial opening (K94), such as a stomy, include infections, hemorrhage, malfunction, and mechanical problems. Stomies for the digestive system include colostomy, enterostomy, gastrostomy, and esophagostomy. Complications from bariatric procedures (K95) such as gastric band procedures include infection or other complication. If the organism causing the infection is known it must also be coded.

DIGESTIVE QUIZ 12

1. What is the code for a patient diagnosed with a peptic ulcer?
2. What are the codes for a patient with a perforated appendix with an abscess?
3. What are the codes for a patient with Crohn's disease?
4. What are the codes for a patient with gastritis and duodenitis?
5. What is the code for GERD?
6. What are the codes for a patient with hemorrhagic alcoholic gastritis?
7. What are the codes for a patient with dysentery and gastritis due to Salmonella?
8. What are the codes for a patient with Crohn's disease of large and small intestines?
9. What are the codes for a patient with acute cholecystitis with bile duct calculus and obstruction?
10. What are the codes for a patient with volvulus with hernia of the intestine with gangrene?
11. What are the codes for a patient with postoperative hernia?
12. What are the codes for a patient with acute gastric ulcer?
13. What are the codes for a patient with gastritis due to alcoholism?
14. What are the codes for a patient with retropharyngeal abscess?
15. What are the codes for a patient with incarcerated inguinal hernia?

CHAPTER 20
ICD-10 INTEGUMENTARY SYSTEM

You will learn the following objectives in this chapter:

A. Integumentary System
B. Infections of the Skin
C. Dermatitis and Eczema
D. Urticaria and Erythema
E. Radiation
F. Disorders of Appendages
G. Other Disorders

Chapter 12 is described as "Diseases of the Skin and Subcutaneous Tissue" and ranges from L00-L99. Many conditions have been removed to other chapters so many changes have been made to this chapter as well as expansions of many codes. Greater specificity has also been added to many codes including a new section (block) for radiation-related disorders of the skin and subcutaneous tissue. There are also some terminology changes.

Section 20.1: INTEGUMENTARY SYSTEM

Integumentary is the skin and its accessory organs which include hair, nails and glands. It is the largest organ of the body. The purpose of the integumentary system is to provide protection, thermoregulation, sensation, and allows secretion. It also prevents the loss of water, salts, and other nutrients.

The first layer of the skin is known as the epidermis and is composed only of squamous epithelium cells. The dermis lies below the epidermis and is composed of blood and lymph vessels, nerve fibers, hair follicles, sweat glands, and the sebaceous glands which are connected through connective tissue. The subcutaneous layer is a layer of connective tissue and also aids in the formation and storage of fat in cells known as lipocytes.

Erythema is reddening of the skin. Ecchymosis is a bluish-black discoloration of the skin, such as a bruise, which occurs due to the loss of blood from its vessels. Petechiae are the same as ecchymosis but smaller. Purpura is when ecchymoses and petechiae grow larger and merge. Vitiligo is loss of pigment (melanin).

Skin neoplasms can be benign or malignant as previously discussed. Benign skin neoplasms include calluses, keloids, nevus, and verruca. A scar is also known as a cicatrix. Verruca are also known as warts and are caused by the human papillomavirus (HPV).

Section 20.2: INFECTIONS OF SKIN AND SUBCUTANEOUS TISSUE

Infections of skin and subcutaneous tissue section (L00-L08) begins with Staphylococcal scalded skin syndrome (L00). Percentage of skin exfoliated should be coded additionally (L49). It is also known as Ritter's disease and staphylococcal epidermal necrolysis. It involves blistering of the skin which results in exfoliation which can vary from a few blisters to affecting the entire body.

Erysipelas is a superficial infection of the skin which is coded as A46 in another section. Impetigo (L01) is a bacterial infection of the skin as evidenced by the presence of pustules and lesions.

Abscesses, furuncles, and carbuncles (L02) are painful bumps formed under the skin. A furuncle (boil) is an infection of the hair follicles. A carbuncle is a composite of several furuncles and is an abscess with pus that is larger and most often due to a bacterial infection. While many anatomic sites are included in this section, there are many exclusions because they are coded in other sections specific to the anatomic site, such as the ear, mouth and nose.

If the organism causing the infection is known it should also be coded. In this section, the anatomic sites coded include face, neck, trunk, buttock, limb, hand, foot, and other sites not listed elsewhere.

An infection of the skin is known as cellulitis (L03) which extends into the subcutaneous tissues and can lead to further sepsis if not treated properly. Lymphangitis (inflammation of the lymph system) is also included in this section. There are many exclusions in this section based on anatomic site such as breast.

Lymphadenitis (L04) is inflammation of the lymph nodes except mesenteric. This is differentiated by anatomic site such as face, head, neck, trunk, and limbs.

Lesions are damaged tissue. There are many types of lesions depending on their appearance and condition. A macule is a discolored flat lesion. This includes freckles and moles. A prominence above the skin would include cyst, polyp, pustule, vesicle, nodule, papule, and wheal.

Pilonidal cysts (L05) are cysts in the buttock area and coded with or without abscess and including sinus or not. Other local infections (L08) include pyoderma.

Bullous disorders (L10-L14) include Pemphigus (L10) which is a chronic autoimmune disease in which blisters appear. There are several types of pemphigus which includes vulgaris, vegetans, follaceous, Brazilian and drug-induced. Pemphigoid (L12) resembles pemphigus in that there are large blisters too. It can be caused by drugs or can be bullous or cicatrical. Other bullous disorders include dermatitis herpetiformis.

Section 20.3: DERMATITIS AND ECZEMA

Dermititis and eczema are terms used interchangeably and are coded as L20-L30. Again, sometimes these conditions are coded in other sections based on anatomic site.

There are many types of dermatitis and it can be due to many things, including contact dermatitis (L23-L27) which includes exposure to various agents such as metals, adhesives, cosmetics, dyes, cement, insecticide, plastic, rubber, and animal dander. Contact dermatitis can also be described as being due to irritants such as detergents, drugs, and solvents which may also be taken internally.

Pruritus (L29) is itching. Eczemas coded as other specified dermatitis (L30) and is inflammation of the skin and may be accompanied by pruritus and formation of lesions.

Papulosquamous disorders (L40-L45) include psoriasis (L40) which is a skin condition characterized by itchy reddened scales. It also includes lichen planus which is an itchy rash on the skin. Psoriasis (L40.5) is an autoimmune disease that appears as red scaly patches on the skin, fingernails, and toenails. The most common type is plaque psoriasis. Psoriasis has been expanded to include manifestations, e.g. psoriatic arthritis mutilans (L40.52).

Section 20.4: URTICARIA AND ERYTHEMA

Urticaria and erythema are coded as L49-L54. Included in this section are codes for exfoliation which can result from erythema and which requires that the condition causing the exfoliation be coded first such as Stevens-Johnson Syndrome. These codes are based on percentage of body affected. Exfoliation (L49) is oftentimes coded with the etiological condition.

Urticaria (L50) is red wheals on the skin due to allergic reactions and are also known as hives. Urticaria can be allergic, idiopathic, dermatographic, vibratory, cholinergic or contact related.

Erythema (L51-L53) is classified as toxic, multiforme, nodosum, rosacea, and lupus. Additional codes should be coded for manifestations such as arthropathy, edema, ulcers, and stomatitis. Toxic erythema is a common rash caused by poisonings, so the drug or toxin should be listed if known. Erythema multiforme can be a minor or major red rash. The most severe form is known as Stevens-Johnson syndrome. Erythema nodosum is an inflammation of the fat cells under the skin (panniculitis).

Section 20.5: RADIATION

Radiation-related disorders (L55-L59) include sunburns (L55) with fourth characters classifying if the burn was first, second, or third degree.

Other radiation-related skin disorders include drug response, solar urticarial, chronic exposure to nonionizing radiation, actinic keratosis (pre-malignant condition of thick scaly skin patches), and radiodermatitis. The source of radiation should also be coded (W89).

Section 20.6: DISORDERS OF THE APPENDAGES

Disorders of the appendages (L60-L75) includes nails. This includes ingrown toenails (L60).

Various types of hair loss are coded in this section including alopecia which is the loss of hair from areas where hair should be, such as the top of the head. It can be due to hereditary conditions, medications, toxins, or trauma. There is a code for male-pattern baldness (androgenic, L64). Hair coloring and hair shaft abnormalities include premature greying. Hypertrichosis includes hirsutism which is excessive hair growth where there normally would not be.

Acne (L70) forms from the buildup of sebum and keratin from the skin in the pores which causes a blockage. It is also known as acne vulgaris. Partial blockage is known as a comedone (blackhead) and complete blockage is known as a whitehead because there is also the collection of the pus. Seborrhea is a scaly, flaky itchy, red skin disorder affecting the scalp, face, and trunk, known as dandruff on the scalp but it is coded as L21.0 and is not in this section.

Rosacea (L71) is facial erythema with inflammation.

Follicular disorders include cysts including a sebaceous cyst (L72.3), acne keloid and eccrine or apocrine sweat disorders. Anhidrosis (L74.4) is the inability of the body to sweat. If a person sweats too much this is known as hyperhidrosis (L74.5).

Intraoperative and postoperative complications are coded as L76 and include hemorrhage, hematoma, puncture, and laceration.

Section 20.7: OTHER DISORDERS

Other disorders (L80-L99) include vitiligo which involves depigmentation of parts of the skin. Other disorders of pigmentation include freckles, café au lait spots, cholasma, and tattoo pigmentation.

Seborrheic keratosis can be either inflamed or other. Corns and callouses are coded as L84. Epidermal thickening (L85) includes ichthyosis and xerosis cutis or dry skin dermatitis.

A break in the skin can occur from a fissure, erosion, or ulcer. Pressure ulcers, which include decubitus ulcers, are coded as L89 and include many sites. Non-pressure ulcers are coded as L97. Decubitus ulcers, commonly known as bedsores, occur when there is continuous pressure on a portion of a skin in the buttock area which results in a breakdown of the skin. Ulcer codes have been expanded significantly with fourth characters indicating the specific site and fifth characters specifying the breakdown of the skin (fat layer exposed, necrosis, and unspecified). The sixth character indicates the stage of the progression of the disease of the ulcer from Stage 1 to Stage 4 which involves necrosis.

INTEGUMENTARY QUIZ 13

1) What are the codes for a patient with severe dermatitis due to her use of pierced earrings?
2) What are the codes for a patient with infected corn on the right big toe with cellulitis with possible sepsis and COPD with diabetes?
3) What are the codes for a 2-month-old baby who presents with a diaper rash?
4) What are the codes for a patient with nonbullous erythema multiforme?
5) What are the codes for a patient with second degree sunburn?
6) What are the codes for a patient with exfoliation on 34% of their body due to erythema multiforme with arthropathy?
7) What are the codes for a patient with pilonidal cyst with abscess?
8) What are the codes for a patient with cheloid scar after an appendectomy?
9) What are the codes for a patient with impetiginous dermatitis?
10) What are the codes for a patient with impetigo simplex?
11) What are the codes for a patient with albinism?
12) What are the codes for a patient with winter's itch?
13) What are the codes for a patient with dermatitis due to allergy to dust?
14) What are the codes for a patient with a stage 2 ulcer that developed from a cast that was applied to their right lower leg for 3 months due to a fracture?
15) What are the codes for a patient with chronic lymphangitis due to staph?

CHAPTER 21
ICD-10 MUSCULOSKELETAL SYSTEM

You will learn the following objectives in this chapter:

A. Musculoskeletal Anatomy
    1. Bones
    2. Muscles
    3. Joints
B. Arthropathies
    1. Pyogenic Arthritis
    2. Crystal Arthropathies
    3. Rheumatoid Arthritis
    4. Juvenile Rheumatoid Arthritis
    5. Osteoarthritis
    6. Other Arthritis
    7. Derangement
    8. Rheumatism
C. Dentofacial
D. Connective Tissue Disorders
E. Dorsopathies
F. Spondylopathies
G. Soft Tissue Disorders
H. Disorders of Synovium and Tendon
I. Osteopathies and Chondropathies
J. Procedural Complications
K. Biomechanical Lesions

Chapter 13 is described as “Diseases of the Musculoskeletal System and Connective Tissue” and ranges from M00-M99. There are many changes, deletions, expansions, and moves within this chapter with almost every code having been changed in some way including designation of laterality.

Section 21.1: MUSCULOSKELETAL ANATOMY

The musculoskeletal system includes the bones, muscles, and joints. Connective tissue includes bones, cartilage, and fibrous tissue. It also includes blood and fat. Bones are organs and are the framework for the body that gives it support, protects the internal organs, and assist in movement.

The middle part of the bone (not to be confused with the inside of the bone) is known as the shaft and is called the diaphysis. The ends of the bone are known as the epiphysis. There is an epiphyseal plate in the bone where the growth occurs which is of importance in the growth of children. The bone is covered by the periosteum.

Cranial bones are the bones of the skull (cranium) and protect the brain. The frontal bone is at the front of the head. Parietal bones (two) are on each side of the skull. Temporal bones (two) are on the lower sides and base of the skull. Occipital bone is at the back and base of the skull. Sphenoid bone is located behind the eyes. Ethmoid bone is behind the nose.

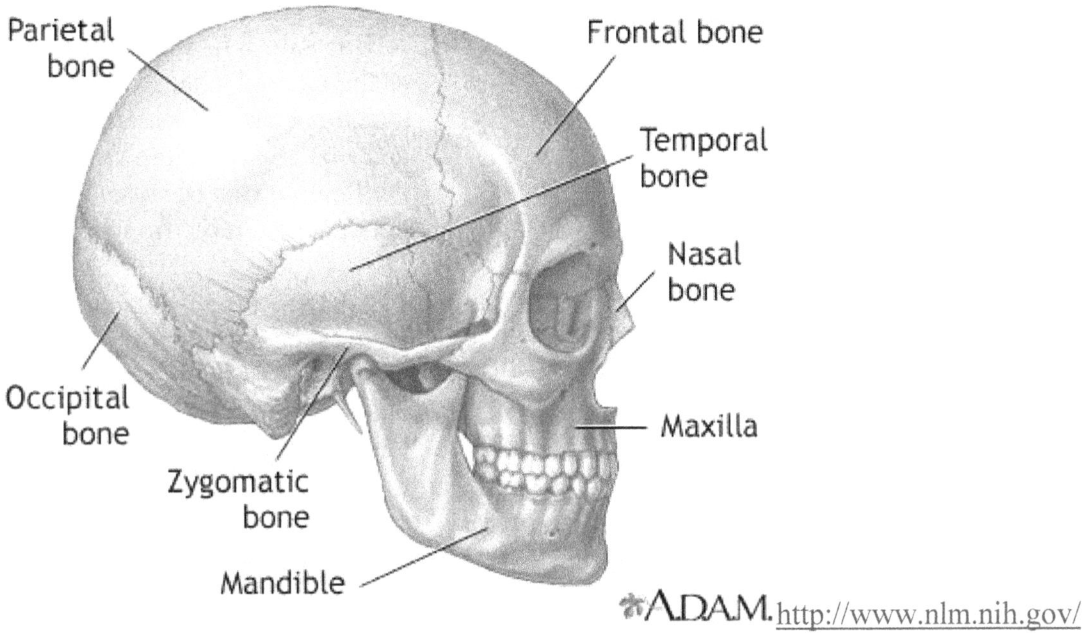

http://www.nlm.nih.gov/

FACIAL: Facial bones include two nasal bones, two lacrimal bones (corner of each eye), two zygomatics (cheeks), vomer (lower part of the nose), two maxillary (upper jaw), and the mandible (lower jaw). The sinuses are located within these areas including the frontal, ethmoidal, sphenoidal, and maxillary sinuses.

SPINE: The bones protecting the spinal cord are known as the spinal column or vertebrae. The vertebrae are separated by cartilage known as intervertebral disks. The spine is divided into five divisions: 7 cervical vertebrae (neck, C1-C7), 12 thoracic (chest & ribs, T1-T12), 5 lumbar (lower back, L1-L5), 1 sacrum, and 1 coccyx (tailbone).

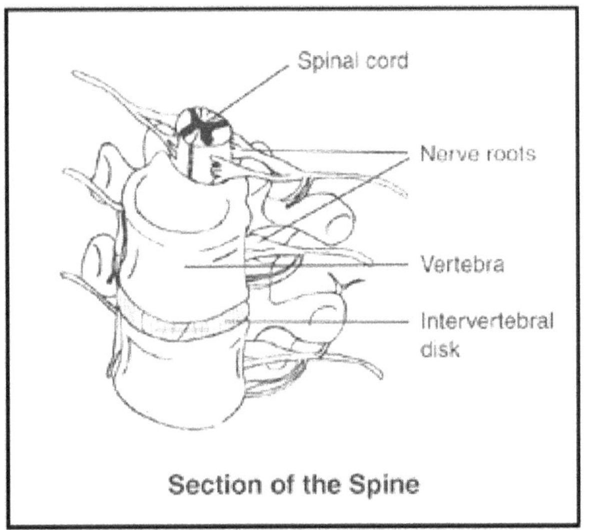

Section of the Spine

The posterior part of the vertebrae is composed of the vertebral arch, spinous process, 2 transverse processes, and 2 laminae.

Nih.gov

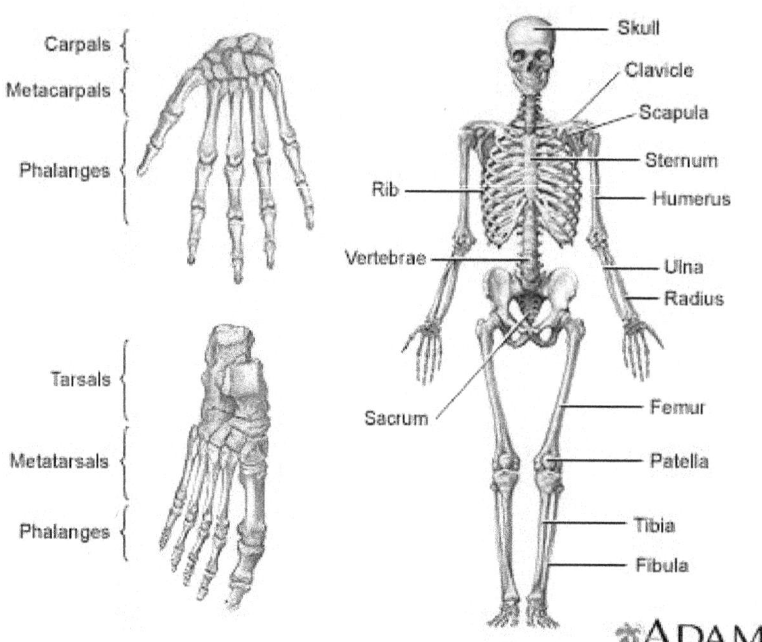

TRUNK: Bones of the trunk include the clavicle (collar bone), scapula (shoulder blade), sternum (breastbone), and ribs (12 pairs).

RIBS: Ribs 8 to 10 are known as the false ribs because they attach posteriorly with the 7th rib and ribs 11 and 12 are known as the floating ribs because they are not attached in the front.

PELVIS: Bones of the pelvis include the pelvic girdle (composed of the ilium, pubis, and ischium).
Nih.gov

EXTREMITIES: The bones of the arms include the humerus (upper), ulna (medial lower which includes the olecranon which is better known as the elbow), radius (lateral lower in line with the thumb), carpals (wrist bones), metacarpals (palm), and phalanges (fingers). The phalanges have three segments, proximal, middle, and distal. The proximal are closest to the palm. For the phalanges, PIP are proximal interphalangeal joints between the first (also called proximal) and second (intermediate) phalanges. DIP are distal interphalangeal joints between the second and third (distal) phalanges.

The bones of the legs include the femur (thigh bone), patella (knee cap), tibia (largest of lower leg bones on the inside), fibula (smallest of lower leg bones on the outside), tarsals (back of foot composed of the calcaneus, heel bone and talus), metatarsals (midfoot), and phalanges (toes).

The femur is the longest bone in the body and its acetabulum fits into the socket of the pelvic girdle.

MUSCLES: Muscles are responsible for movement which consists of contractions and relaxation. There are over 600 muscles. They can be attached to bones, organs, and blood vessels.

There are three types of muscles: striated, smooth, and cardiac. Striated muscles are voluntary (skeletal) muscles. They move the bones and are consciously controlled. Smooth muscles are involuntary (visceral) muscles. They move the internal organs and are controlled by the autonomic nervous system. Cardiac muscles are the muscles of the heart.

A muscle can extend or flex. Flexion is a muscle movement in which the angle between the bones is decreased (bending). Extension is a muscle movement in which the angle between the bones is increased (straightening out). Dorsiflexion is the decreasing of the angle of the ankle joint. Plantar flexion is the increasing of the angle of the ankle joint (pointing of toes).

A muscle can move away from the midline of the body (abduction) or move towards the midline of the body (adduction).

Rotation is circular turning. Supination if the turning of the palm up and pronation is the turning of the palm down.

JOINTS: Joints are the attachment point where bones come together which is known as articulation. The ends of the bones are covered with the articular cartilage so that the bones do not come directly together, otherwise this would be very painful to have bones rubbing on each other. The articular cartilage provides a cushion for the joint to move painlessly and smoothly.

Joints can be movable or immovable. Joints that are immovable include the suture joints of the skull. Joints that are very movable are known as synovial joints which include the ball-and-socket and hinge type. Movable joints include the knee and spine. Synovial joints are surrounded by fibrous tissues known as the joint capsule. The synovial fluid and membrane within it constitute the bursa (bursae).

LIGAMENTS: Ligaments (connective tissue) anchor the bones together. While ligaments connect bones together, tendons connect muscles to bones.

Rheumatism include disorders of the muscles and tendons and their attachments. Enthesopathies are disorders of the peripheral ligamentous or muscular attachments.

Section 21.2: ARTHOPATHIES

Arthropathies (M00-M25) include many types of arthropathies and arthritis. Arthritis is inflammation of the joints which can lead to joint pain, stiffness, and swelling to the point that it becomes difficult to do anything. Arthropathies/arthritis codes specify manifestations, sites, and laterality with the fourth, fifth and sixth characters.

Infectious arthropathies are coded as M00-M02. Infectious arthropathies can be either direct or indirect infections. Indirect infections can be either reactive or postinfective. Reactive arthropathies is when there was infection by an organism but it could not be identified.

Pyogenic (producing pus)/septic arthritis (M00) is caused by an infection such as staph, pneuomococcal or strep. If arthritis develops from an infection, then the codes for organism should also be coded.

Postinfective and reactive arthropathies are coded as M02 with a note to code first the underlying disease such as hepatitis. These arthropathies can occur after intestinal bypass, dysentery, immunization, and Reiter's disease.

Inflammatory polyarthropathies (M05-M14) include rheumatoid arthritis (RA). This is a chronic debilitating autoimmune disease of the joints. Scarring can occur on the bones which then can lead to ankylosis (stiffness of a joint that may result in bones fusing together, making movement difficult and painful) so that movement becomes painful and highly limited. Manifestations, such as myopathy or polyneuropathy, should be coded additionally as indicated in the codes. Notice that rheumatoid arthritis of the spine and rheumatic fever should be coded with codes from other sections as indicated in the codes.

Juvenile rheumatoid arthritis (JRA) (M08) begins before a person is 16 years old. The codes are distinguished as polyarticular, pauciarticular and monoartiuclar. Oligoarticular (pauciarticular) JRA affect four or fewer joints. Polyarticular JRA affects five or more joints. Monoarticular JRA affects one joint.

Crystal arthropathies (M1A) result from an accumulation of crystals in the joints. The accumulation of crystals in joints can be caused by gout which is caused by deposition of uric acid crystals in the joint, causing inflammation and is now included in these codes for arthropathies. High uric acid levels are related to gout. Gout conditions can be idiopathic (origin unknown), drug-induced, lead-induced, with renal impairment, as well as being secondary to other conditions such as myeloma and anemia. Other crystal arthropathies include hydroxyapatite deposition disease and familial chondrocalcinosis.

Other types of arthropathies include Felty's syndrome, lung disease, vasculitis, heart disease, myopathy, polyneuropathy, bursitis, nodules, enteropathies (digestive system disorders), and involvement of various organs, with or without organ involvement, Kaschin-Beck disease, villonodular synovitis, palindromic, transient, allergic, traumatic, and in other diseases such as Charcot's joint. .

Many of these codes have six characters. There is a seventh character for some of the codes such as M1A which is based on whether there is tophus or not present. Some of the codes require additional codes for other conditions present such as calculus and cardiomyopathy.

Gout has been expanded significantly (M1A) and has an unusual combination of letters and numbers for codes. It is differentiated by cause, laterality, etiology, anatomic site, and acute or chronic.

OSTEOARTHRITIS: Osteoarthritis (M15-M19) is inflammation of the bones and joints with erosion of cartilage and is also known as degenerative joint disease. This results in bone rubbing on bone. The most common form of arthritis, osteoarthritis (degenerative joint disease), is a result of trauma or other similar condition to the joint, infection of the joint, or age. Osteoarthritis is further specified by fourth characters for type (e.g. polyosteoarthritis) and fifth characters for laterality.

Polyosteoarthritis occurs in multiple sites. Post-traumatic osteoarthritis occurs after trauma (M19.1). Primary osteoarthritis is a chronic degenerative disorder related to but not caused by aging. Secondary osteoarthritis is caused by another condition, such as an infection or trauma. Localized osteoarthritis affects only the one site where it is located, while generalized affects multiple sites.

Section 21.3: OTHER JOINT DISORDERS

Other joint disorders (M20-M25) include acquired deformities although some deformities are coded in other sections as noted in the exclude note.

Deformities of fingers include mallet finger, Boutonniere, and Swan-neck.

Deformities of the feet include hallux valgus, otherwise known as a bunion. A bunion is a deformity of the bones and the joint between the foot and big toe caused by a swollen bursae and/or a bone deformity on the joint known as the medial eminence. Hallux valgus is when the big toe points away from the rest of the toes and is also commonly called a bunion. Hallux rigidus is a deformity of the great toe that causes pain upon flexion which limits motion.

Hammer toe is a deformity of the proximal interphalangeal joint of the second, third, or fourth toe causing it to be permanently bent. Claw toe is when a toe is contracted at the PIP and DIP joints (middle and end joints in the toe) which can lead to severe pressure and pain.

There are also wrist and foot drop and flat foot. If a person is flat-footed, that is coded as talipes planus

Similar deformities can occur in other anatomic sites, such as valgus and varus of the forearm (wrist, elbow, hand, etc.). Club hand is when the axis of the wrist is permanently deviated and the hand is usually closed.

Unequal limb lengths are specified by anatomic site of the arms and legs and by laterality.

Conditions of the patella are highly differentiated including dislocation, subluxation (partial dislocation), involving the femur, derangements, involving chondromalacia (softening of cartilage).

Internal derangement of the knee refers to disorders involving disruption of the normal functioning of the ligaments or cartilages (menisci) of the knee joint. Derangement of the knee (M23) includes degeneration, loose bodies in the traumatized area, softening, tear, or rupture of cartilage or meniscus of the knee, including an old bucket tear.

There are various disorders of the ligaments including spontaneous disruption, instability, and laxity. Dislocation of joints due to other diseases (pathological) is coded as M24.3 and differentiated by anatomic site and laterality. Dislocation of joints can also be recurrent. Other conditions of the joins include contracture, ankylosis (stiffness and immobility of joint with possible bone fusion), hemarthrosis (bleeding into joint space), fistula, flail (loss of function of joint due to destabilization), effusion, pain, stiffness, and osteophyte (bone spurs).

Section 21.4: DENTOFACIAL

Dentofacial anomalies (M26-M27) include various anomalies associated with teeth and the jaw such as malocclusion of the maxillae or mandible, macrogenia, microgenia, excessive tuberosity, asymmetry, reverse articulation, abnormal jaw closure, deviation in opening and closing of mandible, insufficient guidance, arthralgia, articular disc disorder, and excessive horizontal overlap. Anomalies of the teeth include crowding, excessive spacing, displacement, rotation, and insufficient distance between teeth.

Other diseases of the jaws include Torus palatinus, Giant cell granuloma, Stafne's cyst, osteitis, periostitis, sequestrum, cysts, overfill, and osseointegration failure of dental implant. Periostitis (M27.2) is inflammation of the periosteum which is the connective tissue surrounding bone.

Section 21.5: CONNECTIVE TISSUE DISORDERS

Connective tissue (mainly composed of collagen) exists in many anatomic sites, so diseases related to them can be found in differing sections of the coding book. Systemic connective tissue disorders (M30-M36) include polyarteritis nodosa, juvenile polyarteritis, Kawasaki's syndrome, granuloma, polyangiitis, and systemic lupus erythematosus (SLE).

SLE is an autoimmune disease wherein the body's immune system turns against itself. Sclerosis is the building up of scar tissue on connective tissue. Scleroderma is systemic sclerosis. Other systemic disorders of connective tissue include Sicca, Sjogren, Behcet, and panniculitis. Additional complications need to also be coded as indicated in the notation under these codes, as well as etiology if known.

Section 21.6: DORSOPATHIES

Dorsopathies (M40-M54) are disorders of the back. This section has been greatly enhanced based on etiology, anatomic site, and type. Various curvatures of the spine include kyphosis (curving that causes bowing like with a hunchback), lordosis (inward curvature) and flatback syndrome. Scoliosis is the curvature of spine from side to side. It can be infantile or juvenile idiopathic, thoracogenic, neuromuscular, or secondary. Torticollis is wry neck which is when the head tilts toward one side, and the chin is elevated and turned toward the opposite side.

Osteochondroses are conditions that affect the growth of the skeleton in that it is a disease that includes both the bone and cartilage bone and is characterized by interruption of the blood supply to the bone.

Section 21.7: SPONDYLOPATHIES

Spondylolysis is osteoarthritis of the vertebrae. Spondylolisthesis involves displacement of the vertebrae so it is classified by section of the spine involved. Spondylopathies (M45-M49) include ankylosing spondylitis which occurs when there is stiffness with possible fusion of the vertebrae which includes rheumatoid arthritis of the spine. Inflammatory spondylopathies include enthesopathy (disorder of bone attachments), osteomyelitis, infection, and discitis which all involve the spine. Spondylosis with radiculopathy and myelopathy are coded as M47.0 - M47.2.

Other spondylopathies include spinal stenosis, ankylosing hypoerostosis, kissing spine (condition in which the spinous processes of adjacent vertebra are touching, also known as Baastrup's disease or syndrome), traumatic, collapsed, and fatigue fracture of vertebrae but not pathological fracture which is coded as M84. There is a seventh character for collapsed and fatigue fracture for the type of encounter such as initial, subsequent, and sequel.

Spondylopathies in other diseases (M49) include various curvatures of the spine (e.g. kyphosis and scoliosis) due to other disease such as brucellosis which should be coded first.

Other dorsopathies (M50-M54) include cervical disc disorders with various other conditions such as myelopathy, radiculopathy, disc displacement, disc degeneration, and spinal instabilities. Dorsalgia is back and neck pain including panniculitis (inflammation of tissue beneath the skin), radiculopathy, sciatica (pain that starts in the sciatica nerve and goes down the leg), lumbago (pain in the lumbar region), low back pain, and backache.

Section 21.8: SOFT TISSUE DISORDERS

Soft tissue disorders of the muscles (M60-M63) include myositis (inflammation of the muscles) which can be infective or interstitial. Foreign bodies can produce granulomas (M60.2).

Calcifications and ossification of the muscles can occur known as myositis ossificans and can be traumatic or progressive. Calcification and ossification can occur with quadriplegia or paraplegia (M61.2). It can also be associated with burns.

Other disorders of the muscles include separation, rupture, and ischemic infarction of muscle nontraumatically (M62). These codes also include contracture of muscle and muscle wasting and atrophy.

Other diseases can also cause disorders of the muscles such as leprosy or neoplasm and are coded with M63 with a code for the disease coded first.

Section 21.9: DISORDERS OF SYNOVIUM AND TENDON

Disorders of the synovium and tendon (M65-M67) include synovitis and tenosynovitis which can involve abscesses, other infection, calcific tendinitis, and trigger finger (M65.3) which is stenosing tenosynovitis. This occurs when the motion of the tendon that opens and closes the finger is limited which causes the finger to lock or catch as the finger is extended.

Spontaneous rupture of the synovium or flexor/extensor tendons as well as other tendons is coded as M66. Rupture of the Achilles' tendon is coded as M67.0.

Other abnormal conditions of the synovium and tendons include hypertrophy, transient, toxic, ganglions (swelling or tumor on joint or tendon), and Plica syndrome (irritation to synovial tissues of the knee).

Other soft tissue disorders (M70-M79) include crepitant synovitis, and various bursitis. Bursitis is inflammation of the bursae which are the fluid-filled sacs around the joints caused oftentimes by repeated irritation or injury to the same location. Other disorders include conditions due to overuse and pressure. Abscesses and infections of bursa are coded with M71 and the organism causing it should also be coded. Synovial cysts of the popliteal space in the knee is also known as Baker's (M71.20). Other conditions of the bursa include other cysts, calcium deposits and other bursopathies.

Fibroblastic disorders (M72) include Dupuytren's Syndrome, knuckle pads, necrotizing fasciitis, and fibromatosis. Plantar fasciitis is inflammation of the foot caused by excessive wear to the plantar fascia that supports the arches of the foot. Dupuytren's disease is fasciitis of the hand which causes the fingers to bend in towards the palm. Necrotizing fasciitis (flesh-eating bacterial disease) is a rare infection of the deeper layers of skin and subcutaneous tissues. The organism should also be coded as indicated in the codes.

There is a section specific to lesions of the shoulder (M75) which includes adhesive capsulitis, rotator cuff tear or rupture (either incomplete or complete), tendinitis (either bicipital or calcific), impingement, and bursitis. .

Enthesopathies (M76-M77) include tendinitis of various anatomic sites such as gluteal, psoas, and iliac as well as epicondylitis (medial or lateral), periarthritis, calcaneal spur, and metatarsalgia. Lateral epicondylitis is also known as tennis elbow and golfer's elbow is medial epicondylitis). An epicondyle is a prominence on the distal part of a long bone serving as the attachment for muscles and ligaments.

Other soft tissue disorders (M79) include unspecified rheumatism, myalgia, residual foreign body, hypertrophy of fat pad, pain, fibromyalgia, and nontraumatic compartment syndrome. neuralgia, neuritis, and panniculitis which is inflammation of subcutaneous adipose (fatty) tissue. Compartment syndrome that is nontraumatic is caused by repetitive and extensive muscle use. This results in increased pressure due most frequently to inflammation within a confined space of the body, such as the lower leg which then impairs blood flow. Compartment syndrome that is traumatic would be coded as T79 as indicated in the codes. A nontraumatic seroma is a collection of fluid in soft tissue and nontraumatic hematoma is a collection of blood in soft tissue.

Section 21.10: OSTEOPATHIES AND CHONDROPATHIES

Osteopathies and chondropathies (M80-M94) include disorders of bone density and structure (M80-M85).

OSTEOPATHIES: Osteoporosis is a disease condition in which the bone mineral density (BMD) is reduced which can result in a greater susceptibility to bone fractures. Various types of osteoporosis include pathological (disease-caused) fracture which requires additional coding of the related osseous defect if known. Osteoporosis can also be age-related, drug-induced, idiopathic, from disuse, post surgical and post traumatic. Age-related (senile) osteoporosis is due to old age. In idiopathic osteoporosis the cause is not known. In disuse osteoporosis the cause is the lack of exercise and movement to utilize the bones.

If there was a previous fracture which has healed, a personal history code should be listed (Z87.310).

Seventh characters are required which designate type of encounter as initial, subsequent or sequela which are:

- A Initial encounter for closed fracture
- D Subsequent encounter for fracture with routine healing
- G Subsequent encounter for fracture with delayed healing
- K Subsequent encounter for fracture with nonunion
- P Subsequent encounter for fracture with malunion
- Q sequela

Softening of the bones is known as osteomalacia (M83) which can occur as an adult including puerperal, senile, due to malabsorption, malnutrition, aluminum bone disease or drug induced.

Other disorders of bones include discontinuity such as stress fractures (M84) such as fatigue, March, and stress. Stress fractures are incomplete fracture in bones caused by unusual or repeated stress to the bone and can occur in various anatomic sites. The cause of the fracture should also be coded, if known.

Pathological fractures (M84.4) are fractures caused by a disease process and not from trauma. They can occur from a variety of conditions including chronic fatigue, neoplastic disease, and other diseases. The disease condition that caused the fracture should also be coded. All of these codes have seventh characters which are the same as previously discussed for osteoporosis.

Other disorders of bone density and structure include fibrous dysplasia, skeletal fibrosis, osteitis condensan, bone cysts, and acquired osteosclerosis.

Other osteopathies (M86-M90) include osteomyelitis (acute, subacute or various types of chronic) which is the inflammation and infection of the bone and/or bone marrow.

Osteonecrosis (M87) can be idiopathic aseptic, due to drugs, previous trauma, or secondary. It occurs when the bone does not get blood and dies.

Osteitis deformans (M88) include Paget's Disease which is a chronic disorder with excessive breakdown and formation of bone tissue that results in enlarged and deformed bones.

Other disorders of bones (M89) include algoneurodystrophy, physeal arrest (e.g. arrest of growth plate), hypertrophy, osteoarthropathy, and osteolysis. Osteolysis is breakdown (degeneration or dissolution) of bone.

Various diseases can cause osteopathies such as polio (M89.6) and rickets (M90.8) which require a code for the condition to also be listed.

CHONDROPATHIES: Chondropathies (M91-M94) are disease conditions of cartilage. This includes juvenile osteochrondrosis, nontraumatic slipped femoral epiphysis, osteochondritis dissecans, chondromalacia, and chondrolysis.

Other disorders of the musculoskeletal system and connective tissue (M95) include acquired deformities such as cauliflower ear.

Section 21.11: PROCEDURAL COMPLICATIONS AND DISORDERS

Intraoperative and postprocedural complications and disorders (M96) include pseudarthrosis after fusion or arthrodesis (fixation of joints), kyphosis, lordosis, scoliosis, postlaminectomy syndrome (continued numbness, tingling and muscle weakness), fracture of bone following insertion of implant, prosthesis or bone plate, hemorrhage, hematoma, puncture, and laceration.

Section 21.12: BIOMECHANICAL LESIONS

Biomechanical lesions (M99) include segmental and somatic dysfunction, subluxation, osseous or connective stenosis or lesions. These codes should not be used if the condition can be classified elsewhere.

MUSCULOSKELETAL QUIZ 14

1) What are the codes for a patient who has traumatic asphyxiation?
2) What are the codes for a patient who has pathological fracture of the vertebra due to osteoporosis?
3) What are the codes for a patient who has SLE with chronic nephritis?
4) What are the codes for a patient who has Achilles tenosynovitis?
5) What are the codes for a patient who has pyogenic arthritis of the hip due to staph?
6) What are the codes for a patient who has nonunion nondisplaced neck fracture of the left radius?
7) What are the codes for a patient who has degenerative joint disease of the knee?
8) What are the codes for a patient who has chronic obstructive asthma and neuropathy due to Type 2 diabetes which required treatment with insulin because it was uncontrolled?
9) What are the codes for a patient who has old bucket tear of the lateral meniscus of the right knee?
10) What are the codes for a patient who has a bone spur?
11) What are the codes for a patient who has acute osteomyelitis of the right ankle and foot?
12) What are the codes for a patient who has osteopathy due to typhoid fever?
13) What are the codes for a patient who has rheumatic polyarthritis with myopathy?
14) What are the codes for a patient who has carpal tunnel syndrome of the left arm?
15) What are the codes for a patient who has Sjogren’s disease?

CHAPTER 22
ICD-10 GENITOURINARY SYSTEM

You will learn the following objectives in this chapter:

A. Genitourinary Systems
B. Glomerular Diseases
    1. Nephritis
    2. Glomerulonephritis
C. Renal Failure Disease
D. Urolithiasis
E. Other Diseases of Urinary System
F. Diseases of Male Genital Organs
    1. Benign Prostatic Hypertrophy
    2. Other Diseases
G. Breast Disorders
H. Disease of Female Genital Organs
    1. Gynecologic Disorders

Chapter 14 is described as "Diseases of the Genitourinary System" and ranges from N00-N99.

Section 22.1: GENITOURINARY SYSTEMS

The urinary system is composed of the two kidneys, two ureters, the bladder, adrenals, and the urethra. The purpose of the urinary system is to produce, store, and eliminate urine. The kidneys are designated by the combining forms nephro and renal. The kidneys' main role is to filter waste products from the blood including urea which secretes rennin, a hormone involved in the control of blood pressure which is why hypertension and chronic kidney disease are always related. The glomerulus are contained within the kidneys and part of the filtration system of the kidneys. The ureters carry urine from the kidneys to the urinary bladder. The adrenals are positioned on top of the kidneys, but they are part of the endocrine system.

Testes are contained within the scrotum. The sperm is produced within the seminiferous tubules which are located within the testes. The perineum is located between the scrotum and the anus. The prostate gland lies where the vas deferens meets the urethra.

The female genital organs include the uterus and the ovaries which are located in the pelvis above the uterus and connected to the uterus through the fallopian tubes. The lower narrow portion of the uterus is the cervix. The vagina extends downward from the uterus to an orifice to the exterior of the body. The perineum is the area between the orifice and the anus. This is the area that may be cut (episiotomy) during delivery to prevent tearing.

Adnexa is sometimes used to refer to appendages of an organ which are anatomical parts attached to that organ. For example, the ovaries and oviducts are the adnexa uteri as they are considered part of the uterus since they are attached.

Section 22.2: GLOMERULAR DISEASES

Glomerular disease (N00-N08) does not include hypertensive kidney failure which is coded as N17-N19. It does include nephritic and nephrotic syndromes (N00-N05) which can be acute, rapidly progressive or recurrent/persistent. It can include various associated glomerulonephritis as described in the specific codes. Glomerulonephritis is inflammation of the glomeruli (small blood vessels in the kidneys). Proliferative indicates that there is an increased number of cells in the glomerulus and this usually leads to end-stage renal disease (ESRD) and failure (ESRF).

Nephrotic syndrome is a condition that results from another condition, such as diabetes, in which the kidneys are damaged, causing them to leak large amounts of protein from the blood into the urine. This condition is demonstrated by labs that indicate proteinuria, hyperlipidemia, edema, and hypoalbuminemia. These codes are also differentiated by the presence of lesions and proliferation.

Recurrent and persistent hematuria is coded as N02. Proteinuria is coded as N06 with various associated conditions such as glomerular lesions and glomerulonephritis. Hereditary nephropathy is coded as N07. Glomerular disorders can occur in diseases (N08) such as amyloidosis, congenital syphilis, gout, sepsis, and sickle cell.

Renal tubule-interstitial disease (N10-N16) include nephritis of these anatomic sites such as pyelonephritis which can be obstructive or not. Pyelonephritis (N10) (also known as pyelitis) is a suppurative infection of the kidney and can be coded as acute and/or chronic and with or without necrosis. It can be coded in various other sections as well depending upon complications and comorbidities.

Uropathy (N13) can also be obstructive such as calculus. This includes hydronephrosis and hydroureter. Strictures or kinking (N13.5) are narrowing of the urethra which may result in incontinence (involuntary leakage of urine) and are differentiated by cause, such as inflammation or scarring. Vesicoureteral reflux is the backflow of urine from the bladder into the ureter which is differentiated as being either unilateral or bilateral and with or without nephropathy.

Other diseases can result from drug and heavy metal exposure (N14) and other diseases (N16) such as brucellosis and leukemia.

Section 22.3: RENAL FAILURE/DISEASE

Renal failure is coded as N17 for acute and N18 for chronic. If the condition is hypertensive renal disease, then it is coded as I12.0 and if there is heart disease involved, then code I13 would be used.

While there is much emphasis on chronic renal failure, renal failure can be acute due to necrosis, lesions, toxins, shock, or injury although acute renal failure due to traumatic injury would be coded as T56.3X1A. The underlying condition should also be coded. Hyperkalemia can occur from this which is elevated potassium in the blood which can result in muscles weakness and cardiac arrest.

Chronic Kidney Disease (CKD) is a gradual progressive loss of renal function that results in end stage renal disease (ESRD). Hemodialysis or peritoneal dialysis are used to help control the effects of chronic kidney disease.

Chronic kidney diseases are classified by stages, ranging from I to V with an additional code for end-stage renal disease (ESRD) (N18.6) and unspecified stage (N18.9). Stage II is mild, Stage III is moderate, Stage IV is severe, and Stage V is the stage before ESRD. If a patient is described as having ESRD and CKD, then only the ESRD needs to be coded.

Be sure to check the notations for this code which include a reminder that hypertension must be coded as part of the code. In addition, there is a note that a code should be listed also to indicate if the patient had a kidney transplant. Another note also directs you to code also the manifestation such as neuropathy or pericarditis.

Section 22.4: UROLITHIASIS

There are new codes for urolithiasis (N20-N23) that specify the site of the calculus.

Calculi (N20) can also occur in the urinary tract organs with common occurrences in the renal pelvis or calyces of the kidneys and are known as nephrolithiasis. These codes are differentiated by anatomic site. If these calculi become placed so they obstruct the flow of urine, this is known as hydronephrosis (N13.1) which can lead to atrophy of the kidney. A calculus can become so large that its fills the pelvis of the kidney completely and blocks the flow of urine which is known as a staghorn calculus and has to be removed surgically. Calculi can also occur in diverticulum of the bladder (N21.0) or in other areas of the lower urinary tract.

Section 22.5: OTHER DISEASES OF URINARY SYSTEM

Other disorders of kidney and ureter (N25-N29) include renal osteodystrophy, diabetes insipidus, secondary hyperparathyroidism of renal origin, contracted kidney, small kidney, ischemia and infarction of kidney, and pyelitis cystica. Renal insufficiency (N28.9) is an early stage of renal impairment when the kidneys cannot function properly or adequately.

Other diseases of the urinary system (N30-N39) include cystitis which is inflammation of the urinary bladder and ureters, oftentimes due to a vaginal infection. Cystitis is classified as interstitial, chronic, trigonitis, or irradiation. Cystitis may also occur with the formation of cysts which is known as cystitis cystica.

There are a wide variety of conditions that can occur with the urinary bladder (N32), including fistulas, obstruction, atony (loss of muscle strength), overactivity, diverticulum, neurogenic (dysfunction in the micturition (voiding) due to diseases of the central nervous system or peripheral nerves) such as flaccid, reflex or uninhibited. If urinary incontinence is present, it should also be coded (N39.4).

Urethritis (N34) is inflammation of the urethra and can be with abscesses, nongonococcal or postmenopausal. Urethral strictures (N35) can be post-traumatic or postinfective. Other disorders of the urethra (N36) include fistulas, diverticulum, caruncle, functional and muscular disorders, false passage and involved in other disease.

Urinary tract infections not otherwise specified (NOS) are coded as N39.0. Additional codes should be listed to identify the infectious organism. Included in this section is stress incontinence which requires that any associated overactive bladder also be coded with N32 codes. Other incontinence includes urge incontinence, post-void dribbling, nocturnal enuresis, continuous leakage and mixed.

Section 22.6: DISEASES OF MALE GENITAL ORGANS

Diseases of male genital organs (N40-N53) include enlarged prostate (N40), better known as benign prostatic hyperplasia (BPH) as well as other similar conditions. BPH is the enlargement of the prostate in men, but this is a misnomer because the enlargement is due to hyperplasia rather than hypertrophy. These codes can include lower urinary tract syndrome and can be either nodular or enlarged. Associated symptoms should also be coded such as nocturia or straining on urination.

These codes do not include neoplasms of the prostate which are coded with neoplasm codes, such as C61.

Prostatitis (N41) is inflammation of the prostate which can be acute, chronic or with an abscess or cyst. If an organism is known to have caused the prostatitis, then the organism should be coded first. Other disorders of the prostate include calculus, congestion, hemorrhage, dysplasia, and cysts.

Hydrocele and spermatocele (N43) are accumulations of fluid in any cavity or duct. They can be encysted or infected. Noninflammatory disorders of testis (N44) include torsion (twisted) and cysts. Orchitis and epididymitis (N45) are inflammation of the testis or epididymis.

Male infertility (N46) includes azoospermia (lack of sperm), oligospermia (reduced number of sperm), or other causes such as drugs, infection, or obstruction.

Disorders of the prepuce (N47) include phimosis (tightness of the foreskin), deficient foreskin, cysts, adhesions, and inflammation.

Disorders of the penis (N48) include balanitis which is inflammation of the penis, leukoplakia, priapism (painful erection), ulcers, and induration. The underlying cause should be coded. Inflammatory disorders (N49) include Fournier gangrene, abscesses, boils, and cellulitis.

Male erectile dysfunction (N52) can be vasculogenic, drug-induced, post-surgical, or other. Other sexual dysfunctions include ejaculatory dysfunction (N53.1) such as retarded, painful and retrograde.

Section 22.7: BREASTS DISORDERS

This section is small but has conditions that apply to men and women. TheN60-N65 codes refer to dysplasias of the female mammaries. This includes cysts, fibroadenosis, and fibrosclerosis.

Other disorders include inflammatory disease, hypertrophy, galactorrhea (inappropriate discharge of milk), mastodynia (pain in the breasts), lumps (not cancerous), and ptosis (drooping of breasts). Hypertrophy of breasts (N62) include gynecomastia which is the development of breasts in men.

Section 22.8: GYNECOLOGIC DISORDERS

There are a wide variety of inflammatory diseases (N70-N77) of the various anatomic sites. Sometimes one code may contain several anatomic sites, such as salpingitis and oophoritis which are coded as N70 and can also include oophoritis. These codes can also be used for abscesses, pyosalpinx and tubo-ovarian inflammatory disease.

Inflammation of the uterus (N71) includes pyometra and endometritis. Cervicitis (N72) is inflammation of the cervix which can be acute and/or chronic. Vaginitis is inflammation of the vagina.

Other female pelvic inflammatory diseases (N73) include parametritis and pelvic cellulitis, peritonitis, and peritoneal adhesions. Peritoneal adhesions are internal scar tissue that forms after infection. If the adhesions are due to surgery then it should be coded as N99.4. This can result in infertility.

Pelvic inflammatory disease (PID) is coded as N73.9. PID in disorders in other diseases is coded as N74. Cysts, abscesses or other diseases of Bartholin's gland are coded as N75. Vaginitis, ulcers, and abscesses of the vagina and vulva are coded as N76.

Noninflammatory disorders (N80-N98) include endometriosis which occurs when endometrial tissue is located outside of the lining of the uterine cavity which can result in painful menstruation (dysmenorrhea). Codes are differentiated by anatomic sites.

Genital prolapse (N81) is the collapse of the uterus and/or vagina from its normal position so that it falls or sinks. It can be incomplete or complete. Prolapse codes are differentiated by the presence of a cele. A cystocele is a herniation in which the bladder enters into the vagina. Urethrocele is when the urethra prolapses into the vagina. Rectocele is a hernia in which there is a tear that allows the rectal tissue to bulge through this tear into the vagina. Cystoceles/cystourethroceles can be midline or lateral.

Fistulas (N82) are differentiated by anatomic sites. Other disorders include cysts (N83), atrophy, torsion of ovaries and fallopian tubes, hematomas, polyps (N84), endometrial hyperplasia (N85), hypertrophy, inversion, or malposition of the uterus. Cervical dysplasia (N87) is the abnormal growth of cells in the cervix which can be a precursory sign of cancer and can be mild or moderate.

Other noninflammatory disorders of the cervix (N88) include leukoplakia, old laceration, stricture, stenosis, incompetence and hypertrophic elongation of the cervix. Other noninflammatory disorders of the vagina (N89) include dysplasia (mild or moderate), dysplasia, leukoplakia, tight hymenal ring or hematocolpos. N90 codes are similar to N88 and N89 codes but are for the vulva and perineum. These also include codes for female genital mutilation, Type 1 to Type IV status.

Absent, scanty, or rare menstruation (N91) can be primary or secondary amenorrhea or oligomenorrhea. Excessive, frequent or irregular (N92) menstruation can occur at different times such as premenopausal or at puberty. Metrorrhagia is bleeding in between menstruation periods.

Dyspareunia (painful sexual intercourse) and primary or secondary dysmenorrhea are coded as N94. Dysmenorrhea is painful menstruation. Menopausal and climacteric states (N95) include flushing, sleeplessness, headache, and lack of concentration. The associated symptoms should also be coded.

If a woman has continued to have miscarriages from (three or more consecutive) pregnancies at approximately the same time, usually before 20 weeks of gestation, then this is known as an habitual aborter (N96); however, if she is pregnant, then O26 should be used as the code instead.

Infertility issues (N97) include the cause, such as lack of ovulation, endocrine complications, and anatomic site of problem. Complications associated with artificial fertilization (N98) include infection, hyperstimulation of ovaries, and various complications.

Intraoperative and postprocedural complications or genitourinary system (N99) include kidney failure, urethral stricture, adhesions, prolapse, complications of stoma of the urinary tract (hemorrhage, infection, and malfunction), hemorrhage, hematoma, accidental puncture or laceration, and others.

GENITOURINARY QUIZ 15

1. What are the codes for a patient with acute pyelonephritis due to E. coli?
2. What are the codes for a patient with oophoritis and salpingitis?
3. What are the codes for a patient with chronic uremia with acute pericarditis?
4. What are the codes for a patient with urinary incontinence and genital prolapse?
5. What are the codes for a patient with orchitis and epididymitis due to diphtheria?
6. What are the codes for a patient with menorrhagia?
7. What are the codes for a patient with post-hysterectomy vaginal prolapse?
8. What are the codes for a patient with acute cholecystitis with bile duct calculus with obstruction?
9. What are the codes for a patient with subacute nonsuppurative nephritis?
10. What are the codes for a patient with renal disease with membranous proliferative glomerulonephritis?
11. What are the codes for a patient with diverticulitis of the ileum with hemorrhage and peritonitis?
12. What are the codes for a patient with vesicoureteral reflux with bilateral reflux nephropathy?
13. What are the codes for a patient with ureteral calculus and renal calculus?
14. What are the codes for a patient with posttraumatic renal failure?
15. What are the codes for a patient with septic UTI due to E. coli?

CHAPTER 23
ICD-10 PREGNANCY

You will learn the following objectives in this chapter:

A. Pregnancy Definitions
    1. Gynecology/Obstetrics
    2. Fertilization
    3. Antepartum
    4. Delivery
B. Indentations
C. Coding Scenarios
    1. Unrelated Condition
    2. Related Condition as Combination Code
    3. Related Condition as Multiple Codes
D. Abortions
    1. Spontaneous
    2. Induced
    3. Ectopic Pregnancies
    4. Molar Pregnancies
E. High Risk Pregnancies
F. Eclampsia
G. Gestational
H. Other Disorders During Pregnancy
I. Multiple Gestations
J. Maternal Care for Other Complications
    1. Malpresentations
    2. Disproportions
K. Placental Conditions
L. Delivery
    1. Outcome of Birth
M. Complications
N. Postpartum
O. Infections
P. Other Conditions
Q. Sterilizations

Chapter 15 is described as "Pregnancy, Childbirth and the Puerperium" and ranges from O00-O9A. Be careful when using these codes because the use of the alphabetical O should not be confused with the number zero.

Section 23.1: GYNECOLOGY/OBSTETRICS

Gynecology is the study of female reproduction and obstetrics. Obstetrics is the study of pregnancy. Neonatology is the study of newborns and will not be covered in this packet because neonates have their own ICD-10 codes; only the mother should be coded from obstetric codes.

The gonads of the male and female produce gametes. The female gonads are the ovaries and the male gonads are the testes. The female gamete is the ovum and the male is the sperm.

When the ovum and a sperm cell unite, then fertilization has occurred and the fertilized ovum is known as an embryo. After two months, it is known as a fetus.

The embryo is fed through the placenta that grows in the wall of the uterus throughout the pregnancy. The unborn child grows within the amnion cavity, which is filled with fluid which is known as the sack of water. As you may remember from our discussion about blood, the mother's and baby's blood never mix.

The hormones, estrogen and progesterone, provide major control over the course of the pregnancy. The placenta also produces a hormone, human chorionic gondadotropin (HCG) whose presence indicates pregnancy.

A pregnancy is also known as gestation. It usually lasts 40 weeks (9 months). Dates are very important to know when coding pregnancy and delivery conditions.

Gravidity (G) refers to the number of pregnancies. Parity (P) refers to the number of viable pregnancies (approximately viable at 22 weeks). With these terms, a woman may be classified as G2 P1 Ab1 which means two pregnancies, one viable pregnancy, and one abortion.

Antepartum is the period preceding the delivery which is usually 40 weeks.

Delivery is the birth of the baby. The expulsion of the placenta is also known as the afterbirth. Delivery is also known as parturition.

Postpartum is also known as puerperium which refers to time beginning immediately after delivery and extending until six weeks following delivery. However, puerperium's true definition is the time required for the uterus to return to its normal size.

Section 23.2: INDENTATIONS

This is one of the most difficult sections to code from in the alphabetical index, similar to neoplasms, because there are so many categories, alternate terms, subterms, and indentations which make it extremely easy to select a wrong code from the wrong terms. As discussed in earlier packets, you must follow the alphabetical order of the sections, particularly since some alternate terms have very long sections within the pregnancy codes, such as "due to", "management affected by", "complicated by", etc. However, perhaps one of the greatest attributes of the ICD10 book is that it uses grey bars in the alphabetical index which indicate indentations so that it is much easier to know if a description is included under a section or if it is under a different section.

In addition, if you do not find a condition listed, it may still be listed in the pregnancy codes but under its own or alternate terms, so be sure to check all of these terms before you decide if the condition is not listed under the pregnancy codes. If you do find the condition under its own or alternate terms then use that code as it will cross-reference to any other descriptions. For example, vomiting in a pregnant patient is selected from the alphabetical index under the terms "complicated by" within the pregnancy codes.

Section 23.3: CODING SCENARIOS

When a patient is pregnant, for any condition a coder should begin searching under the terms pregnancy, delivery, or labor depending upon the stage of the pregnancy for that condition. There are several coding scenarios that can occur:

UNRELATED CONDITION: The first scenario for coding when a patient is pregnant is demonstrated in the fracture scenario. Since fracture is not listed under the term "pregnancy", then the fracture should be coded in addition to Z33.1 (incidental pregnancy).

RELATED CONDITION AS COMBINATION CODE: For the second scenario, as demonstrated in the UTI scenario, the coding becomes more complicated. If a condition is found under pregnancy, such as excessive vomiting, then the pregnancy code with the condition should be listed (O21). These codes include both the pregnancy and the condition and does not have any notations requiring the use of another code, so this one code includes both.

RELATED CONDITION AS MULTIPLE CODES: For the third scenario, if, and only if, there is a notation in the tabular index under the code that says another code must also be listed, such as another condition, then additional codes must be listed. For example superficial thrombophlebitis in pregnancy would be coded as O22.2 which requires the additional coding of the thrombophlebitis as I80.0.

Section 23.4: ABORTIONS

Abortion is defined as the termination of a pregnancy by the expulsion of the fetus. Abortions are natural (spontaneous) or induced (legally or illegally).

Ectopic pregnancy is when the embryo implants in a site other than the uterus. Most of these occur within the fallopian tubes and, therefore, are also known as tubal pregnancies. Other sites for ectopic pregnancies include the ovaries and other specified sites. Ectopic pregnancies are coded as O00 with a fourth character for the site.

Molar pregnancies (O02) are an abnormal growth in pregnancy in which a hydatidiform mole is formed from the fertilization of the egg and sperm but no viable fetus is formed due to a lack of the nucleus in the egg. They are also known as gestational trophoblastic disease (GTD).

Other types of abnormal conception products include blighted ovum, molar pregnancy, missed abortions and inappropriate change in HCG during pregnancy. Associated complications should be coded additionally with codes O08.

If complications occurs from these types of pregnancies or abortions, such as septic shock, sepsis, hemorrhage, damage to organs, renal failure, or embolism, then these should be coded from the O08.0 codes.

A missed abortion (O02.1) occurs when fetus dies before 20 weeks gestation in utero but this was not known and the fetus remained in the uterus. If this occurred after 22 weeks, then it is coded as O36.4. If the fetus remains in the uterus for more than 6 weeks it is known as dead fetus syndrome and it is included in the O02.1 and O36.4 codes.

Codes O03 are for the type of abortion, spontaneous, medical, or other. The fourth character indicates if the abortion was complete or incomplete and if there are any complications.

In a spontaneous abortions (O03) the codes are differentiated as to whether they are complete or incomplete and by associated complications and conditions such as genital tract or pelvic infection, hemorrhage, embolism, shock, renal failure, metabolic disorder, damage to pelvic organs, sepsis, and cardiac arrest. Incomplete means some products of the pregnancy are retained in the uterus after the abortion.

If a woman has continued to have miscarriages from (three or more consecutive) pregnancies at approximately the same time, usually before 20 weeks of gestation, then she should be coded as a habitual (recurrent) aborter (N96). However, if she is pregnant and it has not resulted in an abortion, then O26.2 should be used as the code instead. It is important to code this condition because it does present a high risk for the mother. In addition, a code for a history of abortions can be listed (O09.29).

An induced abortion can occur at any time including up until the birth of the baby as long as a portion of the baby remains within the mother. If an abortion fails, then it would be coded as O07. A therapeutic abortion is performed for reasons related to the health of the mother. An elective abortion occurs for other reasons. These codes are differentiated by associated complications and conditions such as infection, hemorrhage, embolism, shock, renal failure, metabolic disorder, damage to organs, cardiac arrest, and sepsis.

If an abortion is performed to reduce the number of fetuses, then it is coded as O31. There is also a code for Encounter for elective termination of pregnancy, Z33.2, which should also be coded when patient presents for an induced abortion. A failed attempted abortion would be coded as O07. Incomplete abortions are not considered failed and should not be coded with these codes. Codes O04 are used when there are complications from the abortion, e.g. termination of pregnancy complicated by embolism (O04.7). Complications following ectopic and molar pregnancies are coded as O08, e.g. shock following ectopic and molar pregnancy (O08.3).

Section 23.5: HIGH-RISK PREGNANCY

Supervision of high-risk pregnancies (O09) now require the specification of history in the fourth character and trimester in the fifth. History can include infertility, ectopic/molar pregnancy, poor past reproductive events, multiparity, elderly gravida, young gravida, and social problems.

Multiparity indicates that mother is or has had deliveries in the past in which more than one baby was born which definitely constitutes high risk. If the mother is expecting multiple births, then O09.4 should be listed in addition to any other pregnancy codes. However, if the mother had presented for delivery then O30 codes can be used to indicate the multiplicity. If a mother has a history of multiple births, then code Z64.1 can be coded as it provides important information about the possibility of future multiple births which are high-risk pregnancies.

If a pregnant woman is 35 years or older for her first pregnancy, then that would be coded as elderly primigravida (O09.51). If this is not her first pregnancy, then the code for elderly multigravida (O09.52) would be used. If a pregnant woman is less than 16 years of age, then it would be coded as O09.6-.

A mother may undergo fetal reduction (O31.3) to reduce the number of fetuses when there is a multiple birth, such as reduction in which one of twins may be terminated while the other twin remains viable.

Section 23.6: ECLAMPSIA

Conditions related to eclampsia are coded as O10-O16. Preeclampsia is pregnancy-induced hypertension and toxemia as indicated by high blood pressure, excessive protein in the urine (proteinuria), and edema. Eclampsia is characterized by tonic-clonic seizures in a patient who had pre-eclampsia. This is a very dangerous condition which is why these conditions are tested regularly during pregnancy.

Eclampsia is preceded by pre-eclampsia which is diagnosed by the presence of hypertension (with heart disease or kidney disease), proteinuria, and edema either alone or in combination (O10-O16) but not all three (which is coded as eclampsia.) Further specification for M10 includes a fourth character for nature of the hypertension, fifth character indicating if the hypertension is affecting the pregnancy, and a sixth character for the trimester involved, e.g. pre-existing hypertensive heart disease complicating pregnancy, second trimester (O10.112).

Section 23.7: GESTATIONAL

Conditions may arise during pregnancy that did not exist when the woman was not pregnant. This includes gestational (transient) high blood pressure (O13) and gestational diabetes (O24) which will disappear after the pregnancy is completed.

Section 23.8: OTHER DISORDERS DURING PREGNANCY

Other disorders that can occur during pregnancy include hemorrhage and vomiting. If vomiting occurs, the code is selected based on when the vomiting began and complications. If it began before the end of 20 weeks' gestation, then it is coded as mild hyperemesis gravidarum (O21.0). If it began before 20 weeks' gestation and involved dehydration, electrolyte disturbance, or carbohydrate depletion, then it is coded as O21.1. If the vomiting began after 20 weeks' gestation, then it is coded as O21.2.

A threatened abortion (O20.0) occurs when there is bleeding before 20 weeks without expulsion of the fetus and without dilation of the cervix. Hemorrhage is coded as O20.

Venous complications (O22) include hemorrhoids, varicose veins, genital varices, thrombophlebitis (superficial or deep), and thrombosis.

Infections during pregnancy (O23) can occur in the kidneys, bladder, urethra and other anatomic sites. The fifth character indicates the trimester when the infection occurs.

Diabetic codes (O24) during pregnancy have also been expanded with the fourth character indicating if the diabetes is pre-existing or gestational. The fifth character indicates when the gestation occurs such as in pregnancy, in childbirth or in the puerperium. The sixth characters indicated trimester involved and if the diabetes is controlled.

Diet and weight conditions affecting pregnancy (O25-O26) include malnutrition and excessive or low weight gain as well as recurrent pregnancy loss and retained intrauterine contraceptive device during pregnancy.

Other conditions (O26) include herpes during the pregnancy, hypotension, liver/biliary tract disorders, subluxation of pubis bone, exhaustion, fatigue, neuritis, renal disease, size-date discrepancy of the pregnancy, spotting, and cervical shortening.

Section 23.9: MULTIPLE GESTATIONS

Multiple gestations (O30) include twin, triplet, quadruplet or other. The fifth characters indicate further define the multiplicity such as if the twins are conjoined, number of placenta and amniotic sacs. Complications due to multiplicity (O31) include papyraceous fetus, pregnancy that continued after spontaneous abortion or death or reduction of one of the fetuses. Seventh characters indicate how many fetus there are. Papyraceous fetus is known as the "vanishing" twin as it is being compressed by the other fetus and dies.

Section 23.10: MATERNAL CARE FOR OTHER COMPLICATIONS

There are various conditions (O32-O47) that require additional maternal care beyond that provided for a normal pregnancy which may require additional observation, hospitalization, or other obstetric care as well as possible cesarean section. . These include malpresentations. Malpresentations (O32) occurs when the baby does not present head first. These include breech, unstable lie, transverse/oblique, face/brow/chin, high head, compound, and footling. A breech birth occurs when the baby's head does not present first but instead the feet do; if one foot is presented first this is known as footling. Usually with malpresentations, the doctor will attempt to correct it by manual manipulation to turn the baby around before delivery. There are other codes to use if the malpresentation complicates delivery with codes O64.

Disproportion (O33) includes problems such as deformity of the mother's pelvic bones, contracted pelvis, outlet contraction, or disproportion between mother and babies. A seventh character indicates how many babies are involved during this pregnancy. Different codes are used if disproportion presents during the delivery with codes O64 codes.

Other conditions include congenital malformations of the mother's uterus, tumors, and scar from previous C-section. Abnormalities of the pregnant uterus can include incarceration, prolapse, and retroversion. There are also abnormalities that occur in the vagina, vulva and perineum. These codes are differentiated by the trimester involved. An incarcerated uterus is trapped in the pelvis. Retroversion is when the uterus has tipped backwards.

Fetal conditions can affect the outcome of the pregnancy as well as the mother's health; therefore, there are pregnancy codes (O35) provided for these conditions but they are codes for the effect or possible effect on the mother, not the fetus. These may include genetic malformations of the baby, damage to the baby, decreased fetal movements, and fetal distress.

Isoimmunizations occurs when there is possible incompatibility between mother and baby which includes the Rh factor (O36) and blood types. Intrauterine death of the baby is coded as O36.4.

Fetal conditions also include if the baby is large or small. If a baby is small, it is known as "light for dates" and is coded as poor fetal growth (O36.5). If the baby is large, it is known as "large for dates" and is coded as excessive fetal growth (O36.6). These conditions must be described by the physician and should not be determined by the coder.

Section 23.11: PLACENTAL CONDITIONS

Various conditions of the amniotic sac and membranes can provide complications (O41-O45). This includes infections and premature rupture of the membranes (water sac breaking) with onset of labor within or after 24 hours after and if this occurs prematurely or preterm. Preterm occurs before 37 weeks gestation. These code are differentiated by trimester involved.

Placental disorders (O43) include transfusion syndrome that can involve the transfer between mother and baby or between babies if multiple births. Other disorders of the placenta include malformation, circumvallate, velamentous insertion of umbilical cord, placenta accrete, placenta increta, placenta percreta, and infarction. Placenta accrete is when the placenta is too deeply and firmly attached in the uterus. Placenta increta is when the placenta attaches in the muscular wall of the uterus. Placenta percreta is when the placenta grows through the uterus.

Placenta previa (O44) is when the placenta is implanted at the lower end of the uterus which can result in a lack of adequate oxygen. These code are differentiated as to with or without hemorrhage.

Abruptio placentae (O45) is when the placenta separates prematurely from the wall and is an emergency. These codes are differentiated by the presence of various conditions such as coagulation defect. Trimester is coded with the sixth character.

Antepartum hemorrhage (O46) is coded with the inclusion of various complications including coagulation defect, afibrinogenemia, or disseminated intravascular coagulation.

Section 23.12: DELIVERY

Gestational age at delivery should be coded additionally if it is not normal (normal is between 37 to 40 weeks). Preterm refers to deliveries prior to 38 weeks gestation and so there should be an additional code listed for early onset (O60) as it does present risks. A pregnancy that ends before 37 weeks of gestation resulting in a live-born infant is known as a premature birth. Preterm labor is threatened labor during this time period which does not result in delivery.

False labor (O47) is known as Braxton Hicks contraction or threated labor. Codes are differentiated as occurring before 37 completed weeks or after and as being in either the second or third trimester. False labor (O47) codes are differentiated by completed weeks of gestation and trimester, either before or after 37 weeks.

Term refers to deliveries between 38 and 40 weeks and do not require any additional codes.

Postterm refers to deliveries between 40 and 42 weeks which are coded as late pregnancies (O48.0) and prolonged is after 42 weeks.

Various conditions can affect delivery. This includes multiple gestations which are coded as O30-O31 and complications due to multiple gestation are coded as O31. Malpresentation of fetus is coded as O32. Vaginal delivery following a previous C-section is coded as O75.7. Single delivery is coded as O80. C-section is coded as O82 if not performed due to any complications; otherwise it is included with the complication precipitating its use. Outcome of delivery is coded as Z37.

Codes for complications of anesthesia during pregnancy have been expanded to include complications during pregnancy (O29), during delivery (O74) and during the puerperium (O89). The complication and trimester are further specified by the fourth and fifth characters. Complications can include aspiration pneumonitis, lung collapse, cardiac arrest or failure, cerebral anoxia, toxic reaction, headache, and failed or difficult intubation.

If induction of delivery is attempted but fails, then it would be coded as O61 and are defined as medical, instrumental, or other. If labor is attempted by fails to deliver this is coded as O66.4 which includes failed attempted VBAC (vaginal birth after previous C-section). If vacuum extractor or forceps are used code O66.5 should be used even if the delivery still occurs with the use of the forceps or by C-section.

Abnormalities of labor forces (O62) include inadequate, arrested, hypotonic, atony, irregular labor, and poor contractions. Labor that is fast is known as precipitate. Prolonged contractions are coded as O62.4. If the labor is prolonged (more than 24 hours) then it would be coded with O63 codes as determined by stages of labor, either first, second, delayed or long.

A normal delivery with the birth of a live born is coded as O82 with no other characters required. If anything else occurs other than an episiotomy, then it is not considered a normal delivery and should be coded from other pregnancy codes that describe other conditions or problems existed.

Cesarean delivery is coded under the complication code such as for disproportion or atony. These can all be found in the alphabetical index under delivery, cesarean. Cesarean delivery occurs when the baby is delivered surgically through the abdomen rather than vaginally. The C-section itself is a procedure and would be coded with the CPT codes.

If a woman delivers, whether it is vaginal or Cesarean (C-section), but had a C-section before, this should be noted with the use of code O34.21. If she has a vaginal birth, but had a C-section before, this is known as VBAC, vaginal birth after Cesarean. The woman may have a vaginal or Cesarean delivery after having had a previous Cesarean section, but this can pose some risks.

OUTCOMES OF BIRTH: When the visit is for delivery, then a code must be listed for the outcome of the births using Z37 codes. A single live born is coded as Z37.0 which constitutes most deliveries. Z37.1 is a single stillborn birth, Z37.2 is for live born twins, Z37.3 is for one live born and one stillborn twins and these classifications culminate in Z37.9 which is for unknown outcome. When a fetus dies in utero after about 20 weeks, or during delivery, it is usually termed stillborn.

Section 23.13: COMPLICATIONS

As described earlier, other than a normal delivery, all other complications must be coded with pregnancy codes other than O80. Complications include medical conditions but can also include labor and delivery issues, such as obstructed labor (O64) or trauma to the perineum or vulva of the mother (O71). Obstructed labor can occur due to the size of the baby, size of mother's pelvis, or other complication. Obstructed labor due to malposition or malpresentations of the baby use codes O64. Physical conditions of the mother's pelvis that complicate delivery are coded as O65 such as deformed or contracted pelvis.

Labor or delivery complicated by hemorrhage is coded as O67. Postpartum hemorrhages (O72) include third-stage hemorrhage with retained placenta, immediate, secondary, delayed, or postpartum coagulation defects.

Various complications with the umbilical cord can complicate delivery (O69). These include prolapse of the cord, cord around the neck of the baby with compression, other types of cord entanglements, short cord, and various conditions of the cord such as hemorrhage, hematoma, bruising, and thrombosis.

If the perineum is lacerated during delivery this is coded as O70. It is differentiated as first, second, third, or fourth degree. There is also a code if the sphincter is torn. Similar complications include rupture of the uterus (O71) either before or during labor, inversion of the uterus, obstetric laceration of the uterus, or hematoma of the pelvis.

Other complications of labor and delivery (O75) include maternal distress, shock, pyrexia, infections, cardiac arrest or failure, cerebral anoxia, maternal exhaustion, and pulmonary edema. If there are abnormalities in the baby's heart rate and rhythm during labor and delivery this is coded as O76 which can include bradycardia (slow), tachycardia (fast), irregularity, or deceleration. Fetal distress is coded as O77.

Section 23.14: POSTPARTUM/PUERPERUM

Complications encountered after labor and delivery (O85-O92) include sepsis and other infections such as cervicitis, vaginitis, pyrexia, and urinary tract infection. Venous complications include thrombophlebitis, hemorrhoids, thrombosis, or embolisms. Embolism can be air, amniotic fluid, pyemic, septic, or thromboembolism. Complications from anesthesia are coded as O89 which includes cardiac or CNS complications or failed intubation. Other complications include disruption/dehiscence of surgical repair such as C-section, hematoma, cardiomyopathy, kidney failure, thyroiditis, and mood disturbance (postpartum blues or dysphoria).

Infections of the breast associated with pregnancy (O91) include infections of the nipples, abscesses, mastitis, retracted nipples, cracked nipples, aglactia, and suppressed lactation.

Sequelae of complications of pregnancy, childbirth and puerperium are coded as O94. The actual condition should be coded first.

Section 23.15: INFECTIONS

Infections or parasitic diseases (O98) complicating pregnancy, childbirth or puerperium include tuberculosis, syphilis, gonorrhea, viral hepatitis, protozoal, and HIV. The organism should also be coded if known.

Section 23.16: OTHER CONDITIONS

Other conditions complicating the pregnancy, childbirth or puerperium (O99) include anemia, other blood problems, obesity, endocrine conditions, mental including alcohol or drug abuse, circulatory and pulmonary conditions, as well as liver and skin. Other conditions also include abnormal glucose levels, Step B carrier, bariatric surgery, malignant neoplasm, injury, poisoning, and physical, sexual or psychological abuse. O9A is for neoplasms, injury, poisonings, and all types of abuse.

Section 23.17: STERILIZATION

Sterilization codes are not coded from either the genitourinary or pregnancy codes, so they will be discussed in a later packet. However, if the reason for the sterilization is either genitourinary or pregnancy, then those codes would be selected from these chapters.

PREGNANCY QUIZ 16

1) What are the codes for a 36-year-old pregnant woman who has a C section due to fetal distress at 39 weeks?

2) What are the codes for a 25-year-old pregnant woman who is 33-weeks gestation, has gestational diabetes and is seen today for dehydration?

3) What are the codes for an 18-year-old pregnant woman who has difficulty in labor due to the birth of a 12 pound baby boy?

4) What are the codes for a pregnant woman who delivered liveborn twins with one normal and the other breech at 32 weeks with both weighing 5 pounds?

5) What are the codes for a pregnant woman who has had three previous miscarriages at approximately 18 weeks and presents today at 20 weeks gestation who is experiencing cramping?

6) What are the codes for a 39-year-old pregnant woman whose baby at 32-weeks gestation is known to have Down's syndrome?

7) What are the codes for a pregnant 23-year-old woman who delivered by C-section a liveborn today at 35 weeks due to severe eclampsia and decreased fetal movement?

8) What are the codes for a pregnant woman who delivered a liveborn girl which required an episiotomy to aid in delivery?

9) What are the codes for a pregnant woman who delivered twins with a normal delivery?

10) What are the codes for a 25-year-old pregnant woman who delivered a 10 pound baby boy but the mother's pelvic was too small and forceps had to be used but when these did not work a C-section was done?

11) What are the codes for a 38-year-old pregnant woman, 37 weeks gestation, who is seen today for her checkup?

12) What are the codes for a pregnant 31-year-old woman who is seen today for deep thrombophlebitis which she developed four days after her delivery of liveborn at 42 weeks?

13) What are the codes for a pregnant woman who had an induced abortion two days ago and is admitted for a severe infection?

14) What are the codes for a pregnant woman who was in a car accident and fractured her tibia?

15) What are the codes for a woman who delivered a liveborn vaginally at 39 weeks and who had a C-section for her previous pregnancy?

CHAPTER 24
ICD-10 PERINATAL

You will learn the following objectives in this chapter:

A. Definitions
    1. Fetal
    2. Perinatal
    3. Newborn
    4. Neonatal
    5. Pediatric
B. Maternal Conditions
C. Malpresentations
D. Other Complications
E. Outcome of Birth
F. Fetal Growth and Malnutrition
G. Birth Trauma
H. Respiratory/Cardiovascular
I. Infections
J. Hemorrhagic
K. Endocrine/Metabolic
L. Digestive
M. Integumentary
N. Other Conditions

Chapter 16 is described as "Certain Conditions Originating in the Perinatal Period" and ranges from P00-P96. There are many new codes and expansions in these codes.

Section 24.1: DEFINITIONS

AGES: The term "fetus" is not used but rather "newborn" is used in the code descriptions. Newborn, therefore, refers to an unborn child up until the 28 days after birth.

Perinatal is the period occurring during pregnancy, specifically from 22 completed weeks of gestation to 28 completed days after birth. Although codes are listed for perinatal conditions which are defined as up until the newborn is 28 days of age, conditions that are diagnosed after this time period but were related to this time period can still be identified as perinatal. For example, if a patient suffers conditions that resulted from anoxia during birth, then associated conditions would be coded as perinatal even if they persist into later years of age.

Pediatric refers to a child who is 24 months of age or less, but older than 28 days. However, the term is also used generally to refer to a child of any age, usually up to the age of 16, but for the purposes of coding pediatric will refer to a child who is 24 months of age or less but older than 28 days.

Section 24.2: MATERNAL CONDITIONS

There may be maternal conditions that influence or affect the care of a newborn (P00). These codes are for the baby and not the mother who has her own codes for related conditions. This includes hypertension, renal and urinary tract problem, infections, nutritional problems (such as malnutrition), injury to the mother, surgical procedure on mother or other conditions.

If a mother undergoes surgery while pregnant, codes P00.7 should be used but damage from amniocentesis is coded as P02.1.

Other maternal conditions that should be coded as they may affect the outcome of care are coded as P01 codes which includes incompetent cervix, premature rupture of membranes, oligohydramnios. Incompetent cervix is when the cervix is weak and begins to open early. Oligohydramnios is inadequate amounts of amniotic fluid in the womb during pregnancy.

Ectopic pregnancies for coding for the baby is coded as P01.4. Multiparity (twins, etc) is coded as P01.5 for the baby. Maternal death is coded as P01.6.

Section 24.3: MALPRESENTATIONS

Malpresentations of the baby before labor is coded as P01.7:

- Normal - the top of the head presents first.
- Brow – the front brow portion of the head presents first.
- Face – the face presents first.
- Frank breech - the baby's bottom comes first.
- Complete breech - the baby's bottom comes first but the feet are down by the buttocks in a cross-legged position.
- Footling breech - one or both feet come first.
- Kneeling breech - the baby is in a kneeling position, with one or both legs extended at the hips and flexed at the knees.
- Compound presentation - more than one part of the baby arrives at the same time.
- Shoulder presentation – when the shoulders present first.
- Transverse – position in which the mother's and the baby's spines make a cross or a "T" shape.
- Oblique - When the baby is positioned at an angle so that the spine is off-center from the mother's.

If there are complications for the newborn during labor due to malpresentation, these are coded as P03.0 or P03.1.

Section 24.4: OTHER COMPLICATIONS

Complications of the placenta, cord and membranes (P02) include placenta previa, placental transfusion syndrome, and prolapsed cord (P02.4). Other problems with the cord include torsion of the cord, the cord wrapped about the baby's neck, knot in the cord, entanglement of the cord, short cord, and varices. If the placenta is retained after delivery without hemorrhaging it is coded as O73 for the mother.

If forceps are required, then a code for the use of forceps should also be coded (P03.2). Codes from P03 should be used to code for other assistive method, such as vacuum extraction and C-section. Precipitate delivery (fast) is coded as P03.5.

If there are complications for the baby during labor and delivery, then these should be coded as P03 such as abnormalities in the heart rate with onset before or during delivery, meconium present, and induction of labor.

Noxious substances, such as alcohol and drugs (P04) should be coded as these can greatly influence the outcome of the baby's care. This includes narcotics, hallucinogens, cocaine, and prescriptions.

Section 24.5: OUTCOME OF BIRTH: When coding for the newborn, Z38 codes must be used to indicate their birth status, such as in the hospital. This code should be listed first when this is the newborn's admission for birth.

Section 24.6: FETAL GROWTH AND MALNUTRITION

Disorders relating to the length of gestation and fetal growth are coded as P05-P08. The codes now distinguish between light for dates (P05.0) and small for gestational age (P05.1). "Light-for-dates" means the baby is underweight for their gestation age which is further classified by the presence or absence of fetal malnutrition. If the newborn is low birth weight but it is not due slow fetal growth or fetal malnutrition, then codes P07 should be used.

Extreme immaturity is coded as P07.2 for less than 28 weeks gestation and other (P07.3) for more than 28 weeks but less than 37 weeks gestation. When both birth weight and gestational age of the newborn are provided, both should be coded with birth weight sequenced first.

Extreme immaturity is when the baby weighs less than 1000 grams. Exceptionally large baby is when the baby weighs more than 4500 grams. "Large-for-dates" or "heavy-for-dates" are babies who weight plots at over 90% for gestational age.

If a baby is born later than 40 weeks of gestation that is coded as post-term infant (P08.21) and these babies are oftentimes not "large-for-dates" because the ability of the placenta to provide sufficient nutrition begins to slow. If the gestation passes 42 weeks, then this is coded as prolonged gestation. The doctor must describe these conditions in his report in order to code them.

Section 24.7: BIRTH TRAUMA

There are many new codes for birth trauma which is coded as P10-P15 and include hemorrhage and injuries to the CNS, scalp, skeleton and peripheral nervous system.

Section 24.8: RESPIRATORY/CARDIOVASCULAR

Respiratory and cardiovascular disorders in the perinatal period are coded as P19-P29. Infant respiratory distress syndrome (IRDS) (P22.0) (also known as hyaline membrane disease) is when a premature infant experiences an insufficiency of surfactant and structural immaturity of the lungs.

Birth trauma can include subdural and cerebral hemorrhage, fracture of the clavicle during delivery, and injuries to various anatomic sites such as spine and scalp.

Other respiratory conditions can include emphysema, pulmonary hemorrhage, atelectasis (when the lungs fail to fully inflate), tachypnea (rapid breathing), apnea (when breathing stops), respiratory failure, aspiration of stomach contents, respiratory arrest, and hypoxemia (absence of oxygen in blood). Various substances can be aspirated into a newborn's lungs (P23.9) that are present at the birth, including meconium, amniotic fluid, and blood.

Section 24.9: INFECTIONS

Infections related to the perinatal period are coded as P35-P39. Infections acquired before or during birth are categorized by organism or anatomic site. This includes rubella (P35.0), cytomegalovirus, herpes, candida, and tetanus. Sites include the umbilicus, breast (P37.5), and eye. If the infection spreads to sepsis/septicemia, this would also be coded as P36. If the sepsis becomes severe, it should also be coded as R65.20. Remember, the organism should also be coded.

Section 24.10: HEMORRHAGIC

Hemorrhagic and hematological disorders of the fetus and newborn are coded as P50-P61 including jaundice and Rh or blood compatibility complications.

Blood loss is coded as P50.0 for fetuses and neonates and is based on cause and/or anatomic site. If the hemorrhage or hematological disorder occurs in the newborn, then it is coded as P53.

With fetuses and neonates, if there is blood loss due to an intraventricular hemorrhage in the heart, it should be coded as P52.2 depending upon the grade. The grades depend upon where the bleeding occurs, whether in the ventricle, cerebral cortex, germinal matrix and if the ventricle is enlarged. If the hemorrhage occurs in the subarachnoid area of the head, then it is coded as P52.5. Hemorrhage of the umbilicus is coded as P51.8. Hemorrhaging evidenced by bruising, ecchymoses, hematoma, or petechiae are coded as cutaneous (P54.5).

Hemolytic disease (P55.0) is also known as erythroblastosis fetalis. It is a condition in which the red blood cells of the fetus are broken down due to the antibodies produced by the mother which were transferred to the fetus and which can result in anemia. This can result from the Rh factor, ABO blood types, and other blood grouping conflicts. Other conditions can result from this, including kernicterus (a serious form of jaundice) and hydrops fetalis (edema in the subcutaneous tissue, pleura, pericardium, or in the abdomen, also known as ascites), and these should be coded additionally, as well as late anemia.

Jaundice (icterus) is yellowish coloration to the skin due to high serum bilirubin levels caused by the breakdown of hemoglobin. Jaundice (P58.8) is coded according to cause, so the underlying condition should also be coded. This includes jaundice due to hereditary hemolytic anemia, excessive hemolysis, preterm delivery, conjugation, hepatocellular damage, and other causes. Jaundice can be conjugated or unconjugated. Unconjugated jaundice is potentially toxic and becomes conjugated when it ties itself to glucuronic acid in the liver.

Section 24.11: ENDOCRINE/METABOLIC

Endocrine and metabolic disorders (P70-P74) include infant of a diabetic mother, diabetes in the newborn, myasthenia gravis (muscle weakness and fatigue), thyrotoxicosis (abnormally high levels of thyroid hormone), hypocalcemia, hypoglycemia, and acidosis (low pH levels and bicarbonate in body fluids of neonate due to excess levels of acid).

Section 24.12: DIGESTIVE

Digestive (P76-P78) disorders in the perinatal period include obstruction by meconium (stools of unborn child), hematemesis and melena due to swallowing the mother's blood, necrotizing enterocolitis (portion of the bowels die), and perforation of the intestine.

Section 24.13: INTEGUMENTARY

Various integumentary conditions of the fetus and newborn (P80-P83) include hydrops fetalis not due to blood types, sclerema, temperature problems including hypothermia, and hydrocele. Sclerema is severe skin condition that is characterized by inflammation of the underlying subcutaneous fat.

If a baby does not obtain sufficient oxygen during delivery (P84), this can cause serious problems such as death, distress, encephalopathy, or asphyxia.

Section 24.14: OTHER CONDITIONS

Other conditions in the perinatal period include convulsions (P90), comas P91.5), feeding problems (P92) (regurgitation and slow feeding), reactions to drugs (P93), failure to thrive (P92.6), muscle tone problems (P94), renal failure (P96.8) and exposure to parental tobacco use (P96.81).

PERINATAL QUIZ 17

1) What is the code for a liveborn whose was delivered with the use of forceps at 34 weeks and weighing 1260 grams due to placentia previa?

2) What are the codes for a newborn whose mother was addicted to cocaine and the newborn is experiencing withdrawal?

3) What are the codes for a newborn at this visit who is diagnosed with neutropenia which is not transient?

4) What are the codes for a newborn with jaundice who was delivered at 34 weeks?

5) What are the codes for a 1-year-old girl who was diagnosed with sepsis due to UTI due to E. coli?

6) What are the neonatal codes for congenital TB?

7) What are the codes for a neonate who is diagnosed with diabetes?

8) What are the codes for a neonate with hyperbilirubinema who was premature at birth and so remained in the hospital with this her third day and weighed 2100 gm at birth?

9) What are the codes for a baby born at 43 weeks who experienced asphyxia due to the cord wrapped around her neck?

10) What is the code for the newborn when her mother dies during childbirth?

11) What are the codes for a patient with a bunion on the right foot?

12) What are the codes for a 1-month old baby who has not gained any weight?

13) What are the codes for a patient with lower respiratory infection?

14) What are the codes for a fetus whose mother has been diagnosed with rubella?

15) What are the codes for a newborn whose mother received an anesthetic during delivery with a C-section performed because the newborn's heart rate slowed and was in fetal distress due to the cord being wrapped about her neck with newborn suffering hypoxia?

CHAPTER 25

ICD-10 CONGENITAL

You will learn the following objectives in this chapter:

A. Congenital Conditions
    1. Acquired Versus Congenital
B. Outcome of Delivery
    1. Sequencing
    2. Congenital
C. Anomalies
    1. Cephalic
    2. Ocular
    3. Auditory
D. Congenital Heart Defects
    1. Acyanotic
    2. Cyanotic
E. Respiratory
F. Gastrointestinal/Genitourinary
    1. Cleft Lip/Palate
    2. Other GI/GU Congenital anomalies
G. Musculoskeletal
    1. Hip
    2. Legs
    3. Feet
    4. Chest
    5. Extremities
    6. Spine
    7. Bone
H. Integumentary
I. Chromosomal
J. Other Congenital Anomalies

Chapter 17 codes are for congenital malformations, deformations and chromosomal abnormalities (Q00-Q99).

Section 25.1: ACQUIRED VERSUS CONGENITAL

Acquired conditions are conditions that arise during life whereas congenital are conditions that arise during gestation and at birth and which are coded with their own codes as distinct from the acquired conditions.

Section 25.2: OUTCOME OF DELIVERY

With the mother, a Z37 code was used to designate the outcome of the birth when coding for the mother during a delivery. For the baby, delivery must be listed with Z38 codes which is always listed first. If a congenital anomaly is identified on the visit when the baby is born, then the anomaly is listed as second and the delivery is first. If the baby is transferred to another hospital or the anomaly is identified at a visit other than delivery, then only the anomaly is listed as the birth did not occur at the hospital at that time.

Section 25.3: ANOMALIES

CEPHALIC CONGENITAL ANOMALIES: Anencephalus (Q00.0) is the absence of a major portion of the brain, skull, and scalp which is due to a neural tube defect during development. Iniencephaly is when the head is bent backwards and the neck is absent due to a neural tube defect also. Encephalocele (Q01) is when a part of the cranial contents protrude through the skull. Microcephalus is a small head. Reduction deformities (Q04.3) are when part of the brain is missing or underdeveloped. Hydrocephalus (Q03.0) is when the ventricles of the brain are filled with fluid.

OCULAR CONGENITAL ANOMALIES

Congenital malformations of the eyelid, lacrimal system and orbit include ptosis, ectropion, and entropion. Ocular congenital anomalies include anophthalmos (Q11) which is the congenital absence of one or both eyes. Cryptophthalmos is when there is skin over the eyeball with absence of eyelids. Microphthalmos is when the eyes are smaller than normal. Buphthalmos is when there is increased intraocular fluid pressure which results in enlargement of the eyes. This includes congenital glaucoma (Q15.0). Cataracts (Q12.0) and other lens congenital anomalies can be congenital. Cataracts are clouding of the lens of the eye. Other congenital anomalies can involve the shape of the eye. Coloboma (Q13.0) is a hole in one of the structures of the eye. Other ocular codes include congenital anomalies of various parts of the eye, including absences and under-development.

AUDITORY CONGENITAL ANOMALIES

Congenital anomalies of the ear (Q16) can include absence of anatomic parts, hypertrophy (excessive growth), or failure to grow properly, or malformation. Atresia can occur when an anatomic site is abnormally closed or absent. There can also be fusion or development of accessory anatomic parts. Macrotia is excessive enlargement and microtia is smaller than normal sizes of part of the ear. Other deformities, such as bat ears or pointed ears are coded as Q17.5.

Section 25.4: CONGENITAL HEART DEFECTS

There are numerous congenital heart defects, some which may correct themselves with age, but others do not. These can be either cyanotic or acyanotic.

ACYANOTIC: Acyanotic means the oxygenated blood is ejected from the heart. These conditions include patent ductus arteriosis, pulmonary stenosis, atrial and ventricular septal defects, and aortic stenosis. Patent ductus arteriosis (Q25.0) is when the blood vessel connecting the ductus arteriosus (vessel connecting the aorta and the pulmonary artery) does not close shortly after birth and allows the blood to bypass the lungs. Ventricular septal defect (Q21.0) is an abnormal connection which allows the blood to pass in the wrong direction from the left ventricle to the right ventricle.

CYANOTIC: Cyanotic means there is right to left shunting of unoxygenated blood which then mixes with oxygenated blood. Common truncus (Q20.0) is a congenital anomaly in which there is abnormal connection between the ascending aorta and the pulmonary artery.

Tetralogy of Fallot (Q21.3) involves four anatomical abnormalities which are ventricular septal defect with pulmonary stenosis or atresia, dextrapostion of aorta, and hypertrophy of right ventricle. Valvular congenital anomalies of the heart include atresia and stenosis. Cor triatriatum (Q24.2) is when the heart has three atrial chambers with there being two left atriums. There can also be congenital malpositioning of the heart.

The great vessels of the heart can be transposed (Q20.3) including the superior and/or inferior vena cavae, pulmonary artery, pulmonary veins, and aorta. Other congenital anomalies can occur with the aorta and great veins, such as coarctation of aorta and anomaly of great veins (Q25.1). There are also congenital anomalies of the peripheral vascular system (Q27.8).

Section 25.5: RESPIRATORY

There are several congenital anomalies related to the respiratory system. This includes choanal atresia (Q30.0) when there is a growth of membrane or tissue over the nasal airways of the newborn. There are also congenital anomalies of missing or additional noses, or deformities to the nose. There can also be congenital anomalies of the larynx, trachea, and bronchus. Congenital cystic lung (Q33.0) can include bronchogenic cysts, benign mass of abnormal lung tissue, lobar emphysema, and pulmonary sequestration which is a mass of nonfunctioning pulmonary tissue.

Section 25.6: GASTROINTESTINAL/GENITOURINARY

CLEFT PALATE/LIP: A cleft is a fissure or opening of the palate or lip which usually occurs within the first couple months of gestation. Cleft palates/lips (Q35) are differentiated within the codes as to whether one or both conditions exist and if they are bilateral or unilateral and complete or incomplete. If the defect extends into the nose, then it is complete, but if it does not extend up into the nose, then it is incomplete.

OTHER GI/GU CONGENITAL ANOMALIES: Aglossia (Q38.3) is the absence of a tongue. Ankyloglossia (Q38.1) is known as tongue tied and is when the frenulum is unusually short which is the membrane connecting the underside of the tongue to the floor of the mouth. Hypertrophy of the tongue is known as macroglossia (Q38.2) and underdevelopment is known as microglossia.

Absence, stenosis, stricture, atresia, or fistulas can also occur of various anatomic sites of the GI/GU systems. A hernia can also be congenital (Q40.1). Meckel's diverticulum (Q43.0) is a small bulge in the small intestine present at birth. Congenital anomalies of the gallbladder, bile ducts, and liver include atresia, absence, duplication, and cysts.

Pyloric stenosis (Q40.0) occurs when there is narrowing of the opening to the stomach and hypertrophy of the pylorus (muscle surrounding the opening of the stomach). This results in severe vomiting in the first few months after birth. Other codes include congenital malformations, atresia, and absences of various parts of the digestive system.

Congenital anomalies of the GU system include conditions with the genital organs (Q50-Q56), such as absences, cysts, accessory anatomic parts, doubling of the uterus, undescended testicles, hypospadias, and indeterminate sex/hermaphroditism (Q56). Hypospadias is when the opening of the penis is located other than at the tip, such as on the underside. Hermaphroditism is having both female and male sex organs.

Polycystic kidney disease (Q61.3) is clusters of fluid-filled cysts in the kidneys which results in enlargement of the kidneys and replacement of kidney tissue which eventually results in uremia and kidney failure. It is further classified by being either autosomal dominant or recessive. To be dominant means that a child need only receive a defective gene from one parent because the gene is dominant and will cause the disease. With autosomal recessive, a child must receive the defective gene from both parents in order for the disease to exist. Another differentiation is if the disease is medullary. Medullary cystic kidney disease (Q61.5) is a hereditary disorder in which cysts in the center of each kidney cause the kidneys to gradually lose their ability to work. Medullary sponge kidney disease is a hereditary disorder in which there is formation of diffuse cysts in the center of the kidney caused by abnormalities in the renal collecting ducts.

Congenital obstruction of the kidneys and ureters are coded as to location (Q62). An ureterocele is a sac caused by the dilation of the ureters at the opening into the bladder. Exostrophy of the bladder occurs when the abdominal wall fails to close properly during development and the urinary bladder protrudes. Other anomalies include atresia and stenosis and fistulas and cysts.

Congenital abnormalities of the diaphragm (Q79.0) can include absence, hernia, or eventration. This code is not used for a congenital hiatal hernia; instead code Q40.1 should be used. Eventration is when all or part of the diaphragmatic muscle is replaced by fibroelastic tissue.

Section 25.7: MUSCULOSKELETAL

HIP: Congenital dislocation of the hip (Q65) are differentiated by being either unilateral or bilateral and defined as a dislocation or subluxation. Subluxation is an incomplete or partial dislocation.

LEGS: There are various curvature deformities of the leg that can occur congenitally. This includes genu extrorsum (bowleg) (Q68.3), genu introrsum (knock-knee) (Q74.1), genu recurvatum (hyperextensibility of the knee joint), genu valgum (knock-knee), and gen varum (bowleg).

FEET: Similar to acquired musculoskeletal deformities, deformities of the feet include talipes varus (Q66.0), talipes equinovarus (downward twisting of the foot), talipes valgus, and pes planus (Q66.5).

CHEST: Congenital chest deformities include pectus excavatum (Q67.6) and pectus carinatum. Excavatum is also known as funnel chest due to the malformation of the sternum and several ribs. Carinatum involves a pronunciation of the sternum. Other deformities can include more or less ribs than normal (supernumerary or absence Q76).

EXTREMITIES: Congenital anomalies of the extremities include polydactyly which is extra fingers or toes and syndactyly (Q70) when the fingers or toes grow together (webbed). Syndactyly can include fusion of bone. Other deformities include having fewer fingers or toes than a person should (reduction). Reduction can also include absence of other anatomic sites of the extremities including hands, feet, humerus, and femur. Reduction can be complete or incomplete depending upon if the entire anatomic site is missing or only partially missing. In addition, while one anatomic site may be missing, anatomic sites distal from that, such as fingers which are distal to the rest of the arm, may still exist. Abnormal growth of cartilage (chondrodystrophy Q77.3) can affect the limbs and affect the growth plates.

SPINE: Spina bifida (Q76.0) is a defective closure of the vertebral column and ranges in severity from occulta with few signs to completely open (rachischisis). In spina bifida occulta the outer part of some of the vertebrae are not completely closed but there is no protrusion of the spinal cord externally. Spina bifida is classified by whether hydrocephalus is involved or not. Hydrocephalus is the accumulation of cerebrospinal fluid within the ventricles of the brain. The affected area is designated by the fifth character. In spina bifida cystica, there is a protruding sac known as meningocele (involves meninges), myelocele (involves spinal cord), or myelomeningocele (involves both meninges and spinal cord). Paralysis can occur if the nerve roots are involved which is frequent. Spondylolisthesis is displacement of vertebrae.

BONE: Osteodystrophies (Q78) are bone anomalies including osteogenesis imperfecta which is when bones break easily. Osteopetrosis is when the bones are denser or harder and is known as stone bone. Osteopoikilosis is an asymptomatic osteosclerotic dysplasia of the bones. Polyostotic fibrous dysplasia of bone is the abnormal replacement of bone with scar-like tissue.

Section 25.8: INTEGUMENTARY

Congenital integumentary anomalies include edema (Q82), ichthyosis (wide variety of skin disorders characterized by dry, thickened, scaly or flaky skin), and dermatoglyphic anomalies which are abnormalities in the creases/prints of fingers, palms, toes, and soles. Birthmarks, strawberry nevus, and port-wine stains on the skin are coded as vascular hematomas (Q82.5).

Other pigmentary anomalies include urticaria pigmentosa, poikiloderma, skin tags and keratoderma. Urticaria pigmentosa is due to an excessive numbers of mast cells in the skin that produce hives. Poikiloderma is extra pigmentation of the skin. Keratoderma is thickening of the skin of the palms and soles, sometimes with painful fissuring.

Congenital anomalies of the hair (Q84) include alopecia (loss of hair), atrichosis and hypertrichosis is the absence or overgrowth of hair, respectively.

Congenital anomalies of nails (Q84.3) include anonychia (absence of nails), clubnail (increased curvature and thickening of nails), koilonychia (also known as spoon nails and the opposite of clubnails in that the nails are thinner and have decreased curvature), pachyonychia (excess keratin in nail beds and thickening of the nails with lesions), and leukonychia (white discoloration of nails).

Other integumentary congenital anomalies can include the absence or accessory breasts.

Section 25.9: CHROMOSOMAL

Chromosomal anomalies (Q90) include Down's syndrome which is also known as Mongolism or Trisomy 21 due to the nature of the genetic defect in which there are three 21st chromosomes, rather than the normal two. There are a wide variety of symptoms which is also true for Patau's syndrome (Trisomy 13) (Q91). Edward's Syndrome is also known as Trisomy E for there are three chromosomes for the 18th.

Other chromosomal anomalies include Cri-du-chat syndrome (Q93.4) and Klinefelter's Syndrome (Q98.4). Klinefelter's Syndrome occurs when a male has two X chromosomes and one Y instead of one Y and one X.

Section 25.10: OTHER CONGENITAL ANOMALIES

Other congenital anomalies include situs inversus (Q89.3) in which all of the major thoracic and abdominal organs are reversed horizontally, conjoined twins (Q89.4), and Prader-Willi syndrome in which there is a defect in the 15th chromosome which results in short stature with mental retardation and obesity. Marfan Syndrome is characterized by very tall stature with long limbs in addition to serious other anomalies of the heart and other organs. Fragile X syndrome (Q99.2) has a wide variety of characteristics also, including a long face and big ears with low muscle tone.

CONGENITAL QUIZ 18

1) What are the codes for a newborn who was born with a hemangioma of the neck?

2) What are the codes for a patient with lateral epicondylitis due to crushing injury?

3) What are the codes for a fetus at 35 weeks gestation who is diagnosed with a myelocele and spina bifida of C2-4 and hydrocephalus?

4) What are the codes for a newborn during this visit with congenital toxoplasmosis with hydrocephalus?

5) What are the codes for a fetus who has been diagnosed with Tetralogy of Fallot?

6) What are the codes for a missed abortion before 22 weeks for the mother?

7) What are the codes for an 8-year-old who is seen today for clubfoot that has developed over time?

8) What are the codes for a pregnant woman whose baby has been diagnosed with Down's Syndrome?

9) What are the codes for a 3-day old baby who remains in the hospital after birth due to a diagnosis of Fallot's triad?

10) What are the codes for a 30-week pregnant woman with aplastic anemia?

11) What at the codes for a patient who has traumatic asphyxiation?

12) What are the codes for a 44-year-old man who has arthritis of his shoulder due to Lyme disease?

13) What are the codes for a 2-year-old child who has been diagnosed with congenital hypothyroidism?

14) What are the codes for a baby born on this visit via C-section with fetal alcohol syndrome due to her mother's alcoholism and occasional cocaine?

1. What are the codes when a 1750 gm baby at 28 weeks gestation is delivered due to hypertonic labor?

CHAPTER 26
ICD-10 SYMPTOMS AND ILL-DEFINED CONDITIONS

You will learn the following objectives in this chapter:

A. Symptoms/ Signs
B. Circulatory/Respiratory
C. Digestive
D. Skin
E. Nervous/Musculoskeletal
F. Genitourinary
G. Emotional/Cognition
H. Speech
I. General Symptoms
J. Abnormal Findings

Chapter 18 is described as "Symptoms, Signs and Abnormal Clinical and Laboratory Findings, not elsewhere classified" and ranges from R00-R99. The symptoms and sign codes are specified by systems, such as R00-R09 is for circulatory and respiratory systems. Abnormal findings are based on content of examination, such as R70-R79 for blood work.

Section 26.1: SYMPTOMS/SIGNS

Symptoms are the descriptions provided by patients about their conditions, in other words they are subjective. In contrast, a sign is objective in that it is a condition that is present and observable.

SCENARIOS: There are three coding scenarios for symptoms and signs:

(1) Symptoms and signs are not coded if a definitive diagnosis is described.
(2) A sign and/or symptom may be coded in addition to a diagnosis that includes them if the sign and/or symptom requires treatment and attention, such as dehydration.
(3) If there is no definitive diagnosis described that would include the signs and/or symptoms, then the signs and/or symptoms would be coded.
(4) If the diagnosis is described as provisional (that is probable, possible, rule out, etc.), then the diagnosis is not coded but the sign and/or symptom would be instead.

Section 26.2: CIRCULATORY/RESPIRATORY

Symptoms and signs associated with circulatory include tachycardia (R00.0) and bradycardia (R00.1). Additional symptoms include palpitations, murmurs, and abnormal blood-pressure readings. Respiratory symptoms include hemorrhages (R04), cough (R05), dyspnea (R06.0) which is difficulty breathing including shortness of breath, stridor, wheezing, hiccoughs and sneezing. Apnea, tachypnea, and snoring are coded as R06.8 codes. Pain in the throat and chest are coded as R07. Asphyxia, hypoxemia, pleurisy, respiratory arrest, and postnasal drip are coded as R09 codes.

Section 26.3: DIGESTIVE

Symptoms and signs associated with the digestive system include abdominal and pelvic pain (R10) which is differentiated by which quadrant the pain is located in. It is important to be sure to be precise in the selection of codes because the codes are specific, e.g. pain in the stomach and abdomen are coded differently. Abdominal tenderness (R10.8) is differentiated by the presence or absence of rebounding. Colic is coded as R10.83. Nausea and vomiting (R11) is differentiated as to type, such as projective or bilious. Heartburn is coded as R12.

Other symptoms of the digestive system include aphagia and dysphagia. Be careful because this is phagia (associated with eating), not phasia (associated with speaking). Flatulence is coded as R14 and includes gas pain, eructation and distension.

Hepatomegaly and splenomegaly are coded as R16 if not classified elsewhere. Ascites is coded as R18. Swelling, mass or lump in the abdominal area is coded as R19.0 and is differentiated by quadrant of the body. Abnormal bowel sounds are coded as R19.1 and include absent or hyperactive. Abdominal rigidity (R19.3) is differentiated by quadrant location.

Section 26.4: SKIN

Symptoms associated with the skin include skin sensation (R20) such as anesthesia (no feeling), hypoesthesia (reduced feeling), paresthesia (tingling feeling), and hyperesthesia (increased feeling). Swelling, mass or lump of the skin is coded as R22 and differentiated by specific location.

Skin changes (R23) can include cyanosis, pallor, flushing or ecchymoses.

Section 26.5: NERVOUS & MUSCULOSKELETAL

Nervous symptoms include abnormal involuntary movements (R25) such as tremors, cramps, spasms, or fasciculations. Mobility symptoms (R26) include ataxic or paralytic gait and unsteadiness. Ataxia is coded as R27.0.

Other symptoms include tetany, clicking hip, repeated falls, facial weakness, loss of height and ocular torticollis.

There are now codes for National Institue of Healths Stroke Scale ranging ins core from 0 to 42 (R29.7) which should be coded with a cerebral infarction code (I63) listed first.

Section 23.6: GENITOURINARY

Symptoms associated with the genitourinary system (R30-R39) include dysuria and painful micturition. Hematuria (R31) is differentiated as gross, benign or other. Retention of urine

(R33) can be due to drugs or other causes such as enlarged prostate. Anuria and oliguria are coded as R34 and polyuria as R35.

Section 26.7: EMOTIONAL AND COGNITION

Symptoms coded in this section (R40-R46) include somnolence, stupor, and coma.

Comas are differentiated by responses and the Glasgow scale. There is a box listing the possible seventh character values similar to the boxes in the ICD-9 book. The coding with the Glasgow coma scale is accomplished by the selection of one code from each of R40.21 (Coma scale, eyes open), R40.22 (coma scale, best verbal response), and R40.23 (coma scale, best motor response). These codes (R40.21 – R40.23) are only used if the individual scores are given for the responses. If only a total score is given for the Glasgow coma scale, then codes R40.24 should be used. Responses can include various levels associated with the following: eyes open, verbal or motor response. A seventh character needs to be added to specify when the coma scale was completed.

Other symptoms include disorientation, amnesia, neglect, age-related, borderline intellectual functioning, and dizziness. Disturbances of smell and taste are coded as R43 and include anosmia, parosmia and parageusia. Hallucinations are coded as R44 and can be auditory, visual or other. Codes for emotional states (R45) include nervousness, unhappiness, restlessness, demoralization, apathy, hostility, irritability, low self-esteem, worries, excessive crying of child, and homicidal or suicidal ideation.

Section 26.8: SPEECH

Symptoms associated with speech and voice (R47-R49) include dysphasia, aphasia, slurred speech, dysarthria, dyslexia, apraxia, dysphonia, aphonia, and hypernasality.

Section 26.9: GENERAL SYMPTOMS

General symptoms (R50-R69) include fever of unknown origin or post-procedural. Headache is coded as R51. Malaise and fatigue are coded as R53 and include functional quadriplegia. Age-related debility is coded as R54 and includes frailty, old age, senile, and senescence. Syncope includes collapse, blackout, or fainting. Convulsions are coded as (R56) and can be febrile or post-traumatic. Shock not coded elsewhere is coded as R57 and include cardiogenic and hypovolemic.

Other general symptoms include enlarged lymph nodes (R59), edema (R60), delayed milestones for development as child (R62.0), failure to thrive as a child (R62.51), short stature ((R62.52), and food/fluid problems such as anorexia, polydipsia, polyphagia, abnormal weight loss or gain and cachexia which is wasting syndrome.

Sepsis codes are coded as R65 codes including systemic inflammatory response syndrome (SIRS) and severe sepsis. Severe sepsis codes list the various associated conditions that would define the sepsis as severe such as shock or organ failure which should also be coded.

Other generalized codes include excessive crying by a baby (R68.11), dry mouth (R68.2) and clubbing of fingers (R68.3).

Section 26.10: ABNORMAL FINDINGS

Nonspecific Abnormal Findings (R70-R79) are codes when labs and tests findings are not normal but not enough information is known to determine a diagnosis.

Abnormal findings codes should not be listed unless the physician states they are abnormal and that no other diagnosis is available for those findings. Other qualified practitioners can also provide valid diagnosis and /or conditions, such as pathologist and laboratory technicians who are qualified. Abnormal findings should be not listed if they are not pertinent to the care of the patient at this visit.

Abnormal findings can include abnormalities in red blood cells (R71), glucose (R73.0), alcohol blood levels (R78.0), inconclusive tests for HIV (R75), increased antibodies (R76), presence of drugs (R78), and blood chemistries (R79).

Abnormal findings on urine tests are coded as R80-R82 and can include proteinuria, biluria (urine which contains bile pigments), hemoglobinuria, and glycosuria.

Other abnormal labs (R83-R89) can include specimens such as from cerebrospinal fluid, respiratory organs, digestive organs, PAP smear, genitourinary, and hemodialysis.

Abnormal findings from diagnostic tests such as x-rays (R90-R94) are differentiated by the anatomic site as well as function tests.

Abnormal tumor markers are coded as R97 and demonstrate presence of antigen such as for cancer and prostate.

SYMPTOMS QUIZ 19

1) What are the codes for a 4-year-old patient with high fever, sore throat, and runny nose who is found to have acute right otitis media with rhinitis?

2) What are the codes for a patient with pathological fracture of the distal radius and COPD with Type I diabetes?

3) What are the codes for a patient who is 82-years-old and broke her right hip and has been severely depressed since?

4) What are the codes for a patient with second and third degree burns covering 25% of her body with 10% being third degree with infection?

5) What are the codes for a pregnant patient who was seen for vaginal bleeding at 20 weeks gestation and she had three prior spontaneous abortions at this same time in the pregnancy?

6) What are the codes for a patient who underwent chemotherapy today for small cell carcinoma lung cancer and is now experiencing vomiting without nausea?

7. What are the codes for a patient who has old bucket tear of the lateral meniscus?

8. What are the codes for a patient with an infected wound of the right humerus which was greenstick fractured with a dislocation and laceration of the axillary nerves?

9. What are the codes for a patient with stage 5 renal disease and hypertension as well as arteriolar nephritis and chronic hypertensive uremia?

10. What are the codes for a 45-year-old man with shortness of breath?

11. What are the codes for a patient with scar tissue of his chest from a third degree burn six months ago?

12. What are the codes for a patient with complaints of dyspnea and tachycardia which the physician believes might be ARDS?

13. What are the codes for a patient with acute and chronic bronchitis with COPD and ASHD?

14. What are the codes for a 72-year-old man who is seen for elevated liver function studies but hepatitis profile and sugar levels were normal? He is also diabetic Type 2 and has cholelithiasis.

15. What are the codes for a 57-year-old man who was admitted to the hospital for possible MI with complaints of chest pain with numbness of the left arm? EKG and stress tests were performed but were negative.

CHAPTER 27
ICD-10 INJURIES, POISONING & CERTAIN OTHER CONSEQUENCES

You will learn the following objectives in this chapter:

A. Injuries
B. Fractures
    1. Closed Fractures
    2. Open Fractures
    3. Malunion/Nonunion
    4. Extensions
    5. Pathological Fractures
    6. Dislocations
C. Sprains/Strains
D. Superficial
E. Open wounds
F. Hemorrhage/Hematoma
G. Vessels/Nerves
H. Head/Skull
I. Neck
J. Thorax
K. Abdomen/Pelvis/Genitals
L. Shoulder/Upper Arms
M. Wrist/Hands/Fingers
N. Hip/Thigh
O. Knee/Lower Leg
P. Ankle/Foot/Toes
Q. Injury/Poisoning/Other
R. Foreign Body
S. Burns
    1. Degrees
    2. Lund Browder Chart
    3. Percentage
T. Frostbite
U. Poisonings/Adverse Effects
    1. Underdosing
    2. Table of Drugs and Chemicals
    3. Coding for Adverse Effects
    4. Coding for Poisonings
    5. Coding for Underdosings
V. Toxic Effects
W. Other Conditions
X. Early Complications of Trauma
Y. Complications of Medical Care

Chapter 19 is described as "Injury, Poisoning, and Certain Other Consequences of External Causes" and ranges from S00-T88. S codes are specific to body regions and T codes are specific to unspecified body regions. There is a significantly increased number of codes in this section. Injuries are now organized according to anatomic site, with injuries listed secondary.

Section 27.1: INJURIES

The first block of codes are first differentiated by anatomic site and then by injury. Injury is bodily damage or injury caused by an external force (trauma). Types of injuries include superficial and open wounds, burns, fractures, dislocation, crushing, bites, rupture, foreign bodies, bruises, sprain/strains, and amputations. Injuries to organs, muscles, tendons, vessels, and nerves are also listed within each anatomic site.

Codes are now highly specific to site such as which finger or toe and laterality (left or right).

If there are multiple injuries, the most severe injury should be listed first.

An extra seventh character is added for injuries and external causes to identify the encounter as initial, subsequent, or sequelae. The extensions are:

- A Initial encounter
- D Subsequent encounter
- S Sequelae

Late effects are coded using the extension S for sequelae.

Section 27.2: FRACTURES

Fractures are a break in the continuity of the bone which can be caused by trauma or a disease process.

- Open fracture is one in which the skin was broken and there is exposure to the outside which creates a possibility of infection or other complications by the entry of foreign materials into the body.
- Closed fracture is when there is no breakage of skin.

- Complete fractures are fractures in which bone fragments separate completely.
- Incomplete fractures are fractures in which the bone fragments are still partially joined.
- Compacted fractures are fractures caused when bone fragments are driven into each other.
- Stress fractures are caused by unusual or repeated stress on a bone.
- Compression fractures are fractures of the vertebrae where the front portion of a vertebra in the spine collapses.
- Le Fort fractures are bilateral horizontal fracture of the maxilla. Le Fort fractures are classified as I, II, or III.

- Monteggia's fracture is a fracture of the proximal half of the shaft of the ulna, with dislocation of the head of the radius.

CLOSED FRACTURES

- Simple fractures are fractures that only occur along one line, splitting the bone into two pieces.
- Depressed fractures are fractures of the skull in which a fragment is depressed.
- Elevated fractures are when fractured portion is elevated above the level of the intact skull.
- Fissured fractures are cracks extending from a surface into, but not through, a long bone.
- Greenstick fracture are fractures in which one side of a bone is broken, the other being bent.
- Impacted fractures are fractures in which one fragment is firmly driven into the other.
- Slipped capital epiphysis fractures are separations of the ball of the hip joint from the femur at the upper growing end of the bone.
- Comminuted fractures are fractures in which there are multiple pieces.
- Linear fractures are fractures that are parallel to the bone's long axis.
- Transverse fractures are fractures that are at a right angle to the bone's long axis.
- Oblique fractures are fractures that are diagonal to a bone's long axis.
- Spiral fractures are fractures where at least one part of the bone has been twisted.

OPEN FRACTURES: The following terms indicate that the skin has been broken:

- Compound fractures are open fractures in which the skin is broken.
- Infected fractures are open fractures in which foreign bodies which gained access through the open wound have caused an infection.
- Missile, puncture, foreign body indicates fractures in which the skin has been broken by an external object.

The seventh character denotes if the fracture is open or closed for an initial encounter or if a subsequent encounter is for routine healing, delayed healing, nonunion, malunion, or sequelae. A malunion means the fracture did not heal together properly. A nonunion means the fracture did not heal together at all.

The fracture extensions are:

- A Initial encounter for closed fracture
- B Initial encounter for open fracture
- D Subsequent encounter for fracture with routine healing
- G Subsequent encounter for fracture with delayed healing
- K Subsequent encounter for fracture with nonunion
- S Sequelae

Subsequent is used for encounters after the patient has received active treatment of an injury whereas sequelae is used for complications or conditions that result from an injury such as scar tissue from a burn.

Like the ICD-9 codes, if there is no description of the fracture being open or closed, it is coded as closed. If the fracture is not described as displaced or nondisplaced, then it should be coded as displaced. In a displaced fracture, the two ends of the bone are separated from each other.

Do not use Z codes for aftercare of injuries as the aftercare for injuries is care provided during the healing process and the regular S or T code should be used for the injury itself.

PATHOLOGICAL FRACTURE: If a fracture is caused by a disease process, then the fracture is described as pathological and this term should be included in the selection of the proper codes which are not coded from these codes but rather from M84 codes.

DISLOCATIONS: While fractures and dislocations can be coded separately, when they occur together as an injury, i.e. fracture/dislocation, the fracture codes are now differentiated based on if there is a dislocation or not. Dislocations (also known as displacements or subluxation) should be coded when present if they are the only injury. A subluxation is a partial dislocation.

Dislocations are classified by anatomic sites and if they are open or closed. Dislocations can be either open or closed based also on the premise that there is a break in the skin which would be open. However, closed dislocations may be described as complete, NOS, simple, partial or uncomplicated. Open dislocations are described as compound, infected, or with foreign body. Dislocation of knees include tears of cartilage or meniscus which includes bucket handle tears. Dislocations of knees are also classified by area, i.e., anterior, posterior, medial or lateral.

Although similar to dislocations, derangements are a chronic condition in which the anatomic site has become disarranged and should be coded with musculoskeletal codes (M codes) because they are not traumatic injuries.

Section 27.3: SPRAINS/STRAINS

A sprain is an injury of the ligaments when they are stretched beyond their normal capacity and possibly torn. Whiplash is a sprain of the cervical spine. Strains are a similar injury to sprains, but they occur to muscles and tendons. Sprains and strains codes also include avulsions, hemarthrosis, laceration, rupture and tears of joint capsules, ligaments, muscles, and tendons. If these occur in an open wound, then this is coded as an open wound. Sprains and strains are classified by anatomic site and part, i.e., ligament, tendon, etc. Whiplash is coded as S13.4.

Section 27.4: SUPERFICIAL

Superficial injuries include abrasions, friction burns, blisters, insect bites, superficial foreign body, and others. An abrasion is superficial damage to the skin not extending beyond the epidermis and is not as severe as a laceration. An avulsion is a traumatic abrasion that removes all layers of skin. Blister is a pocket of fluid in the epidermis and dermis oftentimes caused by friction, burning, infection, freezing, and chemical exposure.

Superficial injuries do not include burns, contusions, foreign bodies, venomous insect bites, and open wound which are coded with T codes and will be discussed later. Superficial injuries are further classified by anatomic site and infected or not infected. Contusions with intact skin include bruising or hematoma without fracture or open wound.

Crushing injury are classified by anatomic site. Any additional injuries should also be coded, such as fracture, internal or intracranial injuries.

Section 27.5: OPEN WOUNDS

Open wounds are also known as lacerations. A wound is an injury to the soft tissue in conjunction with an interruption of the skin. Wounds may be described as incising, puncturing and penetrating. Penetrating indicates the passage of an object into or through the body. If there is an accumulation of blood in a body cavity due the wound, this is known as a hemothorax, hemopericardium, hemoperitoneum, or hemoarthrosis based on which cavity is involved. Open wounds include animal bites, avulsions, cut, laceration, punctures, amputations, and trauma.

Wounds are not coded if they are associated with a more serious injury, such as a fracture or internal injury.

A complicated wound is indicated as having delayed healing, delayed treatment, foreign body, or infection present. Infection of wounds is now coded as an additional code rather than included as part of the description of the wound as complicated.

Section 27.6: HEMORRHAGE/HEMATOMA

Hemorrhage is bleeding. Hematoma is a collection of blood outside the blood vessels, otherwise known as internal bleeding. A subdural hematoma occurs between the dura and the leptomeninges of the brain. Subarachnoid hematoma or hemorrhage occurs directly beneath the arachnoid.

Contusions are soft tissue injuries in which the skin is not broken but there is bleeding within which results in a hematoma. Hemorrhages and hematomas are specified according to the part of the brain involved, type of injury, and level of consciousness.

Section 27.7: VESSELS/NERVES

Traumatic injury to vessels and nerves are coded within each anatomic site. This includes avulsions, hematomas, laceration, rupture, fistula, and aneurysm. These codes are classified by the vessel and nerve involved. Remember that with the spinal cord, injuries are classified by the interspace between two vertebrae, i.e., C1-C3 is two interspaces, C1-C2 and C2-C3.

Section 27.8: HEAD/SKULL

Injuries to the head are coded as S00-S09. There should be an additional code listed if there is an infection also. This section also includes traumatic injuries to the eye, ear, nose, and lips. Any injuries to nerves or vessels should be coded in addition. Superficial foreign body injuries and bites by nonvenomous insects are coded in these sections. These types of injuries are included in each anatomic site within the injury codes

Superficial injuries of the head and all areas including eyes and ears are coded as S00. Open wounds of the head are coded as S01 which includes bites, puncture wounds, and lacerations.

A laceration (wound) is when there is a traumatic disruption of skin. A contusion is a closed wound and is more serious than a concussion as it is damage to the brain in the form of a bruise with bleeding.

Fractures of the skull (S02) are differentiated by anatomic site of the skull, and type of encounter. Additional codes (S06) should be coded if patient was unconscious. A blowout fracture is a fracture of the walls or floor of the orbit (eye socket) with fragments possibly pushed into the paranasal sinuses.

The section of codes (S06) for intracranial injuries do not include those with skull fractures which were coded with S02 codes. All intracranial injuries are classified by loss of consciousness within each type of traumatic injury. They are differentiated by the length of time the person experiences loss of consciousness, i.e., less than 30 minutes (S06.0X1) or 31 to 59 minutes (S06.0X2) and so forth for longer periods of time using S06 codes. Seventh digits indicate if it is initial encounter (A), subsequent encounter (D) or sequela (S).

A concussion is coded as S06.0. Edema of the brain caused by trauma is coded as S06.1. Other types of brain injury include diffuse, focal, contusions, lacerations, and hemorrhage and are highly differentiated by specific anatomic site.

Crushing injuries of the head are coded as S07 and include face and skull. Amputations are coded as S08. Injuries to blood vessels, tendons, and muscles of the head are coded as S09 and specific to anatomic site and laterality.

Section 27.9: NECK

Codes for the neck and trunk (S10 – S19) include the vertebrae. Superficial injuries and open wounds are coded as S10-S11. Spinal cord injuries should be coded additionally as well as infection.

As with most spinal cord codes (S12), the location of the fracture on the spinal column should be coded for cervical in this section. These codes are also further differentiated by whether the fracture is open or closed and displaced or nondisplaced. Remember to code as closed or displaced if type not known. If there is spinal cord injury, then the codes are differentiated by what part of the cord is involved, that is the anterior or central cord. The codes also distinguish if there is a lesion or not (lesion is damage or injury).

Dislocation and sprain of joints and ligaments are coded as S13. This includes avulsions, lacerations, sprains, hemoarthrosis, rupture, tear, and subluxation. These codes are differentiated by the two vertebrae involved and comprising the intervertebral space, such as C1-C2 which counts as one diagnosis.

Injuries of nerves and spinal cord in the neck area are coded as S14. This includes concussion, edema, lesions, cord syndrome, and injuries. Injuries of blood vessels are coded as S15 as differentiated by specific artery involved. Injury of muscles, fascia and tendons are coded as S16 which include strains and lacerations.

Crushing injuries of the neck area are coded as S17.

Section 27.10: THORAX

Pneumothorax is also known as a collapsed lung when air or gas is able to enter the pleural cavity due to trauma or disease. Hemothorax is when blood accumulates in the pleural cavity. Injuries to the thorax area (S20-S29) include superficial, contusions, blisters, abrasions, superficial bites, nonvenomous insect bites, and external constrictions. With open wounds (S21) any associated injury should be coded such as hemopneumothorax or fractures. Some of these codes are differentiated as to whether there was penetration into the thoracic cavity.

Fractures of the ribs, sternum, and thoracic spine are coded as S22. Again, if the type is not known, then fractures should be coded as closed and/or displaced. As with the cervical vertebrae, the specific vertebrae should be listed. Flail chest (S22.5) occurs when there are multiple fractures of the ribs and sternum which causes the chest to be unstable.

Dislocation and subluxation of joints and ligaments of the thorax, as well as injuries to nerves and spinal cord are coded as S23 and differentiated by intervertebral space, i.e. T1-T2. Injuries to blood vessels are coded as S25 and differentiated by vessel involved.

Injuries to the heart are coded as S26 and any hemothorax and/or pneumothorax should be coded additionally.

Injuries to other intrathoracic organs are coded as S27 including lungs, bronchus, thoracic part of the trachea and esophagus, pleura, and diaphragm.

Crushing chest injuries are coded as S28.0. Traumatic amputation of part of the thorax is coded as S28.2 and can include the breast.

Injuries to muscles and tendons are coded as S29.

Section 27.11: ABDOMEN/PELVIS/GENITALS

Injuries to the abdomen, lower back, lumbar spine, pelvis and external genitals are coded as S30-S39. These include blisters, contusions, external constriction, and superficial foreign body and bites by nonvenomous insects. Open wounds are coded as S31.

Injuries to the liver (S30) are classified based on the extent of the wound (minor, moderate or major) and if there is a hematoma and/or contusion. A laceration is considered minor if it extends less than 1 cm deep. A laceration is considered moderate if it extends to less than 3 cm deep but more than 1 cm. A laceration is considered major if it extends to more than 3 cm deep which significantly disrupts the parenchyma (functional parts of an organ).

Fracture of the lumbar spine and pelvis are coded as S32. They are differentiated by zones and types. Zone I is the most distal from the spinal cord and Zone III is the most proximal, central portion of the spinal cord. Types vary according to whether they are flexion or extension and with posterior or anterior displacement.

Dislocation and sprain of joints and ligaments of lumbar spine and pelvis are coded as S33 and include subluxation. Injury of lumbar and sacral spinal cord and nerves in the abdominal/pelvic area are coded as S34. All of these codes are differentiated by intervertebral segment involved which is denoted by the vertebrae involved such as L1-L2. Injuries of blood vessels in the abdominal/pelvic area are coded as S35.

Injury to internal organs in the abdominal area are coded as S36 and include spleen, gallbladder, bile ducts, pancreas, stomach, colon, rectum, and peritoneum. Codes for injury to the urinary and pelvic organs are coded with S37 codes and include the kidneys, ureter, ovary, bladder, urethra, fallopian tubes, uterus, and prostate.

Crushing injuries to abdominal/pelvic areas are coded as S38. Amputations are coded as S38.2. Injuries to muscle, fascia, and tendons are coded as S39.0.

Section 27.12: SHOULDER/UPPER ARM

Injuries of the shoulder and upper arm are coded as S40-S49. These include contusions, superficial foreign body, nonvenomous insect bites, wounds, laceration, dislocation, subluxation, sprain, and fractures. Injuries to the nerves are coded as S44 for the shoulder and S54 for the upper arm. Injury to blood vessels is coded as S45 for shoulder and S55 for the forearm. Injuries of muscles, fascia, and tendons are coded as S46 for the shoulder and S56. Crushing injuries are coded as S47 for the shoulder and S57 for the upper forearm. Amputations are coded as S48 for the shoulder and S58 for the upper forearm. Notice there are significantly more codes in these sections as they are very specific to exact anatomic sites and laterality.

Fractures of the forearm are coded as S52 and open fractures are differentiated by the Gustilo open fracture classification which is based on wound size, soft tissue contamination and damage, as well as if the fracture is comminuted or not.

Section 27.13: WRIST/HAND/FINGERS

Injuries to the wrist, hand and fingers are coded as S60-S69. As in the previous sections it includes codes for contusions, blisters, abrasion, nonvenomous insect bite, superficial foreign bodies, external constriction, open wound, amputation, fracture, dislocation, subluxation, traumatic rupture, crushing, and damage to nerves, vessels, tendons, muscles, fascia and tendons. The fracture codes also include the use of the Gustilo open fracture classification system.

Section 27.14: HIP/THIGH

Injuries to the hip and thigh are coded as S70-S79. As in the previous sections it includes codes for contusions, blisters, abrasion, nonvenomous insect bite, superficial foreign bodies, external constriction, open wound, amputation, fracture, dislocation, subluxation, traumatic rupture, crushing, and damage to nerves, vessels, tendons, muscles, fascia and tendons. The fracture codes also include the use of the Gustilo open fracture classification system.

Section 27.15: KNEE/LOWER LEG

Injuries to the knee and lower leg are coded as S80-S89. As in the previous sections it includes codes for contusions, blisters, abrasion, nonvenomous insect bite, superficial foreign bodies, external constriction, open wound, amputation, fracture, dislocation, subluxation, traumatic rupture, crushing, and damage to nerves, vessels, tendons, muscles, fascia and tendons. The fracture codes also include the use of the Gustilo open fracture classification system.

Section 27.16: ANKLE/FOOT/TOES

Injuries to the ankle, foot and toes are coded as S90-S99. As the previous sections it includes codes for contusions, blisters, abrasion, nonvenomous insect bite, superficial foreign bodies, external constriction, open wound, amputation, fracture, dislocation, subluxation, traumatic rupture, crushing, and damage to nerves, vessels, tendons, muscles, fascia and tendons. The fracture codes also include the use of the Gustilo open fracture classification system.

Section 717: INJURY, POISONING & OTHER

Injury to unspecified body regions are coded as T14 and include abrasions, contusions, fracture, and crushing. If there are multiple unspecified sites they are coded together as T07.

Section 27.18: FOREIGN BODY

Foreign bodies entering the body through a natural orifice are coded as T15-T19. T15 codes are for the eye, T16 for the ear, T17 for the respiratory tract, T18 for the alimentary tract (esophagus, stomach, intestine, colon, anus and rectum), and T19 for the genitourinary tract (urethra, bladder, vulva, vagina, uterus, and penis).

Section 27.19: BURNS

Burns are injury to the layers of the skin but can extend into other parts of the body, including muscles, bones, and blood vessels. Burns can occur due to many reasons, including chemical agents, trauma, radiation, and electrical currents.

DEGREES: Burns are classified by the extent of damage to the skin and underlying tissues.

- FIRST DEGREE: A first degree burn only involves the epidermis with no blisters.
- SECOND DEGREE: A second degree burn includes the epidermal and dermal layers (known as partial-thickness) of the skin and can include blistering and hyperesthesia.
- THIRD DEGREE: A third degree burn includes all layers of the skin with necrosis of the epidermis and dermis layers and damage to the subcutaneous layer.
- NECROSIS: Necrosis is the death of tissue which results from a serious burn.

If there are multiple degrees of burn at the one site, then the highest degree burn should be coded. A non-healing burn is coded as an acute burn. Necrosis is also considered a non-healing burn. If an infection is present, be sure to code it also. If the organism causing the infection is known, code that also.

LUND-BROWDER CHART: The Lund-Browder Chart is also known as the Rule of Nines which is the division of the parts of body into multiples of nine so that the percentage of the total body surface area burned can be determined. Percentages for an adult are: 9% for the head/neck (front and back), each arm 9%, each leg 18%, anterior trunk 18%, posterior trunk 18%, and genitalia 1%. With a child these percentages change because a child's head is bigger in comparison to their body with 17% for the head/neck (front and back), each arm 9%, each leg 13%, anterior trunk 18%, posterior trunk 18%, and genitalia 1%. For a child less than 10 kg, the total body surface area burned percentages are 20% for the head/neck (front and back), each arm 8%, each leg 16%, anterior trunk 16%, posterior trunk 16%, and genitalia 1%.

Injuries due to burns and corrosion are coded as T20-T32. These can occur due to electricity, flame, friction, hot air and gases, lightning, radiation and chemicals. Seventh characters are based on if the encounter is initial, subsequent, or if it is a sequela.

The external source of the burn, place and intent should also be coded using X00-X19, X75-X77, X96-X98, and Y92.

If the extent of the body surface burned is known, then codes T31 or T32 should also be listed.

Burns of unspecified degree are coded to specific anatomic sites. T20.0 are codes for burns of the head, face and neck. First degree burns of the head, face, and neck are coded as T20.1, second degree as T20.2, third degree as T20.3 and corrosion as T20.4. For the trunk, unspecified degree is coded as T21.0, first degree as T21.1, second as T21.1, third degree as T21.3, and corrosion as T21.4. Unspecified degrees of shoulder and arms (not including hands and wrist) are coded as T22.0, first degree as T22.1, second degree as T22.2, third degree as T22.3, and corrosion as T22.4. Unspecified degrees of wrist and hand are coded as T23.0, first degree as T23.1, second degree as T23.2, third degree as T23.3, and corrosion as T23.4. Unspecified degree burns of the leg except ankle and foot are coded as T24.0, first degree as T24.1, second degree as T24.2, third degree as T24.3, and corrosion as T24.4.

Burns of the eye and adnexa are coded as T26 and are differentiated by specific anatomic part of the eye and laterality and not degree. Burns of the respiratory tract are coded as T27 by specific anatomic site and laterality also and not degree.

PERCENTAGE: Extent of body surface burned is coded as T31 and is based on percentage of body burned. The fourth character indicates the percentage of total body surface burned including all degrees. The fifth character indicates the percentage of body surface that was third degree burns.

Section 27.20: FROSTBITE

Frostbite is coded as T33-T34. It is differentiated by anatomic site, laterality, and if it is superficial or involving necrosis of tissue.

Section 27.21: POISONINGS/ADVERSE EFFECTS

Poisonings, adverse effect and underdosing are now included together in one code so no additional codes are needed. Poisonings are differentiated as accidental, intentional self-harm, assault, undetermined, or underdosing. They are coded as T36-T50 and are specific to drug, medicaments or biological substances involved. If the intent in the taking of the substance is not known, then it should be coded as accidental.

POISONING: Poisoning and underdosing codes are differentiated by the same methods as in the ICD-9, i.e. if the substance was taken as a poisoning or if it was taken properly but the patient suffered an adverse effect.

A poisoning occurs when a toxic substance, such as drugs or chemicals, is swallowed, inhaled, or comes in contact with the skin, eyes, or mucous membranes, resulting in harmful effects but the substance was not taken according to a physician's recommendations. Poisonings can occur due to numerous reasons:

- First, the patient may have chosen to overdose, possibly in an attempt to commit suicide.
- Second, the patient may have taken another person's prescriptions.
- Third, a wrong dosage may have been given erroneously by medical care personnel.
- Fourth, someone may have provided the substance to a person for the reasons of murder.
- Fifth, the patient may have mixed up medications, whether their own or someone else's.
- Sixth, the patient may have taken a prescription drug in combination with alcohol as alcohol with any prescription is not in accordance with medical advice.

- Seventh, the patient may have taken a prescription with an over-the-counter which they did not tell the physician they were taking, and the combination has detrimental effects.
- Eighth, the patient may have taken the wrong amount.
- Ninth, wrong dosage given by a non-medical person.

ADVERSE EFFECT: An adverse effect is when a patient takes a substance, such as drugs, in accordance with doctor's orders, but the patient still experiences a harmful reaction. Adverse effects can occur due to numerous reasons.

- First, this include toxicity wherein the patient took the substance or drug as recommended but for various reasons it was too strong for the person and caused an adverse effect. This may be due to an inappropriate level prescribed for the patient or the occurrence of a cumulative effect in which previous drugs or substances compounded the strength of the substance.
- Second, the patient may have suffered a hypersensitivity, allergic reaction, to the substance.
- Third, a synergistic effect may have occurred in which one substance heightens the effect of another substance.
- Fourth, one substance may interact inappropriately with another substance.
- Fifth, various side effects are always associated with substances.

UNDERDOSING: Underdosing occurs when a person takes less of a medication than prescribed or instructed by manufacturer or healthcare provider. Additional codes should be provided for all manifestations and for intent such as failure in dosage during medical care (Y63.61, Y63.8-Y63.9) and patient's underdosing of medication regime (Z91.12, Z91.13).

TABLE OF DRUGS AND CHEMICALS: The Table of Drugs and Chemicals follows the Alphabetical Index and Neoplasm Table. It is known as Alphabetical Index to Poisoning and External Causes of Adverse Effects of Drugs and Chemical Substances. It is broken into columns for poisonings, underdosing, and adverse effects with T codes. It contains a listing of drugs and chemicals with categories based on their means of introduction into the body. The headings are: Poisoning Accidental, Poisoning Intentional, Poisoning Assault, Poisoning Undetermined, Adverse effect and Underdosing.

This table lists various substances that can adversely affect someone, including legal and illegal drugs, toxins, cleaning supplies, poisons, chemicals, prescriptions, environmental toxins, etc.

The substances are listed by generic and brand names, but not all brand names are listed. In such a case when the brand name cannot be found, generic name must be used. Generic names are the scientific names for the drugs and the brand names are the names provided by manufacturers to distinguish their product from other manufacturers' products. The first letter of a brand name drug is capitalized, but not for a generic name.

There are several ways to find the generic name for a brand name drug that is not listed.

- First, if you know the generic name is ibuprofen for the brand name Advil, then you can look for ibuprofen in the Table of Drugs and Chemicals.

- Second, if you do not know the generic name, you can search for it in Appendix C which is the Classification of Drugs by AHFS List.
- Third, and perhaps an easier way, is to find the brand name in a drug book, such as the PDR, or search for it on the internet and the generic will be listed there.

CODING FOR ADVERSE EFFECTS: Adverse effect scenarios are only used when the patient has taken the substance in accordance with medical advice and experienced side effects. . When a patient has taken a substance properly and in accordance with medical advice, yet they experienced an adverse effect, then the adverse effect is listed first (such as gastritis) which is a regular code. Then the T code for the drug would be listed. Code as many substances involved.

CODING FOR POISONINGS: For coding of poisonings, the poisoning code should be listed first. Remember, you will provide codes for each substance involved. There are several coding scenarios for poisonings:

- First, a condition may be described as well as the substance causing the poisoning. In this case, the condition is listed first and then the poisoning code.
- Second, a condition may be present in addition to a prescription drug, but the person may have ingested over-the-counter drugs without informing the physician; therefore, this is against medical advice and so a poisoning code is assigned to each substance. Be sure to code the over-the-counter drug as well.
- Third, a condition may be present in addition to a prescription drug as well as alcohol which is always against medical advice and so this should be coded as a poisoning for both the prescription and the alcohol.

Poisoning codes include T36-T50. The various codes are differentiated by type of drugs, medicaments and biological substance. T36 is to be used for poisonings involving antibiotics. Poisonings by hormones is coded as T38. Poisonings by narcotics is coded as T40. Poisonings by anesthetics is coded as T41. Poisonings by agents affecting the gastrointestinal system are coded as T47.

CODING FOR UNDERDOSING: Under-dosing is described as taking less of a medication than is prescribed by physician either purposely or by mistake. Intent of the underdosing should be also be coded such as failure in dosage during medical care (Y63.61) or patient's underdosing (Z91.12).

Section 27.22: TOXIC EFFECTS

Codes for toxic effects due to a substance include T51 to T65. T51 is for toxic effect of alcohol. Toxic effects of corrosive substances is coded as T54. Toxic effects of soap and detergents is coded as T55. Toxic effects of metals is coded as T56. Toxic effects of gases and fumes is coded as T59. Toxic effects from contact with venomous animals and plants is coded as T63.

Section 27.23: OTHER/UNSPECIFIED EFFECTS OF EXTERNAL CAUSES

Other and unspecified effects of external causes is coded as T66-T78. This includes radiation sickness (T66) and effects from heat and light (T67) which includes heat syncope, heat cramps, sunstroke, and heat exhaustion. Hypothermia is coded as T68. Effects from differences in air and water pressure (T70) includes barotrauma, anoxia due to high altitude, and Caisson disease (decompression sickness). Barotrauma are conditions that occur due to rapid changes in atmospheric pressure, such as otitis and aerosinusitis.

Note that there are many exceptions in these codes.

Asphyxiation is coded as T71 but, again, there are many exceptions. Asphyxiation can be due to plastic bags, smothered by a pillow, trapped in bed linens, smothered by another person's body, hanging or trapped in something such as a car or refrigerator.

Other deprivations are coded as T73 and include starvation, deprivation of water, and exhaustion due to excessive exertion.

Confirmed abuse and neglect of children and adults are coded as T74 including abandonment, physical or mental abuse, sexual abuse, and shaken infant syndrome. Suspected abuse is coded as T76.

Other effects from external causes include effects of lightning (T75.0), effects from vibration (T75.2), motion sickness (T75.3), and electrocution (T75.4).

Anaphylactic shock due to reaction to food is coded as T78.0. Other allergic responses such as allergic shock and anaphylaxis are coded from other T78 codes. Anaphylactic shock is the most severe type of anaphylaxis which is the body's allergic response which causes a sudden drop in the blood pressure, edema, difficulty breathing, and possibly death.

Section 27.24: EARLY COMPLICATIONS OF TRAUMA NEC

Early complications from trauma NEC are coded as T79. This includes air and fat embolism, hemorrhage, traumatic shock, anuria, ischemia and emphysema. Traumatic compartment syndrome (T79.A) occurs when there is increased pressure within an anatomic site, usually due to inflammation, that has been confined due to injury, surgery, or other medical condition.

Section 27.25: COMPLICATIONS OF MEDICAL OR SURGICAL CARE

Codes T80-T88 indicate complications of medical or surgical care with an extensive exclude note at the beginning since many of these complications are now coded under the codes for each anatomic system. These codes include complications following infusion, transfusions and injections (T80). Air embolisms following infusions, transfusions and injections are coded as T80.0 and infections as T80.2. Blood and Rh incompatibility are coded as T80.3.

Postprocedural shock is coded as T81.1. Disruption of wounds are coded as T81.3. Infection following a procedure is coded as T81.4. A foreign body left in the body after a procedure is coded as T81.5. T81.51 are for adhesion complications. Other complications from foreign bodies left in the body include perforation and obstruction. T82-T85 are for complications due to mechanical devices and implants, e.g. displacement of breast prosthesis and implant (T85.42).

INJURIES QUIZ 20

1) What are the codes for a patient who is diagnosed with pneumothorax due to gunshot wound?

2) What are the codes for a patient who is diagnosed with a laceration of the right patella with dislocation?

3) What are the codes for a patient who is diagnosed with a third degree burn of the chest area?

4) What are the codes for a patient who is diagnosed with comminuted fracture of the shaft of the left humerus with dislocation?

5) What are the codes for a patient who is diagnosed with pneumothorax due to stab wound in the chest?

6) What are the codes for a patient who is diagnosed with swelling of right thumb due to a non-venomous spider bite?

7) What are the codes for a patient who is diagnosed with a sprain of the lateral medial collateral ligament of the right knee?

8) What are the codes for a patient who is diagnosed with swelling and fever due to rattlesnake bite on her right ankle?

9) What are the codes for a patient who is diagnosed with second degree burns of the upper right arm?

10) What are the codes for a patient who is diagnosed with a pathological fracture of the femur?

11) What are the codes for a patient who is diagnosed with frostbite with necrosis of the right ear?

12) What are the codes for a patient who is diagnosed with a sprain of the posterior cruciate ligament of the left knee?

13) What are the codes for a patient who is diagnosed with crushing injury of the left lower leg and foot?

14) What are the codes for a small child who was seen for a bean in his right ear?

CHAPTER 28
ICD-10 EXTERNAL CAUSE CODES

You will learn the following objectives in this chapter:

A. Alphabetical Index
B. Transport Accident
C. Accidents
D. Exposure to Inanimate Mechanical Devices
E. Exposure to Animate Mechanical Devices
F. Nontransport Drowning
G. Exposure to Electrical Current/Radiation
H. Exposure to Fire/Hot Substances
I. Exposure to Forces of Nature
J. Harm
K. Medical Complications
L. Supplementary Factors

Chapter 20 are the former E codes and are described as "External Causes of Morbidity" and ranges from V00-Y99. As previously noted, poisoning and adverse effects from substances are no longer included in these codes but are coded in the previously discussed injury section. E codes answer the questions, how, why and where an injury or condition occurred. External causes (E codes) include codes for "environmental events, circumstances, and conditions as the cause of injury, poisoning, and other adverse effects".

Section 28.1: ALPHABETICAL INDEX

External cause codes are not found in the Alphabetical Index for the regular codes but rather have their own alphabetical index which follows the Drugs and Chemical Table.

Section 28.2: TRANSPORT ACCIDENT

Transport accident codes include V00-V99. Definitions of all types of transport vehicles are provided in this section.

Transport accident is "any accident involving a device designed primarily for, or being used at the time primarily for, conveying persons or goods from one place to another".

Farm and construction machines are considered to be machinery unless they were on a highway and used for transportation, not work.

A device which can travel by more than one means, such as water and highways, is coded with regards to where it was being used at the time of the accident, so if it was being used on a highway then it is considered a motor vehicle.

When people are injured by a transport device that is being used for purposes other than transportation, then it would not be coded as a transport accident, such as maintenance work, other injuries unrelated to transport (such as a fight on a plane), industrial work, and sports when the device was not involved in the injury.

Pedestrians injured by a transport device are coded as V00 which includes roller-skating, skateboarding, scooter, ice skates, sleds, snowboarding, skiing, wheelchair, and baby stroller. Injuries sustained by a pedestrian by a pedal bicycle are coded as V01. Pedestrian injury caused by a two- or three-wheeled motor vehicle are coded as V02 which includes various modes of transportation by the pedestrian at the time such as walking, roller skates and skateboarding.

Pedestrian injured in a collision with a car, truck or van is coded as V03 with reference to pedestrian's mode of transportation such as walking, roller skates or skateboarding.

Pedestrian injured in collision with a train is coded as V05. Pedestrian injured in collision with other non-motor vehicle such as animal-drawn vehicle is coded as V06.

Injuries sustained by a person on a pedal bicycle is similar to the pedestrian codes as differentiated by what object the bicyclist collided with (V10-V19). Motorcycle riders sustaining injuries are differentiated by what object the rider collided with such as animal or car (V20-V29).

Injuries sustained by an occupant (driver or passenger) in a three-wheeled motor vehicle are differentiated in the same manner as the previous codes as to what it collided with (V30-V39). Codes for occupants in a car, truck or van are coded in the same manner according to what the car collided with (V40-V59). If the vehicle is a heavy transport vehicle, then the codes are V60-V69. Occupants of buses involved in an accident are coded in the same manner (V70-V79). Other means of transport are coded as V80-V89 and include animal-riders, train, streetcar, industrial vehicle, agricultural vehicle, and off-road vehicles.

Injuries sustained during an accident involving a water transport vehicle (V90-V94) include drowning, crushing, burn, falling, struck, and submersion while on various vehicles such as a boat or ship. Injuries sustained from an accident involving an air and space transport vehicle (V95-V97) include helicopters, gliders, private or commercial planes, and spacecraft.

Section 28.3: ACCIDENTS

Accidental falls, tripping, slipping, and stumbling (W00-S19) are classified by how the patient fell, such as from stairs or ladder, if it was from one level to another or not, and if there were other factors involved. This includes falls due to icy conditions or from objects such as chairs, bed, tree, cliff, and playground equipment. Codes are also differentiated by falls into certain places such as a swimming pool, well, dock, and bathtub. These codes are much more detailed than they were in the ICD-9 codes.

Section 28.4: EXPOSURE TO INANIMATE MECHANICAL FORCES

Exposure to inanimate mechanical forces (W20-W49) include being struck or thrown from an object such as piece of machinery or sports equipment. Being caught, crushed or jammed between objects is coded as W23.

Injuries sustained by contact with glass is coded as W25. Contact with tools is differentiated by whether they are powered or not (W27). Injuries caused by accidental discharge of guns is coded as W32 to w33.

Injuries caused by explosions (W35-W40) can be caused by rupture of a boiler or pressurized pipe or hose. It can also occur due to fireworks, blasting materials and explosive gases. Exposure to loud noises are coded as W42.

Foreign body or object entering through the skin is coded as W45 and is differentiated by what the foreign body or object was, such as paper or nail. Contact with needles is coded as W46.

Section 28.5: EXPOSURE TO ANIMATE MECHANICAL FORCES

Exposure to animate mechanical forces (W50-W64) include being hit, struck, kicked, bitten, twisted, scratched, crushed, pushed, or stepped on by another person. Contact with rodents is coded as W53 including mice, rats, and squirrels. Being bitten or struck by a dog is coded as W54. Contact with other animals (W55) include cats, horses, cows, and pigs. Contact with marine animals (W56) includes dolphins, whales, or sharks. Contact with crocodiles or alligators is coded as W58. Contact with nonvenomous reptiles is coded as W59. Contact with birds is coded as W61.

Section 28.6: NON-TRANSPORT DROWNING

Non-transport drownings (W65-W74) include while in bath-tub, pool, or lake.

Section 28.7: EXPOSURE TO ELECTRICAL CURRENT/RADIATION

Exposure to electrical current, radiation and extreme ambient air temperature and pressure (W85-W99) include exposure to electric transmission lines or current, radiation, UV light, lasers, excessive cold or heat, and excessive air pressure changes.

Section 28.8: EXPOSURE TO FIRE/HOT SUBSTANCES

Accidents due to fire and flames (X00-X08) include fires, smoke, explosion, fumes, and burns occurring in different types of structures and on clothing. Contact with heat and hot substances (X10-X19) include hot drinks, fats, water, gases, appliances, tools, and metals.

Section 28.9: EXPOSURE TO FORCES OF NATURE

Exposure to forces of nature (X30-X39) include cold, sunlight, earthquake, volcanoes, hurricanes, blizzards, dust storms, tidal waves, and floods. Exposures to other specified factors (X52, X58) include being in a weightless environment.

Section 28.10: HARM

Various types of harm by various means include intentional self-harm (X71-X83), assault by someone else (X92-Y08), terrorism, wars and military operations (Y35-Y38). These codes have been greatly expanded to include many reasons and involvement within these codes.

Section 28.11: MEDICAL COMPLICATIONS

Complications due to medical and surgical care that are not coded elsewhere are coded as Y62 to Y84. Misadventures to patients during surgical and medical care (Y62-Y69) include failure to properly sterilize, wrong dosage of drugs, contaminated medical substances, and non-administration of surgical and medical care. Complications with medical devices (Y70-Y82) include devices involved with anesthetic, cardiovascular, otorhinolaryngological, gastroenterology, neurological, obstetric, gynecological, ophthalmic, radiological, and orthopedic procedures. Abnormal reactions by patients to healthcare (Y83-Y84) include responses that did not occur at the time of the procedure and include amputation and removal of organs or body parts, cardiac catheterization, dialysis, radiological, and aspiration of fluids.

Section 28.12: SUPPLEMENTARY FACTORS

Supplementary factors related to cause of morbidity classified elsewhere (Y90-Y99) include blood alcohol level (Y90), place of occurrence (Y92), activity codes (Y93) which include swimming, ice skating, climbing, and baseball. External cause status (Y99) include status as a civilian, military, or volunteer.

LATE EFFECTS/POISONINGS QUIZ 21

1) What is the code for a patient with an embolism due to their pacemaker?

2) What is the code for a patient with gastritis after ingesting Percodan with alcohol and OTC antihistamines?

3) What is the code for a patient with scar tissue due to a second and third degree burn on both legs six months ago?

4) What is the code for a patient with dislocation of an artificial hip joint?

5) What is the code for a patient with CMV infection due to transplanted liver?

6) What is the code for a patient with joint pain of the knees from rickets a year ago?

7) What is the code for a patient with a pressure ulcer with necrosis from her cast of the left lower leg due to a fractured upper tibia?

8) What is the code for a patient with esophageal reflux due to ingestion of drain cleaner as an attempted suicide?

9) What is the code for a patient with failure of skin graft of the left upper arm sustained after a burn six months ago when boiling water fell on her?

10) What is the code for a right-handed patient with hemiparesis of the left side due to a CVA four months ago?

11) What is the code for a patient with mental retardation due to viral encephalitis more than 5 years ago?

12) What is the code for a patient with ataxia due to alcohol and carbamazepine?

13) What is the code for a patient with an infection and pain due to his peritoneal dialysis catheter?

14) What is the code for a patient with sequelae from a gunshot wound of the right leg a month ago?

15) What is the code for a patient with dihescence of a mastectomy wound a week ago with infection?

CHAPTER 29
FACTORS INFLUENCING HEALTH STATUS AND CONTACT

You will learn the following objectives in this chapter:

A. Medical Necessity
B. Sequencing
C. Alphabetical Index
D. Examinations
E. Retained Foreign Body
F. Communicable Diseases
G. Reproduction
    1. Contraception
    2. Procreative
    3. Pregnancy
    4. Outcome of Delivery
    5. Liveborn
H. Prophylactic Care
I. Artificial Openings
J. Aftercare
K. Donors
L. Procedures Not Completed
M. Living Conditions
N. Blood Type
O. Body Mass
P. Other Circumstances
Q. History
R. Status
S. Dependence on Machines

Chapter 21 are the former V codes and are described as "Factors Influencing Health Status and Contact with the Health Services" and range from Z00-Z99. There are three conditions under which a V code may be applied:

(1) When a person who is not currently sick encounters the health services for some specific purposes.
(2) When a person with a known disease or injury, whether it is current or resolving, encounters the health care system for a specific treatment of that disease or injury.
(3) When some circumstance or problem is present which influences the person's health status but is not in itself a current illness or injury.

Section 29.1: MEDICAL NECESSITY

Because of the nature of the Z codes, they provide ICD-10 documentation of the necessity of services provided either because there is no documented diagnosis or symptom which can be coded or as supplementation to other codes to ensure that reimbursement will be provided.

Section 29.2: SEQUENCING

Most Z codes are secondary codes and should be listed second to the codes for the diagnosis or symptoms. There are some exceptions, however, when Z codes would be listed first. These exceptions are based on when the Z code describes the main reason for the healthcare visit, such as therapy codes. For example, a patient may have carcinoma and is being seen for chemotherapy. The coding guidelines in the front of the coding book outlines these issues of sequencing.

Section 29.3: ALPHABETICAL INDEX

Finding the Z codes in the alphabetical index can be challenging because they are listed under a large number of general terms including:

Admission
Aftercare
Attention to
Boarder
Care
Carrier
Checking
Contact
Contraception
Convalescence
Counseling
Delivery outcome
Dependence
Donor
Encounter
Examination
Exposure
Family history
Fitting
Follow-up
Maintenance
Maladjustment
Observation
Personal history
Problem
Prophylactic
Replacement
Screening
Status
Supervision
Transplant

For this reason, it is recommended that you familiarize yourself with the contents of the Z code section to see what types of categories are listed. If you are familiar with the sections you will be able to find codes in the tabular Z listings rather than in the alphabetical index.

Section 29.4: EXAMINATIONS

Patients are seen by healthcare providers for a wide variety of examinations which are coded as Z00-Z13. Z00 is for visits in which the patient had no complaint or suspected diagnosis. Z00.0 is for a general adult exam, otherwise known as a well check.

A well check for a child is also now included in this same area of codes which is Z00.1 and is differentiated by age of the child. Newborns are up to 28 days and are coded as Z00.11-. For older children codes Z00.12 are used who are over 28 days of age. One code is used to indicate abnormal findings and another indicates without abnormal findings. Visit for a child experiencing rapid growth is coded as Z00.2. Delayed growth is coded as Z00.7 codes.

Examination and encounters for someone who may be a possible donor is coded as Z00.5. Exams for other reasons, such as for vision, hearing, dental, and blood pressure are coded with Z01 codes. Gynecological exams are coded as Z01.4 including a PAP test. Encounters to test patients prior to a surgical procedure (pre-procedural) are coded as Z01.8. Encounters for other reasons, such as admission to schools, armed forces, jobs, paternity testing, and blood-alcohol levels are coded with Z02 codes.

Encounters for observation are coded as Z03. Encounters for suspected maternal and fetal conditions that are eventually ruled out after testing and examination are coded with Z03 codes.

Examinations and encounters following transports or work accidents are coded with Z04 codes as well as for alleged rape, alleged physical abuse, and psychiatric evaluation.

Follow-up codes are now described as "Encounter for follow-up examination after completed treatment for malignant neoplasm" which is much clearer than it was in the ICD-9 codes. Codes Z08 are for follow-up after completed treatment for neoplasm. For follow-up of other conditions that are not related to neoplasm, code Z09 should be used.

Exams and encounters for screening for infectious and parasitic diseases are coded with codes Z11. Encounters for screening for malignant neoplasms are coded with codes Z12. Encounters for screening of other diseases (Z13) include blood disorders, diabetes mellitus, developmental disorders, metabolic, genetic, eyes and ears, cardiovascular, and other anatomic sites.

Genetic carriers and genetic susceptibility to diseases (Z14-Z15) include hemophilia A (asymptomatic or symptomatic), and cystic fibrosis.

Resistance to antimicrobial drugs (Z16) include resistance to antibiotics which are specifically listed by drug name, and antimicrobial drugs.

Estrogen receptor status (Z17) is differentiated as to negative or positive status.

Section 29.5: RETAINED FOREIGN BODY

The presence of a foreign body can be coded from various sections including S and T. However, if a foreign body remains in the body it is coded as Z18. This can include fragments that are radioactive, metal, plastic, organic such as a tooth or wood or other such as glass or stones.

Section 29.6: COMMUNICABLE DISEASES

If a person has been exposed and it has been confirmed that the organism is present in their system but they are not exhibiting symptoms, then they are carriers or suspected carriers. Patients with potential health hazards related to communicable diseases (Z20-Z28) include contact and possible exposure to communicable diseases is coded by anatomic site or type such as intestinal infectious diseases (Z20.0) and rabies (Z20.3).

Patients diagnosed as being asymptomatic with HIV are coded as Z21. HIV positive NOS is also included in these codes. B20 is used if the patient tested positive for the virus and has displayed symptoms related to it, otherwise known as AIDS which is the disease process. Z21 indicates that the patient tested positive but has not displayed any symptoms related to HIV and, therefore, does not have AIDS.

If a patient seeks healthcare to receive vaccinations or inoculations, then these are coded as Z23. These can be for single vaccinations or combinations. If they are provided during a well check for a child, the well check should be listed first.

If immunizations are not completed which can be for a variety of reasons, it would be coded with Z28 codes. Reasons for immunizations not being done or patient not receiving a full regimen for a vaccination include when it is contraindicated due to illness in the patient, allergic reaction, patient refusal, patient had the disease, or patient not returning.

Section 29.7: REPRODUCTION

Codes Z30 to Z39 include Persons Encountering Health Services in Circumstances Related to Reproduction and Development.

CONTRACEPTION: Contraceptive measures, such as devices, counseling, prescriptions, and surveillance of contraceptive measures are coded in this category of codes (Z30.0). Prescriptions such as for contraceptive pills, injectable and intrauterine are coded as Z30.01 codes. Counseling for instruction on their use is coded as Z30.018 and Z30.09. If a patient is being observed due to their contraception it is coded as Z30.4.

Encounter for an actual sterilization procedure is coded as Z30.2. For reversal of a sterilization procedure, code Z31 should be used.

PROCREATIVE MANAGEMENT: Procreative investigation and testing (Z31.0) includes healthcare services relating to infertility and aftercare of contraception such as reversal of sterilization. Counseling for procreation is coded as Z31.6 and Z31.8 codes.

PREGNANCY: Codes Z32 are for encounters for pregnancy testing or childbirth or childcare instruction. Z33 codes indicate if the patient is pregnant. Incidental pregnancy is coded as Z33.1 which is used when a pregnant patient is receiving medical care but the care is not related to the pregnancy such as a fracture. Two codes would need to be coded in this instance, the fracture and Z33.1.

Codes Z33.2 are used if the patient elects to terminate their pregnancy. Other codes for supervision of a normal pregnancy are Z34. These codes are divided by trimester and if this is the first pregnancy or not. The number of weeks of gestation (pregnancy) are coded as Z3A for each week from less than 10 weeks up to more than 42 weeks.

Postpartum care for the mother is coded as Z39.

OUTCOME OF DELIVERY: We discussed Z37.0 in an earlier chapter which referred to outcome of delivery when coding for the mother as the patient. This code is only used for the hospital visit for the mother in which delivery occurred to indicate the outcome of the birth and should be coded in addition to the pregnancy codes previously discussed earlier. These codes are differentiated by stillborn or liveborn and number of children. Complications of pregnancy should be coded first and outcome of delivery after.

Supervision of high risk pregnancies are now coded as O09 codes and are not included in this chapter. As a reminder, high-risk pregnancies include conditions that may increase the risk to the pregnancy, such as history of infertility, history of previous abortions, multiparity, insufficient prenatal care, and preterm labor. These codes may also include elderly primigravida (first pregnancy in a woman over 35), elderly multigravida (second or later pregnancy in an older woman over age 35), young primigravida (first pregnancy in a female less than 16 years of age), and young multigravida (second or later pregnancy in a female younger than 16 years of age).

LIVEBORN BIRTHS: Codes Z38 describe Liveborn Infants According to place of birth and type of delivery. These are codes used in the newborn's chart, not the mother's chart, in reference to the type of birth which includes a single birth or part of a multiparous birth and liveborn or stillborn. Deliveries include vaginally or cesarean. There are also codes if the baby is born outside of the hospital.

This code should always be listed FIRST and is only listed for the visit in which delivery occurred. If the newborn is transferred after birth to another hospital, even if it is on the same day, these codes would not be used at the hospital to which the newborn is transferred as delivery did not occur at the other hospital.

Section 29.8: PROPHYLACTIC CARE

Z40-Z53 codes are used to code for patients who are receiving aftercare or prophylactic care, or care to consolidate the treatment or to deal with a residual state after having previously received treatment for specific conditions. Prophylactic measures are treatments aimed at preventing a disease. Encounters for removal of parts of the body due to malignant neoplasms are coded with Z40.0 codes.

Codes for procedures performed for reasons other than remedying a health condition are coded as Z41 and include cosmetic surgery, circumcision, and ear piercing. Reconstructive and plastic surgery are coded with Z42 codes such as for breast reconstruction.

Section 29.9: ARTIFICIAL OPENINGS

Codes Z43-Z46 are for medical care provided for prosthetic devices. Codes Z43 are for various services provided for artificial openings which include tracheostomy, gastrostomy, colostomy and ileostomy. Care includes closure of openings, removal of catheter, or cleansing.

Fitting and adjustment of external prosthetic devices (Z44) can be provided for artificial arms, legs, eyes, and breast. These codes are differentiated by laterality and if the device was partial or complete.

Adjustment and management of implanted devices (Z45) include removal or replacement of implanted devices such as cardiac pacemakers, defibrillator, infusion pump, visual, hearing, VAD (vascular access device), neuropacemaker, breast implant, and myringotomies.

Fitting and adjustment of other devices (Z46) include spectacles, contact lenses, hearing aids, dental, orthodontic, and insulin pump.

Artificial opening status (Z93) indicate the presence of a surgical opening, not the actual operation to create one. Artificial openings include tracheostomy, colostomy and cystostomy.

Section 29.10: AFTERCARE

Orthopedic aftercare (Z47) are provided for removal of internal fixation devices and joint replacements.

Other postprocedural aftercare (Z48) include attention to dressings, sutures, and drains such as changing or removal.

Aftercare visits following organ transplants (Z48.2) include for heart, kidney, liver, lung or multiple organs.

Encounter for renal dialysis (Z49) is differentiated by what type of care is provided, whether preparatory or adequacy testing. ESRD (end stage renal dialysis) should also be coded (N18.6).

Encounters for antineoplastic aftercare such as radiation therapy is coded as Z51.0, Z51.1 for chemotherapy and immunotherapy, Z51.5 for palliative care and Z51.81 for therapeutic drug level monitoring.

Section 29.11: DONORS

Codes for people who donate blood are Z52.0. Skin donors are coded as Z52.1, bone as Z52.2, bone marrow as Z52.3, kidney as Z52.4, and liver as Z52.6. Donation of eggs for procreation are coded with A52.81 codes and differentiated by type of donor (anonymous or designated) and age of donor (over or under age 35). If a patient received a donated organ in the past but is not currently undergoing a procedure to implant a donated organ, this is known as status post transplanted organ and is coded as Z94.

Section 29.12: PROCEDURES NOT COMPLETED

Procedures or treatment may not be completed for various reasons (Z53) such as patient elects not to or other contraindications.

Section 29.13: LIVING CONDITIONS

Living conditions should also be reported when they may affect the management or outcome of the patient's care utilizing codes Z55-Z65. Problems related to education and literacy (Z55) include illiteracy, school failure, and discord with teachers. Problems related to employment (Z56) include unemployment, change of job, threat of job loss, stress at work, or hostile work place. Exposure to occupational risks (Z57) include noise, radiation, dust, smoke, toxic agents, extreme temperatures, and vibrations.

Problems relating to housing (Z59) include homelessness, poor surroundings, neighbor difficulties, lack of adequate food and safe drinking, poverty, loan foreclosure and creditor problems. Problems within the social environment (Z60) include empty nest syndrome, social exclusion, living alone, discrimination and migration. Problems with upbringing (Z62) include negative life events in childhood such as inadequate parental supervision or overprotection, living in foster homes, scapegoating of child, and inappropriate parental pressure. It also includes history of physical, sexual and psychological abuse. Parent-child conflict, neglect, and estrangement are also included.

Other family difficulties (Z63) include problems with spouse or partner or in-laws, military deployment or other parental absences, divorce, death of family members, alcoholism, and drugs. Psychosocial circumstances (Z64) include unwanted pregnancy, multiparity problems, problems with counselors, criminal convictions, incarceration, victim of crime, and exposure to disasters or war.

Do not resuscitate status (DNR) is coded as Z66.

Section 29.14: BLOOD TYPE

Blood types are coded as Z67 for all types, A, B, AB and O and differentiated as to Rh being negative or positive.

Section 29.15: BODY MASS

Body mass index (Z68) varies by patient's weight in kilograms for adults and percentile for children (Z68.5).

Section 29.16: OTHER CIRCUMSTANCES

Other circumstances (Z69-Z76) include encounters for mental health for child abuse (Z69.0). Abuse by spouse or partner is coded as Z69.1. For other abuse, code Z69.8 is used. Counseling related to sexual issues (Z70) include concerns about impotence, promiscuity, and sexual orientation.

Worried well is coded as Z71.1 which means the patient had good reason for concern regarding their health and so they received medical examination. Dietary counseling and surveillance is coded as Z71.3. Counseling for issues with alcohol is coded as Z71.4, for drugs as Z71.5, tobacco Z71.6, and HIV as Z71.7.

Problems related to lifestyle (Z72) include tobacco use, lack of physical exercise, inappropriate eating habits, high risk sexual behavior, gambling Z72.6, antisocial behavior as Z72.81, and problems sleeping Z72.82. Problems related to life management include burn out (Z73.0), lack of leisure (Z73.2, stress (Z73.3), different types of insomnia (Z73.81), reduced mobility (Z74.0, and need for assistance in the home (Z74.2).

Issues relating to medical facilities include patient waiting for admission to facility, unavailability of help, and holiday relief care (Z75). Malingerer (Z76.5) is someone who feigns illness.

Section 29.17: HISTORY

There are two types of histories that can be coded and are important in the provision of healthcare services which are personal and family histories (Z77-Z99). Do NOT confuse the two when selecting codes. History indicates that the condition no longer exists so do not code a personal history for a condition for which a patient is still being treated.

Histories include cancer, mental disorders, diseases, fractures, congenital malformations, allergies, surgeries, poisonings, injuries, and conditions of the circulatory, urinary, digestive, genital, skin, or other system including nutritional deficiencies. These codes also include history of drug, tobacco, or alcohol abuse and exposure to toxic substances such as asbestos and lead.

There are codes for exposure to substances (Z77) such as hazardous chemicals such as arsenic and lead, environment hazards such as mold, or bodily fluids from someone else that may be hazardous such as a person who has HIV.

Z79 codes are for long term drug therapy which are currently being taken such as anticoagulants, insulin, antibiotics, and steroids.

Allergic reactions to drugs such as penicillin are coded as Z88. Food allergies are coded as Z91 for various food items, insects, latex, and radiographic dye.

Z89-Z90 indicate a person having had replacement of organ or tissue by transplant (animal or human) (status post) such as hands, legs, organs, or genitalia.

Failure to comply with medical recommendations are coded as Z91 and include noncompliance and underdosing.

History of psychological trauma (Z91.4) include abuse of adult and self-harm.

Z92 codes indicate history of use of contraceptives, drug therapy (e.g. chemotherapy and estrogen), irradiation and failed moderate sedation.

Presence of implanted devices or organs are coded as Z94-Z97 and are known as status post, meaning that the device or organ was previously implanted. These codes include cardiac grafts, heart valves, pacemakers, intraocular lens, orthopedic joint implants, and artificial eyes or limbs.

Section 29.18: STATUS

Postprocedural status (Z98) indicates that a patient received surgery in the past. This is important because it can influence decisions regarding the patient's healthcare such as intestinal bypasses, and collapsed lung.

Removal of cataracts in the past is coded as Z98.4. If patient was sterilized previously, they would be status post sterilization (Z98.5). If a patient received an angioplasty in the past it is coded as Z98.6. Breast implants are coded as Z98.82. If breast implants were removed they are coded as Z98.86.

Section 29.19: DEPENDENCE ON MACHINES

Dependence on machines while under medical care (Z99) includes aspirator, respirator, renal dialysis, wheelchair and oxygen.

SUPPLEMENTARY CODES QUIZ 22

1) What are the codes for a patient seen for follow-up exam of breast cancer which was removed a year ago and treated with chemotherapy?

2) What are the codes for a patient seen who had a replacement of their colostomy?

3) What are the codes for a patient seen today for prophylactic administration of Nolvadex for breast cancer which metastasized from skin cancer on the back which was removed a year ago with positive estrogen receptor status?

4) What are the codes for a woman who delivered a newborn who was 550 grams at 34 weeks with hyperbilirubinemia?

5) What are the codes for a patient who is leaving the country and needed a cholera vaccination?

6) What are the codes for a patient seen today for counseling regarding instructions in the use of an insulin pump for her diabetes Type I and high blood pressure?

7) What are the codes for a patient seen today for cataracts and diabetic neuropathy Type II with long term use of insulin and ASHD?

8) What are the codes for a 3-year-old child during a well check who was to receive DTP vaccination but was uncontrollable and so the vaccine was not administered?

9) What are the codes for a patient who was seen today for laparoscopic resection of the small intestine with anastomosis which had to be changed to an open procedure for cancer?

10) What are the codes for a patient seen today for routine PAP test with no findings?

11) What are the codes for a patient who is a bone marrow donor?

12) What are the codes for a patient seen today for adjustment of peritoneal dialysis catheter during dialysis?

13) What are the codes for a patient seen today for possible gout due to complaints of stomach pain but tests were negative?

14) What are the codes for a patient seen today for exercise therapy after suffering a severe crushing injury to the left lower leg four months ago?

15) What are the codes for a patient seen today for drug resistant pulmonary TB?

CHAPTER 30
ICD-10 PCS OVERVIEW PROCEDURAL CODES

You will learn the following objectives in this chapter:

- ICD-10 PCS Coding System
- Characters
  1. First Character: Section
  2. Second Character: Body System
  3. Third Character: Root Operation
  4. Fourth Character: Body Part
  5. Fifth Character: Approach
  6. Sixth Character: Device
  7. Seventh Character: Qualifier

ICD-10 Procedure Coding System (PCS) is used only for inpatient hospital procedural code and therefore, physician-based coders do not need to know this as they will be using CPT codes instead. This is a brief overview so any curious coder can gain some understanding of the coding system.

Section 30.1: ICD-10 PCS CODING SYSTEM

The goal in developing the ICD-10-PCS system is to provide completeness unique definitions, expandability, structural integrity, and is multiaxial with standardized terminology. Completeness means having unique codes for procedures that are able to expand to accommodate the growth in healthcare in procedures and services.

Section 30.2: CHARACTERS

ICD-10-PCS codes are seven characters which represent some aspect of the procedure. They are not specifically listed as one code but rather require the selection of each character one by one based on what the character represents as it relates to the procedure.

The second through seventh characters mean the same thing within each section, but may mean different things in other sections. Each character can be any of 34 possible values the ten digits 0-9 and the 24 letters A-H, J-N and P-Z may be used in each character. The letters O and I excluded to avoid confusion with the numbers 0 and 1.[2] There are no decimals in ICD-10-PCS.

Character 1 represents the section.
Character 2 represents the body system.
Character 3 represents the root operation
Character 4 represents the body part.
Character 5 represents the approach.
Character 6 represents the device.
Character 7 represents the qualifier.

For example, code 0U524ZZ is for destruction of the both ovaries which was done percutaneously with a scope but no devices or additional qualifiers were involved.

There are 16 sections in the ICD-10-PCS.

The first character represents the section which are broad such as Medical and Surgical. There are 16 sections as denoted by 0 through 9 and letters B through D and F through H.

The second character represents the body system (physiological/anatomical) such as respiratory system.

The third character represents the root operation which is the procedure or services provided.

The fourth character represents the body part which is much more specific such as the left upper leg.

The fifth character represents the approach used to gain access to the surgical site such as the procedure being open or performed with a scope.

The sixth character represents a device, if implanted although some procedures may not involve a device which would be coded with a "Z". There are four categories for devices: grafts/prosthesis, implants, simple or mechanical appliances, and electronic appliances.

The seventh character represents a qualifier which describes any special attributes of the procedure. If there is no qualifier "Z" would be used.

Section 30.3: FIRST CHARACTER

The first character represents the section which are broad such as Medical and Surgical. There are 16 sections as denoted by 0 through 9 and letters B through D and F through H.

The following is a table for the values of the first character:

SECTION VALUE	DESCRIPTION
1	Obstetrics
2	Placement
3	Administration
4	Measurement and Monitoring
5	Extracorporeal Assistance & Performance
6	Extracorporeal Therapies

7	Osteopathic
8	Other Procedures
9	Chiropractic
B	Imaging
C	Nuclear Medicine
D	Radiation Oncology
F	Physical Rehabilitation & Diagnostic Audiology
G	Mental Health
H	Substance Abuse Treatment

Placement characters are for procedures in which a device is used to protect, immobilize, stretch, compress, or pack a site.

Administration characters indicate procedures in which there is administration of a substance such as infusions, injections or transfusions.

Extracorporeal assistance refers to the use of devices to assist a patient such as mechanical ventilation.

Section 30.4: Second Character

The second character is the physiological or anatomical system where the procedure is performed. Body systems include:

VALUE	DESCRIPTION
0	Central Nervous System
1	Peripheral Nervous System
2	Heart & Great Vessels
3	Upper Arteries
4	Lower Arteries
5	Upper Veins
6	Lower Veins
7	Lymphatic & Hemic System
8	Eye

9	Ear, Nose, Sinus
B	Respiratory
C	Mouth & Throat
D	Gastrointestinal
F	Hepatobiliary & Pancreas
G	Endocrine
H	Skin & Breast
J	Subcutaneous Tissue & Fascia
K	Muscles
L	Tendons
M	Bursae & Ligaments
N	Head & Facial Bones
P	Upper Bones
Q	Lower Bones
R	Upper Joints
S	Lower Joints
T	Urinary System
U	Female Reproductive
V	Male Reproductive
W	Anatomic Region, General
X	Anatomic Regions, Upper Extremities
Y	Anatomic Regions, Lower Extremities

Section 30.5: Third Character

The third character describes the actual procedure. There are 31 different root operations. There are nine groups:

- Procedures that take out some/all of a body part.
- Procedures that take out solids/fluids/gases from a body part.

- Procedures involving cutting or separation only.
- Procedures that put in/put back or move some/all of a body part.
- Procedures that alter the diameter/route of a tubular body part.
- Procedures that always involve a device.
- Procedures involving examination only.
- Procedures defining other repairs.
- Procedures defining objectives.

Procedures that take out some/all of a body part include excision, resection, detachment, destruction or extraction.

Procedures that take out solids/fluids/gases from a body part include drainage, extirpation, and fragmentation.

Procedures involving cutting or separation only include division or release.

Procedures that put in/put back or move some/all of a body part include transplantation, reattachment, transfer, and repositioning.

Procedures that alter the diameter/route of a tubular body part include restriction, occlusion, dilation and bypass.

Procedures that always involve a device include insertion, replacement, supplement, change, removal and revision.

Procedures involving examination only include inspection and mapping.

Procedures defining other repairs include repair and control.

Procedures defining other repairs include fusion, alteration and creation.

Section 30.6: Fourth Character

The fourth character represents the specific anatomical site where the procedure is performed including laterality such as left lower leg.

Section 30.7: Fifth Character

The fifth character represents the approach used to get to the procedural site. Various approaches include open (0), percutaneous (3), percutaneous endoscopic (4), via natural or artificial opening (7), via natural or artificial opening endoscopic (8), via natural or artificial opening endoscopic assistance (F), and external (X).

Open involves cutting through the skin and membranes. Percutaneous means puncturing the skin or any other layer. Percutaneous endoscopic means puncturing the skin or any other layer to insert a scope. Via natural or artificial opening is an approach that uses an opening to gain access, one with a scope involved and one without. This type of approach which is also described as assistance means that additional instrumentation was inserted through the opening. External indicates that the procedure was performed on top of the skin and not cutting was involved.

Section 30.8: Sixth Character

The sixth character describes the device inserted into the body during the procedure. "Z" should be used if there is no device inserted. The types of devices are biological or synthetic material that takes the place of all or portion of body part, biological or synthetic material that assists or prevents a physiological function, therapeutic material that is not absorbed by, eliminated by, or incorporated into a body part, and mechanical or electronic appliances used to assist, monitor, take the place of or prevent a physiological function.

Values differ by procedures. Some examples include:

VALUE	DESCRIPTION
0	Drainage Device
2	Monitoring Device
3	Infusion Device
4	Internal Fixation Device
7	Autologous Tissue Substitute
8	Zooplastic Tissue
9	Autologous Venous Tissue
A	Autologous Arterial tissue
C	Extraluminal Device
D	Intraluminal Device
J	Synthetic Substitute
K	Nonautologous Tissue Substitute
L	Artificial Sphincter
M	Bone Growth Stimulator
Q	Implantable Heart Assist System
R	External Heart Assist System
T	Radioactive Intraluminal

	Device
Y	Other Device
Z	No Device

Section 30.9: Seventh Character

The seventh character provided additional information about the procedure but is not always applicable which is known as a qualifier. "Z" should be used if there is no qualifier.

Values differ by procedures. Some examples include:

VALUE	DESCRIPTION
0	Allogeneic
1	Syngeneic
2	Zoolastic
3	Monoplanar
4	Ring
5	Hybrid
6	Ureter, Right
7	Ureter, Left
8	Colon
9	Colocutaneous
A	Pacemaker Lead
B	Skin & Subcutaneous Tissue
C	Ileocutaneous
D	Cutaneous
G	Pressure Sensor
S	Biventricular
T	Ductus Arteriosus
X	Diagnostic
Z	No Qualifier

TEST 2
ICD-10 CHAPTERS 1 - 30

1. What are the codes for a patient with senile dementia?

2. What are the codes for a patient who has sickle cell anemia Hb-SS with acute chest syndrome?

3. What is hemolysis?

4. What are the codes for a patient who is diagnosed with anemia due to a chronic gastric ulcer?

5. What are the codes for a patient with benign CKD stage 4 and ASCVD due to hypertension?

6. What are the codes for a pregnant woman who has had three previous miscarriages at approximately 18 weeks and presents today at 20 weeks gestation who is experiencing cramping?

7. What are the codes for a patient with Crohn's disease?

8. What is the term for painful menstruation?

9. What are the codes for a patient with oophoritis and salpingitis?

10. What are the codes for a patient with cellulitis with possible sepsis and COPD with diabetes?

11. What are the codes for a 2-month-old baby who presents with a diaper rash?

12. What is the code for a patient with gastritis after ingesting Percodan with alcohol and OTC antihistamines?

13. What is the code for a patient with scar tissue due to a second and third degree burn on both legs six months ago?

14. What are the codes for an anemic patient due to hemorrhaging of a lower leg wound caused by a car accident?

15. What are the codes for a patient with a stage 2 ulcer of the ankle that developed from a cast that was applied to their left lower tibia for 3 months due to a transverse fracture of the shaft?

16. What are the codes for a patient who has pyogenic arthritis of the hip due to staph?

17. What are the codes for a patient with acute and chronic pericarditis?

18. What are the codes for a patient with amebic carditis?

19. What are the codes for a patient who has right heart failure?

20. What are dilated, swollen, painful veins in the anus or rectum known as?

21. What are the codes for a patient with COPD and emphysema?

22. What are the codes for a Type II diabetic patient with neuropathy and pneumonia due to MRSA and a fever?

23. What are the codes for a patient with asthma that was precipitated by exercise?

24. What are the codes for a patient with a perforated appendix with an abscess?

25. What are the codes for a patient with RAD?

26. What three things must occur for a woman to be diagnosed as having preeclampsia?

27. What are the codes for a 36-year-old pregnant woman who has a C section due to fetal distress at 39 weeks?

28. What is another term for delivery?

29. What is considered a high blood pressure?

30. What are the codes for a patient who has mitral valve stenosis with aortic valve insufficiency?

31. What are the codes for a patient who was diagnosed nine weeks ago with chronic coronary insufficiency?

32. What are the codes for a 25-year-old pregnant woman who is 33-weeks gestation, has gestational diabetes and is seen today for dehydration?

33. What are the codes for an 18-year-old pregnant woman who has difficulty in labor due to the birth of a 12 pound baby boy?

34. What are the codes for a pregnant woman who delivered liveborn twins with one normal and the other breech at 32 weeks with both weighing 5 pounds?

35. What are the codes for a patient with ASHD and chest pain due to an MI that was treated 10 weeks ago?

36. What are the codes for a patient with second degree sunburn?

37. What are the codes for a patient with pilonidal cyst with abscess?

38. What are the codes for a patient experiencing septic shock due to UTI?

39. What are the codes for a patient with goat's milk anemia?

40. What are the codes for a patient who metastatic cancer of the uterus?

41. What are the codes for a patient who has nonunion fracture of the left humerus?

42. What are the codes for a patient who has degenerative joint disease of the knee?

43. What are the codes for a patient who is seen today for a high fever and chest congestion due to the common cold?

44. What are the codes for a patient who has right heart failure?

45. What are the codes for a patient who is diagnosed with pneumothorax due to gunshot wound?

46. What are the codes for a patient who has old bucket tear of the lateral meniscus?

47. What are the codes for a newborn who was born with a hemangioma of the neck?

48. What are the codes when a 1750 gm baby at 28 weeks gestation is delivered due to hypertonic labor?

49. What are the codes for a neonate who is diagnosed with diabetes?

50. What are the codes for a baby born at 43 weeks who experienced asphyxia due to the cord wrapped around her neck?

51. What is the code for the newborn when her mother dies during childbirth?

52. What are the codes for a patient with second and third degree burns covering 25% of her body with 10% being third degree with infection? T31.21, T79.8XXA

53. What causes essential hypertension? CAUSE UNKNOWN

54. What is reactive airway disease? ASTHMA

55. What are the codes for a patient with lower respiratory infection? J22

56. What are the codes for an asthmatic patient with status asthmaticus and COPD? J44.0

57. What is the code for a patient with dislocation of an artificial hip joint?

58. What is the code for a patient with CMV infection due to transplanted liver?

59. What is the code for a patient with anoxic brain damage resulting from their bypass graft surgery for an MI?

60. What is the code for a patient with failure of the battery of the pacemaker after two years requiring replacement?

CHAPTER 31
CPT STRUCTURE

You will learn the following objectives in this chapter:

A. HCPCS
B. CPT
   1. Structure
   2. Alphabetical Index
   3. Modifiers
C. NOTATIONS
   1. Symbols
   2. Guidelines/Notes
   3. Semicolon
   4. Add-on Codes
   5. Multipliers
D. REPORTING
   1. Special Reports
   2. Unlisted Procedures
E. SELECTION OF CODES
   1. Significant Procedure
   2. Global
   3. Unbundling
   4. Downcoding
   5. Upcoding
   6. Separate Procedure
   7. Each/Separate/Additional

Section 31.1: HCPCS

HCPCS are known as Healthcare Common Procedure Coding System (National Codes). There are two levels to the HCPCS. The first level are the CPT codes as discussed below. The second level are what are listed in the HCPCS coding book and are developed and adopted by the Centers for Medicare and Medicaid Services which is a division of the Health and Human Services Federal Department. HCPCS provide alphanumeric codes for coding many items and services not included in the CPT coding book, such as ambulance services, durable medical equipment, and supplies. HCPCS will be discussed further in a later packet.

Section 31.2: CURRENT PROCEDURAL TERMINOLOGY (CPT)

The CPT coding book is known as the Current Procedural Terminology and is developed by the American Medical Association with changes every year and is a listing of services provided by healthcare providers. This book was first developed in 1966. The CPT coding book contains codes and descriptions of medical services and procedures provided by healthcare providers in any setting. Hospitals do not use these codes for coding services since they are charging for services, such as nursing, tests, therapies, etc., that are provided during a hospital stay so they use Volume 3 of the ICD-10-CM coding book. However, physicians or other healthcare providers who provide services to a patient whether in the hospital will still use CPT/HCPCS codes and do not use Volume 3 hospital procedural codes.

The CPT coding book is composed of the tabular and an alphabetical index in addition to appendices. The book begins with an Introduction which describes important notes. Remember this – when you are studying for your national exams and/or coding on the job, the notes in the CPT book are critical.

If you have a professional edition of the CPT coding book (which is definitely the most highly recommended edition), anatomical illustrations are provided which are extremely helpful when coding and taking the tests.

Remember, as with the ICD-10 coding book, when you are studying and preparing for the national exams you can write in your coding books, so be sure to write notes by applicable codes, but remember also to not put too many notes or you will have trouble finding the information.

SECTIONS: There are six sections to the CPT coding book:

Evaluation and Management
Anesthesia
Surgery
Radiology
Pathology and Laboratory
Medicine

All of these codes are five numbers.

After the six sections, there are the Category II codes which are used to track patient care through the use of performance measures, such as physical exams and follow up. These codes are composed of four numbers followed by a letter of the alphabet.

Category III codes are listed next which are temporary codes for new and emerging technologies and are composed of four numbers and a letter following, similar to the Category II codes.

The next section in the CPT coding book are the appendices which include:

Appendix A: Modifiers
Appendix B: Summary of Additions, Deletions, and Revisions
Appendix C: Clinical Examples
Appendix D: Summary of CPT Add-on Codes
Appendix E: Summary of CPT Codes Exempt from Modifier 51
Appendix F: Summary of CPT Codes Exempt from Modifier 63
Appendix G: Summary of CPT Codes That Include Moderate (Conscious) Sedation
Appendix H: Alphabetic Index of Performance Measures by Clinical Condition or Topic
Appendix I: Genetic Testing Code Modifiers
Appendix J: Electrodiagnostic Medicine Listing of Sensory, Motor, and Mixed Nerves
Appendix K: Product Pending FDA Approval

Appendix L: Vascular Families
Appendix M: Summary of Crosswalked Deleted CPT Codes
Appendix N: Summary of Resequenced CPT Codes
Appendix O: Multianalyte Assays with Algorithmic Analyses

ALPHABETICAL INDEX: The alphabetical index in the CPT coding book is not as clearly defined and specific as in the ICD-10 book. For this reason, it can be more difficult to find the correct code.

Codes in the alphabetical index are classified by anatomic site, general or specific procedure or service, synonyms, eponyms and abbreviations which can be very helpful.

MODIFIERS: Modifiers consist of two digits (either numeric or alphanumeric) and are attached to a regular CPT code at the end of the code by a dash and then the two-digit modifier, e.g. 11201-51. Modifiers indicate changes in the status of the main code which may result in changes in reimbursement but it does not alter the definition of the code. Modifiers can be found in Appendix A of the CPT book or in the HCPCS book. The modifiers in Appendix A are numeric and the modifiers in the HCPCS are alphanumeric.

Section 31.3: NOTATIONS

SYMBOLS: The meaning of these symbols can be found at the bottom of each page or in the Introduction at the front of the book.

a. A solid dot next to a code indicates that it is new.
b. A circle with a dot inside of it next to a code indicates that the code includes conscious sedation.
c. A triangle next to a code indicates that a code has been changed substantially in the new book.
d. Two triangles pointing towards each other next to a code indicates new and revised text other than the procedure's description.
e. A plus sign indicates that the code is an add-on code which will be discussed in another packet.
f. A circle with a slash through it indicates that the modifier 51 does not need to be used with this code which will be discussed in another packet.
g. A hashtag means that the code is out of order, so you need to look a little more for it as it does not follow numerically but it will be in the general area.

GUIDELINES/NOTES: The most important part of physician coding and the national exams are the guidelines/notes in the coding books which are listed at the beginning of each section and interspersed throughout the entire book.

SEMICOLON: The semicolon is a very important concept in the proper utilization of the CPT coding book. When there is a semicolon within a coding description in the CPT book, there are additional indented codes listed underneath the main code. The semicolon, therefore, indicates that everything before the semicolon in the first original code should be retained and applied as part of the description for the additional indented codes underneath the main code;

however, the part of the description that follows the semicolon should be discarded and replaced with the information provided in the additional indented code. This also implies that any description following the semicolon of one code is not included in other additional indented codes, so selection of an indented code will not include the description following the semicolon of another code.

ADD-ON CODES: Add-on codes are indicated by a "+" sign. The guidelines (notes) indicate that these codes cannot be coded by themselves but must be listed in addition to other codes as specified. Add-on codes are used to code for additional services, e.g., additional units of service, such as second ten whereas the first ten were coded with the first code.

MULTIPLIERS: When coding for additional separately billable individual services, the additional units can be designated in the unit block on the CMS1500 form or if written as times the unit (i.e. x3 for 3 units). This may not be true if the code is described as containing multiple units, such as next 10 lesions. Be careful to read the descriptions as coding for multiples can vary across codes.

SEPARATE PROCEDURE: Some procedures in the CPT coding book are indicated as "separate procedures". "Separate procedures" means that these codes can be coded by themselves only if they are not included as part of a larger global packaged procedure.

REQUIRED CODING: Some primary or other selected relevant codes may require the coding of other codes. *Follow the instructions.* If the codes direct you to "code also," then code also the additional required code. Be careful of "excludes" and "includes." *Read the details carefully.*

RELEVANT CARE: All care relevant to the care of the patient and the outcomes should also be coded if it is not bundled in another primary code.

Section 31.4: REPORTS

SPECIAL REPORTS: In some circumstances, a payer may request additional information, such as a special report to demonstrate the need for charges. This oftentimes occurs with the use of unspecified ICD-10 codes which do not clearly demonstrate the medical necessity for the services provided. This may also occur if an "unlisted" procedure code is selected or if extra services are charged in addition to the main procedure code due to comorbidities or complications which have resulted in the provision of additional medical care. Again, the ICD-10 codes must demonstrate medical necessity for these additional charges.

UNLISTED PROCEDURES: Unlisted procedures are procedures that do not currently have specific codes for them, usually because they are new or unusual procedures. When utilizing these codes, a special report is required to be sent with the claim. However, it is not preferable to use these codes and another acceptable code should be chosen instead if possible.

Section 30.5: SELECTION OF CODES

LINKAGE: No claim can be sent without both a diagnostic code (ICD-10) and a CPT/HCPCS codes. It is the linkage of the ICD-10 code to the CPT/HCPCS codes on the billing form that demonstrates medical necessity and, therefore, ensures proper payment. CCI edits can also assist with proper linkage because it delineates which codes can be used together. Oftentimes, reimbursement errors are due to improper linkage due to ICD-10 codes being assigned to CPT/HCPCS codes that are not consistent with each other and/or the ICD-10 code does not prove medical necessity for the use of the CPT/HCPCS code that it is linked to.

Coding is not black and white, but has gray areas, particularly with CPT coding as there are two types of codes in the CPT book – (1) highly specified codes in which a specific procedure is well described and (2) general descriptions of a group of procedures. Therefore, it is clearly understandable if there is not a specific code for a procedure, then you need to pick the more generalized code that includes the procedure but does not exceed what occurred in the procedure. You can never select a code that includes details that were not performed. For example, if a patient has an oophorectomy, you cannot code it as a total hysterectomy because only the ovaries were removed.

NOT DOCUMENTED NOT DONE: Remember also – NOT DOCUMENTED NOT DONE! Do not code what the doctor does not describe in his report.

USE OF ALPHABETICAL INDEX: The CPT alphabetical index is not as detailed as it was in the ICD-10 book, so sometimes you may find that you are not sure where to find a code. In this instance, you may want to try to get as close as you can to the section of the coding book where the correct code may be. There may sometimes be several codes listed – you should check them out. Sometimes you can even go to the codes themselves because the codes are listed in a consistent manner by anatomic site and then procedures, so there is a pattern to the listing of the codes.

When are you searching for a code, it is critical with the CPT coding book that you take a few extra minutes and check above and below the area of codes you believe are correct because you may find that another code is more applicable.

ABSTRACTING: Abstracting is the extraction of documented data from a patient's report for selection of proper ICD-10 and CPT/HCPCS codes; sometimes there may only be one report to use for abstracting of codes, but sometimes it can involve several reports.

Abstracting can be accomplished in several steps:

(1) The first step in selecting a code is to determine who you are coding for – a radiologist, surgeon, primary care, consultant, etc. When you have recognized which healthcare provider you are billing for, then you will only code for the services they provided.
(2) What services and procedures were provided must be coded with a CPT or HCPCS code, and then linked to the ICD-10 codes on the billing form.
(3) It is important to indicate where services were provided. Some services are payable only in the hospital and some are only payable in other settings, therefore

it is important that the claim properly indicate where the services were provided. Some codes differ according to where services are provided.

SIGNIFICANT PROCEDURE: A significant procedure is a procedure that has risks or requires special training in order to treat it and which is usually the primary code listed. The significant procedure code usually contains all typical services associated with it so no additional codes would be listed which is known as bundling of services and the period of time in which typical services are considered to be a part of the significant procedure is known as the global period.

GLOBALS: Codes that are global include all services provided including pre and post office visits for a specific procedure for a specified length of time determined by how long it typically takes patient to become well which can range from a couple of days to several months.

With globals, there is a time frame established for the postoperative care which is different for different procedures, such as one week to 30 or 60 days, which is known as the POSTOPERATIVE PERIOD. These time frames are established by the government and related health organizations and do change frequently. Until that time frame has expired, no postoperative care can be billed because it is included in the global package with some exceptions which include services extraordinary to the global or for other diagnosis, such as infection or other complications.

To list additional codes for services that are included in a global code is known as unbundling. Bundled services include:

5. Preoperative visits.
6. Intraoperative services that are a usual and necessary part of a surgical procedure;
7. All additional medical or surgical services during the postoperative period of the surgery for complications.
8. Follow-up visits during the postoperative period of the surgery.
9. Postsurgical pain management;
10. Certain supplies and miscellaneous services (e.g., dressing changes; wound care, removal of sutures or staples or other device including catheters; insertion and care of tubes).

DOWNCODING/UPCODING: Downcoding is the selection of a lower-paying code than what is justified by the services provided to a patient. Downcoding demonstrates poor practices and raises other questions of why lower-paying codes are being selected. Upcoding is the selection of a higher-paying code than what is warranted by the services provided. Upcoding can be considered abuse or fraud.

HOW TO SELECT PROPER CODES:

(2) You should first examine several headings – the discharge diagnosis and procedure are the first headings you should examine. At this point, you should find the codes for these diagnosis and procedures. You should find these codes first because then you will know what you are looking for in the report based on how codes are differentiated.

(3) You can find the codes by first checking in the alphabetical index; however, if you cannot find anything there you can always check under other related terms or go directly to the codes as they are listed in an orderly fashion by anatomic site and then by procedures.
(4) Return to the codes themselves and select the proper code. Take your time to check for the correct codes as some codes are very similar and some are more general while others are more specific.
(5) Once you have completed this, you should check the admit diagnosis heading and see if there is additional information or if the discharge diagnosis are confirmed by the admit diagnosis heading.
(6) After this, you should check any other heading to determine if any additional information is available. You can also search the body of the reports for additional information. Sometimes other headings can indicate important information, such as laboratory findings can indicate findings of involved organisms. Radiology tests can indicate if a lesion is malignant or benign.

CHAPTER 32
EVALUATION AND MANAGEMENT

You will learn the following objectives in this chapter:

A. Evaluation & Management Codes
    1. Guidelines/Notes
    2. Components
B. Service Areas
    1. New Patient
    2. Areas
C. Components
    1. Seven Components
    2. Counseling
    3. Coordination of Care
    4. Nature of Presenting Problem
    5. Time
    6. Key Components
        a. Levels
        b. History
        c. Exam
        d. Medical Decision Making
        e. Meeting of Levels
        f. Bell Curve
        g. Undercoding
        h. Overcoding
        i. Appendix
D. Who, What, Where
E. Selection Criteria
F. Visits
    1. Office Visits
    2. Hospital Observation
    3. Hospital Visits
    4. Consultations
    5. Emergency Department Services
    6. Critical Care Services
    7. Nursing Facility Services
    8. Domiciliary, Rest Home or Custodial Care Services
    9. Home Services
    10. Physician Standby Services
    11. Case Management and Oversight Services
    12. Preventive Medicine Services
    13. Other Codes
    14. Newborn Care Services
    15. Inpatient Neonatal and Pediatric Intensive/Critical Care Services.

16. Chronic Care Management

G. Time
    1. Higher Level Code
    2. Prolonged Services

H. E/M Criteria

I. Globals

J. Modifiers

Section 32.1: EVALUATION AND MANAGEMENT CODES

Evaluation and Management codes, known as E/M codes, are used by healthcare providers to bill for their services. This includes physicians, anesthesiologists, laboratory and radiology technicians, etc. At this point, it becomes critical to remember that you must code only for the services your healthcare provider performs and none other. This means that if a surgery is done with x-rays and you are coding for the surgeon you will code for the surgery and not the x-ray tests, but if you are coding for the radiologist you will only code for the x-rays that the radiologist performed. This also means that a surgeon would not bill for the hospital's services, such as room, tests, medications, etc, because the hospital provides these services and not the surgeon.

Guidelines/notes are critical to proper selection of CPT codes – this definitely applies to the proper selection of E/M codes.

Section 32.2: SERVICE AREAS

E/M codes begin with services provided in the Office/Other Outpatient. This is followed by Hospital Observation, then Hospital Inpatient Services, Consultations, Emergency Department, Critical Care, Nursing Facility, Domiciliary and Rest Homes, Home Services, Prolonged Services, Case Management, Care Plan Oversight, Preventive Medicine, Non-Face-To-Face Physician Services, Special E/M Services, Newborn Care, and Inpatient and Pediatric Neonatal. At the front of the professional edition of the CPTs, there is a listing of the two-digit numbers for the service area which would be listed on the CMS-1500 form.

Section 32.3: COMPONENTS

There are seven major components used to determine many of the E/M codes. These include history, exam, medical decision making, counseling, coordination of care, nature of presenting problem and time. These E/M codes are used for patients presenting with a problem, or chief complaint. Other E/M codes are determined by other factors, such as time and age.

We will defer discussion of the first three components as they are the key components used to determine the selection of the E/M codes for most visits. The other four components are:

1. Counseling: Counseling involves the time spent by a physician talking to and advising patient and family/friends as necessary for proper care of the patient.
2. Coordination of Care: Coordination of care includes review of previous and

current medical reports from other healthcare providers and consultations with other healthcare providers.

3. Nature of Presenting Problem: Presenting problems can be classified as minimal, self-limited/minor, low severity, moderate severity, and high severity which will be discussed later in this packet.
4. Time: Time is a complicated component in several ways in its use to determine the proper level of E/M code.

First, some E/M codes are determined solely on the amount of time the healthcare provider spent with the patient, such as urgent care, which will be discussed later.

Second, although the other E/M codes that use the components to determine the levels do list a specified time, these times are not used to determine the proper level of E/M service.

Third, time is measured by the time a healthcare provider provides face-to-face with the patient for some of the codes, such as office visits. However, visits that involve hospitalization are based on healthcare provider services that were face-to-face or unit/floor time. Face-to-face time is direct time the physician spends with the patient. Unit/floor time is the time a healthcare provider spends on a unit relative to a patient's care, such as review of charts and reports; however, for this the healthcare provider must be on the patient's unit and available to the patient if necessary.

Fourth, typically time can be accounted for by the selection of a code based on the three key components; however, if a healthcare provider spends more time with the patient in legitimate services than what was provided for in the key components, he can be reimbursed extra for that extended time. This additional reimbursement for the extended time of services can be achieved in several ways which will be discussed in the next packet.

THREE MAJOR COMPONENTS: Of the seven components, only three are primarily used to determine the selection of some E/M codes; these are history, exam, and medical decision making. Many CPT codes, including the professional edition, list these three components in the description of the each code for visits.

For this section, please access the auditing form provided in the Appendix.

There are several levels of service within each E/M code group as distinguished by area of service, i.e. office, hospital, etc. The levels proceed from the lowest level (e.g. 99201), which indicates the lowest level of service provided and which pays the least, to the highest level (e.g. 99205) which indicates the highest level of services provided and which pays the most.

HISTORY: The first key component is history which is defined by the chief complaint and then further differentiated as History of Present Illness (HPI), Review of Systems (ROS), and Past Family Social History (PFSH).

The following information are guidelines that have been adopted based on Medicare and other payers and healthcare providers' interpretations of what constitutes these levels of care, therefore, there is flexibility in interpretation of how to determine the proper levels.

All History components must begin with a chief complaint because that is why the patient presents for healthcare so this is the basis for the visit.

The next component is the History of Present Illness (HPI). This is the information the patient provides when they are queried as to the reason for their visit. Oftentimes this information can be collected on a form prior to the patient being seen by the physician; however, any information collected on a form must be confirmed by the doctor by his querying the patient as to the validity of the information.

HPI would include elements relating to their complaint such as location, quality, severity, duration, timing, context, modifying factors, and associated signs and symptoms. There is flexibility in how these elements may be described by the physician.

The levels of HPI are brief and extended. For a brief HPI, 1 to 3 elements must be provided; for extended more than 4 elements must have been described in the patient's report.

Review of Systems (ROS) is the collection of the patient's history, particularly relevant to medical history. The level of ROS is determined by the number of systems of the body for which information was gathered and reviewed by the physician. ROS includes the systems typically examined in a general exam, including constitutional, HEENT, cardiovascular, respiratory, GU, GI, musculoskeletal, psychiatric, integumentary, neurological, etc. This information is typically collected from the patient so the physician needs to review it and confirm it with the patient. Also, if there is something not normal this information should be described in the patient's report and not stated only as "positive". A shorthand method for describing normal systems which will account for a multitude of system examined is "HEENT, cardio, respiratory, GU, and GI system are all negative," which indicates that five systems have been reviewed.

The levels of ROS are pertinent, extended, and complete. Again, it is important for the physician to include this information in the report because not documented, not done, so if he does not report it then a lower level of code will be selected and the physician will lose reimbursement. From this perspective, a pertinent ROS would include information on one system. An extended ROS would include information on 2 to 9 systems and a complete ROS would include information on 10 systems.

Past, Family and Social History (PFSH) has three elements as stated, past, family and social history. All that is needed to qualify any of these elements is one statement, such a "Patient has a long history of smoking" or "Mother has diabetes".

A pertinent PFSH is one that includes descriptions of only one or two of these elements. A complete PFSH usually contains descriptions of all three elements.

The selection of the History level is determined by combining all three of these together as demonstrated on the auditing sheet. Based on these three components, a History can be the lowest level beginning with problem-focused (PF), or expanded problem-focused (EPF), or detailed (D), or the highest level comprehensive (C). Problem focused History contains a brief HPI and no information for ROS and PFSH. An expanded problem-focused History contains a brief HPI, pertinent ROS, and no PFSH. A detailed History contains an extended HPI, extended ROS, and pertinent PFSH. A comprehensive History contains an extended HPI, complete ROS, and complete PFSH.

		Problem Focused	Exp. Prob. Focused	Detailed	Compre-hensive
1	**CHIEF COMPLAINT:**				
2	**HISTORY** **HPI** (history of present illness) elements: ☐ Location ☐ Severity ☐ Timing ☐ Modifying factors ☐ Quality ☐ Duration ☐ Context ☐ Associated signs and symptoms	Brief 1-3 Elements	Brief 1-3 Elements	Extended ≥ 4 elements or status of ≥ 3 chronic or inactive conditions	Extended
3	**ROS** (review of systems): ☐ Constitutional (Wt. Loss, etc.) ☐ Ears, nose, mouth, throat ☐ GI ☐ Integumentary (skin, breast) ☐ Edno ☐ Eyes ☐ Card/Vasc ☐ GU ☐ Neuro ☐ Hem/Lymph ☐ Resp ☐ Musculo ☐ All/Imm ☐ Psych ☐ All others negative	None	Pertinent to problem 1 system	Extended 2-9 systems	Complete ≥ 10 systems, or some systems with statement "All Others Negative"
4	**PFSH** (past medical, family, social history) areas: ☐ Past history (the patient's past experiences with illnesses, operations, injuries and treatments) ☐ Family history (a review of medical events in the patient's family, including diseases which may be ☐ hereditary or place the patient at risk).	None	None	Pertinent 1 or 2 history areas	Complete 2 or 3 history areas
5	Circle history type within appropriate grid under Level of Service				

When selecting the level of History, the levels of all three components must be met in order to select the level of History, so if one level is lower than the others, then the lowest level determines the overall level. For example, if a physician provides documentation for an extended HPI, an extended ROS, but provided no PFSH, then the highest level of History that can be selected is the EPF. If the physician had documented at least two elements of the PFSH, the highest level of History that could be selected would have been Detailed.

However, if some of the History elements cannot be determined because the patient is not able to provide the information nor can anyone else, the physician is not necessarily penalized by having to select the lowest level of code. Instead, the physician must demonstrate that reasonable effort was made to obtain the information but it was not possible due to factors such as the patient being unconscious and no family members available. This must be documented in the patient's report.

The following represents a sample History from a report:

> HPI: The patient presents with complaints of stomach pain which has been worse after eating. The pain is localized to the right upper quadrant and has been occurring for the past two weeks. ROS: All systems are negative. No history of angina or MI. Recent bronchitis. PFSH: The patient smokes. His father died from alcoholism and his mother is diabetic. The patient has had problems with alcoholism and COPD.

EXAM: The exam is the actual exam performed by the physician at the time of the patient's visit. Like the ROS, the selection of the exam level is based on the body systems, i.e. constitutional, HEENT, cardiovascular, GU, GI, respiratory, neurological, etc. or can be based on elements that would be examined during specialty exams, such as dermatology.

There are basically two types of Exams that can be performed and either one may be selected as the criterion for determining the level of the exam. These are known as the 1995 multisystem exam or 1997 specialty exams. With the multisystem exam, all of the systems as previously mentioned in the ROS are the basis for determining how many elements have been demonstrated. With the specialty exam, various aspects of the particular system are used to determine the level of exam. It is important to know the difference between these two types of exams so that proper application can be used to determine the proper code because if a physician performs a specialty exam then he will probably not meet the criteria of having examined all the body systems because his focus will be on the specialty area. On the other hand, if the multisystem exam is not utilized for a general exam and the criteria for a specialty exam is used, then again the physician will probably not be able to meet the criteria for the proper level of code because he will not be providing enough information about one specialty area. For example, while a physician who performs a multisystem exam may examine the eyes, ears, nose and throat, during a specialty exam of this area other elements might include hearing and speech, inspection of nasal mucosa, exam of all of the throat and mouth areas, use of equipment for testing and visualization, and examination of other areas of the HEENT not otherwise examined in a multisystem exam. Templates for multi-system and specialty exams can oftentimes be found in various resources.

The levels of exam are problem focused (PF), expanded problem focused (EPF), detailed (D), and comprehensive (C). The following guidelines are listed in the chart below as to how many elements must be included in the patient's medical record as it does differ by type of exam.

EXAM	GENERAL MULTI-SYSTEM EXAM		SINGLE ORGAN SYSTEM EXAMS
	1-5 elements identified by bullet (*)	Problem Focused	1-5 elements identified by bullet (*)
	≥ 6 elements identified by bullet (*)	Exp Problem Focused	≥ 6 elements identified by bullet (*)
	≥ 2 elements identified by bullet (*) from 6 areas / systems OR ≥ 12 elements identified by bullet (*) from ≥ 2 areas / systems	Detailed	≥ 12 elements identified by bullet (*) EXCEPT ≥ 9 elements identified by bullet (*) for eye and psychiatric exams
	Perform all elements identified by bullet (*) from ≥ 9 areas / systems AND document ≥ 2 elements identified by bullet (*) from 9 areas /	Comprehensive	Perform all elements identified by bullet (*): document all elements in shaded boxes; document ≥ 1 element in unshaded boxes

Circle exam type within appropriate grid under Level of Service

Remember, again, that a report can describe negative systems as "HEENT, GU, GI all negative" which constitutes three systems to be used in the determination of the level of exam and subsequently the code. However, if there is a positive finding, it is not adequate for a physician to report this as "GU positive", instead the reason why it is positive needs to be described.

The following is an example of an exam that constitutes 10 systems:

> PHYSICAL EXAM: GENERAL: The patient is a 23-year-old white female who is well-developed and well-nourished and is in no acute distress. Temperature is 98.8 and weight is 120 pounds. Blood pressure is 110/80. HEENT: PEERLA. EOMs intact. Sclerae are clear. NECK: Supple. No adenopathy. Thyroid not palpable. No JVD. HEART: Normal S1 and S2. Normal sinus rhythm. CHEST: Lungs clear to percussion and auscultation. ABDOMEN: Soft, nontender, with no organomegaly. PELVIC/RECTAL: Deferred because they have recently been done by her primary care physician. MUSCULOSKELETAL: No tenderness of the spine. INTEGUMENTARY: Some scarring on the right arm from a previous burn. NEUROLOGICAL: Nonfocal. Cranial nerves II-XII intact.

MEDICAL DECISION MAKING: Medical Decision Making (MDM) is much more complex but provides the justification for medical necessity for services provided; therefore, it is critical to the selection of the proper E/M codes. Many templates today, including computerized, facilitate the completion of the previous two components, history and exam, but oftentimes neglect the impact of MDM, so remember that although a template may be completed fully with reference to history and exam, the selection of a higher E/M code is dependent upon the demonstration of medical necessity through the proper use of codes, Including coding of complications and comorbidities. Complications and comorbidities are conditions that conditions that can influence the outcome of the patient's care, thus possibly resulting in the provision of greater services. Examples include diabetes and AIDS.

Levels of MDM are Straight Forward (SF), Low (L), Moderate (M), and High (H). These levels are determined by the diagnosis, complications, comorbidities, and services provided.

The diagnosis for the reason for the services provided demonstrates medical necessity, therefore, MDM is critical in the selection of proper codes. For example, if a patient presents with a laceration which requires several sutures, then it is not reasonable that the highest level of E/M code should be selected and that extensive tests and labs should be conducted because they simply are not needed and there would be no medical necessity for extensive services. Even if a physician provides extensive services for a minor problem, again, the diagnosis drives the proof of medical necessity and, therefore, the physician would not be reimbursed for additional services that were not warranted by the medical necessity of the diagnosis. This is, again, where the linkage on the billing form between diagnosis and CPT/HCPCS codes is critical in achieving proper reimbursement.

There are several elements used to determine the level of MDM which include number of diagnosis, risk of complications, and amount and/or complexity of data reviewed to which points are attributed as indicated in the chart above. Review the various categories used to determine the data reviewed as there are several factors involved, such as review of lab tests and x-rays. When these three elements are combined, the level of the MDM can be determined. In a straightforward MDM, 1 or less points would result in the lowest level which would be for self-limiting with minor risks. A low complexity MDM would have elements with 2 points and these are two or more self-limited or minor conditions or one stable chronic illness. A moderate complexity MDM would have elements totaling 3 points and the risk would be for one or more chronic illnesses with mild exacerbation, two or more stable chronic illnesses, new undiagnosed problem, acute illness with symptoms, or acute chronic head injury. In a high MDM, there would be 4 or more points and the risk would be one or more acute or chronic illnesses with acute exacerbation with possible threat to life or an abrupt change in neurological status, i.e. unconscious.

A Number of Diagnoses of Treatment Options

Problems to Exam Physician	Number X Points = Results	
Self-limited or minor (Stable, improved or worsening)	1	Max = 2
Est. problem (to examiner): stable, improved	1	
Est. problem (to examiner): worsening	2	
New problem (to examiner): no additional workup planned	3	Max = 3
New prob. (to examiner): add, workup plannec	4	
	TOTAL	

Bring total to line A in Final Result for Complexity

C Amount and/or Complexity of Data to Be Reviewed

Data to Be Reviewed	Points
Review and/or order of clinical lab tests	1
Review and/or order of tests in the radiology section of CPT	1
Review and/or order of tests in the medicine section of CPT	1
Discussion of test results with performing physician	1
Decision to obtain old records and/or obtain history from someone other than patient	1
Review and summarization of old records and/or obtaining history from someone other than patient and/or discussion of case with another health care provider	2
Independent visualization of image, tracing or specimen itself (not simply review of report)	2
TOTAL	

Bring total to line C in Final Result for Complexity

COMPLEXITY

Final Result for Complexity

A	Number diagnoses or treatment options	≤1 Minimal	2 Limited	3 Multiple	≥ 4 Extensive
B	Highest Risk	Minimal	Low	Moderate	High
C	Amount and/or complexity of data	≤ 1 Minimal or Low	Limited	Moderate	≥ 4 Extensive
	Type of decision making	Straight Forward	Low Complex	Moderate Complex	High Complex

Circle exam type within appropriate grid under Level of Service

B Risk of Complications and/or Morbidity or Mortality

Level of Risk	Presenting Problems(s)	Diagnostic Procedure(s) Ordered	Management Options Selected
MINIMAL	One self-limited or minor problem, e.g. cold, insect bite	Laboratory tests requiring venipuncture • Chest X-rays • EKG / EEG • Urinalysis • Ultrasound • KOH prep	• Rest • Gargles • Elastic bandages • Superficial dressings
LOW	• Two or more self-limited or minor problems • One stable chronic illness, e.g. well controlled hypertension, non-insulated dependent diabetes, contact, BPH • Acute uncomplicated illness or injury, e.g. cystitis	• Physiologic tests not under stress, e.g. function tests • Non-cardiovascular imaging studies with contrast, e.g. barium enema • Superficial needle biopsies • Clinical laboratory tests requiring arterial puncture • Skin biopsies	• Over-the -counter drugs • Minor surgery with no identified risk factors • Physical therapy • Occupational therapy • IV fluids without additives
MODERATE	• One or more chronic illnesses with mild exacerbation, progression, or side effects of treatment • Two or more stable chronic illnesses • Undiagnosed new problem with uncertain prognosis, e.g. lump on breast • Acute illness with systemic symptoms, e.g. pyelonephritis • Acute complicated injury, e.g. head injury with brief loss of consciousness	• Physiologic tests under stress, e.g. cardiac stress test, stress test • Diagnostic endoscopies with no identified risk factors • Deep needle or incisional biopsy • Cardiovascular imaging studies with contrast and no identified risk factors, e.g. arteriogram, cardiac cath • Obtain fluid from body cavity, e.g. lumbar punction, thoracemtesis,	• Minor surgery with identified risk factors • Elective major surgery (open percutaneous or endoscopic) with no identified risk factors • Prescription drug management • Therapeutic nuclear medicine • IV fluids with additives • Closed treatment of fracture or dislocation without manipulation
HIGH	• One or more chronic illnesses with severe exacerbation, progression • Acute or chronic illnesses or injuries that may pose a threat to life or badily function, e.g. trauma, acute MI, severe respiratory distress, progressive severe rheumatoid arthritis, psychitatiric illness with potential threat to self or others, acute renal failure • An abrupt change in neurologic status, e.g. seizure, TIA, weakness, or sensory loss	• Cardiovascular imaging studies with contrast with identified risk factors • Cardiac electrophysiological tests • Diagnostic endoscopies with identified risk factors • Discography	• Elective major surgery (open, percutanepus or endoscopic) with identified risk factors • Emergency major surgery (open, percutanepus or endoscopic) • Parenteral controlled substances • Drug therapy requiring intensive monitoring for toxicity • Decision not to resuscitate or to de-escalate care because of poor prognosis

FINAL SELECTION OF E/M CODE: First, it must be determined what type of visit the encounter was, e.g. hospital or office visit.

Second, it must be determined if the patient is new or established. A new patient is defined as the patient having not been seen in the practice for the past three years. There are various statements a physician can make that indicate if a patient is new or established, such as "this patient returns today" which would indicate that the patient is established and "this patient was referred by Dr. ?" which indicates that this patient is new.

Third, Notice that many of the E/M codes list the three components and the level associated with each code for History, Exam, and MDM. Notice in the description of the E/M code that for new patients it states that all three levels for each component must be met in order to select the code; however, with established patients' only two levels must be met. For example, for code 99203 the history and exam must be at least detailed level and MDM must be at least low complexity. Therefore, if a physician report demonstrates that the history was comprehensive, the exam was comprehensive, but the MDM was low then code 99203 for a new patient would be correct. However, if this same scenario was applied to an established patient, then a higher level code, 99215, can be selected because the code states that only two components must be met, so the fact that the MDM was not high enough does not prevent the selection of a higher level code, which is higher-paying.

Medicare and insurance companies are capable of running a computerized report which demonstrate the distribution of the various E/M charges that a healthcare provider has charged. This distribution typically should resemble a Bell Curve with the two ends of the E/M codes being less than the middle where most of the E/M codes should be located. Therefore, there should not be as many 99201 and 99205 E/M visits charged as there are 99202, 99203, and 99204.

UNDER/OVER CODING: Choosing E/M codes lower than the correct level as justified by the medical report is known as undercoding. Choose E/M codes higher than the correct level as justified by the medical report is known as overcoding.

APPENDIX C: Appendix C provides clinical examples of appropriate situations for selecting the proper level of E/M code. However, these are not extensive medical reports and, therefore, very limited as to information provided and thus the ability to properly select the right E/M code.

Section 32.4: OFFICE VISITS

For proper selection of E/M codes, it must be remembered that a physician can only bill for:

ONE E/M PER DAY PER PATIENT PER PRACTICE PER DIAGNOSIS

If anything changes in the above statement, then another E/M can be charged which will be discussed thoroughly below.

Time charged for during an office visit must consist of face-to-face time between the patient and the healthcare provider.

As mentioned in the previous packet, the three levels of the major components of History, Exam, and MDM are listed underneath each code. Remember that with new patient office visits, as described in the notes with the code, all three levels of the components must be met. With established patients only two of three levels of the components must be met in order to select a code.

There is a note within each code which describes a typical timeframe for that level of code, but we do not use this time to justify the selection of the code with few exceptions which will be discussed later.

There are five levels to each section. With new patients, the levels are 99201, 99202, 99203, 99204, and 99205. For established patient, the levels are 99211, 99212, 99213, 99214, and

99215. Sometimes these will be referred to as levels 1, 2, 3, 4, and 5 in discussion but the entire code must always be listed for reimbursement purposes.

Note that with code 99211 there is a note that this code can be used if someone under the supervision of a physician provides services.. All other levels require that a physician provide the services although others may assist them.

Section 32.5: HOSPITAL OBSERVATION VISITS

Sometimes patients are admitted to the hospital for observation only. A patient admitted as "observation" to a hospital do not have to be in an area specified as "observation."

Observation admissions are typically for time periods up to 24 to 48 hours. After this amount of time it is typically expected that the observation should have resulted in either the discharge from the hospital or admission as inpatient.

There are two types of codes for hospital observation services: observation care discharge services (99217) and initial observation care (99218-99220) with only three levels of E/M components used to determine the proper code with no distinction between new and established patients.

On the day when a patient is discharged from the hospital observation, then code 99217 would be used if it occurs on a separate day from the admission. If the admission and discharge occur on the same day, then codes 99234-99236 should be used instead.

Section 32.6: HOSPITAL VISITS

Hospital visits supercede all other E/M visits, so if a patient is seen in the office but then admitted to the hospital by the same physician, then only the hospital admit code could be coded because there can only be one E/M per day per patient per diagnosis per practice. If services are provided in the office in addition to the services provided at the hospital, then the services provided at both locations are included in the development of the report, thus providing additional documentation for the selection of the level of code.

Time charged for during a hospital visit may consist of face-to-face time between the patient and the healthcare provider or unit/floor time at which time the healthcare provider must be on the unit the patient is on and performing duties related to the patient's care.

Hospital visits consist of initial hospital care and subsequent hospital care with no distinction between new and established patients. Initial represents the first day when the patient is admitted and subsequent are all other days except for discharge, which is also coded separately, so for a hospital visit a patient will have charges for at least the initial admit, subsequent day(s), and discharge. Initial hospital care (99221-99223) are used for the admission of the patient to the hospital. Subsequent hospital care (99231-99233) consists of all other days that the patient remains in the hospital. This does not include the day of admission nor the day of discharge. Note that these services have only three levels of codes to select from with regards to the main components. Discharge on a separate day would be coded as 99238-99239. These codes are based only on time with code 99238 for discharge times less requiring less than or equal to 30 minutes of time to complete or 99239 for time requiring more than 30 minutes.

When a patient is admitted and discharged from the hospital on the same date, then codes 99234-99236 should be used.

Section 32.7: CONSULTATIONS

A consultation occurs when an appropriate request is made for a healthcare provider to provide additional examination of a patient. Appropriate requests can only be made by other healthcare providers including physicians, physician assistant, nurse practitioner, chiropractic doctor, physical therapist, occupational therapist, speech-language pathologist, psychologist, social worker, lawyer, or insurance company as described in the CPT book.

A consultation in which the patient and/or family request a second opinion does not qualify as a consultation but is considered a second opinion and is charged as an office or hospital visit.

With a consultation several things must occur in order for a visit to qualify as a consultation. First, the patient needs to be referred by an appropriate requester. This referral source needs to be indicated on the CMS-1500 billing form in box 17.

Second, the consultant cannot take over the care of the patient. The difference between referral and consultation is that in a referral the doctor the patient is referred to will take over the care of the patient. With a consultation, the consultant does not take over the care of the patient. While the consultant is not allowed to assume the care of the patient, there are services the consultant can provide as part of the process to determine the patient's diagnosis and therapeutic care, such as diagnostic tests and procedures.

Third, there must be communication in the patient's chart from the referring agency indicating that this visit is a request for consultation in addition to subsequent communication from the consultant to the referring agency indicating the findings and opinion of the consultant so that the referring physician can make decisions regarding the care of the patient.

After a consultation has been properly completed, the referral physician can recommend to the patient that the consultant take over the care of the patient.

There are two categories for consultations, either office or other (99241-99245) and inpatient hospital (99251-99255). These are all determined in the same manner as office and inpatient hospital with the three key components of History, Exam, and MDM. There is no distinction between new and established patients.

Section 32.8: EMERGENCY DEPARTMENT SERVICES

An emergency department is described in the CPT coding book as "an organized hospital-based facility for the provision of unscheduled episodic services to patients who present for immediate medical attention. The facility must be available 24 hours a day."

There are five levels of Emergency Services from codes 99281 to 99285 which are classified by the three key components of History, Exam, and MDM. The codes are not differentiated as new or established patients.

A patient may receive critical care services while in the Emergency Department, but the services would be coded as critical care and not emergency services. The doctor must determine what type of service the patient is receiving.

Section 32.9: CRITICAL CARE SERVICES

Critical care is described in the CPT coding book as "the direct delivery by a physician of medical care for a critically ill or critically injured patient" with critical illness or injury described as an illness or injury that "acutely impairs one or more vital organ systems such that there is a high probability of imminent or life threatening deterioration". The determination that a patient is receiving critical care is not to be determined by the coder but by the physician and does not need to occur in an area designated as critical care.

Critical care services may be coded in addition to other E/M codes and are not to be added into another E/M code, so a patient may receive inpatient hospital services in addition to critical care and both of these services would be billed separately.

Critical care time by a physician does not have to be consecutive times but can be an accumulation of various times over the period of a day consisting of services provided to one patient. The time can be face-to-face or unit/floor time, so other services the physician provides, such as reviewing charts and research, can also be included in the determination of the time; however, in order to charge for these additional services the physician must be present on the unit where the patient is located and involved in services related to the patient.

In addition, the accumulation of time cannot overlap between patients with the time spent with another patient by the same physician. For example, if a physician spends from 9 am to 10:30 am with a patient, then returns and spends more time from 11:30 to 12:00 noon, then the total amount of time spent with the patient is 2 hours. During the times 9 am to 10:30 am and 11:30 am to 12 noon, the physician cannot charge for time spent with another patient.

Critical care codes are based on time. If a patient receives less than 30 minutes of critical care, then this service would be billed as the appropriate E/M code, such as inpatient hospital. If the patient receives anywhere from 30 to 74 minutes of critical care service, this would be coded as 99291. Additional increments of time are coded with the add-on code 99292 with a "times multiplier" for each additional unit. These increments progress by 30 minutes, i.e. when an additional 30 minutes are provided then additional codes and units are applied. However, the converse of this is that while the 30 minutes starts a new unit of time for critical care, this means the previous unit has to end at 29 minutes. For example, the next increment would be from 75 to 104 minutes and would be coded as 99291 and 99292. The increment after that is from 105 to 134 minutes and is coded as 99291 and 99292 x 2. Rather than trying to understand the concept of the first increment ending at 29 minutes, it is much easier to simply use the table in the CPT coding book.

Services included in critical care and, therefore, not billed separately are listed in the notes of the CPT coding book and include interpretation of cardiac output measurements, X-rays, pulse oximetry, blood gases, gastric intubation, temporary transcutaneous pacing, ventilatory management, and vascular access procedures.

Section 32.10: NURSING FACILITY SERVICES

Nursing facility E/M codes are for services provided in nursing facilities (formerly known as Skilled Nursing Facilities SNF), intermediate care facilities, psychiatric residential treatment center, or long-term care facilities. These facilities conduct comprehensive assessments of each resident upon admission using a data set called Minimum Data Set (MDS) which is contained within the assessment known as Resident Assessment Instrument (RAI). Also included in this instrument are the Resident Assessment Protocols (RAPs) and utilization guidelines.

Nursing facility E/M codes are differentiated as initial or subsequent y the three key components of History, Exam, and MDM, but not on new or established patient. There are only three levels of service though, 99304-99306 for the initial and 99307-99310 for subsequent visits. There are also codes for discharge services with codes 99315-99316 based on time of 30 minutes or less or greater than 30 minutes.

Section 32.11: DOMICILIARY, REST HOME, OR CUSTODIAL CARE SERVICES

These codes include services provided in a facility that provides room and board with personal assistive services, such as a living facility. These codes are differentiated by new patient (99324-99328) and established patient (99334-99337) and by the three key components of History, Exam, and MDM.

Section 32.12: HOME SERVICES

Home services are services provided in a private home. These codes are differentiated by new patient (99341-99345) and established patient (99347-99350) and by the three key components of History, Exam, and MDM.

Section 32.13: PHYSICIAN STANDBY SERVICES

Physician standby services occur when another physician requests that a physician standby to assist in surgery but then the physician's services are not required. If the physician is on standby and does then assist in the surgery, the physician would charge for the surgery and not the standby services. During this time the standby physician cannot be providing services to the patient or any other patient.

The code for standby services is 99360 and requires that the standby is at least 30 minutes in length of time to be an allowed charge. The increments in units for this code are 30 minutes, however, it must be a full 30 minutes to be charged. For example, if a physician is on standby for 85 minutes for a C-section but then his services are not required, then the codes would be 99360 x 2 as there are two full 30 minutes segments but the remaining 25 minutes cannot be charged.

Section 32.14: CASE MANAGEMENT AND OVERSIGHT SERVICES

Various case management services include anticoagulant management (99363-99364) which is based on days, medical team conferences (99366-99368) which are based on time, and care plan oversight services (99374-99380) which are based on time and place of service.

Section 32.15: PREVENTIVE MEDICINE

These visits are better known as "well checks" in which the patient is seen for a regular checkup. These codes are differentiated by age and new or established patient. What is unique to these codes in contrast to the other E/M codes is that patient does not have a chief complaint that initiated the visit, therefore the three key components cannot be used to select the E/M code level.

New patient well checks are coded as 99381-99387 ranging in age. Established patient well checks are coded as 99391-99397 ranging in age.

Section 32.16: OTHER CODES

Other E/M codes include counseling risk factor reduction and behavior change intervention (99401-99429), non-face-to-face physician services include telephone services 99441-99443, on-line medical evaluation 99444, and special evaluation and management services 99450-99456.

There are codes (99490 - 99489) for chronic care management services requiring at least 20 minutes of service for 99490 and at least 60 minutes for the remaining codes with multiple required elements as listed in the code's description.

Code 99497 is for advanced care planning such as for proxies, advanced will directives, power of attorney, and living wills.

Section 32.17: NEWBORN CARE SERVICES

There are E/M codes for newborn care separate from other E/M codes. A newborn is age up to 28 days. These codes are for initial care and discharge for the first days after birth. These codes are based on days and type of care: initial hospital per day (99460), care other than in a hospital per day (99461), subsequent hospital care per day (99462), and admit and discharge on same day (99463). There are also codes for a physician's attendance at the birth (99464) and resuscitation at delivery (99465).

Section 32.18: INPATIENT NEONATAL AND PEDIATRIC INTENSIVE/CRITICAL CARE SERVICES

Neonatal codes are for babies up to 28 days after birth and pediatric codes are for children 24 months of age or less. Physician services provided during the transporting of a neonate or pediatric patient is coded as 99466-99467 and is based on time in increments of 30 minutes. Critical care codes are differentiated by age, day and initial or subsequent using codes 99468-99482 including treatment of hypothermia.

Sections 32.19: CHRONIC CARE MANAGEMENT

Codes 99487-99489 are for complex chronic care management services who demonstrate need for coordination of care, inability to perform daily activities, comorbidities, and need for social support. It is based on time. Transitional care management (99495-99496) are also coded by time and include a wide variety of services that can be considered transitional.

Section 32.20: TIME

Although typically time is not a factor considered in the selection of E/M codes, there are several exceptions when it can be considered.

HIGHER LEVEL CODE: Time can be used to select the proper E/M code when more than half of the time spent with the patient was for services other than those involved in the exam. If the extra time spent by the physician in providing allowable service to the patient is more than 50% of the time requirement of a higher level code, then the higher level code can be selected.

For example, if a patient receives services consistent with a level 1 new office E/M visit, code 99201, but the physician spends an additional 15 minutes providing counseling to the patient, the physician would be able to use the higher level E/M code, 99202. This is because the time requirement for the 99202 code is 20 minutes. Half of 20 minutes is 10 minutes, so the physician would need to provide more than 10 minutes of counseling to justify selecting the higher level E/M code of 99202, which he has. Therefore, although the three key components may only justify coding a 99201 office visit, the extra time spent the physician constitutes more than half of the time requirement for the 99202 code so the higher level 99202 can be selected.

PROLONGED SERVICES: Additional time spent by the physician can also be charged with the prolonged services codes. There are two types of prolonged services series of codes: direct (face-to-face) and nondirect and further divided by either inpatient or outpatient visits. These codes are based on time similar to the Critical Care codes with segments of 30 minutes. Prolonged services less than 30 minutes cannot be charged as an additional code. For prolonged time from 30 to 74 minutes for direct outpatient services, code 99354 is listed. For prolonged times of 75-104 minutes code 99354 and 99355 would be listed. For each additional 30 minutes 99355 would be used again and again. For example, if a physician provides prolonged services of 110 minutes, this would be coded as 99354 and 99355 x 2. Inpatient direct services are coded as 99356 and 99357. Indirect prolonged services are coded as 99358 and 99359 which are for both inpatient and outpatient services.

Notice that both prolonged codes are add-on codes so the prolonged code is coded in addition to any level of E/M code when the physician provides services that extend beyond the expected time for the E/M code, so there would need to be two codes listed when a prolonged code is used, the E/M code and the code for prolonged services.

Section 32.21: ADDITIONAL E/M CODING SCENARIOS

Remember, only one E/M is allowed per day per patient per diagnosis per practice for reimbursement purposes; however, if any of those factors change additional E/Ms can be coded for reimbursement on that day or during a global period.

CHANGE IN PATIENT: Only one E/M can be charged per patient per day per practice per diagnosis; however, if a different patient receive services clearly this is a different visit which is charged separately from visits with any other patients.

CHANGE IN DAY: Only one E/M can be charged per day per patient per practice per diagnosis; however, if the E/M visit occurs on a different day from another visit then clearly this E/M on a new day can be charged separate from the previous day as long as it is not part of a global package as discussed earlier, because a global package code includes all services and visits during the global period.

CHANGE IN DIAGNOSIS: Only one E/M can be charged per diagnosis per patient per practice; however, if the patient is seen for a different diagnosis on the same day then this additional visit can be charged since there is a different reason for the visit, so the same patient on the same day could be seen by a physician for different reasons and both visits would be reimbursed. The important aspect to these criteria is that different diagnosis must be listed on the billing form and linked to the different E/M visits. If two E/M visits performed on the same day are linked on the billing form to the same diagnosis, then the second E/M will not be paid. This reasoning also applies to other services provided on the same day in which the E/M might be assumed to be included as part of the other services provided, thus if the diagnoses linked to each service or E/M are not different, then reimbursement may be denied with the reason that is may be a duplicate, not medically necessary, or part of a global. Modifiers 24 and 25 can be used to indicate this which will be discussed below.

CHANGE IN PRACTICE: Only one E/M can be charged per practice per diagnosis per patient; however, if the practice is not the same practice that provided the initial E/M visit then both practices can charge for their E/M services on the same day for the same patient for the same diagnosis. However, the practice must meet the criteria of being separate from the other practice and there are several scenarios in which this is so.

i. One of the easiest ways to demonstrate that practices are separate is the use of separate tax ID numbers. This can be important particularly in clinics where there may be different specialties to ensure that the separateness of the practices is clear.

ii. In a clinic there may be different practices based on different specialties which can be considered to be separate and can, therefore, bill separately.

iii. The arrangement between healthcare providers/physicians may be delineated as separate or not, whether as single providers or multiple providers. Providers can either decide to create a practice together and bill together in which case a patient cannot visit any of these physicians on the same day for the same diagnosis as they did for another physician within that practice. However, several physicians may agree to work within the same offices yet retain their own separate practices and, therefore, a patient can see both of them on the same day for the same diagnosis and both physicians would be able to bill separately. This retention of separate practices remains even if the physicians have an agreement to provide coverage when the other physician is absent; however, when a patient sees the other physician under the circumstances that the physician is covering for the other, then the charges and billing remain under the principal physician and not the physician providing coverage during the absence of the other physician.

Section 32.22: MODIFIERS

Modifiers consist of two digits (either numeric or alphanumeric) and are attached to a regular CPT code at the end of the code by a dash and then the two-digit modifier, e.g. 11201-51. Modifiers indicate changes in the status of the main code which may result in changes in reimbursement but it does not alter the definition of the code.

Modifiers are listed in Appendix A. Notice that some of these modifiers are described as only being applied to certain codes, such as E/M codes only. We will be discussing those modifiers used only for E/M codes or related to their use and the reason and impact they have on reimbursement.

a. **Modifier 24** is described as “Unrelated Evaluation and Management Service by the Same Physician During a Postoperative Period.” Remember that in a global package there is a postoperative period which is different for different procedures. During this postoperative period, no services that are typically included in the procedure can be charged because they are included in the code for the procedure. Remember, a physician or practice can only charge for one E/M per day per patient per diagnosis.

   However, during that global period a patient may certainly need healthcare for a different reason by the same physician or practice group which would not be included in the payment for the global package, in other words the diagnosis changes so another E/M service can be charged. However, if a claim is submitted the payer may believe that the charges are for services included in the global and will not pay. To ensure that payment is made for services performed for reasons other than the global package by the same physician or practice, this modifier should be attached to the procedural code, which is the purpose of this modifier, in addition to the linkage of the different diagnosis on the billing form. This modifier is explaining that the patient had an E/M visit for reasons other than the globally packaged procedure and that this E/M was not a postoperative visit for the procedure and, therefore, is reimbursable.

For example, if a patient had a fracture package for a broken tibia which is still in the postoperative global period but the patient is seen today for an office visit due to complaints of severe stomach pains which is not related to the fracture care and, therefore, the visit can be billed as an E/M code with this modifier attached, i.e. 99203-24. Notice that this modifier can only be attached to E/M codes.

b. **Modifier 25** is described as "Significant Separately Identifiable Evaluation and Management Service by the Same Physician on the Same Day of the Procedure or Other Service." This modifier is applied in the same way as the previous modifier, 24, except this modifier is applied to an E/M service that is provided on the same day by the same physician or practice but which has a diagnosis different from the a previous E/M service or procedure on the same day. Again, the diagnosis changes so the same physician or practice can charge for another E/M service on the same day. To ensure that payment is made for services performed for reasons other than the other E/M on the same day by the same physician or practice, this modifier should be attached to the procedural code, which is the purpose of this modifier, in addition to the linkage of the different diagnosis on the billing form.

   For example, if a patient is seen earlier in the day by the same physician or practice for complaints of GI bleeding, but then returns later that day for complaints of uncontrolled diabetes then there are two different diagnosis so two visits can be charged for that day but the modifier must be attached to the E/M code. This also applies to if a service is provided earlier in the day at the same physician or practice's office, such as a wound repair, but then the patient returns later that day to the same physician or practice for complaints associated with uncontrolled diabetes. The first visit would be the procedural code for the wound repair and the second code would be for the E/M visit with the modifier 25 attached.

   However, if the patient returns later in the day and the diagnosis remains the same then an additional E/M visit cannot be charged because the diagnosis remains the same; however, if any additional services are provided these can be combined together with the services from the earlier visit to determine the level of the visit. This is also true if the patient is admitted or seen in the hospital earlier in the day by one physician from a practice and then the patient is seen later in the day by another physician from the same practice, such as for rounds or complications; again, only one E/M can be charged for the day despite there being two different physicians because they are from the same practice and the visits are on the same day for the same diagnosis, but in both of these scenarios only one E/M can be charged for the day which is linked to the same diagnosis.

c. **Modifier 32** is described as "Mandated Service." This modifier is attached to an E/M service or procedure that was required by a third party, such as an insurance company or government agency, e.g. if a patient is required to have a worker's compensation evaluation.

d. **Modifier 54** is described as surgical care only; **modifier 55** is described as postoperative management only; and **modifier 56** is described as preoperative management only. Although these codes are only attached to surgical codes, they will be discussed because they are used to code for office visits. Remember in a global all pre and postoperative care (which includes office visits) is included as well as any other related services that are included as part of a major procedure for the physician who provides the major procedure.

While the physician who performed the major procedure cannot be reimbursed for any pre and postoperative office visits as it is included in the global, a different physician who provides an office visit either before or after a global procedure has been performed should be reimbursed for their services since they did not receive any reimbursement for the performance of the procedure – this is where these modifiers assist in reimbursement. If a physician provides an office visit before a procedure which is performed by another physician, then the physician providing the preop office visit will list the code for the operative procedure followed by the modifier 54. If the physician only performs the surgical procedure, then they should list the procedural code followed by the modifier 55. The physician providing a postoperative office visit would list the procedure followed by the modifier 56.

It is important that physicians use these modifiers if they know they are going to be providing pre and/or postoperative care, otherwise other physicians who provide the pre and/or postoperative care will be denied reimbursement, and usually this translates into the patient will be denied any follow-up care unless they return to the physician who performed the procedure which is not always possible.

For example, if a patient is visiting relatives in another state and sustains a fracture which is treated in that state, when the patient returns, maybe a week later to his home state he will need follow-up care for the fracture.

E/M CODES QUIZ 23

1) What are the codes for a patient who received IV infusion of non-chemotherapeutic drugs for 3 hours for septicemia?

2) What are the correct codes for a 32-year-old patient, well known to the physician, presents with complaints of fever, backache, and blood in urine. Patient states that the backache began a week ago, but the blood appeared last night with the pain worsening overnight. ROS is negative for all systems except for GI for which the patient has had ulcers in the past which were treated with prescriptions. Exam today found the patient to be malnourished as he has not been eating for several days now due to the pain. HEENT is negative and PERRLA. Head is normocephalic. Throat is clear. No adenopathy. Heart shows normal S1 and S2. No syncope or murmur. Lungs are clear to P&A. Extremities move well with no edema. Patient is ordered to get x-rays and blood labs were sent and patient was given a prescription. Patient is to return if pain continues after a week.

3) What would the codes be for a patient who was seen today at the doctor's office for their regular checkup for their diabetes Type I which is exacerbated with a high blood sugar so the history is PF and the exam is EPF. The physician conducts further testing and counseling including discussion with patient for further evaluation and treatment which was 50 more minutes?

4) What are the codes for a new patient who is having difficulty breathing and is seen today in the office? The patient's father had a history of asthma as does the patient. The patient does have COPD. The patient states that the breathing became more difficult after a long afternoon of playing basketball but has not been alleviated by his asthma medication and has only become more difficult overnight. The ROS is negative except for the history of breathing problems. During the exam, the patient's condition worsened and he was admitted to the hospital by the physician with the exam finding that GU, GI, skin, and HEENT normal. The patient does have hypertension which is treated with medication. Extremities move well with no edema. Cranial nerves are intact.

5) What are the codes for a patient who was admitted to the hospital at 9 pm due to various trauma from a car accident with numerous facial lacerations as well as a possible concussion when they hit the windshield with the patient having lost consciousness in the ambulance? Patient was intoxicated so it was difficult to get a history and the exam was detailed. The patient then left AMA at 11:30 pm.

6) What are the codes for a patient who was admitted yesterday and seen today in the hospital for various testing due to difficulty breathing and pain to determine if the patient was a candidate for surgery to remove carcinoma of the left lung, but the patient is not a good candidate with history being detailed and exam detailed?

7) What are the codes for a 30-day old newborn who was admitted to the hospital for complications due to withdrawal due to mother's use of cocaine during the pregnancy

which included anoxia, failure to thrive, and seizures requiring critical care. The history is EPF and the exam is detailed.

8) What are the codes for a physician who was on standby for 45 minutes to assist with a C-section at which time he did assist for a successful C-section of a single liveborn male?

9) What are the codes for a 65-year-old patient who was referred to a cardiologist by their PCP due to possible CVA with hemiplegia on the left side with an EPF history and exam and Moderate MDM?

10) What are the codes for this new patient who is seen today in the office as referred by his PCP for possible AIDS with the patient's labs positive for HIV and tests are positive for Kaposi's sarcoma as was suspected with EPF History and Exam and moderate MDM so the physician spent 25 minutes counseling the patient and his family?

11) What are the codes for a patient who is required by the insurance company for a consultation for a work-related injury when the patient fell from the roof and injured his back with a comprehensive History and Exam and Moderate MDM?

12) What are the codes for a 2-year-old who is seen today for a well check as part of continuing pediatric care with the office?

13) What are the codes for an alcoholic patient who was admitted to the hospital at 9 pm due to possible concussion in a car accident with acute intoxication but who was transferred to another hospital at 11 pm for further treatment with a PF history and exam and moderate MDM?

14) What are the codes for a patient who was admitted to the hospital with a Detailed History and Exam and moderate MDM due to possible kidney failure, which was later diagnosed as kidney failure and the patient was provided critical care from 10:30 to 12:30 and 2:30 to 4:00?

15) What are the codes for a 3-year-old child who is seen in the emergency room after hitting their head on the fireplace that required sutures with PF History and EPF exam with SF MDM?

16) What are the codes for a premature baby born at 32 weeks who was in NICU an. received services from the physician from 9:30pm to 11:00 pm and then from 11:30 pm to 1:00 am?

17) What are the codes for a patient who is seen today in the office for follow-up after repair of a greenstick facture of the shaft of right radius with manipulation that occurred a week ago with a PF history and exam with SF MDM?

18) What are the codes for a well-known patient who was seen in the office for checkup of COPD and asthma due possibly to pneumonia with the History PF history, EPF exam,

and SF MDM, but the patient was found to be experiencing a severe headache and hemiparesis so the patient was admitted to the hospital for possible CVA with an EPF history and EPF exam and moderate MDM? Later that day another physician from the practice visited the patient on rounds and found that the patient's condition had deteriorated with neurological disturbances and further tests were ordered with a Detailed History and Exam and high complexity MDM.

19) What are the codes for a patient well known to this doctor who is seen today for a check of his diabetes Type I who cut his toe a week ago and which is now infected with a PF history, EPF exam, and moderate MDM and who had removal of a 1.5-cm lesion from her right hand? The patient was also examined for a suspicious neoplasm on his back which was removed and specimen sent to path.

20) What are the codes for a patient who was admitted to the hospital for observation for 24 hours due to complaints of chest pains after having undergone a CABG for ASHD and MI a month before but tests were negative?

CHAPTER 33
HCPCS

You will learn the following objectives in this chapter:

A. HCPCS
   a. CPT
   b. DME
   c. DMEPOS
B. Format
   a. Sections
   b. Selection of Codes
   c. Durable Medical Equipment
   d. Administration of Drugs
C. Modifiers
D. Codes

Section 33.1: HCPCS

The HCPCS are known as the Healthcare Common Procedural Coding System. Remember, level I HCPCS are the CPT codes and level II are the codes contained within the HCPCS book and are also known as the national codes. These codes are alphanumeric and are used to bill for the many services that are not included in the CPT book, such as durable medical equipment and supplies. HCPCS include codes for durable medical equipment (DME) and durable medical equipment, prosthetics, orthotics, and supplies (DMEPOS).

Section 33.2: FORMAT

HCPCS are produced by CMS and are used to code for supplies, materials, and injectable material in addition to certain procedures and services that are no listed in the CPT codes. These codes embrace over 4000 categories for millions of products.

There are three types of HCPCS codes Level II which are permanent national codes which are the majority of the codes, dental codes, temporary codes, and miscellaneous codes which provide a means of coding materials and supplies that do not have an applicable code.

Temporary codes are used to code for several types of materials and supplies that have not yet been assigned a permanent code. This includes C codes for pass-through payments for outpatient hospital claims which are not relevant to physician coding. G codes are for services that would otherwise be listed in CPT but are not. Q codes are for services that would not be given a CPT code, such as drugs. K codes are for DMEs that are currently not listed in the code book. S codes are for use by private insurers for materials and services when there are no national codes available. H codes are for Medicaid agencies for mental health services. T codes are for use by Medicaid for services or items for which there are no national codes.

HCPCS codes are required for use on Medicare claims, and most other payers now require their use too.

Sometimes CMS will not accept certain CPT codes and will require the use of HCPCS codes instead such as G0001 is used to code for venipuncture instead of CPT code 36415.

Remember that services and supplies that are an inherent part of a larger procedure or service are bundled into the larger procedure and cannot be coded separately, which applies to HCPCS supplies and materials as well, so a surgical tray, for example, would not be coded in addition to the surgery.

HCPCS codes are updated quarterly by CMS. Like all coding materials produced by CMS, it is a public domain and free to download which you can find at the http://www.cms.hhs.gov/. Otherwise, it can be purchased from publishers who create various versions of the book for sale.

Section 33.3: FORMAT:

HCPCS codes are alphanumeric and composed of five digits with the first being an alphabetical character and the other digits are numbers.

SECTIONS: The following are the sections within the book:

Transportation Services Including Ambulance	A0021-A0999
Medical and Surgical Supplies	A4206-A8004
Administrative Miscellaneous and Investigational	A9150-A9999
Enteral and Parenteral Therapy	B4034-B9999
Outpatient PPS	C1300-C9728
Dental Procedures	D0120-D9999
Durable Medical Equipment	E0100-E8002
Procedures/Services Temporary Codes	G0008-G9036
Oncology Demonstration Project	G9050-G9139
Alcohol and Drug Abuse Treatment Services	H0001-H2037
Drugs Administered Other Than Oral Method	J0120-J8999
Chemotherapy Drugs	J9000-J999
Temporary Codes for DME Regional Carriers	K0001-K0899
Orthotic Procedures	L0112-L4398
Prosthetic Procedures	L5000-L9900
Medical Services	M0064-M0301
Pathology and Laboratory Services	P2028-P9615
Q Codes (Temporary)	Q0035-Q9964
Diagnostic Radiology Services	R0070-R0076
Temporary National Codes (Non-Medicare)	S0012-S9999
National T Codes Established for State Medicaid Agencies	T1000-T5999
Vision Services	V2020-V2799
Hearing Services	V5008-V5364

Section 33.4: SELECTION OF CODES

These codes are very easy to use and resemble a typical catalog of supplies and materials, so the format to using them is simple. To select the proper code, the alphabetical index should be checked. For selection of drugs, there is a Table of Drugs available.

DURABLE MEDICAL EQUIPMENT: Durable Medical Equipment (DME) is composed of various equipment and services provided by a company which is a durable medical equipment company that has obtained their own provider number and is approved by Medicare. If they are not approved by Medicare, then Medicare will not provide any payment and patients must be informed of this through and Advanced Beneficiary Notice (ABN). These companies include companies that provide durable medical equipment, orthotics, and supplies (DMEPOS). Claims for these services are processed by durable medical equipment regional carriers (DMERCs).

Be careful when selecting the codes to ensure that the number of units are properly charged. Most HCPCS codes describe if the materials and supplies are charged per unit, as each or separate.

ADMINISTRATION OF DRUGS: Drug materials that are administered by the physician (other than oral method of administration) are coded with J codes. These are only charged when the physician has purchased the medication and administered it in addition to the charge for administration by a physician which will be discussed in a later packet. If the physician does not purchase the medication but does administer it, then only the administration code can be charged.

Medications are listed in the HCPCS book by name, dosage, and route of administration so there can be multiple codes for the same medication but in different dosages and by different route of administration.

Sometimes a medication will be administered in a dosage that does not equate to a specific dosage in the HCPCS codes. In this case you must be sure to select a code that includes enough of the medication to ensure that the physician received full payment and the excess is not considered. For example, if a patient receives a 400 mcg injection of filgrastim, the HCPCS codes indicate that it is only administered by injection. There are two dosages listed: J1440 for 300 mcg, J1441 for 480 mcg. Since 400 mcg was injected so neither code has the correct dosage, the code J1441 should be listed since it contains enough of the material, i.e. 480 mcg although the entire dose is not administered. However, if 500 mcg were administered, then both codes would be listed to ensure that enough material has been charged.

Sometimes several doses of a medication may be given. In this case, you must list the code for the medication and use a multiplier for the additional units. For example, if 100 mg of amphotericin B is injected, then code J0286 (50 mg) would be listed twice as J0286 x 2.

Medication codes are listed in milliliters (mL) or in cubic centimeters (cc). Therefore, it is possible that you would have to convert the amount of medication if the physician does not describe in the units under which the code is describe, so remember that one cc equal one mL.

Section 33.5: MODIFIERS

HCPCS modifiers can be used for both CPT and HCPCS codes. They are composed of two digits, either alphanumeric or numeric. HCPCS modifiers are used to describe anatomic site, dressings, healthcare provider, additional information about procedures and services, type of healthcare program, reason for healthcare, funding agency, regulations on DMEPOS, physical status of patient, findings, anesthesia, opinions, and level of Medcaid care.

Some major HCPCS modifiers are listed in the front of the CPT coding book.

HCPCS modifiers include:
A1: Dressing for 1 wound
A2: Dressing for 2 wounds
A9: Dressing for 9 or more wounds
AG: Primary physician
AX: Item furnished in conjunction with dialysis services
BO: Orally administered nutrition, not by feeding tube
E1: Upper left, eyelid
E2: Lower left, eyelid
E3; Upper right, eyelid
E4: Lower right, eyelid
ET: Emergency services
F1: Left hand, second digit (beginning with index finger)
F2: Left hand, third digit
F3: Left hand, fourth digit
F4 Left hand, fifth digit
F5: Right hand, thumb
F6: Right hand, second digit
F7: Right hand, third digit
F8: Right hand, fourth digit
F9: Right hand, fifth digit
FA: Left hand, thumb
GH: Diagnostic mammogram converted from screening mammogram on same day
H9: Court ordered
HF: Substance abuse program
KI: DMEPOS item, second or third month rental
LC: Left circumflex coronary artery
LD: Left anterior descending coronary artery
LT: Left side
M2: Medicare secondary payer
NU: New equipment
P1: Normal healthy patient

P6: Declared brain-dead patient whose organs are being removed for donor purposes
QS: Monitored anesthesia care service
QW: CLIA waived test
RC: Right coronary artery
RT: Right side
SA: Nurse practitioner rendering service in collaboration with a physician
SC: Medically necessary service or supply
T1: Left foot, second digit (great toe is the first digit)
T2: Left foot, third digit
T3: Left foot, fourth digit
T5: Right foot, great toe
T9: Right foot, fifth digit
TA: Left foot, great toe
TC: Technical component
UE: Used durable medical equipment

There are also single digit modifiers that can be applied to ambulance services which indicates where the ambulance is coming from with the patient:
H: Hospital
N: Skilled nursing facility
P: Physician's office
R: Residence
S: Scene of accident

Section 33.6: CODES

Following is a listing of some HCPCS codes:

A4206: Syringe with needle, sterile 1 cc or less, each
A4222: Infusion supplies for external drug infusion pump per cassette or bag (list drugs separately)
A4250: Urine test or reagent strips or tablets (100 tablets or strips)
A4301: Implantable access total catheter, port/reservoir)
A5501: For diabetics only, fitting (including follow-up) custom preparation and supply of shoe mold from casts of patient's foot per shoe
A6216: Gauze, non-impregnated, non-sterile, pad size 16 sq. in or less without adhesive border, each dressing
A9560: Technetium Tc-99m labeled red blood cells, diagnostic, per study dose, up to 30 mCi
B4087: Gastrostomy/jejunostomy tube, standard, any material any type, each
B4220: Parenteral nutrition supply kit; premix, per day
E0100: Cane, includes canes or all materials, adjustable or fixed with tip
E0110: Crutches, forearm, includes crutches of various materials adjustable or fixed pair, complete with tips and handgrips
E0424: Stationary compressed gaseous oxygen system, rental
E0607: Home blood glucose monitor
E1050: Fully reclining wheelchair, fixed full-length arms, swing away detachable elevating leg

rests

H0001: Alcohol and/or drug assessment
J1440: Injection, filgrastim 300 mcg (Neupogen)
J1630: Injection, haloperidol, up to 5 mg (Haldol)
J1631: Injection, haloperidol decanoate, per 50 mg (Haldol deconoate)
J7030: Infusion, normal saline solution, 1000 cc
J7070: Infusion D-5-W 1000 cc (Dextrose 5% in water)
J7609: Albuterol, inhalation solution, compounded product, administered through DME, unit dose 1 mg (Ventolin, Proventil)
J9070: Cyclophosphamide 100 mg (Cytoxan, Neosar)
J9080: Cyclophosphamide, 200 mg (Cytoxan, Neosar)
L5000: Partial foot, shoe insert with longitudinal arch, toe filler
L5200: Above knee molded socket, single axis constant friction knee, shin, SACH foot
V2100: Sphere, single vision, plano to plus or minus 4.00, per lens
V2623: Prosthetic eye, plastic, custom
V5254: Hearing aid, digital, monaural CIC

CHAPTER 34
ANESTHESIA

You will learn the following objectives in this chapter:

A. Types
   1. General
   2. Block
   3. Regional
   4. Epidural
   5. Conscious (Moderate) Sedation
   6. Monitored Anesthesia Care (MAC)
   7. Local
B. Format
   1. Classification
   2. Package
   3. Time
C. Modifiers
   1. Surgeon
   2. HCPCS
   3. Physical Status
D. Qualifying Circumstances
E. Pain Management

Section 34.1: ANESTHESIA

Anesthesia codes are for services provided by a licensed healthcare provider to provide for the removal or blocking of sensation which includes pain.

TYPES: Anesthesia can be provided as general, block, regional, epidural, and monitored anesthesia care.

1. General: General anesthesia occurs when the patient experiences loss of consciousness due to the introduction of drugs, usually inhalation, which create a state wherein patients are not arousable even by painful stimulation. Patients generally need maintenance of an airway as they cannot breathe on their own.
2. Block: A block occurs when a small volume of local anesthetics are injected into the spinal canal which results in loss of sensation to a specific area of the body.
3. Regional: Regionals occur when a local anesthesia is administered to specific peripheral nerves which results in loss of sensation to a specific area only.
4. Epidural: Epidurals are regional anesthesia that is performed by the injection of local anesthetic into the epidural space of the spinal canal.
5. Conscious (Moderate) Sedation: A moderate level of anesthesia provided by a physician to allay patient anxiety and control pain as opposed to a deep level and in which the patient remains able to respond to verbal commands and light tactile stimulation.
6. Monitored Anesthesia Care (MAC): MAC is the anesthesia which is part of a planned procedure in which the patient undergoes local anesthesia together with

sedation and analgesia so that the patient is awake and able to provide feedback to the physician in addition to faster recovery for the patient as opposed to a slower recovery with general anesthesia. MAC differs from Conscious Sedation in that a qualified individual must be responsible for administration who can convert to general anesthesia and restore the airway immediately if needed or compromised. The use of sedatives, hypnotics, and analgesics that are used in general anesthesia are also used.

7. Local: Local anesthesia is similar to regional but a much smaller defined area of the body is anesthetized.

Section 34.2: FORMAT

If you are coding for an anesthesiologist, then you will not use surgical codes but will use the codes listed in the Anesthesia section of the CPT book.

Anesthesia must be provided by a licensed healthcare provider, including anesthesiologists, physicians, certified registered nurse anesthetists (CRNSa) or anesthesiologist assistants.

Two types of anesthesia codes will be discussed in this packet. First are the codes described within the Anesthesia section of the CPT codes. Second are the pain management codes described within the Surgery section of the CPT codes.

Anesthesia codes range from 00100 to 01999. Only one anesthesia code can be used per session, which should be the anesthesia code for the most difficult and, therefore, time consuming and costly procedure.

CLASSIFICATION: Anesthesia codes are primarily classified by anatomic site. As this is very clear cut and the Anesthesia section is so small, you can just as easily find the anesthesia code in the section by looking under the anatomic site, as well as by looking in the alphabetical index.

Anesthesia codes are further classified by some specific procedures which are listed underneath general codes for procedures and services. If an anesthesia code is not listed for a specific procedure, then the general code must be selected. For example, code 00700 is for anesthesia for procedures performed on the upper anterior abdomen, but there is a specific code for percutaneous liver biopsy (00702) underneath the 00700 code.

PACKAGE: Codes for anesthesia are packages which contain other services including anesthesia during the procedure, administration of fluids, and monitoring (ECG, temperature, oximetry (oxygen), capnography (carbon dioxide). Unusual types of monitoring are not included and should be coded separately, such as arterial catheters, central venous lines, and Swan-Ganz catheters.

TIME: In addition to the code for the anesthesia, the time should also be reported which begins with the preparation of the patient and ends when the patient is placed under postoperative supervision. Time is measured in units with one unit being equal to 15 minutes. If several procedures are performed, only one anesthesia code is listed which is the most difficult and time-consuming procedure, and all of the time spent in surgery (which is an accumulation of the time spent on all procedures) are added and used as the time for the anesthesia.

Section 34.3: MODIFIERS

MODIFIERS 47: If a surgeon performs the anesthesia in addition to the procedure, then only the procedure code is listed with a modifier 47 attached; however, most types of anesthesia that are performed are usually included in the procedural code, e.g. if a patient receives sutures the anesthesia by the physician is included.

MODIFIER 23: This modifier is for "unusual anesthesia". This means that a type of anesthesia that is more extensive in time and cost was used for a procedure for which it would normally not be used, e.g., if a patient is mentally handicapped it may be more difficult to treat them so they need to receive a general anesthesia, such as tooth removal.

HCPCS MODIFIERS: HCPCS modifiers that are used for anesthesia include AA for anesthesia services performed personally by anesthesiologist; AD for medical supervision by a physician for more than four concurrent anesthesia procedures (when the surgeon or anesthesiologist are overseeing more than one other person who is providing the anesthesia, such as anesthetists); G8 for monitored anesthesia care (MAC) for deep complex, complicated or markedly invasive surgical procedure; G9 for monitored anesthesia for patient who has history of severe cardiopulmonary condition; QK for medical direction of two, three or four concurrent anesthesia procedures involving qualified individuals; QS for monitored anesthesia care (MAC) service and QY for medical direction of one CRNA by anesthesiologist.

PHYSICAL STATUS MODIFIERS: Physical status modifiers are used to indicate certain physical statuses of the patient that may affect the administration and complexity of anesthesia. Not all carriers recognize the use of these modifiers and will not provide additional reimbursement due to the increased complexity of a higher level physical status for a patient. These modifiers are attached the same as other modifiers with a dash after the anesthesia code, followed by the two digit alphanumeric modifier as described below:

1. P1: A normal healthy patient. This modifier can be attached to all healthy patients; otherwise, if no physical status modifier is attached to an anesthesia code, then it would be assumed that the patient's status was a P1.
2. P2: A patient with mild systemic disease. The anesthesiologist must provide the documentation and make the determination if the patient is P2, as is true of the remaining modifiers.
3. P3: A patient with severe systemic disease.
4. P4: A patient with severe systemic disease that is a constant threat to life.
5. P5: A moribund patient who is not expected to survive without the operation.
6. P6: A declared brain-dead patient whose organs are being removed for donor purposes. Anesthesia is still provided as this time because it is not known what such a patient may be undergoing during the process and so it is considered humane to do so.

Section 34.4: QUALIFYING CIRCUMSTANCES

Qualifying circumstances are codes listed in the medicine section but which are used as additional codes for anesthesia services because they represent unusually difficult situations that may affect the administration of anesthesia and its outcomes. In addition to being listed in the medicine section, these codes are also listed in the notes in the beginning of the anesthesia section. They are marked as add-on codes and must be used in conjunction with an anesthesia code.

These codes can only be listed if the patient's record describes the condition.

Code 99100 is for anesthesia administered to a patient of extreme age, either younger than one year or older than 70.

Code 99116 is for anesthesia administered to a patient whose health is compromised by total body hypothermia.

Code 99135 is for anesthesia administered to a patient whose health is compromised by controlled hypotension.

Code 99140 is for anesthesia administered to a patient whose health is compromised by an emergency condition and the condition must be specified also.

Section 34.5: PAIN MANAGEMENT

Other than for anesthesia during a procedure, anesthetic procedures are also provided for other reasons, particularly for pain management and provided by physicians. No physical status modifiers or qualifying conditions are used with these codes.

Examples of anesthesia used for control of pain include epidurals for labor and delivery (CPT 62319 continuous lumbar epidural infusion) or placement of an epidural during surgery to control postoperative pain (62318-62319) which is billed separately from the anesthesia during the surgery. If an epidural is used for postoperative pain management for more than a day and the anesthesiologist must check it, this can be coded as 01996 (daily management of epidural).

Other pain management codes include epidurals for control of pain in other parts of the body which may be coded from the anatomic site sections or from other codes which can be found in the alphabetical index under "pain" or "injection". For placement of epidurals, codes 62350-62351, 62360-62362, or 99601-99602 could be used or for IVs codes 96374-96379.

Trigger point injections are used to treat pain in muscles due to the presence of a knot formed when a muscle fails to relax. An injection is the introduction of a local anesthetic through a needle into the muscle which inactivates the trigger point, thereby alleviating the pain. Trigger injections would be coded as 20550-20553. Codes are differentiated also on if ultrasound guidance was used.

ANESTHESIA QUIZ 24

1) What are the anesthesia codes for a patient who had a lobectomy of the right lung due to small cell carcinoma which metastasized to the kidney and who was admitted to the hospital with severe difficulty breathing which was also complicated by pneumoniae pneumonia?

2) What are the anesthesia codes for a patient who was given an epidural during her delivery due to prolonged delivery because of a large baby at 42 weeks?

3) What are the anesthesia codes for a 75-year-old patient who had emergency amputation of their left leg below the knee due to gangrene and sepsis after the patient was experiencing septic shock?

4) What are the anesthesia codes for a patient who has an esophagectomy performed due to esophageal cancer that has metastasized to the liver and brain?

5) What are the anesthesia codes for removal of an infected dental molar from a 3-year-old which required general anesthesia?

6) What are the anesthesia codes for a 1-year-old child who had tubes placed in her ears for suppurative otitis media?

7) What are the anesthesia codes for a patient who required a C-section due to fetal distress at 34 weeks?

8) What are the anesthesia codes for a patient who had two left toes removed due to frostbite after the patient was lost in a snowstorm and experienced hypothermia?

9) What are the anesthesia codes for a patient who had a rectal endoscopy with biopsy due to bleeding?

10) What are the anesthesia codes for a patient who had a pacemaker implanted due to ventricular fibrillation and hypertension?

CHAPTER 35
CPT MODIFIERS

You will learn the following objectives in this chapter:

A. Modifiers
B. Bilateral
A. Multiple
B. E/M
C. Anesthesia
D. Surgical

Section 35.1: MODIFIERS

CPT modifiers are two-digit alphanumerical codes that follow the CPT code and are separated from it with a hyphen. There are additional modifiers as listed in the HCPCS that can contain alphanumerical or alphabetical letters, for example, E1 for upper left eyelid and T1 for left foot, second digit. Modifiers indicate when there are additional circumstances influencing the CPT or HCPCS code that may alter reimbursement; therefore, they help ensure accurate payment for services. Some modifiers can be used with all CPT codes, but some can only be used with certain ones, as will later be discussed with each modifier. Some modifiers can only be applied to certain codes, such as E/M or surgery, and not to other codes. Modifiers are listed in Appendix A but also in some of the information sections of major headings of the code book, such as "Anesthesiology."

More than one modifier can be attached to a code (e.g., 73580-59-50).

Section 35.2: BILATERAL

Bilateral refers to the performance of the same procedure on both sides, such as ears or eyes; however, in order to use the bilateral modifier the sides must be mirror images of each other. With the heart and lungs, the two sides are not the same so the bilateral modifier cannot be used for these anatomic sites.

If a code is described as bilateral and the procedure is bilateral, you do not need to use a modifier. If, however, the code is described as unilateral, or does not say bilateral, then unilateral is assumed. If a unilateral code is used for a bilateral procedure, then you must use the modifier 50. Using the modifier 50 is preferable in coding bilateral procedures or services because it is more descriptive and familiar than billing twice or placing a 2 in the unit box on the billing form.

If a procedure is described as bilateral, but only a unilateral procedure is done, then use modifier 52, which is for reduction of service.

WARNING: Procedures done on both sides of the body are not always necessarily considered bilateral, but rather multiple procedures. For instance, a heart catheter is not listed as bilateral even if it goes through both sides of the body because the course of the catheter is the intent of the code, not whether it is done on opposite sides or not. Another example would be lacerations repaired on both sides of the face. None of these are considered bilateral procedures. However, mastectomies on both sides of the breasts would be considered bilateral. Also, the two sides have to be mirror images of each other as previously described.

Section 35.3: MULTIPLE

Modifier 51 is used for multiple services provided during the same visit.

Do not use modifier 51 on codes that are listed as separate, each, additional, or add-ons, or that have a 51 exempt notation. Modifier 51 is not used with E/Ms or pathology codes. Instead, when listing an E/M code with other services, use a 25 modifier to indicate that the E/M service is provided at the same time as another service but is separate and distinct and not associated with the other services (i.e., not part of a global package). Modifier 51 is not used when there are separately distinct diagnoses for each service or procedure or when the services or procedures are provided at different visits. A 59 must be attached to indicate the difference for the services (e.g., preoperative and postoperative x-rays for a procedure, so code for procedure and both x-rays with modifier 59).

Section 35.4: E/M MODIFIERS

The following three modifiers are used with E/M codes only.

Modifier 21 is for prolonged E/M services. This modifier can only be used on the highest level of E/M service because if services are higher than a -low-level code, you would simply move up in the levels of E/M codes until you reached the highest level.

Modifier 24 is for unrelated E/M services by the same physician during a postoperative (global) period. Payment for such a service would be questionable because the patient is in a postoperative period, but this modifier signals that this service was not related to the global service and should, therefore, be paid. In addition, the diagnosis should verify the distinction.

Modifier 25 is for significant, separately identifiable E/M services by the same physician on the same day of another service. This modifier is important because normally only one E/M can be charged per physician practice per day, but if a patient does visit later that day for a different diagnosis, the physician will be providing additional E/M services that certainly should be paid. The diagnosis should verify this.

Modifier 57 is used with an E/M code when the physician makes the decision for surgery during an E/M visit but cannot be as a part of the E/M for hos-pital admission.

Section 35.5: ANESTHESIA MODIFIERS

Modifier 23 is used for unusual anesthesia, that is, anesthesia that is not the usual type of anesthesia for that service, such as the provision of general anesthesia for repair of teeth in a person with handicaps, which makes them unable to have dentistry otherwise.

Modifier 47 is used when the surgeon administers the anesthesia rather than an anesthesiologist.

Do not forget the physical status modifiers for anesthesia, that is, P1, P2, P3, P4, P5, and P6, as mentioned earlier.

Section 35.6: SURGICAL MODIFIERS

While the following modifiers are used frequently with surgical codes, some of them can certainly be used with other types of codes. Do not forget modifiers 50 and 51, which were previously discussed.

Modifiers 47 and 52 can also be used for surgical codes, as described earlier.

Modifier 22 is used for unusual procedural services that may require more extensive services than are normally anticipated and compensated for in the codes. A special report would be necessary to be submitted with the use of this modifier.

Modifier 26 is to indicate when a physician provides professional services and includes the reading and interpretation of results, documentation in a report, and supervision. The professional component is in contrast to the technical component, which is the actual performance of the service and can be designated with the modifier TC. The use of these modifiers is dependent, however, on the description of the code because some codes will delineate professional services only (supervision and interpretation) and would, therefore, not need a modifier.

Modifier 32 is for mandated services as requested by a -third-party, such as for second opinions.

Modifier 52 is used for reduced services based upon physician's discretion, such as a procedure listed in the codes as bilateral but service is only unilateral.

Modifier 53 is used for a discontinued procedure as determined by the physician due to the extenuating circumstances, such as the deteriorating condition of the patient. This is not used when it is electively decided to cancel a procedure before surgical preparation or the administration of anesthesia.

Modifiers 54, 55, and 56 are used to indicate the provision of only a portion of the care for a procedure; 54 is for surgical care only, 55 is for postoperative care, and 56 is for preoperative care. This can occur if a patient receives surgical care from one physician while on vacation in another state, then returns to his home state and is followed up by his own physician. His own physician will bill using the procedure code (although he or she did not perform the surgery) and then attach the 55 modifier to indicate that he or she only provided the postoperative care. These modifiers are necessary because otherwise the procedural code is assumed to include all of the preoperative and postoperative care associated with the procedure (global). Do not use these modifiers if the code already specifies the level of care, that is, preoperative or postoperative care only. These modifiers are attached to the procedure code.

Modifier 58 is used for staged or related procedures that were either planned, more extensive than the original, or for therapy after a procedure. This modifier must be attached even to a code that states it is staged. This modifier will be added to the procedure each time it is performed.

Modifier 59 is used to bill for a distinctly different procedure or service performed on the same day that is not a part of the bundled package of another procedure or service. The procedure or service may be distinct due to different anatomical site, different session, or different encounter. Linking of the CPT codes with proper ICD-10-CM codes become critical in such instances because the diagnoses can indicate the difference. The use of this modifier also ensures that full payment will be received for the procedure or service and not reduced due to the provision of the other service or procedure.

Modifier 62 is used when there are two surgeons involved with the service or procedure. Both surgeons will bill using the same code with the addition of the modifier 62. Reimbursement is then split between the two surgeons.

Modifier 63 indicates that a procedure was performed on an infant that weighs less than 4 kg and is used primarily for surgical codes, and not E/Ms, anesthesia, radiology, pathology/laboratory, or medicine.

Modifiers 76 and 77 are used to bill for the provision of the same procedure within a global period. Modifier 76 is used when the physician is the same and modifier 77 is used when the physician is not the same. Without this modifier, payment would be denied because the code would be viewed as a duplicate bill.

Similar to modifiers 76 and 77, modifier 78 is used when an additional procedure that is related to a prior procedure still in its global period is performed on a patient. Payment will depend on the global period and specifics of the codes.

Modifier 79 indicates that a procedure was performed on a patient by the same physician during a global period but is not related to the global procedure.

Modifiers 80, 81, and 82 refer to assistant surgeons.

Modifiers 90 and 91 refer to the use of outside laboratory and repeat of tests.

Modifier 99 is used to indicate the use of more than one modifier to one code.

When the patient is on Medicare, there may sometimes be reasons to bill Medicare when you know that they are not going to pay for the service. However, to bill Medicare for charges that are not allowable can create problems because it could be considered a false claim. To remedy this situation, there are two modifiers, GY and GZ, which accommodate this. GY is for services or procedures that you bill Medicare that are not payable because they are either excluded or not a benefit, such as cosmetic surgery. GZ is for services or procedures that are expected to be denied.

CHAPTER 36
RADIOLOGY

You will learn the following objectives in this chapter:

A. Positions
B. Directions
C. Techniques
   1. Scans
   2. Contrast Materials
   3. Fluoroscopy
   4. X-rays
   5. Imaging
      a. MRI
      b. PET
   6. Ultrasound
      a. Doppler
      b. Color Flow
      c. Nuclear Medicine
D. Therapies
E. Oncology
F. Contrast Materials
G. Supervision and Interpretation
H. Format
   a. Subsections
   b. Code Selection
   c. Diagnostic Radiology (Diagnostic Imaging)
   d. Diagnostic Ultrasound
   e. Radiologic Guidance
   f. Breast, Mammography
   g. Bone/Joint Studies
   h. Radiation Oncology
   i. Nuclear Medicine
I. Modifiers

Section 36.1: POSITIONS

POSTEROANTERIOR (PA): Posteroanterior view is when the person is facing the detector (film) and the source of radiation is located to the posterior and projected onto the film as it passes through the body from the posterior to the anterior. This is the most commonly used type of x-ray.

ANTEROPOSTERIOR (AP): Anteroposterior view is when the person's back is towards the detector (film) and the patient is facing the source of radiation so the radiation travels from front to back.

LATERAL: Lateral view is when one side is facing the machine and the other side the film (detector).

OBLIQUE: Oblique view is when the patient is facing the machine at an angle.

SAGITTAL: A sagittal plane divides the body into two halves dividing the body into right and left sides.

CORONAL: Coronal (frontal): A coronal plane cuts the body into two halves, a front and a back.

TRANSVERSE: A transverse plane cuts the body into two halves, a top and bottom.

PRONE: Prone is when the patient is laying on their belly (face down).

SUPINE: Supine is when the patient is laying on their back (face up).

RECUMBENT: Recumbent is any position when the patient is laying down (either supine or prone).

Section 36.2: DIRECTIONS

Radiological tests can be performed from several directions.

IPSILATERAL: From the same side or affecting the same side.

CONTRALATERAL: On the opposite side.

ANTEGRADE: Extending or moving forward.

RETROGRADE: Moving backward against the normal flow.

Section 36.3: TECHNIQUES

SCANS: Scans are general terms for the visualization of anatomic images through the production of a picture such as through x-rays or imaging which can then be used to determine and provide treatment.

CONTRAST MATERIALS: Contrast materials are radiopaque materials (do not allow the passage of light) that are introduced into the body and allowed to circulate which then provides a picture of problems within the body since some structures, such as neoplasms and obstructions, will appear as a solid white on a radiological test where there should not be any solid structures.

They are used for x-rays, CT and MRI scans, such as cystogram, barium enema, angiography, retrograde pyelogram, fistulogram, and endoscopic retrograde cholangiopancreatogram.

Oral materials include a variety of materials including iodine, barium, barium sulfate, and gastrografin.

If several tests are done together with some being without and then with contrast, then a code should be listed that includes both, not listed as separate codes, e.g. 70553.

A double contrast study uses both a contrast medium to provide highlight of both radiopaque and radiolucent structures, such as the stomach being coated with barium and the lumen being filled with air.

Contrast materials may be administered in several ways. First, they can be administered intravenously through a vein in the arm or hand which helps highlight the blood vessels to increase the visibility of structures like the brain, spine, liver and kidney.

Second, they can be administered orally with two of the most common contrast materials being barium sulfate and gastrografin of which the patient must drink up to 48 ounces after having fasted for several hours before the scan. The contrast material then highlights the gastrointestinal organs.

Third, they can be administered rectally through an enema with the use of barium sulfate or gastrografin which highlights the large intestine and lower gastrointestinal organs. Prior to the CT scan, the patient must fast for several hours, and cleanse the colon by enema the night before the scan.

Fourth, they can be administered through inhalation of xenon gas which is used for specialized brain or lung tests which are not readily available.

Oral and rectal contrast administration is not coded as "with contrast."

FLUOROSCOPY: Fluoroscopy is used to observe the flow of materials by means of the introduction of a contrast agent into the body which then appears on x-rays or can be used to guide a medical procedure, such as insertion of catheters due to its ability to glow or fluoresce. Fluoroscopy performed on the cardiovascular system is known as an angiography.

GRAPHY: "Graphy" is the process of producing an x-ray images that provide visualization of anatomic sites or objects. Arthrography provides visualization of joints, angiography provides visualization of the blood vessels, myelography provides visualization of the spinal column, and cholangiography provides visualization of the bile ducts. Graphies are what a radiologist or physician interpret as part of the professional component of these tests and include:

Section 36.4: THERAPIES

MODALITY: Modality is a treatment method, such as radiotherapy.

RADIOTHERAPY: Radiotherapy is when radiation is used to treat illnesses or disease.

STEREOTACTIC RADIOTHERAPY: Stereotactic radiotherapy involves the use of an external beam that focuses high doses of radiation within the body.

TELETHERAPIES: Teletherapies are therapies administered from far away.

BRACHYTHERAPIES: Brachytherapies are therapies administered up close to the patient.

3-DIMENSIONAL CONFORMAL RADIOTHERAPY (3DCRT): 3DCRT is a virtual simulation test in which each radiation beam is shaped to fit the target.

INTENSITY-MODULATED RADIATION THERAPY (IMRT): IMRT is an advanced type of high-precision radiation that utilizes computer controlled accelerators to control the administration of radiation.

Section 36.5: SUPERVISION AND INTERPRETATION

Normally a radiology test is performed by a licensed practitioner, such as a radiologist. When the radiologist conducts the test, this is known as the technical component (TC) and these reports are known as "graphies", for example, an arthrography would provide visualization of joints and angiography would provide visualization of the blood vessels. The radiologist will then interpret the results, which is known as supervision and interpretation (S&I). Most radiology codes include both the technical and supervision and interpretation services.

However, sometimes a physician may read and interpret a radiological report which, again is known as supervision and interpretation and this service should be coded. There are several ways to code for S&I.

First, some Radiology codes indicate that they are only for supervision and interpretation. In this case, only this one code is necessary to code for the physician reading and interpreting the results.

Second, most Radiology codes include both the technical and supervision and interpretation portions of a radiological procedure. If a radiologist performs both the TC and S&I which is typically the case, then only this one code is necessary. However, if a physician provides only the S&I and there is no code for just the S&I, then the code which contains both the TC and S&I services would be listed with modifier 26 (professional component) which indicates that the physician only did the S&I portion of the services for that code.

Section 36.6: FORMAT

SUBSECTIONS: The subsections of radiology are:

Diagnostic Radiology (Diagnostic Imaging):	70010-76499
Diagnostic Ultrasound:	76506-76999
Radiologic Guidance:	77001-77022
Breast, Mammography	77051-77059
Bone/Joint Studies	77071-77084
Radiation Oncology	77261-77799
Nuclear Medicine	78012-79999

The radiology codes are differentiated by anatomic sites within the sections which are based on types of tests performed. The radiation oncology section is differentiated by type and method of treatment. Codes in the nuclear medicine section are differentiated by whether they are diagnostic or therapeutic.

Multiple tests can be coded even if performed during the same procedure and/or visit. However, do not unbundle and code separately tests that involve several tests which are combined together under one code.

Section 36.7: DIAGNOSTIC RADIOLOGY (70010-76499)

Diagnostic radiology includes x-rays, computed tomography (CT) scans, and Magnetic resonance imaging (MRI) which oftentimes uses contrast material. However, CT and MRI are imaging and not x-rays.

X-RAYS: X-rays are tests that use ionized and non-ionized electromagnetic radiation (invisible waves of energy) such as X-rays to view objects and may use contrast materials.

Radiolucent materials allow the passage of x-rays so they appear clear on the x-ray. Radiopaque materials do not allow as much passage of x-rays which can vary in how much x-rays are allowed through so these objects may appear a solid white on the x-ray and may indicate a tumor in this way.

Computed tomography (CT, formerly known as CAT) uses a high amount of x-rays in conjunction with a computer to create images of both soft and hard tissues with contrast materials oftentimes used. Mammographies are x-rays of the breasts. DEXA is a bone densitometry which utilizes x-rays to check for osteoporosis.

Imaging tests do not use ionized radiation, like x-rays. Magnetic resonance imaging (MRI) uses electromagnetic energy rather than x-rays.

X-rays testing includes upper GI series with ingestion of barium sulfate for visualization of the esophagus, stomach, and duodenum. A lower GI series visualizes the large intestine. To code for these services, the test performed and number of views is important for the selection of the correct code.

Angiographies, lymphangiographies, and venographies are component codes in that they are used as part of a procedure which is coded in another section of the CPT coding book, such as surgical or medicine. These codes are used to report the supervision and interpretation of cardiac procedures, such as catheterizations and injections. There are four directions from which the radiological service can be provided in these cases: ipsilateral, contralateral, antegrade, and retrograde. In addition to the direction, placements can be either nonselective or selective.

Nonselective means that it goes directly into the one location, i.e. directly into a vein or artery. Selective means that it is guided into other vessels (other than the original vessel). These terms are oftentimes used to refer to catheter placement. If both a nonselective and selective catheterization of the same site was performed, then only the selective would be coded.

With this type of coding, as well as cardiovascular surgical coding, it becomes important to know the vascular system, which resembles a tree with branches coming from the main branches or trunk. In consideration of these branches, vascular families are defined as a group of vessels that extend from a primary branch. Each vascular family should be coded separately with the code being selected from the highest level of the family that is first order family extending immediately from the main line, with corresponding extensions comprising second, third and so forth as orders of the family. This type of coding is also used in the medicine and surgical codes for cardiovascular procedures. The branches and families can be found in Appendix L of the CPT coding book.

Section 36.8: DIAGNOSTIC ULTRASOUND (76506-76999)

An ultrasound uses high-frequency inaudible sound waves that bounce off body tissues, thereby providing a picture of anatomy and any unknown masses and do not use ionizing radiation like x-rays do. Ultrasound uses a powerful magnetic field to produce an image with much greater contrast than an x-ray can. Contrast materials may be used. The record produced is called a sonogram.

Doppler is an ultrasound technique based on the Doppler effect which is a change in frequency of a wave based on its movement away from another object which can measure blood flow.

Color flow is an ultrasound technique which illustrates velocity shifts in blood flow by color coding with blood flowing in one direction appearing red and blood flowing in the opposite direction appearing blue which also allows for measurement of flow and pressures within the heart and the calculation of stroke volume.

There are four types of ultrasound:

1. A-mode refers to a one-dimensional ultrasound procedure.
2. M-mode refers to a one-dimensional ultrasound procedure which also shows movement which records amplitude and velocity of structures.
3. B-scan refers to a two-dimensional ultrasound procedure with display.
4. Real-time scan refers to two-dimensional ultrasound scanning procedure showing both structure and motion relative to time.

Ultrasounds during pregnancy are coded as 76801-76817 according to extent of the ultrasound as described in the codes.

If radiological guidance is used to assist with a surgical procedure, such as a biopsy or catheter, then codes should be listed for the procedure and for the radiological guidance (76942).

Color Doppler studies are included in the codes but color and spectral Doppler performed at the same time are coded separately from the radiological codes and are coded with medicine codes (93875-93990).

Ultrasounds can be either complete or limited. The CPT code book describes what anatomic sites must be included to constitute a complete exam; if these sites are not included then it is limited.

Section 36.9: RADIOLOGIC GUIDANCE (77001-77022)

Radiologic guidance codes include the use of fluoroscopic guidance when used to assist in the implantation of access devices, such as catheters, computed tomography and magnetic resonance to assist with guidance, such as with needles and radiation therapy fields, and other types such as stereotactic localization.

Section 36.10: BREAST, MAMMOGRAPHY (77051-77059)

There are two types of mammographies: screening and diagnostic. A screening is a checkup used to confirm that there are no abnormal masses or if the screening determines there is, then a need for further testing as a diagnostic mammography. A diagnostic mammography is used for determination what a suspicious mass is. A diagnostic mammography occurs whenever there is a suspicious growth.

A mammogram can be coded as either a unilateral procedure (77055) or a bilateral procedure 77056). If the mammogram is diagnostic and bilateral it would be coded as 77057.

Section 36.11: BONE/JOINT STUDIES (77071-77084)

Various procedures are included in this section which are used to test for bone and joint problems, which includes bone age studies (77072), bone length studies (77073), osseous survey (77074-77076), absorptiometry (DXA) bone density scan (77080), bone marrow imaging (77084).

Section 36.12: RADIATION ONCOLOGY (77261-77799)

There are four types of treatment for cancer: surgery, radiation therapy, chemotherapy and biological therapy, which can be administered singularly or together. Radiation therapy can be either curative, palliative, or adjuvant in that they can be administered as follow-up to another treatment either because the other treatment was not able to remove all of the cancer, to assist in more thorough and successful treatment, or as prophylaxis. For example, a patient may receive surgery to remove a cancerous growth and then receive chemotherapy for another six months to ensure that that all cancer has been removed.

Terms used in radiation oncology are:

1. Rad: A rad is the dosage absorbed in radiation treatment for cancer.
2. Fraction: A fraction occurs when cancer treatment is divided into small repeated dosages rather than one or two large dosages.
3. Palliative: Palliative treatments are used to relieve symptoms rather than being curative.
4. Adjuvant: Adjuvant therapy is a treatment that is an aid to surgery.

Radiation oncology is used to treat diseases and neoplasms which include the administration of radiation, oftentimes through teletherapies and brachytherapies. The purpose of radiation therapy is to destroy the cancer but as little of the healthy surrounding tissue as possible; therefore, therapies that can be isolated to the cancer only are highly effective.

Radiation oncology codes include various services which are initial consultation, clinical treatment planning, simulation, medical radiation physics, dosimetry, treatment devices, special services, clinical treatment management procedures, and follow-up care for three months following completion of treatment which are described more thoroughly in the CPT code book.

Clinical treatment planning are differentiated by simple, intermediate, and complex which are described in the CPT book (77261-77263). Basically, simple involves the treatment of a single area with simple or no blocking. Intermediate involves the simulation of three or more ports, two separate treatment areas and multiple blocks. Complex simulation involves simulation of three or more treatment areas with complex blocking and several other factors. Three-dimensional (3-D) computer-generated imaging provide as 3-D image of the tumor.

Other tests and treatment include medical radiation physics, dosimetry, treatment devices, and special services (77295-77370) and stereotactic radiation treatment (77371-77373).

Treatment with radiation is coded as 77401-77425 and the number of treatment areas, number of ports, number of shielding blocks and total volts administered need to be known to select the proper code. Neutron beam treatment is coded as 77422-77423. Proton beam treatment is coded as 77520-77525 and is highly-focused high-energy irradiation.

Management of radiation treatment is coded as 77427-77499. This includes review of films, review of dosimetry and dose delivery, review of patient treatment set-up and examination of patient for management. These codes are differentiated by treatment sessions or in units of five fractions which do not have to be performed on the same day.

Hyperthermia (77600-77615) is the use of heat to treat the disease by ultrasound, microwave, radiofrequency and probes. There are three types: external, interstitial, and intracavity. External is applied from outside the body, interstitial is placed within tissues, and intracavity is placed within body cavities. These codes include planning, insertion of sensors, and follow-up care for three months after completion.

Brachytherapy (77750-77799) involves the temporary and permanent implantation of natural or man-made radioelements that are applied around or into the cancer area as interstitial, (directly into tumor), intracavitary (in close proximity to the tumor), or on the surface of the patient. There are three levels of service which include simple (one to four sources/ribbons); intermediate (five to ten sources/ribbons); and complex (greater than 10 sources/ribbons). Sources refer to permanent placement of radioelements either intracavitary or interstitial and ribbons refer to temporary placement of radioelements interstitially.

Section 36.13: NUCLEAR MEDICINE (78012-79999)

Nuclear medicine involves the use of radioisotopes to detect abnormalities, not radiation and not contrast material. As the isotopes deteriorate, gamma rays are released which appear on the scan and, therefore, visible.

There are several types of nuclear medicine tests.

1. Scintigraphy is the process to produce an image from the nuclear test is scintigraphy and the captured image is the scintiscan.
2. PET: PET (positron emission tomography) are scans which can be used to test various parts of the body with the introduction of radioisotopes (not contrast material) which emit positrons which can be recorded.
3. SPECT: Single photon emission computed tomography (SPECT) is performed by the injection of a radioactive tracer into the body which then creates a 3-D image
4. Technetium Sestamibi: Radioactive Techneitum is intravenously introduced into the body and used to test the heart for problems. A form of this test is the MUGA (multiple gated acquisition scan) which studies the motion and ejection fraction of the heart.

Some radioisotopes are absorbed only by specific organs or tumors which help in viewing and identification. Various nuclear scans include bone, cardiac, (e.g. thallium 201 and technetium), lungs, biliary system, renal, and thyroid.

There are codes for tests and codes for therapy using radioisotopes. Oral and intravenous administration for therapy are included in the codes but all other methods must be coded additionally, such as intra-arterial, intracavity, and intra-articular.

Nuclear tests can be in vitro or in vivo. In vitro means that the test is performed in the test tube and in vivo beans that it is performed in the body. RIA (radioimmunoassay) is an in vitro tests which is the combination of blood and radioactive material in the test tube and can measure substances that may be present in the blood. In vivo tests trace the presence of radioactive materials that are purposely introduced into the body and that will collect (uptake) into certain areas which can then be tested.

Nuclear scans include bone, gallium (tumors), liver and spleen, PET, SPECT, Technetium sestabibi, thallium, and thyroid.

HCPCS codes should be used to code for materials used, that is the isotopes.

Section 36.14: MODIFIERS

MODIFIER 26: Modifier 26, Professional Component, represents the professional services performed during a radiological exam that is the supervision and interpretation. Remember that most often, radiology codes include both the technical (TC) and the professional (S&I) services; however, if only the professional component is performed by a healthcare provider, then the code for the radiology exam should be listed with the modifier 26 attached to indicate that only the professional component was provided and not the technical. However, there are some radiology codes that state they only include the S&I services, so modifier 26 would not need to be added to this type of code since the code only includes the S&I service, e.g. 75989.

MODIFIER TC: HCPCS modifier TC represents the provision of the technical component of a radiology service only and not the S&I. As stated above, most radiology codes include both the technical and professional (S&I) services, so if only the technical component was provided by the healthcare provider, the modifier TC would need to be attached to the code for the test.

MODIFIER 59: Modifier 59 is for Distinct Procedural Service and is applied to a CPT code to indicate that the service was distinct from any other services listed and that it should be paid in addition to other listed codes. This is important with radiology codes because the same type of x-ray may be done prior to surgery and then following surgery to check the outcome of the procedure, so two x-rays were done on the same time at the same visit but both x-rays should be paid.

MODIFIER GH: Modifier GH is a HCPCS modifier and is used to indicate that a diagnostic mammogram was changed from a screening mammogram on the same day.

MODIFIERS BODY SIDES: LT is for the left side; RT is for the right side.

RADIOLOGY QUIZ 25

1. What are the codes for a 48-year-old patient who had a computed axial tomography of T1-T3 with contrast material for severe back pain and difficulty breathing?

2. What are the codes for a 26-year-old patient who has gastroparesis and had a study for gastric emptying of the stomach?

3. What are the codes for a 66-year-old patient with ASHD who had angiography with noncardiac vascular flow imaging with cardiac stress test with treadmill with continuous monitoring and supervision by physician of the internal mammary artery?

4. What are the codes for a 37-year-old patient who is suspected of having lymphoma of the abdominal lymph nodes because of ongoing constipation and abdominal pain and today receives a whole body bone marrow imaging?

5. What are the codes for a 48-year-old patient who had hysterosonography with color Doppler with introduction of saline and found to have septate uterus?

6. How would you indicate that someone only did S&I?

7. What are the codes for a 48-year-old patient who had MRI of the ankle due to extreme pain and inflammation which demonstrated acute distal tibiofibular syndesmotic injury of the left ankle?

8. What contrast materials are not coded as separate from the test?

9. What are the codes for a 45-year-old patient who had imaging for carcinoma of the thyroid with urinary recovery which was found to be positive?

10. What are the codes for a 48-year-old patient who had CT of the head with oral contrast materials after falling from the roof and was unconscious for approximately 10 minutes but results were negative?

CHAPTER 37
PATHOLOGY/LABORATORY

You will learn the following objectives in this chapter:

1. Laboratory
   a. Blood Draw
   b. CLIA
   c. Qualitative Studies/Quantitative Studies
   d. Drug Screening
   e. Panels
   f. Evocative/Suppression Tests

B. Pathology

C. Format
   1. Subsections
   2. Code Selection
   3. Testing Site

D. Types of Laboratory Services
   1. Evocative/Suppression Tests
   2. Hematology and Coagulation
   3. Immunology
   4. Transfusion Medicine
   5. Microbiology

E. Pathology Tests

F. Other Lab Procedures

G. Modifiers

H. HCPCS

Section 37.1: FORMAT

SUBSECTIONS: The subsections of Pathology and Laboratory are:

Organ and Disease-Oriented Panels	80047-80076
Drug Testing	80100-80104
Therapeutic Drug Assays	80150-80377
Evocative/Suppression Testing	80400-80440
Consultations (Clinical Pathology)	80500-80502
Urinalysis	81000-81099
Molecular Pathology	81161, 81200-81479
Multianalyte Assays/Algorithmic Analyses	81500-81599
Chemistry	82000-84999
Hematology and Coagulation	85002-85999
Immunology	86000-86849
Tissue Typing	86805-86849
Transfusion Medicine	86850-86999
Microbiology	87001-87999
Anatomic Pathology	88000-88099
Cytopathology	88104-88199

Cytogenic Studies	88230-88299
Surgical Pathology	88300-88399
In Vivo Transcutaneous Procedures	88720-88749
Other Procedures	89049-89240
Reproductive Medicine Procedures	89250-89398

Section 37.2: TESTING

For purposes of coding, it is important to determine who can charge for the pathology or laboratory services; this of course depends on who provided the services, so it must be determined which healthcare provider is providing the services and, therefore, allowed to charge for the services. There are two scenarios that can occur with regard to the provision of pathology and laboratory services:

ON-SITE: On-site provision of pathology or laboratory services indicates that the pathology or laboratory services were provided by the healthcare provider who collected the specimen, i.e. a physician collected the sample and his office tested it as well; a separate agency did not perform the pathology or laboratory services. Most healthcare providers send their specimens to an outside laboratory because most practices do not have the capability or authorization to provide pathology or laboratory services. However, some practices do have the capability and authorization to provide certain laboratory services. In order to provide these services, the practice must possess a Clinical Laboratory Improvement Act (CLIA) license.

1. When a healthcare provider performs the test, they can charge using the codes for the pathology or laboratory service. They cannot, however, charge for collection or preparation/handling of the specimen since they did not send it to an outside laboratory.
2. Practices can acquire CLIA waivers for certain tests which do not require formal education as described above.

The CLIA (Clinical Laboratory Improvement Act) of 1988 requires that an office or practice must be approved by CLIA in order to perform laboratory tests or to obtain a waiver. Practices can acquire CLIA waivers for certain tests which do not require formal education, such as dipstick urines, finger stick glucose and home pregnancy testing, so they can then perform these tests in their office and report the results. Modifier –QW must be listed after the procedure code. An office or practice that receives this approval is known as a physician office laboratory (POL).

OFF-SITE: A healthcare provider may collect a specimen and send it to an outside lab for evaluation.

1. In this scenario, the healthcare provider can charge for the collection of the specimen and the preparation/handling of it to submit to the outside laboratory, so two codes can be listed as described below.
2. Collection of specimens can occur in several ways so various codes can be used to charge for these services.
3. Blood draws can be collected by venipuncture (needle) 36415, puncture (finger, heel or ear stick) 36416, and arterial puncture 36600. Only one blood draw can be charged per day per patient per practice. These codes should not be confused with a therapeutic blood draw (99195) which is performed for purposes of treating a condition rather than

collection of blood for testing. Medicare requires the use of code G0001 for venipunctures.

4. Urinalysis (81000-81099) is the testing of urine for substances. Typical urinalysis is performed by a dipstick or collection of urine in a bottle. There are several types of urinalysis based on numerous factors: (1) with or without automation; (2) quantitative or semi-quantitative, (3) with or without microscopy and (4) purpose for test (pregnancy, volume measurement, and bacteriuria screening.
5. Preparation/Handling: Preparation and handling codes can be found in the medicine section of the CPT book and are 99000-99002.
6. Billing form: On the billing form, Box 20 must be checked if the specimen was sent to an outside laboratory, in addition to the listing of the procedure codes and their linkage to the diagnostic codes which will be discussed later.
7. There is a table listing the codes for molecular pathology for specific genes which can be very helpful.
8. Some books will have a listing of definitions and acronyms for various drugs in the pathology/laboratory section.

Section 37.3: PANELS

Panels (80047-80076) are a series of laboratory tests that are routinely performed together to assist in diagnosis and treatment and, therefore, can all be coded with one code, which is the panel code rather than having to code each test separately. These are:

1. Basic metabolic panel (calcium ionized) 80047
2. Basic metabolic panel (total calcium) 80048
3. General health panel 80050
4. Electrolyte panel 80051
5. Comprehensive metabolic panel 80053
6. Obstetric panel 80055
7. Lipid panel 80061
8. Renal function panel 80069
9. Acute hepatitis panel 80074
10. Hepatic function panel 80076

Examine some of these panels and notice what tests are included in each one. For example, a lipid panel contains tests for total serum cholesterol, lipoprotein, and triglycerides and is coded as 80061. Notice that within the panel the code for each test if performed singly is listed, such as total serum cholesterol if performed singly would be coded as 82465.

There are three important functions to know about these series of tests.

11. These panel codes can only be used if all of the tests contained in the panel are performed. If even one test is not performed, then the panel code cannot be used. In this case, each test would have to be coded separately.
12. If all of the tests in a panel are performed but there is an additional test performed that was not included in the panel, then the panel and the additional tests should be coded separately. All tests must be coded either as included in the panel or with its own code.

13. These panels change yearly as to what tests are performed in them so a coder must be careful that they do not assume a test is included.

Section 37.4: ASSAYS, QUALITATIVE & QUANTITATIVE

Assays are now broken into different codes based on the purpose, drug class, and type of results obtained.

DRUG CLASSES: There are two types of drug classes, presumptive and definitive.

Presumptive drug class assays (80300-80304) are used to determine the use or non-use of a drug or drug class. The drug classes are either A or B. A listing of which drugs are included in which class are listed in the CPT book. For example, Class A includes alcohol, barbiturates, methadone and opiates and are coded as 80300 for multiple tests and 80302 for single. Class B includes nicotine, fentanyl and acetaminophen and are coded as 80303 for single or multiple and 80304 is for a procedure not specified.

Definitive drug testing (80320-80377) is able to identify individual drugs and may be either qualitative or quantitative, or a combination of both.

Sometimes a test is done to determine what substance is present and if so, how much. A qualitative test is most oftentimes performed first to determine a particular substance is present in the specimen (such as a blood draw or urinalysis), so these tests are usually described as positive or negative. These codes are listed in the Drug Testing subsection (80150-80377) and are differentiated by how many substances are being tested for, i.e. 80100 should be used when testing the presence of more than one drug class. Code 80101 is used when only one drug class is being tested for its presence. If the presence of a drug class is found, then code 80102 is used to confirm the presence of the drug. Tests that are typically conducted as qualitative are for alcohol, amphetamine, barbiturates, benzodiazepines, cocaine, methadone, opiates, and tricyclic antidepressants.

Once it has been determined that a substance is present, a quantitative test can be performed to determine how much of the substance is present. These codes are listed in the subsection Therapeutic Drug Assays (80150-80299) or the Chemistry subsection (see below).

Section 37.5: EVOCATIVE/SUPPRESSION TESTS

Evocative suppression tests occur when a substance is administered to a patient and the reaction recorded in order to determine the effect the substance has on the patient which aids in the determination of the diagnoses, e.g. giving insulin or sugar to determine a diagnosis of diabetes.

There are four codes that must be coded together when these types of tests are administered: first the administration code from the Medicine section of the CPT code book (90765-90779), second the test (80400-80440), third a HCPCS code from the J section for the substance, and fourth an E/M code for the office visit with the physician who oversees the monitoring of the test.

Section 37.6: URINALYSIS

There are only several codes for different types of urinalysis procedures (81000-81099) based on various services such as automated or non-automated.

Section 37.7: MOLECULAR PATHOLOGY

This is a newer section of the CPT book (81161-81479) which codes for procedures involving analyses of nucleic acids of genes to determine genetic conditions. Multianalyte Assays with Algorithmic Analyses are coded as 81500-81599 which use multiple procedures to derive multiple results of a specimen. Each code lists procedures contained within codes and are sorted as to Tier 1 and Tier 2. Genomic sequencing is coded as 81410 to 81471.

Section 37.8: CHEMISTRY

Chemistry tests (82000-84999) are most often quantitative tests collected from any bodily fluid although some codes will indicate that they are for qualitative in nature. Examples include arsenic, total bilirubin, and qualitative or quantitative codes for the presence of fasts in the feces (82705-82706). The codes are differentiated by the substance (analyte) being tested or test.

Codes 83890-83913 are for molecular diagnostics, such as DNA testing.

The same test can be conducted more than once on the same day either at a different time or different body location and each test can be coded separately with the use of modifier 91 to indicate that these are multiple chemistry tests. In addition, different tests may be conducted on the same substance and all of these tests can be coded separately.

Section 37.9: HEMATOLOGY AND COAGULATION

Blood tests include various tests including for bleeding time (85002), numerous blood count (85004-85049), clotting (851700-85421), and RBC counts. However, bone marrow aspiration or biopsy is not located in this section but is located in the Surgery section (38220 and 38221).

Section 37.10: IMMUNOLOGY

Immunology tests are used to check the patient's immune system, e.g. allergens (86000-86005), presence of antibodies or antigens to specific disease agents, such as hepatitis and AIDS. Many of these tests report as negative or positive.

Section 37.11: TRANSFUSION MEDICINE

Transfusion medicine (86850-86999) performs lab tests to ensure compatibility of blood to ensure there are no negative reactions by the patient, such as blood typing and paternity testing.

Section 37.12: MICROBIOLOGY

Microbiology (87001-87999) includes tests to determine the presence of certain bacteria, fungus, parasites, and viruses usually through the growth of colonies on a media in a dish and include tests such as Gram stains. Each result should be coded separately with modifier 59 attached to indicate that the result was different from other results.

Section 37.13: PATHOLOGY TESTS

Pathology is the study of a specimen (anatomic part) in order to determine a diagnosis of what disease may exist. If it is performed on an entire body, then it is considered an autopsy (or post-mortem exam or necropsy).

A specimen is a tissue that is obtained and submitted for examination either visually (gross) or microscopically.

POSTMORTEM EXAMINATION: Postmortem exams (88000-88099) are performed on a person who has died and is also termed necropsy or autopsy. Codes are differentiated by the presence or absence of a brain, if it is an infant, stillborn, or adult, and if it is visual (gross) or both visual and microscopic. There are also codes for if only an organ is examined (88036-88037).

CYTOPATHOLOGY: Cytopathology (88104-88199) examines cells for disease and can be collected in several ways including washings, brushings, with enhancement or concentration.

Cervical and vaginal cytopathology codes are different from cytopathology performed on other specimens and are coded as 88141-88167 with many variations in the type of specimen and testing. The variations include first the traditional method of preparation or a thin-layer method, second the reporting of results as using the Bethesda method or other method, or third the level of screening (manual, computer-assisted, or automated) . The Bethesda method reports on specimen adequacy, general categorization, and diagnosis. There is an additional code if the physician provides professional services (supervision and interpretation) which is coded as 88141, if a hormonal evaluation was performed.

It needs to be remembered that these codes should be used for diagnostic pap smears, such as when a physician is performing regular pap smears to determine if the diagnosis of cancer is present in a patient who had cancer before. When a physician performs regular pap smears to ensure that cancer has not returned, this not a screening but a diagnostic pap smear and code 88141 should be used for the physician' services.

CYTOGENIC STUDIES: Cytogenetic studies (88230-88299) are performed to determine the existence of oncologic or genetic disorders including testing of chromosomes.

SURGICAL PATHOLOGY: Surgical pathology is performed on specimens and each specimen constitutes a unit for coding and billing.

Surgical pathology is differentiated by levels as determined by type of specimen and if the exam is gross only (visual) or gross and microscopic. There is only one code for gross pathology of any specimen (88300). The remaining levels II-VI (88302-88309) are described by specimen, e.g. hemorrhoids are coded as Level III (88304).

There are numerous add-on codes (88311-88314) that can be used with these codes. These add-on codes describe various methods such as stains.

There are also codes for consultations by the pathologist (88321-88334).

Other tests can also be coded with codes 88342-88399.

Section 37.14: OTHER LAB PROCEDURES

There are a wide variety of other laboratory tests that are performed including cell count (89050) and sweat collection (89230). Reproductive procedures are also included here, such as with fertility services, including embryo hatching (89253), preparation for embryo transfer (89255), and sperm evaluation (89329).

Section 37.15: MODIFIERS

Many of the modifiers discussed in previous packets can be applied to laboratory and pathology services. For example, if a test is repeated, then modifier 59 would need to be applied to indicate that the test had to be repeated; if the test is a repeat lab test then modifier 91 could be applied. Modifier 90 should be used if a physician sends the specimen or substance to an outside laboratory.

Section 37.16: HCPCS

Various HCPCS codes can be used with laboratory and pathology codes. These include the following:
G0123-G0148: Variations of screening cytopathology, cervical or vaginal.
P3000-P3001: Screening pap smear.
P9612-P9615: Catheterization to collect specimen.
Q0091: Collection of specimen by pap smear to send to outside lab.

PATHOLOGY/LABORATORY QUIZ 26

1) What are the codes when a physician tests to determine how much Lithium an 8-year-old patient ingested?

2) What are the codes for a 42-year-old male who has a blood count smear with manual WBC count and bleeding time is also tested and the patient is found to be positive for von Willebrand's?

3) What are the codes for a path exam of a PAP smear that required physician interpretation due to patient complaints of erratic vaginal bleeding but there were no abnormal findings?

4) What are the codes for the gross examination of a wedge from the liver of a 43-year-old patient which is found to be cancerous?

5) What are the codes for a semiquantitative immunoassay test for chlamydia with a reagent strip which is found to be negative?

6) What are the codes for a 77-yo patient who had a blood draw and a finger stick on his office visit with complaints of fatigue?

7) What are the codes for a 67-year-old patient who has tests for carbon dioxide, potassium, bilirubin, chloride, sodium, and glucose for a well check?

8) What are the codes for when a physician tests a 17-year-old female to determine if she has taken barbiturates because of general fatigue?

9) What are the codes when a 37-year-old female is tested for histoplasm antibody which is found to be positive for histoplasmosis?

10) What are the codes for a hamster penetration test which was found to be negative for insterility?

11) What are the codes for measurement of hemoglobin performed transcutaneously and is positive for polycythemia?

12) What are the codes for microscopic and gross examination of a left breast of a 48-year-old woman which includes the lymph nodes which is found to be cancerous?

13) If I was checking for the presence of antibodies, why type of test would I use?

14) The substance being chemically tested is known as what?

15) What are the codes for testing for cocaine and meth?

CHAPTER 38
MEDICINE

You will learn the following objectives in this chapter:

A. Immunizations
B. Psychotherapy
C. Biofeedback
D. Dialysis
E. Gastroenterology
F. Ophthalmology
G. Cardiovascular
H. Injections, Infusions & Chemotherapy
I. Dermatology
J. Chiropractic
K. Allergy & Immunology
L. Injections, Infusions, & Chemotherapy
M. Nutritional Therapy

Section 38.1: FORMAT

This section of the CPT book provides codes for those services and procedures not coded in other sections (similar to the V codes), so there includes a great variety of services and procedures.

SUBSECTIONS: The Medicine section can be likened to the V codes of ICD-10 in that they contain a great variety of service and procedures. The subsections of Medicine are:

Immunoglobulins	90281-90399
Immunization Administration For Vaccines/Toxoids	90460-90474
Vaccines, Toxoids	90476-90749
Psychiatry	90785-90899
Biofeedback	90901-90911
Dialysis	90935-90999
Gastroenterology	91010-91299
Ophthalmology	92002-92499
Special Otorhinolaryngologic Services	92502-92700
Cardiovascular	92920-93799
Noninvasive Vascular Diagnostic Studies	93880-93998
Pulmonary	94002-94799
Allergy & Clinical Immunology	95004-95199
Endocrinology	95250-95251
Neurology & Neuromuscular Procedures	95782-96020
Medical Genetics & Genetic Counseling Services	96040
Central Nervous System Assessments/Tests	96101-96125
Health & Behavior Assessment Intervention	96150-96155

Hydration, Therapeutic Prophylactic, Diagnostic Injections & Infusions and Chemotherapy & Other Highly Complex Drug or Highly Complex Biologic Agent Administration	96360-96549
Photodynamic Therapy	96567-96571
Special Dermatological Procedures	96900-96999
Physical Medicine & Rehabilitation	97001-97799
Medical Nutrition Therapy	97802-97804
Acupuncture	97810-97814
Osteopathic Manipulative Treatment	98925-98929
Chiropractic Manipulative Treatment	98940-98943
Education & Training for Patient Self-Management	98960-98962
Non-Face-to-Face Nonphysician Services	98966-98968
On-Line Medical Evaluation	98969
Special Services, Procedure/Reports	99000-99091
Qualifying Circumstances for Anesthesia	99100-99140
Moderate (Conscious) Sedation	99143-99150
Other Services & Procedures	99170-99199
Home Health Procedures/Services	99500-99602
Medication Therapy Management Services	99605-99607

Section 38.2: IMMUNIZATIONS

Immunization is a process by which a person's immune system is activated and fortified against an immunogen which assists in the body's attack against the immunogen and its subsequent removal from the body in addition to the ability of the body to fight future attacks by the immunogen. Immunogen is an antigen that is a foreign body that activates the body's production of antibodies so that the body can remove it.

A vaccination is a type of immunization in which a vaccine is administered to the patient to produce immunity to a disease prior to the patient being exposed to the disease. There are two types of vaccines: attenuated or dead. Attenuated vaccines are composed of live weakened immunogens which are administered to the patient to produce an immunological response by the body for future protection against the immunogen. These vaccines tend to be more effective and do not require boosters as frequently since. Dead vaccines are composed of immunogens that are grown and then killed using a method such as heat or formaldehyde.

A toxoid vaccine is a bacterial toxin which has been weakened which induce an immune response to the toxin, such as for exposures to tetanus or diphtheria. Antitoxins are made within organisms by injecting them with a safe amount of the toxin to which their body produces an immunological response and produces an anti-toxin which can then be injected into a patient who has been exposed to the toxin.

There are a variety of reasons why a patient may receive immunizations. We most frequently think of children who receive vaccinations during a well check; however, a person traveling to another country or exposed to a disease may need immunizations.

When a patient receives an immunization, there are several codes that can be charged. First, the administration of the immunization is coded, then the substance itself is charged of which there could be several components to one administration or there would be several administrations at the same time.

Codes 90281-90399 are for the immunoglobulin product only and should always be coded with code for the administration of the immunoglobulin using codes 96365-96379. Notice that these administration codes are not the same as the administration codes for vaccine and toxoids. Note that the immunoglobulin codes are differentiated by method of administration and the type of immunoglobulin, such as antitoxins for botulism or diphtheria.

The next section of the Medicine codes are for administration of vaccines and toxoids (90460-90474). Pay close attention to the details in the descriptions of these codes. These administration codes should be coded in addition to the vaccine or toxoid material as listed in codes 90476-90749.

The administration codes are differentiated by age of patient. Types of administration include oral, intranasal, percutaneous, intradermal, subcutaneous, or intramuscular.

For adults, administration codes are coded for each administration, so if there are multiple administrations of vaccines then each administration by its type should be coded separately. If several vaccines are included in injection, then only one administration and one vaccine is coded. However, with children each component of the vaccine is coded for administration even if they are combination vaccines.

For adults, the most commonly used administration code is 90471 which is for one percutaneous, intradermal, subcutaneous or intramuscular injection for anyone not 18 or younger. If a second administration is performed through any of these means, then the add-on code 90472 can also be listed. If a different means of administration as used, either oral or intranasal, then code 90473 should be used which also has an add-on code 90474 in case there is another administration by these means. However, if there are two administrations, for example, one intramuscularly and the other orally, then codes 90471 and 90473 would be listed. The add-on codes are only used if there is a second administration by the same method. For adults, you can only charge on administration code for a vaccine even if contains several vaccines, such as DTP.

If a patient is 18 or younger and the physician or other qualified healthcare provider providing counseling, then codes 90460-90461 should be used in the same manner as noted above for the 90471-90474 series of codes excepting that each component of a combination vaccine are coded separately for administration. There is also no other code specified for nasal or oral route of administration; all types of administration are included in the same code.

The various types of vaccines and toxoids that can be coded in addition to the administration codes and are listed with codes 90476-90749.

Notice that some vaccine and toxoids are differentiated by age, method of administration, and combination of vaccines and toxoids.

The most important detail to recognize in these codes is that there are vaccines and toxoids listed singly or in combination with other vaccines and toxoids, so you must be careful to code administration of a combination vaccine or toxoid as only one administration and be sure to select the proper vaccine toxoid code, e.g. 90710 is one code that includes vaccine for measles, mumps, rubella and MMRV administered subcutaneously so only one administration code would be used for this (either 90471). Otherwise, if there is not a correct combination code for the vaccines and toxoids administered, then separate codes must be listed with separate administration codes for each vaccine or toxoid administered.

In addition to coding for administration and the substance, an office visit may be charged at the same visit if more services other than the immunization were provided, such as a well check.

Section 38.3: PSYCHIATRY

The psychiatric codes (90785-90899) include an add-on code for interactive complexity (90785). There are also codes for general clinical psychiatric interview procedures (90791-90802), special clinical psychiatric procedures, and therapeutic procedures. Psychiatric therapeutic procedures (90832-90853) are differentiated by type of psychotherapy, such as insight oriented or interactive either in the office or in the hospital and are based on time. Psychoanalysis is included in this category as 90845, as well as family therapy (90846-90847) and group therapy (90853). Management of psychiatric drugs is coded as 90863. ECT (electroconvulsive therapy) is coded as 90870.

"Psychotherapy is the treatment for mental illness and behavioral disturbances in which the clinician establishes a professional contract with the patient and, through definitive therapeutic communication, attempts to alleviate the emotional disturbances, reverse or change maladaptive patterns of behavior, and encourage personality growth and development" (CPT Coding book definition).

1. Interactive Psychotherapy: "Interactive Psychotherapy involves the use of physical aids and nonverbal communication to overcome barriers to therapeutic interventions" and is most often used with children (CPT coding book).
2. Insight-oriented Psychotherapy: Insight-oriented Psychotherapy is a form of treatment that helps people through understanding and expressing feelings, motivations, beliefs, fears and desires through a therapeutic relationship.
3. Behavior Modification Psychotherapy: Behavior Modification Psychotherapy involves the positive change of behaviors through techniques by altering person's reactions to stimuli through positive and negative reinforcement and reduction of maladaptive behavior through punishment and/or therapy.

If a healthcare provider provides a hospital or office visit in addition to psychiatric services, an E/M can also be charged if validated by the documentation; however, do note that some psychiatric codes cannot be coded in addition to E/M visits as noted in the CPT coding book, i.e. 90805, 90807, 90809, 90811, 90815, 90817, 90819, 90822, 90824, 90827, and 90829. E/Ms cannot be coded with these codes because these codes include "medical evaluation and management services."

Section 38.4: BIOFEEDBACK

Biofeedback only has two codes, one for training by any modality (90901) and training of perineal muscles or urethral sphincter (anorectal) (90911). Biofeedback is when bodily functions such as blood pressure, heart rate, skin temperature, sweat gland activity, and muscle tension, are measured and conveyed to the patient via a machine so that the patient can learn to gain control of those functions.

Section 38.5: DIALYSIS

Hemodialysis codes include the E/M services performed on the day dialysis is provided, whether they are provided as inpatient or outpatient. The insertion or declotting of cannulas or catheters used in order to provide dialysis are not included in the dialysis codes and should be coded separately using appropriate surgery codes which will be discussed later in the surgery packets.

Dialysis is the separation of nitrogenous waste materials from the blood stream due to kidney failure and is used to treat kidney failure, notably ESRD (end-stage renal disease). There are several types of dialysis:

1. Hemodialysis: Hemodialysis (HD) removes the waste materials from the blood stream through the use of an artificial kidney machine which passes the blood through the machine where it is filtered and returned to the body which may be done several times a week. Blood that has been cleaned is known as being dialysed.
2. Peritoneal Dialysis: Peritoneal dialysis (PD), with one version known as CAPD (continuous ambulatory peritoneal dialysis), removes the waste materials from the blood stream by the introduction of fluid (dialysate) through a catheter into the peritoneal (abdominal) cavity where it remains for several hours. During this time, the waste from the capillaries then passes out of the bloodstream and into fluid which is then removed via the catheter many hours later. PD is usually preferred when the patient wishes to perform the dialysis at home.
3. Hemofiltration: Hemofiltration is similar to hemodialysis but involves the pumping of blood through a dialyzer or "hemofilter" by means of a pressure gradient and no dialysate used. The pressure gradient allows the water to pass into the bloodstream and pull substances out of the bloodsteam. Sometimes hemodialysis and hemofiltration can be combined in one process.

There are several types of dialysis services:

1. Hemodialysis: These hemodialysis codes are differentiated by how many evaluations the physician provides on the same day, i.e. one for 90935 and more than one for 90937.
2. Other dialysis: Peritoneal dialysis and hemofiltration are differentiated by the number of evaluations performed on the day of the dialysis and is coded with 90945 for a single evaluation and 90947 for more than one evaluation.
3. Home Visits: Home visits to assist with dialysis by nonphysician personnel is coded as 99512.
4. End-Stage Renal Disease (ESRD) Services: When a person has been diagnosed with ESRD, they receive dialysis services several times a week, in addition to other services, so the codes for these services reflect the extensive care that is provided with codes differentiated by length of time in receiving ESRD services.

If a patient has received ESRD services for one month, then codes 90951-90962 should be used which are further differentiated by age of the patient and number of face-to-face physician encounters.

If a patient has received ESRD dialysis at home, then codes 90963-90966 should be used as differentiated by age of patient.

If the patient does not receive a full month's of ESRD services due to either just beginning or discontinuing, then codes 90967-90970 should be used based on patient's age. These codes are for each day so a multiplier should be attached to the code for the number of days ESRD service are provided, such as 90967 x 5 for 5 days of service.

Dialysis training is coded as either 90989 or 90993 when the patient and a helper are provided training on how to perform dialysis.

Section 38.6: GASTROENTEROLOGY

The Medicine Section for Gastroenterology (91010-91299) provides codes for non-surgical gastroenterological procedures and services. Be careful when using these codes because many of them may already be included (bundled) into a larger procedure and would, therefore, not be separately billable, such as intubation and gastric studies. Gastric intubation (43753) is used to code for stomach pumping when poisons have been ingested. Gastric reflux tests are coded as 91037-91038.

If fluoroscopy is used for studies or placement, code 76000 should also be coded.

Section 38.7: OPHTHAMOLOGY

Ophthalmology (92002-92499) is the branch of medicine which deals with the diseases and surgery of the eyes and associated functions.

Professional ophthalmological CPT codes are differentiated by level of service and new or established patient. Professional services have their own E/M codes and are differentiated as intermediate or comprehensive for new and established patients; however, an ophthalmologist can choose to use these codes or they can use the E/M office visit or consultation codes instead. Like any other office visit, professional services are defined as face-to-face contact between physician and patient.

Intermediate professional services (92002 for new patient; 92012 for established patient) include "history, general medical observation, external ocular and adnexal examination and other diagnostic procedures as indicated and may include use of mydriasis" (CPT coding book) in addition to ophthalmoscopy. If ophthalmoscopy is performed by itself then it would be coded as 92225. There is a notation by the code 92225 which describes it proper usage. The provision of lens service is not included in a general exam and should be coded separately.

Comprehensive ophthalmological professional services (92004 for new patient; 92014 for established patient) include an examination of the complete visual system which can occur over several visits. The service includes "history, general medical observation, external and ophthalmoscopic examinations, gross visual fields, and basic sensorimotor examination and can include biomicroscopy, exam with cycloplegia or mydriasis and tonometry and always includes initiation of diagnostic and treatment programs" (CPT coding book) in addition to ophthalmoscopy. If ophthalmoscopy is performed by itself then it would be coded as 92225. There is a notation by the code 92225 which describes it proper usage. The provision of lens service is not included in a general exam and should be coded separately.

Notice that there are additional services which can be coded if performed in addition to the exams and which are listed under the Special Ophthalmological Services, such as the CCT (computerized corneal topography) 92025, fitting of contact lens for treatment of disease (92071-92072), visual field exam (92081-92083), and extended ophthalmoscopy including retinal drawing (92225-92226).

Fluorescein angiography is a procedure used to examine the circulation of the retina using the dye tracing method. Fluorescein angiography is coded as 92230-92235. Extended color visions test are coded as 92283. Special ophthalmological services include codes for ophthalmological exams done under anesthesia (92018-92019) which is not the norm but in some cases anesthesia may be necessary to complete the exam. No modifiers are needed because the code actually states that the service was performed with anesthesia.

Gonioscopy is a viewing of the angle where the cornea and iris meet with the use of a gonioscope and slit lamp or microscope to check for eye conditions, such as glaucoma. If a gonioscopy is performed by itself, then it can be coded with 92020, but if it is part of another procedure then it would not be coded as it would be included in the other procedure (bundled) which is indicated by the terms “separate procedure” following the code. Tonometry is the measurement of intraocular pressure (IOP) of the eye. Tonometry (92100) is also considered a separate procedure and would only be coded if performed by itself, otherwise it is included in more significant procedures.

Notice that some of the codes are described as unilateral or bilateral. In this case, whether the service was provided to one or both eyes, these codes would be used without any modifier attached since they are acceptable for either a unilateral or bilateral procedure, e.g., 92081.

Notice also that some codes include the professional components of supervision and interpretation, e.g. 92133. In these cased no modifier 26 would need to be attached to the code if the ophthalmologist provided the professional component.

PRESCRIPTION FOR LENSES: Determination of refractive state (92015) is used to code for prescription of spectacles. Fitting of spectacles and supply of materials are coded separately though with supplies coded from the HCPCS.

The prescription, fitting, and replacement of contact lens (92310-92326) are billed separately from other procedures, including exams. Follow-up of fitting is part of a general exam.

Remember that the prescription of spectacles is included in code 92015 as previously discussed for the determination of refractive state. Fitting of the spectacles, repair, refitting, prosthesis service and supply of materials are coded separately, however. Materials would be coded with the HCPCS codes and the fitting would be coded as 92340-92355. Prosthesis service would be coded as 92358 and repair and refitting would be coded as 92370-92371.

There are two HCPCS codes for glaucoma screening which can be used to bill for Medicare patients, G0117 and G0118. Some corneal procedures are also coded with S0800-S0812 codes. In addition, HCPCS codes for supplies include S05000-S0590 for contact lens and V2020 for frames.

Section 38.8: OTORHINOLARYNGOLOGIC

Otorhinolaryngologic services (92502-92700) are for ENT (ear, nose, throat) services. Many ENT services are included as part of an E/M code, which includes otoscopy, anterior rhinoscopy, tuning fork test, and removal of cerumen, so they would not be coded separately from the E/M code.

Special ENT service that are coded separately include an exam under anesthesia (92502), binocular microscopy (92504), evaluation and treatment of speech, language and auditory processing (92506-92507), function tests (92512-92524), and treatment for swallowing dysfunctions (92526). Note that treatment of speech, language and auditory processing are differentiated by whether the services are for an individual or group.

Vestibular function tests are used to determine problems of the inner ear (vestibules) to determine if there are other disorders causing dizziness. These function tests codes include test for nystagmus and vestibular test (92531-92548).

AUDIOLOGIC FUNCTION TESTS: There are very specific tests included in this section, Audiologic Function Tests (92550-92597). Some hearing tests, such as tuning fork and whispered voice, are included in the E/M code for the exam and not coded separately from the E/M code. Hearing aid exams are included in this section (92590-92593).

All audiologic test codes are described as being performed on both ears (binaural), so if a procedure is done only one ear (monaural), then modifier 52 for Reduced Services need to be attached to the CPT code for the service.

EVALUATIVE AND THERAPEUTIC SERVICES. Services associated with external devices are included in evaluative and therapeutic services, e.g. cochlear implants 92601-92604, speech-generating devices 92605-92609, swallowing function tests 92610-92618, and auditory function tests 92620-92633. Notice that there are codes for the test and the professional component (supervision and interpretation) which are followed by a code for the professional component only.

Section 38.9: CARDIOVASCULAR

With cadiovascular, definitions are important to know to understand the codes.

1. CPR: Cardiopulmonary resuscitation; CPR is physical intervention to provide artificial circulation through chest compressions and artificial respiration.
2. Cardioversion: Cardioversion is the conversion of a rapid heart or cardiac arrhythmia to a normal rhythm through the use of a device or drugs.

3. Thrombectomy: A thrombectomy is the excision of an abnormal or dangerous thrombus (blood clot) by the use of a balloon catheter which is inserted into the vessel.
4. Thrombolysis: Thrombolysis is the breakdown of blood clots by pharmacological means.
5. Stents: stent is a man-made tube inserted into a natural passage in the body to prevent, or counteract, a disease-induced, localized flow constriction. The term may also refer to a tube used to temporarily hold such a natural conduit open to allow access for surgery.
6. PTCA: Percutaneous transluminal coronary angioplasty; Angioplasty is the surgical procedure to widen an obstructed blood vessel usually due to atherosclerosis.
7. Atherectomy: Atherectomy is a minimally invasive method of removing plaque and blockage from an artery with subsequent widening of the artery.
8. Cardiac Rhythm: Cardiac rhythm includes the heart rhythm, ST analysis, heart rate variability, and T-wave alternans.
9. Cardiography: Cardiograph is the production of a report/rhythm strip to evaluate the presence of arrythymias, and cardiography is the process of reading the report.
10. EKG/ECG: Electrocardiography is a recorded test of the electrical activity of the heart over time.
11. ICM: ICM is an implantable cardiovascular monitor which is a "device used to assist the physician in the management of non-rhythm related cardiac conditions such as heart failure" (CPT code book). Cardiovascular data is collected via internal and external sensors placed on the body.
12. ICD: ICD is an "implantable cardioverter-defibrillator" which is an "implantable device that provides high-energy and low-energy stimulation to the heart" in order to slow rapid heart rate or speed up slow heart rates as well as fibrillation (CPT code book).
13. ILR: ILR is an "implantable loop recorder" which is an "implantable device that continuously records" the rhythm of the heart with this information then transferred to the physician either locally or remotely (CPT code book).
14. Pacemaker: A pacemaker is "an implantable device that provides low energy stimulation" to the heart to initiate contractions when necessary (CPT code book). A pacemaker can be single lead or dual lead which refers to the placement of the electrodes on one or two chambers.
15. Echocardiography: Echocardiography, like its terms, refers to the use of 2-dimensional and/or use of color Doppler ultrasounds to view the heart and arteries. This is not the same as an electrocardiogram which is a noninvasive recording transthoracic interpretation of the electrical activity of the heart over time as recorded by skin electrodes.

THERAPEUTIC SERVICES AND PROCEDURES: CPR (cardiopulmonary resuscitation) is coded as 92950 which is not considered part of critical care so it could be coded as an additional code. If cardioversion is performed using a defibrillator it is coded as 92960 as long as it is not included within any other procedure, so be careful if coding for another procedure because the cardioversion may be included.

As with most procedures, lesser procedures that are typically part of the procedure are considered part of the global package and not coded separately. For example, a PTCA is considered to be part of procedures that involve atherectomy; an atherectomy and/or PTCA are considered to be a part of the procedure for stenting, which is the most complex of the three procedures and all inclusive of the others, so if all three procedures are performed, only the stenting procedure would be coded.

A PTCA is a percutaneous transluminal coronary angioplasty. This procedure involves the use of a catheter with a balloon on the end which is inflated after it is passed into an artery. The purpose of the inflation of the balloon is to crush and flatten the plaque (which caused narrowing (stenosis) in the arteries so that blood can once again flow through the arteries. However, there are other procedures that are usually done at the same time as the PTCA which includes implantation of stents, atherectomy and brachytherapy (radioactive material used to inhibit restenosis. A stent is a mesh tube which is inserted into the artery to keep it open.

Be careful when coding for placement of stents because this too may be part of a larger procedure. In addition, some other procedures may be included in the stent code so only the stent code would be coded, but this is explained in the notes for this section of the CPT code book. For example, an atherectomy or angioplasty of the same artery is "considered part of the stenting procedure and is not reported separately" (CPT code book). However, a thrombectomy, brachytherapy or ultrasound are coded in addition to other procedure codes and are not included in other codes.

Notice that there are several add-on codes for additional vessels, whereas the first code is for the initial vessel. If several blockages are treated within the same coronary artery, then this procedure is coded only once. HCPCS modifiers should be added also, LC for left circumflex artery, LD for left anterior descending artery, and RC for right coronary artery.

Notice that many of these codes also mention the inclusion of the professional component (supervision and interpretation).

CARDIOGRAPHY: Cardiographies involve the use of equipment, such as EKG/ECGs to test for arrhythymias by producing a report/rhythm strip. These tests can be read and interpreted either by a technician present at the time or remotely by a telephone signal.

The correct code is determined by the number of leads applied to the patient for the EKG/ECGs, e.g. 12 leads. These codes are further differentiated by the services provided, whether the entire service is performed or if only a part is, e.g. tracing or interpretation and reporting (93000-93010).

If the patient is fitted with an EKG/ECG which they wear then this would be coded as 93224-93272 which is differentiated by what type of additional services are included and the length of time.

Cardiovascular stress test, which is a common testing procedure, is coded as 93015-93018 with differentiation by which services were provided, tracing, supervision, reading, and interpretation.

DEVICE MONITORING: "Cardiovascular monitoring services are diagnostic medical procedures using in-person and remote technology to assess device therapy and cardiovascular physiologic data" (CPT code book) and it is not the insertion of the devices which is coded from the surgical section. This includes ICM, ICD, ILR, pacemaker, cardioverter-defibrillators, and loop recorders. In-person and remote cannot be coded at the same time because the physician can only be performing in one mode at a time.

The time period listed in some of the codes (e.g. 93295) is to be described by the physician but is based on when the remote monitoring begins or at the 91st day after the insertion of a pacemaker or cardioverter-defibrillator and extends for 90 days or 31 days for loop recorder or cardiovascular monitor which extends 90 days.

The codes in this section are also dependent on what type of device is being monitored and/or programmed, in addition to the number and placement of leads.

ECHOCARDIOGRAPHY: Echocardiography (93303-93352) involves the use of ultrasound utilizing two-dimensional image and/or Doppler color to examine the heart and the arteries. These codes are differentiated by anatomic site involvement, type of imaging, such as M-mode or real time, and if they are complete or limited exams. Limited exams do not evaluate or document all structures that are part of the echocardiographic exam.

Echocardiographies are oftentimes used to collect data when patients are performing a stress test, such as walking on a treadmill, using a bicycle, or administration of drugs to evoke a response.

Contrast materials are coded separately, in addition to the echocardiography code.

CATHETERIZATION: A catheterization coded from the Medicine section are coded as right or left heart catheterization in addition to codes for the injections and supervision and interpretation. Cardiac catheterization is a specialized study of the heart during which a catheter (small hollow flexible tube) is inserted into the artery of the groin or arm and introduced into various vessels so that the insides can be visualized for any blockage. Contrast material (dye) that has been previously introduced allows the x-ray visualization of the vessels which is known as an angiogram.

These codes from the Medicine section are used if the procedure is described as a left or right heart catheterization; if not, cardiovascular injection codes from the Surgery section (36011-36015; 36215-36218) are used.

There are two groups of cardiac-related codes that may be confusing in reference to catheters. The 36000 codes are injection procedures used for treatment or diagnostics and involve injections only. In contrast, cardiac catheterization codes are used for left and right heart catheterizations to provide more indepth diagnostics and services, such as angioplasties and use codes 93451 through 93572. In addition, radiology codes can also be reported for angiographies, or the technical portion of this type of cardiovascular service. These radiological codes may be provided by the physician or by a radiologist.

Sometimes insertion of a catheter into the venous system allows access to veins for administration of drugs, IV fluids, and other materials or to obtain blood samples, known as Port-a-Cath, PICC, and Hickman. These are known as Central Venous Access Devices (VADs or CVDs) and there are two types: completely implanted or partially implanted. Insertion can be either central or peripheral. For central lines, access is usually through the subclavian or jugular veins of the neck. One type of central, known as a peripheral venous catheters (PICC) are placed peripherally in the veins of the arms, legs, feet or head. CVDs are known as implantable CVDs and allow for vascular access without repeated needle sticks, such as for total parenteral nutrition (TPN), chemotherapy, dialysis, etc. Ports are implanted VADs which supply medication or materials and is composed of an injection port (placed in a pocket) and a catheter which is tunneled from the vein into the subcutaneous tissue to the port.

Catheterization codes (93451-93462) include introduction, positioning, and repositioning of catheter(s), recording of intracardiac and intravascular pressure, obtaining blood samples, and final evaluation as described in the CPT coding book. A right heart catheterization usually is performed with the insertion of the catheter into the venous system and a left heart catheterization is usually performed with the insertion of the catheter into the arterial system.

For coding purposes, the first code to be listed is for the right (93451) or left heart (93452) catheterization. There are also codes for combined left and right catheterizations, e.g. 93453. There are different codes for the right or left heart catheterization when the procedure is performed due to congenital anomaly (93530-93533). Second, additional codes include vascular injection codes (93561-93568). These codes describe the progression of the catheter into other vascular sites which includes arterial conduits, aortocoronary venous bypass grafts, and angiographies for the pulmonary artery, or right or left ventricular and atrial.

Notice that some of these codes are marked as being acceptable for the additional coding for conscious sedation, if performed.

Other codes in this section include the use of dilution studies or Doppler (93561-93572). As described in the CPT book, dilution studies are not to be coded in addition to the catheterization codes as they are globally contained within the catheterization code and can only be coded if there were no other service performed that they are a part of. Repair of a skeptical defect with the use of a transcatheter is also coded here (93580-93583).

ELECTROPHYSIOLOGICAL STUDIES: Electrophysiological studies involve the insertion and repositioning of a catheter to collect cardiovascular data used to diagnose arrhythmias which can be assisted by the induction of an arrhythmia.

These codes are differentiated by the vascular anatomic site, such as Bundle of His or right ventricle. Notice that many of these codes can involve conscious sedation and are 51 modifier exempt.

If ablation and mapping are also performed in addition to the electrophysiological studies, then they should be coded separately. Mapping (93609-93613) is the development of a picture that demonstrates where the problems areas are as evidenced by the electrophysiological data. Ablation (93655) is the destruction of problem areas from where the arrhythmias originate.

REHABILITATION & PHYSIOLOGIC STUDIES: Treatment for PAD (peripheral vascular disease (93668) are coded per session which usually lasts about 45 to 60 minutes and can involve the use of various equipment, such as a treadmill or track. Noninvasive physiologic studies (93701-93799) include plethysmography and temperature gradient studies.

Section 38.10: PULMONARY

VENTILATOR MANAGEMENT: Mechanical ventilation is a method to mechanically assist or replace spontaneous breathing with the use of a ventilator machine or can be done manually by a physician using a bag to force air into the patient and are either termed negative-pressure ventilation, where air is essentially sucked into the lungs, or positive pressure ventilation, where air (or another gas mix) is pushed into the trachea.These services are provided in the hospital or a nursing home with the codes differentiated by initial or subsequent days (94002-94004) or at home which requires training for oversight which is coded by time (94005).

Other important terminology is Spirometry which is a test using an instrument that tests the patient for difficulty in breathing, such as for asthmatic patients. CPAP is continuous positive airway pressure performed by a device which delivers a stream of compressed air via a hose to a nasal pillow, nose mask or full-face mask, to promote unobstructed breathing, thereby reducing and/or preventing apneas and hypopneas.CNP is continuous negative pressure ventilation when air is sucked into the lungs.

OTHER PROCEDURES: Other procedures include laboratory procedures and interpretation of test results, such as spirometry (94010-94060), lung capacities (94070-94200), gas collections (94250), determination of pulmonary volumes (94375), responses (94400-94450), high altitude simulation test (94452), administration of surfactant for the lungs (94610), pulmonary stress tests (94620- 94621), inhalation treatment including nebulizer treatments (94640-94645), CNP & CPAP ventilation (94660-94662), chest wall manipulation to facilitate lung function (94667-94668), analysis of oxygen uptake and saturation (94680-94762), carbon dioxide measurement (94770), and measurement of apnea and circadian respiratory pattern (94772-94799).

Section 38.11: ALLERGY & IMMUNOLOGY

Allergy testing codes are differentiated by type of test. Each test is coded separately and so additional tests with the same code would be indicated by an increased number of units on the CMS 1500 billing form.

Allergy tests include percutaneous tests (commonly known as scratch, puncture or prick tests) (95004) and include interpretation by the physician.

Intracutaneous (intradermal) tests are coded as 95017-95028. Patch, application, or photo tests are coded as 95044-95071. Codes 95076-95079 for ingestion challenge test can only be billed once no matter how many times it is performed. For inhalation bronchial change testing, two codes need to be coded: one for the inhalation bronchial challenge test and one for the pulmonary testing which is used to document the results.

ALLERGEN IMMUNOTHERAPY: Allergen immunotherapy (95115-95199) is the process of desensitization or hyposensitization to an allergen. This is achieved by the "parenteral administration of extracts of the allergen at periodic intervals, usually on an increasing dosage scale to a dosage which is maintained as maintenance therapy" (CPT code book). To code this treatment, two codes are required: first, the coding of the preparation of the extract and second, the administration which are based on the type of allergen being desensitized.

These codes are administered by injected dosages contained with a vial which are billed as separate and additional units. A dose is defined as the "amount of antigen(s) administered in a single injection from a multiple dose vial" (CPT code book).

Similar to immunizations and vaccinations, office visits can be charged if the additional services other than just the administration of the extract is performed and documented. However, the interpretation and supervision of the administration are not considered a separate E/M service and cannot be billed separately.

Section 38.12: NEUROLOGY AND NEUROMUSCULAR PROCEDURES

There are a variety of codes contained within this section, including sleep testing, EEG, muscle and range of motion testing. These codes include both the technical and professional components are included so if the physician does not conduct the test, he must attach a modifier 26 to indicate that he only provided the professional component of supervision and interpretation.

SLEEP TESTING: Sleep testing services are the "continuous and simultaneous monitoring and recording of various physiological and pathophysiological parameters of sleep for 6 or more hours with physician review, interpretation, and report" (CPT code book). These codes are used to test for sleep disturbances and to evaluate patient responses to treatments.

Actigraphy is a method of monitoring human rest/activity cycles for gross motor activity to produce data to be analyzed. Polysomnography is the monitoring of the patient's airflow through the nose and mouth, blood pressure, ECG, oxygen level, brain wave pattern, eye movement, and the movement of respiratory muscle and limbs to evaluate sleep disorders.

Sleep testing and polysomnography are distinguished from each other although they are contained with this same section because the polysomonography (95782-95783) includes sleep staging which must be recorded. These codes are differentiated by the number of parameters performed including EEG, EOG, and EMG and examine other sleep parameters including ECG, airflow, ventilation and respiratory effort, gas exchange, transcutaneous monitoring, end tidal gas analysis, extremely muscle activity, motor activity-movement, penile tumescence, gastroesophageal reflux, continuous blood pressure monitoring, snoring, body positioning and more (CPT code book).

Sleep testing codes are differentiated by attendance of technologist (95807), type of test and length of the test. For example, an actigraphy test (95803) is a minimum of 72 hours up to 14 consecutive days of recording. Note that the CPT code directs that if the actigraphy test is less than 6 hours, then modifier 52 for reduction of services needs to be attached to the code 95803.

EEG: Electroencephalogram (EEG) is a test that measures and records the electrical activity of your brain. Electrooculogram (EOG) is a record of the difference in electrical charge between the front and back of the eye associated with eyeball movement which is recorded by electrodes placed on the skin near the eye. Electromyogram (EMG) is a test to test the activation signals of the muscle in addition to the nerves that control them. Electroencephalogram (EEG) codes are differentiated by length of monitoring (95812-95813) and types of recordings (95816-95827), such as awake, sleep, coma, cerebral death, or all night. If the EEG is performed during surgery it is coded as 95827. Additional EEG tests are coded from 95950 to 95967, such as for localization of seizures, EEG during nonintracranial surgery, testing of brain hemispheric activity, brain mapping, and magnetoencephalography (MEG).

MUSCLE/RANGE OF MOTION TESTING: Muscle and range of motion testing are differentiated by anatomic site and by either being manual testing (95831-95834) or the measurements and reporting (95851-95857). These codes also include a tensilon test for myasthenia gravis.

ELECTROMYOGRAPHY: Electromyography is the study of the electrical responses of the muscles as recorded by electrodes. These codes are differentiated by number of extremities involved (95860-95864), other anatomic sites (95865-95866), or cranial or paraspinal nerves (95867-95869).

MUSCLE TESTING: Muscle testing codes (95831-95857) are mostly add-on codes and are used when there is electrical stimulation or EMG performed in addition to the primary procedure as described in the CPT code book.

NERVE CONDUCTION TESTS: Nerve conduction tests (95905-95913) code for nerve conduction tests which can be motor, sensory, or amplitude and latency/velocity studies. Appendix J should be utilized to assign the proper code as this describes which nerves are included under which codes.

INTRAOPERATIVE NEUROPHYSIOLOGY: There is only one code for intraoperative neurophysiology, 95940-95941, which is based on hours. This is an add-on code which should be used in conjunction with the primary procedure. Be sure to read the notes in this section which describes which codes can and cannot be used together and what other codes should be coded.

AUTONOMIC FUNCTION TESTS: Autonomic function tests (95921-95943) are tests of the autonomic nervous system based on testing of cardiovagal, vasomotor, and sudomotor.

EVOKED POTENTIALS & REFLEX TESTS: Evoked potential studies (95925-95937) are differentiated on anatomic sites and if they are visual, central motor, or somatosensory. Reflex tests (95933-95937) are for blinking, knee, and neuromuscular junctions.

NEUROSTIMULATOR ANALYSIS & PROGRAMMING: Neurostimulators are low levels of electricity to the nerves that provide treatment in which pain is blocked so that it is not received by the brain. The two types of neurostimulation are spinal cord stimulation and peripheral nerve stimulation. Autonomic: The autonomic nervous system (ANS) is known as the visceral nervous system which controls the visceral functions such as heart rate, digestion, and respiration. It is part of the peripheral nervous system and divided into the parasympathetic nervous system and sympathetic nervous system. An evoked potential is an electrical response from the nervous system as a response to a stimulus. This is distinctly different from spontaneous potentials that are detected by EEGs or EMGs.

Neurostimulators consists of a generator and electrodes. After they are implanted, there needs to be analysis and programming so that data can be received and interpreted. Neurostimulators can be either simple or complex. A simple neurostimulator affects three or less areas of study while a complex neurostimulator affects more than three. These areas of study include pulse amplitude, duration or frequency, electrode contacts, cycling, stimulation train duration, train spacing, number of programs or channels, alternating electrode polarities, and dose time as described in the CPT code book.

These medicine codes are differentiated by analysis of either single or complex neurostimulators with or without programming and which nerves are involved (95970-95982) with analysis also differentiated by time.

Additional codes must be used for the insertion of the neurostimulator pulse generator which is part of the neurostimulator utilizing codes such as 61885, 63685, or 64590. Revision or removal of a generator is coded separately as 61888, 63688, or 64595. There are a variety of codes to select from for the implantation of the electrodes which includes 61850-61875 or 64553-64580, which are listed in this section of the Medicine codes.

Brain mapping only has one code (96020) and includes the administration of the test and review of data by the physician or psychologist for testing of language, memory, cognition, movement, sensation and other neurological functions.

MOTION ANALYSIS: Motion analysis codes (96000-96004) are used for procedure and services for patients with complex movement problems such as associated with cerebral palsy, stroke, and spina bifida. This code can only be listed once as described in the CPT code book.

Section 38.13: CENTRAL NERVOUS SYSTEM

Codes in this subsection of central nervous system (96101-96125) are for testing of cognitive functions of the CNS. Codes 96101-96103 are for psychological tests (such as MMPI, WAIS, and Rorschach). Code 96105 is for assessment of aphasia. Codes 96110-96111 are for developmental testing. Code 96116 is for neurobehavioral status exam, codes 96118-96120 are for neuropsychological testing, and code 96125 is for standardized cognitive testing. All of these codes include the administration of the test and the interpretation and reporting of the results. The Minnesota Multiphasic Personality Inventory (MMPI) is a personality test that assists in identifying personality structure and psychopathology. The Wechsler Adult Intelligence Scale (WAIS) is a test used to measure intelligence quotient (IQ). The Rorschach test is also known as the inkblot test. It is a psychological test in which patients provide their interpretation of the inkblots which are then interpreted to examine the patient's personality and any possible mental disorders.

Section 38.14: HEALTH & BEHAVIOR ASSESSMENTS & INTERVENTION

"Health and behavior assessment procedures are used to identify the psychological, behavioral, emotional, cognitive, and social factors important to the prevention, treatment, or management of physical health problems" (CPT code book). This subsection of Medicine codes (96150-96155) focuses on biopsychosocial factors relating to physical problems and not on mental health issues. Psychiatric services would be coded instead with codes 90785-90899, so these codes should be not coded in addition to the health and behavior assessment codes (96150-96155). E/M visits should also not be coded in addition to these codes since these codes represent the purpose for the visit.

Health and behavior assessment and intervention codes are based on time and type of group involved.

Section 38.15: INJECTIONS, INFUSIONS & CHEMOTHERAPY:

Administration Routes are enteral or parenteral.

ENTERAL: Administered through the intestines.

1. Oral: Some drugs are given by mouth, then absorbed into the bloodstream through the stomach of the intestinal wall, such as oral polio.
2. Rectal: Some drugs are inserted by suppositories or solutions into the rectum.
3. Enteral feeding tube: Gastric feeding tubes placed into the body so that nutrition can be administered via the tube, also known as PEG (percutaneous endoscopic gastrostomy tube).

PARENTERAL: Administered through a means other than the digestive tract.

1. Intradermal: Intradermal injections occur when an injection is made into the upper layers of the skin.
2. Intracavitary: Intracavitary injections are made directly into a body cavity, such as the pleural cavity.
3. Intravenous: Intravenous (IV) injections are placed directly into a vein.
4. Percutaneous: Injections through the skin.
5. Subcutaneous: Subcutaneous injections are placed into the subcutaneous tissues under the skin.
6. Intrathecal: Intrathecal injections are placed into the space under the meninges surrounding the brain and spinal cord.
7. Transdermal: Transdermal are usually patches that are placed on top of the skin and deliver the drugs through the skin.
8. Sublingual: Some drugs are placed under the tongue and then are dissolved by the saliva, such as nitoglycerin tablets.
9. Intranasal: Some drugs are given by inhalation through the nose, such as the flu vaccine, which are known as aerosols.
10. Intramuscular: Intramuscular (IM) injections are usually placed into the buttocks or upper arm directly into the muscle.

ADMINISTRATION: Once an IV has been established, other injections or infusions may be provided through that site but these are coded as subsequent, not initial. Only one initial service can be coded, even if other services are provided that are not the same but are a part of the treatment plan. Other than the original initial service code, all other services are coded as subsequent services. The original initial service is the service that is described by the physician as being the primary reason for the visit. For example, if a patient has received an IV infusion and then there is an IV push later, even though they are not the same, only the IV infusion is coded as an initial service. The push is coded as a subsequent service.

Services included as part of the global for injections, infusions, and chemotherapy codes are local anesthesia, IV start, access to indwelling IV, flush at conclusion of infusion, and standard supplies.

Separate E/M visits that are for additional services/exam beyond the injections, infusions and chemotherapy can also be coded with a different diagnosis linked to it to indicate that the exam was for more reasons than just these services and a modifier 25 should be attached to the E/M code.

HYDRATION: Dehydration is the significant depletion of body water and electrolytes and can require differing levels of treatment. When a physician provides the services, treatment can consist of IV replacement of fluid and electrolytes. Hydration (96360-96361) is an IV infusion of pre-packaged fluid and electrolytes (such as saline solution or D5W). These codes are based on time. Both the hydration infusion and the materials should be coded with using the Medicine codes and HCPCS J codes, respectively. The infusion of drugs or substances for purposes other than hydration are coded separately.

INJECTIONS/INFUSIONS: Infusions are the introduction of a solution into the body usually through a cannula into a vein for therapeutic purposes which can be performed over various times frames. An infusion of less than 15 minutes is coded as a push (see below).

There are several types of infusions: Continuous infusion is small units of materials (drugs) administered at set time intervals. Intermittent infusion are more rapid programmed administrations of larger doses of materials (drugs) which is then alternated with low doses. Patient-controlled infusions are regulated by the patient as on-demand, usually for pain medication. Total parenteral nutrition infusions usually follow a dietary schedule for feeding the patient. Infusions are administered by a pump which infuses fluids, medication or nutrients into a patient's circulatory system.

An IV or intra-arterial push is described as "an injection in which the health care professional who administers the substance/drug is continuously present to administer the injection and observe the patient or an infusion of 15 minutes or less" (CPT code book).

This subsection of the Medicine codes includes codes for IV infusions, subsequent and concurrent infusions, and diagnostic or therapeutic injections administered as subcutaneous, IM, intra-arterial, and IV which are based on time and whether the service was the first service (initial), subsequent, or concurrent. An increment must be more than 30 minutes in order to qualify for coding of an additional hour.

IV infusions are coded as 96365-96371. Injections are coded as subcutaneous or IM (96372), intra-arterial (96373), IV or push (96374-96376). These do not include injections for allergic immunotherapy which were previously discussed.

If the pushs, injections, and infusions are part of another larger procedure, then do not code these services separately, such as the administration of a contrast material during a study in which only the code for the x-ray test would be coded.

Using HCPCS J codes, the materials need to be coded in addition to the code for the injection or infusion codes. Remember that one cc is equal to one mL since the description of the dosage by the physician may differ from the description of the dosage in the HCPCS book. If a brand name is used and this cannot be located in the HCPCS book, then a reference book may help in finding the generic name of the drug.

Prolonged services codes cannot be coded additionally to these codes.

CHEMOTHERAPY: Chemotherapy administrative codes are differentiated by time, administration method, and type of technique. Each technique should be coded. This includes subcutaneous or IM (96401-96402), intralesional (96405-96406), IV or push (96409-96411). IV infusion of a chemotherapeutic agent is coded as 96413-96417 and is differentiated by time. Intra-arterial (which also includes regional/isolation chemotherapy) is coded as 96420-96425 and is based on time. Other types of administration and chemotherapeutic services are coded as 96440-96549. This includes refilling and maintenance of the pumps used to administer the chemotherapeutic agent.

Preparation of the chemotherapeutic material is included in these codes and not coded separately. However, using the J codes from the HCPCS book, the chemotherapeutic material should be coded in addition to the chemotherapy codes.

Surgical procedures to insert or remove catheters, pumps or reservoirs used to administer the chemotherapeutic material should be coded separately with the proper surgical codes.

If other drugs are administered before or after chemotherapy, this administration and material can be coded additionally.

Section 38.16: PHOTODYNAMIC THERAPY

Photodynamic therapy (96567-96571) is used to destroy premalignant or malignant lesions on the skin and adjacent mucosa by the application of light and is based on time.

Section 38.17: DERMATOLOGY

Various types of dermatological procedures include actinotherapy (96900), microscopic examination of hairs (96902), whole body photography (96904), photochemotherapy (96910-96913), and laser treatment for disease (96920-96922) based on area to be treated in square centimeters. Photochemotherapy is the administration of oral medication followed by skin treatment with UV light, such as PUVA. Actinotherapy is the treatment of disease (especially cancer) by exposure to a radioactive substance

Section 38.18: PHYSICAL MEDICINE/REHABILITATION

Various codes are included in this section including physical or occupational therapy and athletic training (97001-97006). Other codes include the following categories which are defined by modality, procedure and time:

MODALITIES: Modality is "any physical agent applied to produce therapeutic changes to biological tissue" and includes modalities that are thermal, acoustic, light, mechanical, or electric energy (CPT code book). A modality can be coded as either with constant attendance which requires face-to-face contact with patient or supervised which does not require face-to-face contact with the patient. Various modalities include hot or cold packs (97010), traction (97012), electrical stimulation (97014), whirlpool (97022), diathermy (97024), or UV light (97028). Notice the use of the semicolon in describing these codes – this means that if several modalities are used, then each one must be coded as the codes only include the one type of modality.

THERAPEUTIC PROCEDURES: Therapeutic procedures (97110-97546) are used to effect positive changes through the application of clinical skill to the body. Only direct (face-to-face) contact is allowable with these codes. These codes are differentiated on time, type of procedure, and number of areas treated. These codes include aquatic therapy (97113) and massage (97124).

WOUND CARE: Wound care codes (97597-97610) are used to remove devitalized or necrotic tissue and does require direct (face-to-face) contact with the patient. These codes are differentiated by number of sessions, and area in square centimeters.

TESTS & MEASUREMENTS: These codes (97750-97755) are used to test progress of physical therapy and treatments.

ORTHOTIC/PROSTHETIC MANAGEMENT: These codes (97760-97762) are used to code for training and management services for patients with orthotics or prosthetics so they can learn to use it properly and fully and is based on time.

Section 38.19: NUTRITIONAL THERAPY

Medical nutrition therapy codes (97802-97804) are based on time and include assessments and interventions, either individually or as a group.

Section 38.20: ACUPUNCTURE

Acupuncture is a procedure in which specific body areas are pierced with needles to achieve pain relief or for other therapeutic purposes. Acupuncture codes (97810-97814) are based on the number of needles used, time, and the use of electrical stimulation.

Section 38.21: OSTEOPATHIC

Osteopathic treatments are a "form of manual treatments applied by a physician to eliminate or alleviate somatic dysfunction and related disorders" through a variety of techniques (CPT code book) based on the musculoskeletal system. Osteopathic manipulative treatment (OMT) is coded as 98925-98929 and is based on the number of body regions receiving treatment. Body regions are defined as head, cervical, thoracic, lumbar, sacral, pelvic, lower extremities, upper extremities, rib cage, abdomen and viscera as described in the CPT code book.

Section 38.22: CHIROPRACTIC

Chiropractic treatments are a "form of manual treatments to influence joint and neurophysiological function" through a variety of techniques (CPT code book) which is based on the assumption that disorders and diseases result from the abnormal functioning of the nervous system with treatment consisting of manipulation of the spinal column and other parts of the body. Chiropractic manipulative treatment (CMT) is coded as 98940-98943 based on the five spinal regions (cervical, thoracic, lumbar, sacral, and pelvic or extraspinal (head, lower extremities, upper extremities, rib cage, and abdomen.

Section 38.23: PATIENT SELF-MANAGEMENT

The services included in these codes (98960-98962) are for training and patient self-management which are prescribed by a physician but can be provided by a non-physician according to specific standards and are differentiated by time and number of patients.

Section 38.24: NON-FACE-TO-FACE NONPHYSICIAN SERVICES

Non-face-to-face nonphysician services (98966-98968) are for telephonic assessment and management and are differentiated by time and online medical evaluations (98969). Oftentimes these services are considered part of a more significant procedure and are, therefore, not reimbursable.

Section 38.25: SPECIAL SERVICES, PROCEDURES & REPORTS

Special services, procedures, and reports include a variety of codes.

Codes 99000-99002 are used to report the preparation and handling of a lab specimens, so if a physician obtains a sample to be sent to an outside lab, he can charge for that in addition to this code. For example, the physician performs a venipuncture to obtain blood for laboratory examination. He can code for the venipuncture and 99000 for the preparation and handling of the blood specimen so that it can be sent to the lab. The physician cannot charge for the laboratory tests though.

Code 99024 is for a postoperative office visit for a condition for which services were provided and it is still within the global postoperative period for the services, e.g., a patient is seen for follow-up exam a week after treatment for a fractured tibia. This code can be listed but there is no payment for it because it is part of the global postoperative care of the patient.

Codes 99026-99027 are for physician time when they are on-call for a hospital and is based on time; however, payers pay per services provided and so these codes may not be billable to payers.

Codes 99050-99060 are for services provided in the office at times other than regularly scheduled office hours or under not normal circumstances; however, most payers will not pay this and it is considered to be part of doing business for a physician.

Code 99070 is for materials and supplies provided during the provision of a service and which are not included as part of the global packaging for the service e.g, a surgical tray is considered part of a surgery. However, it is usually better to use HCPCS codes so that materials and supplies are charged per item because this 99070 pays a one-time fee and does not compensate for the cost of each item.

Code 99071 is used for the provision of educational materials to the patient. The provision of educational information by the physician in a group setting is coded as 99078.

Code 99075 is for medical testimony performed by the physician.

The preparation of special reports is coded as 99080 but usually this is not reimbursable but considered a part of other services.

Section 38.26: QUALIFYING CIRCUMSTANCES FOR ANESTHESIA

These codes were already discussed in the Anesthesia section. For review, they are codes 99100-99140 for circumstances that may affect the outcome of anesthesia services, such as age, hypothermia, hypotension, and emergency condition.

Section 38.27: MODERATE (CONSCIOUS) SEDATION

Moderate (conscious) sedation codes (99143-99150) are differentiated by time, physician performing the service, and patient's age. Time begins when the sedation agent is administered and is completed at the end of the recovery.

When moderate (conscious) sedation is used with certain procedures by the same physician performing the procedure, it cannot be coded as it is included in the codes which is typical. These procedures are marked in the Surgery section with a hollow circle with a small black circle in the middle of the hollow circle and are also listed in Appendix G. If, however, a different physician performs the conscious sedation, then the physician providing the conscious sedation can bill for his services which is in addition to the surgeon billing for his procedure. However, this is not typical in which another physician performs the conscious sedation, as described by the terms in the CPT book that this should be unusual.

The following services are included in the code for moderate (conscious) sedation and so cannot be billed separately: assessment of patient, IV access and fluids, administration of agent, maintenance of sedation, monitoring of oxygen levels, and recovery (CPT code book).

Section 38.28: OTHER SERVICES

Other services include visual tests (99170-99174), administration of ipecac for poisoning (99175), provision of hyperbaric oxygen therapy (99183), operation of oxygenator pump (99190-99192), and phlebotomy (99195). Usually phlebotomy is part of a more significant procedure.

Section 38.29: HOME HEALTH

Home health services (99500-99600) are used by non-physician healthcare providers as physicians use codes 99341-99350 for home visits. Reasons for home visits include prenatal care, newborn care, respiratory care, stoma care, injections, maintenance of catheters, hemodialysis, and activities of daily living.

Section 38.30: MEDICATION THERAPY

Medication therapy (99605-99607) are used to code for services, such as assessment and intervention, provide by a pharmacist and is based on time.

MEDICINE QUIZ 27

1) What are the codes for a patient who had training for the use of a TENS unit?

2) What are the codes for a 52-year-old patient with ESRD who had monthly dialysis services with only 13 days of services this past month?

3) What are the codes for a 43-year-old patient with complaints of severe abdominal pain who has an IVP with KUB study for possible kidney stones?

4) What are the codes for a 3-year-old patient who is seen today for her well-check and received oral polio and DTP whole cell IM with flu vaccine which were administered by the nurse?

5) What are the codes for a 27-year-old patient who is hospitalized at this time for depression and suicide watch who was counseled by the psychiatrist concerning proper use of her prescriptions?

6) What are the codes for a 22-year-old patient who is seen today in the office for yellow fever vaccine before leaving the country?

7) What are the codes for a 23-year-old OCD patient whose parents had a therapy session with her psychiatrist?

8) What are the codes for a 51-year-old patient who suffers from SSS and whose dual lead pacemaker is evaluated and programmed after implantation?

9) What are the codes for a 49-year-old patient who had a TEE for possible dysrhythmia due to fatigue and difficulty breathing?

10) What are the codes for 48-year-old patient who had a lymphangiography of both legs due to restless leg syndrome?

11) What are the codes for 62-year-old patient who had an audiological screening of both ears due to tinnitus?

12) What are the codes for a 32-year-old patient who receives 45 minutes of electrical stimulation and acupuncture to help relieve chronic neck and back pain?

13) What are the codes for a 34-year-old patient who was treated today for sepsis due to MRSA with an antibiotic injection of Avelox?

14) What are the codes for a 73-year-old diabetic patient with a history of COPD and emphysema who was admitted to the hospital due to her diabetes Type I being uncontrolled at this time resulting in a diabetic coma? She was placed on a ventilator at this time and spirometry and testing of thoracic gas volume.

15) What are the codes for a 17-year-old patient who purposely overdosed on Xanax and Lithium and was treated in the ER with gastric intubation, aspiration, and lavage with history and exam being EPF?

16) What are the codes for a 48-year-old patient who is seen today for IM nonhormonal chemotherapy with Xolair due to small cell carcinoma of the left lung?

17) What are the codes for a 15-year-old patient who had three scratch allergy tests of which two are extracts and the other is drug which were negative?

18) What are the codes for a 29-year-old patient of a sleep study with attendant which was staged with ventilation, respiratory effort, EEG, ECG and oxygen saturation for sleep apnea?

19) What are the codes for a 59-year-old patient seen today for electrical stimulation and hot packs due to rotator cuff syndrome?

TEST 3
ICD-10 AND CPT CHAPTERS 1 - 38

1. What are the seven components used to determine the E/M levels?

2. What are the codes for a patient who is admitted to the hospital at 11 pm for a gunshot wound but leaves AMA at 12:30 am with a Detailed History, EPF exam, and moderate MDM?

3. What are the codes for a 51-year-old patient who suffers from SSS and whose dual lead pacemaker is evaluated and programmed after implantation?

4. What are the codes for a 49-year-old patient who had a TEE for possible dysrhythmia due to fatigue and difficulty breathing?

5. What are the codes for a computerized ophthalmic diagnostic imaging of the posterior segment that is computerized for both eyes which includes professional services?

6. What are the codes for a patient who is required by the insurance company for a consultation for a work-related injury when the patient fell from the roof and injured his back with a comprehensive History and Exam and Moderate MDM?

7. If a report states that the patient is a smoker and his father died of lung cancer from smoking, what level of PFSH is this?

8. What are the correct codes for a patient who had an electromyography of two extremities in the paraspinal areas for paresis?

9. What type of HPI would the following be: The patient presents with complaints of chest pain with possible MI. The patient states that it began last night after eating and has not lessened over the night.

10. What level of exam would the following be: The patient is a well-developed well-nourished white male whose GI and GU are negative. He has COPD but otherwise his respiratory is negative. He does present with complaints of chest pains today but otherwise his S1, S2 are normal. PEERLA and head is normocephalic. EOMs are intact. Neck is supple. Skin does present with some lesions which should be checked in the future.

11. What are the codes for a patient seen for COPD and chronic bronchitis who is new to this doctor and the history was EPF, Exam was PF and MDM was SF?

12. What are the codes for a patient who was admitted to the hospital at 9 pm due to various trauma from a car accident with numerous facial lacerations as well as a possible concussion when they hit the windshield with the patient having lost consciousness in the

ambulance? Patient was intoxicated so it was difficult to get a history and the exam was detailed. The patient then left AMA at 11:30 pm.

13. What are the codes for a physician who was on standby for 45 minutes to assist with a C-section at which time he did assist for a successful C-section of a single liveborn male?

14. What are the codes for a patient who is seen today for a second opinion consultation regarding possible renal cancer which was diagnosed by his PCP a week ago due to complaints of suspicious renal mass with an EPF history and exam and moderate complexity MDM?

15. What are the key components for determining a history portion of the office visit?

16. What are the codes for an established 78-year-old patient seen today for a well check and follow-up for her emphysema and diabetes Type I?

17. What are the codes for a patient who was seen today by his regular PCP for fracture follow-up care of his left tibia a week ago when he was out of town visiting his ex-wife which was repaired with ORIF?

18. What level of Exam would the following report constitute: General: Patient is well-developed, well-nourished. HEENT is normal with PERRLA. Respiratory, GI and GU are negative. Cardiovascular and skin are positive.

19. What is the code for a new patient whose visit consisted of a PF history, Detailed Exam and moderate MDM?

20. What are the codes for a new patient who is having difficulty breathing and is seen today in the office? The patient's father had a history of asthma as does the patient. The patient does have COPD. The patient states that the breathing became more difficult after a long afternoon of playing basketball but has not been alleviated by his asthma medication and has only become more difficult overnight. The ROS is negative except for the history of breathing problems. During the exam, the patient's condition worsened and he was admitted to the hospital by the physician with the exam finding that GU, GI, skin, and HEENT normal. The patient does have hypertension which is treated with medication. Extremities move well with no edema. Cranial nerves are intact.

21. What are the codes for a patient who received IV infusion of non-chemotherapeutic drugs for 3 hours for septicemia?

22. What is the code for a patient who is an established patient whose visit consisted of a PF History, EPF exam and SF MDM?

23. What are the codes for a 3-year-old child who is seen in the emergency room after hitting their head on the fireplace that required sutures with PF History and EPF exam with SF MDM?

24. What are the codes for a patient well known to this doctor who is seen today for a check of his diabetes Type I who cut his toe a week ago and which is now infected with a PF history, EPF exam, and moderate MDM and who had removal of a 1.5-cm lesion from her right hand? The patient was also examined for a suspicious neoplasm on his back which was removed and specimen sent to path.

25. What is a DMERC?

26. If a patient is given 500 mcg of filgrastim by injection, what are the codes for this?

27. What HCPCS codes are used for outpatient prospective payment system?

28. If a patient in the hospital after a procedure is given IV pain medication, what type of codes will the physician use to charge for this?

29. What does HCPCS mean?

30. If a wheelchair is being charged for a second month rental, how should this coded?

31. What is the first level of HCPCS?

32. What HCPCS codes are used for ambulance services?

33. If a patient has repair of three wounds, what HCPCS modifier would be attached?

34. If a patient is admitted to the hospital and given 1500 cc of D5W to treat dehydration, how would this be coded?

35. If the patient is given medication by IV and IM, will the same HCPCS code be used? Why or why not?

36. When assigning HCPCS modifiers to fingers and toes, where does the counting begin?

37. What are the anesthesia codes for a patient who had a lobectomy of the right lung due to small cell carcinoma which metastasized to the kidney and who was admitted to the hospital with severe difficulty breathing which was also complicated by pneumoniae pneumonia?

38. What physical status modifier would be applicable to a patient who is hospitalized for septicemia with shock?

39. What are the anesthesia codes for a patient who has an esophagectomy performed due to esophageal cancer that has metastasized to the liver and brain?

40. What are the anesthesia codes for removal of an infected dental molar from a 3-year-old which required general anesthesia?

41. What are the anesthesia codes for a 1-year-old child who had tubes placed in her ears for suppurative otitis media?

42. What are the codes for a 48-year-old patient who had a computed axial tomography of T1-T3 with contrast material for severe back pain and difficulty breathing?

43. What are the codes for a 26-year-old patient who has gastroparesis and had a study for gastric emptying of the stomach?

44. What are the codes for a 66-year-old patient with ASHD who had angiography with noncardiac vascular flow imaging with cardiac stress test with treadmill with continuous monitoring and supervision by physician of the internal mammary artery?

45. What contrast materials are not coded as separate from the test?

46. What are the codes for a 45-year-old patient who had imaging for carcinoma of the thyroid with urinary recovery which was found to be positive?

47. What are the codes for a 67-year-old patient who has tests for carbon dioxide, potassium, bilirubin, chloride, sodium, and glucose for a well check?

48. What are the codes for a patient who had training for the use of a TENS unit?

49. What are the codes for a 52-year-old patient with ESRD who had monthly dialysis services with only 13 days of services this past month?

50. What are the codes for a 43-year-old patient with complaints of severe abdominal pain who has an IVP with KUB study for possible kidney stones?

51. What are the codes for a 3-year-old patient who is seen today for her well-check and received oral polio and DTP whole cell IM with flu vaccine which were administered by the nurse?

52. What are the codes for a 27-year-old patient seen in ICU by his PCP after having emergency CABG by a cardiologist due to ASHD? The patient is seen by the PCP from 10:30 am to 11:15 am and then from 1:40 pm to 2:20 pm and pulse oximetry is provided

53. What are the codes for 62-year-old patient who had an audiological screening of both ears due to tinnitus?

54. What are the codes for a 2-year-old who is seen today for a well check as part of continuing pediatric care with the office?

55. What are the codes for a patient who was seen today for ORIF of his compound fracture of his right humerus in the emergency room. After this procedure, the patient is driving back to his hometown five hours away and won't be seen again by this physician?

56. What are the codes for a patient who is seen for the first time today as a referral from his PCP for possible anemia due to extreme fatigue with the history being PF, exam EPF and moderate MDM?

57. What are the codes for a 32-year-old patient who receives 45 minutes of electrical stimulation and acupuncture to help relieve chronic neck and back pain?

58. What are the codes for a 34-year-old patient who was treated today for sepsis due to MRSA with an antibiotic injection of Avelox?

59. What are the codes for a 15-year-old patient who had three scratch allergy tests of which two are extracts and the other is drug which were negative?

60. Define which of the following scenarios are unit/floor time, face-to-face or neither:
   a. Discussion with nurses on the patient's floor about schedules for staff.
   b. Phone call to patient's parents from doctor's office.
   c. Family consultation at nurse' station on patient's unit.
   d. Review of patient's chart at nurse's station.
   e. Review of research at doctor's office relative to patient's care.

CHAPTER 39
SURGERY INTEGUMENTARY

You will learn the following objectives in this chapter:

A. Integumentary
   1. Surgical Package (Global)
   2. Separate Procedures
   3. Laparoscopic Procedures
   4. Notes
   5. Add-On Codes
   6. Moderate Sedation
   7. Introduction and Removal
B. Incision and Drainage
C. Excision
D. Debridement
E. Dermabrasions
F. Biopsy
G. Lesions
H. Wound Repair
   1. Simple
   2. Intermediate
   3. Complex
I. Graft
   1. Flap
   2. Free Graft
   3. Adjacent Graft
   4. Pinch Graft
J. Destruction
K. Biopsies
   1. Incisional
   2. Excisional
   3. Core Needle
   4. Fine Needle Aspiration
   5. Wire Localization
B. Pressure Ulcers
C. Burn Treatment
D. Destruction
E. Mohs Surgery
F. Breast
G. HCPCS

Section 39.1: SURGICAL PROCEDURES

As previously discussed in other chapters, a surgical package is a concept in which all related services to a major procedure are included in the one code for the major procedure. There is a designated time frame for these services, which can vary from days to months depending on the major procedure which is known as the global period. During this global period services included in the surgical package cannot be billed since they were already reimbursed for in the payment for the major procedure or service.

The surgical package includes

a) All minor related procedures as well.
b) Local infiltration, metacarpal/metatarsal/digital block or topical anesthesia
c) Subsequent to the decision for surgery, one related E/M encounter on the date immediately prior to or on the date of the procedure (history and physical)
d) Immediate postoperative care, including dictation, post operative notes, talking with the family and other physicians
e) Writing orders
f) Evaluating the patient in the post anesthesia recovery area
g) Typical postoperative care
h) Supplies and materials

The above mentioned services cannot be coded separately, i.e. in addition, to the primary procedure. If they are coded separately, this is known as unbundling and can be considered fraud.

Pre and post-op E/M visits are included in the surgical package as mentioned. Although not necessary, code 99024 can be used to designate when the patient comes in for a post-operative visit during a global period. Although there is no reimbursement for this code, it does provide the means to enter a code into the patient's record to indicate a visit did occur, but it is not necessary to do so.

However, any services or procedures that may be provided during this time period that are not usual and/or require treatment greater than what is typically provided or planned can be coded in addition to the surgical package but must be justified as medically necessary by the linkage of the ICD-10 codes to the CPT/HCPCS services or procedures.

SEPARATE PROCEDURES: Services or procedures that are considered to be integral, in other words a part, to another major procedure or service and should not be coded in addition to the code for the major procedure or service. These codes are designated by a statement "separate procedure" following the code. When coding, if a procedure or service is described as separate and is being coded with a major procedure, this should warn you that this service or procedure is probably considered part of the major procedure and should, therefore, not be coded separately, i.e. in addition to the code for the major procedure or service. However, if the separate procedure is performed without a major procedure or service or is not related to another procedure or service, then it can be coded separately.

LAPAROSCOPIC PROCEDURES: In all of the surgery sections there are separate codes for laparoscopic procedures and open procedures, i.e. laparoscopic procedures involve the use of a scope to perform the procedure whereas an open procedure involves opening (tomy) up the body. There are two primary types of surgeries and they are coded differently – open and with a scope. Some procedures may start out as scopic procedure but then have to be changed to an open procedure due to complications. Remember there are V codes (V64.41-V64.43) indicating that a scopic procedure was changed to open and this should be linked to this procedure to indicate the change.

There are two things must be remembered when coding surgeries with regards to the use of scopes: (1) if a procedure is initially begun as a scopic procedure but is changed to an open procedure, then only the open procedure can be coded and charged; (2) It must be remembered with these codes that if a scope is used to perform a diagnostic procedure it can be coded separately if it is not combined with any other procedure or use of scope; however, if the use of the diagnostic scope turns into a surgical procedure performed with the scope, then the diagnostic code is not coded, only the surgical procedure with the scope.

NOTES: Notes are listed at the beginning of each section and subsection of the CPT book. They are critical to read and understand. There are also notes listed in various other places through the CPT book and they are equally important to read and understand. Much of the questions on the national exams are based on these notes. There are also notes included within codes, which again are equally as important.

ADD-ON CODES: There are add-on codes which are services or procedures that are not included in the surgical package or are additional units and, therefore, can be coded in addition to the code for the major procedure or service. These codes are designated by a plus sign and there is a note within the description of the code that explains the use of this code as an additional code and what types of codes it can be coded in addition to. For example, composite grafts (35681-35683) can be coded in addition to the major procedure.

MODERATE SEDATION: In the anesthesia and medicine packet we discussed types of anesthesia including moderate (conscious sedation) so please review that packet. Moderates sedation is now billed with its own codes, 99151 to 99157 in addition to the procedure. They are billed by time and age of patient as well as if it is the same physician or a different physician. There is no longer a separate appendix for them and some codes are not excluded anymore from charging for conscious sedation.

Section 39.2: INTEGUMENTARY

The integumentary system includes the skin (dermis and epidermis), subcutaneous and areolar tissues, hair follicles, glands, nails and breasts. These procedures are classified by anatomic site and procedures. These include I&Ds, excision of lesions, burn treatment, wound repair, grafts and flaps.

It is important to remember when coding that diseases and conditions can occur in various aspects of one site, such as abdominal may be referring to the skin, organs, tissues, muscles, tendons, nerves, vessels, etc. in that area. Also, not all procedures related to integumentary conditions and diseases will be included in this section of the CPT codes but may be found in other sections, such as genitalia since it must be remembered that the codes in this section refer to the integumentary system.

Section 39.3: INTRODUCTION AND REMOVAL

Codes 10030-10036 are for introduction and removal of image guidance including localization devices such as clips, needles or seeds to help ensure procedures are performed exactly where they need to be, such as removal of lesions.

Section 39.3: INCISION AND DRAINAGE (I&D)

Incision and drainage (I&D) is the making of an incision in the skin which allows the drainage of fluids, such as pus, to drain through the incision.

I&D codes (10040-10180) are only used when no other service or procedure is provided because typically I&D are included in more significant procedures and are, therefore, usually not coded unless they are the only procedure performed. These codes are distinguished by what is being treated and if the procedure is simple or complicated. The physician needs to define the procedure as complicated and if there is any question about the classification then the physician should be queried. Examples of I&Ds that are complicated include infection, delayed treatment, and patient condition.

I&D codes include drainage accomplished by puncturing and aspiration (10160). I&D of a postoperative wound which has become infected is also coded in this subsection (10180).

Removal of a foreign body from the integumentary system is coded in this subsection as 10120 but not if the removal requires deep penetration.

Section 39.4: EXCISION-DEBRIDEMENT

Excision is the removal of part of the body by cutting, also known as a resection. Debridement is the removal of dead, damaged, or infected tissue.

Excision and debridement codes (11000-11047) are used for debridement of the skin, subcutaneous tissues, muscle, and bone. Usually debridement is included in a more significant procedure and would, therefore, not be coded separately. However, if the debridement is more extensive than would typically occur, then it can be coded additionally. There are several ways, however, to code debridement in addition to a more significant procedure, so be sure to read the notes in the CPT book (although these circumstances will be discussed in this packet in this and other sections).

Debridement codes are differentiated by area of body and type of material being removed. For example, codes 11000-11001 are to be used for debridement of eczematous or infected skin and are determined by percentage of the body surface. Note that code 11001 is an add-on code which must be used as a secondary code to code 11000. Code 11000 is for the first 10% of the body and the add-on is for the additional body surface based on 10% increments. Remember, that if only partial percentages are described, then code 11001 must be listed in sufficient quantities to include all body surfaces. For example, if there was excision and debridement of 32% of body surfaces, then the proper codes would be 11000 and 11001 x 3 because 11000 was for the first 10% but that leaves an additional 22% to be coded with 11001. Listing code 11001 once will include the first 10% of the extra 22%, but that still leaves 12%, so a second listing of 11001 is necessary to code for the next 10%, but this still leaves 2%, so a third listing of the 11001 code is necessary, or it can be listed as 11000 and 11001 x 3.

These excision/debridement codes are not used for burns (16000) or nails (11720-11721). Dermabrasions are also not coded from this subsection but are coded as 15780-15783. Dermabrasion is the removal of the surface of the epidermis of the skin by abrasion, e.g. sanding.

Section 39.5: REMOVALS

There are many different means for removal that are described throughout the various sections of the CPT coding book. In the integumentary section, the series of codes 11055-11057 is for paring or cutting of benign lesions, such as corns, which is simply the cutting away of the lesion.

Code 11200 is for removal of skin tags (benign lesions) by any sharp method which includes ligature, strangulation, and electrosurgical. There is also an add-on code that accompanies code 11200 which is 11201. The first code, 11200, is for "up to and including" the first 15 lesions, which means if 1 tag is removed, then the code 11200 is listed; if 10 are removed then code 11200 is listed, but only once because the codes says it is for up to the first 15 lesions. If more than 15 lesions are removed, then the add-on code, 11201, would be listed. Notice, however, that the description of this code is for "each additional" lesion; therefore, this code would be listed for the removal of each lesion greater than 15. Therefore, code 11200 can never be listed more than once and code 11201 could be listed as many times as there are more lesions than 15. For example, if 18 tags are removed, then it would be coded as 11200 and 11201x3.

Be especially careful when coding that you read the notes in the CPT book and pay particular attention to the description of how specimens or units are coded. If a code's description says "each, additional" this means that the code is coded each time for each specimen or unit. If there is no description of how to code for each specimen or unit, then it is assumed that you code once for each specimen or unit.

Section 39.6: BIOPSIES:

There are several types of biopsies: incisional, excisional, core needle, wedge, and fine aspiration needle. A biopsy is the removal of cells or tissues (specimen) which is examined for the presence of disease, usually microscopically. There are two types of biopsies: excision and incisional.

An incisional biopsy (11100-11101) is when only a portion of a specimen or tissue is removed and no other procedure is performed. If other procedures are performed related to the incisional biopsy, then there is a strong probability that the incisional biopsy is part of the global package for the larger procedure and would not be coded separately, e.g. if an excision is performed then the biopsy is part of the excision. An excisional biopsy involves the removal of the complete specimen and, therefore, is a resection or removal (ectomy) and is coded as an excision or resection and not as a biopsy. Fine needle aspiration is when a sample of tissue or fluid is removed by a needle. Fine needle aspiration has its own codes, 10021-10022.

Biopsies are sent to pathology for examination as previously discussed in the Pathology section of the codes. These codes usually include both the technical and S&I (supervision and interpretation) services, which means the pathologist prepares and examines the specimen and then makes interpretations based on the findings. However, sometimes physicians may wish to conduct their own S&I services to ensure proper interpretation of the findings. In this case, modifier 26 needs to be attached to the pathology code and billed for the physician; therefore, in addition to the pathologist billing for his services, the physician will also be billing for his S&I services. The pathologist's code would not include the use of the modifier. However, if the pathology code is for S&I only, then this one pathology code would be used to bill for the physician's S&I services in addition to the biopsy code (as discussed in the prior pathology packet).

Section 39.7: LESIONS

There are several types of lesions and there are several ways to remove them, all which are indicated in the codes.

All lesions are measured by the greatest measurement of the diameter of a defect area plus the narrow margin on both sides. For coding purposes, the physician's measurements when he removes the lesion is used, not the measurements from the pathology report since the lesion may have shrunk by the time it is measured by the pathologist. Each lesion is coded separately and lesions are not added together when determining codes.

Lesions can be removed by shaving which is the "sharp removal by transverse incision or horizontal slicing or by excision. Shaving (11300-11313) includes cauterization, is not full-thickness, and does not require suturing. The codes do state that the codes are for single lesions, so the code would be listed for each lesion that is shaved in centimeters. The shaving codes are differentiated by anatomic site and size.

The behavior of a lesion is either benign (11400-11471) or malignant (11600-11646) which can be determined from the physician's report, if provided, or the pathology report. The pathology report can be used to support behavior because the pathologist is a physician and qualified to make the determination.

Simple single-layer suture repair is included in the CPT code for the excisions and there is no need for repair with shaving. If an excision of a lesion requires layered closure (intermediate repair) or complex repair and not just single layer suturing, then this should also be coded from the intermediate wound repair codes (12031-12057) or complex (13100-13160). If a graft is required to repair the defect area caused by the removal of the lesion, then the graft should be coded separately unless the excision is part of the graft procedure that is with an adjacent graft. This will be discussed later in the grafting section. Also, the size of the excision of the lesion may not be the same as the size of the wound repair because the physician may need to make the defect area larger in order to properly repair it.

Sometimes with excision of malignant lesions, it may be found that the excision was not large enough to remove all of the malignancy and so the physician must perform another excision to remove more of the area surrounding the original excision site. If so, then the second procedure must be coded as a separate procedure because it is larger than the first and modifier 58 should be attached to the second procedural code to indicate that the second procedure was more significant than the first procedure.

Other types of removal of lesions are coded with other CPT codes which will be discussed later.

Section 39.8: NAILS/PILONIDAL CYST

CPT codes with regards to nails include trimming (11719), debridement (11720), avulsions (11730-11732), evacuation of a hematoma (11740), excisions (11750) without an amputation and 11752 with an amputation, biopsies (11755), repair (11760), reconstruction (11762), and wedge excision (11765). Avulsions are a tearing away. A wedge is when a portion is removed.

Be sure to read the notes and descriptions accurately because the units vary by code. For example, code 11719 for trimming is for any number, so this code can only be used once no matter how many nails are trimmed. The code for debridement (11720) is for 1 to 5 nails but if 6 or more nails are debrided, then code 11721 should be used. Notice that 11721 is not an add-on code to be used with 11720 but rather is used by itself and includes 6 or more nails and can only be coded once no matter how many nails are debrided. In contrast, avulsion codes are coded for each separate nail with the first nail being coded with 11730 and any other nail being coded with the add-on code 11732 and multiplied for each extra nail. Notice the reference in the add-on code to “each additional” and remember that whenever the words, each, separate or additional are described then each additional nail is coded with its own code. For example, if there was avulsions of 3 nails, then the codes would be 11730 and 11732 x 2.

It is very important with nail codes that proper diagnostic codes be linked to them because otherwise Medicare will not pay for the service unless it is provided for a patient with a qualifying diagnosis, such as diabetes.

A pilonidal cyst is an abscess or cyst near the buttocks. Codes for pilonidal cysts include simple (11770), extensive (11771), or complicated (11772) excisions which must be described by the physician as such.

Section 38.9: INTRODUCTION

Introductions (11900-11983) in the skin include insertion, replacement, injection, implantation, or removal of lesions, tattoos, filling materials (such as collagen), tissue expanders (but not for breasts which are coded elsewhere), prosthesis, contraception, and drug delivery systems.

Section 39.10: WOUND REPAIRS: Wound repairs are also known as closures and includes the use of sutures, staples, and tissue adhesives. The use of adhesive bandages/strips only is not considered wound repair and is included in the coding of an office visit with an E/M code.

SIMPLE: A simple repair involves closure of one layer of the skin. Local anesthesia and cauterization is included.

INTERMEDIATE: There are two criteria for selecting intermediate repair. First, a wound that requires closure of more than one layer is to be coded as an intermediate repair because the wound extends deeper into the layers of the skin (into the subcutaneous layers) than it does on the simple repair. Second, if excessive debridement is provided for a wound that required simple repair then it would be coded as an intermediate repair.

COMPLEX: Complex repair is for repair of wounds that require more than layered closure such as those requiring extensive undermining, stents, retention sutures, and scar revisions.

DEBRIDEMENT & DECONTAMINATION: Debridement and decontamination are usually included the codes for repair and are not coded separately. However, if the debridement and decontamination performed are extensive, then these can be coded as additional codes. Notice again, however, that extensive debridement or decontamination of a wound requiring simple repair is coded as an intermediate repair and not as two codes (one for simple repair and one for decontamination and debridement, rather just coded as one code for intermediate repair.)

OTHER INVOLVEMENT: If there is involvement of other parts of the anatomic site, then there are several coding scenarios that may exist.

First, if there is extensive debridement and decontamination of deeper tissues, such as the subcutaneous tissues, muscle, muscle and/or bone, then the codes for these sites are used, i.e. 11010-11012.

Second, simple ligature of blood vessels and simple exploration of blood vessels, nerves, or tendons during a wound repair is included in the code for the repair and should not be coded separately.

Third, if there is wound exploration that is more extensive and requires increasing the size of the wound, extensive debridement, or removal of foreign body, then this should be coded as exploration of the wound (20100-20103).

Fourth, if the involvement of the vessels, nerves, and/or tendons is more extensive and requires its own repair, then this is what should be coded from the appropriate surgical section, i.e. the nervous system for repair of the nerves, the vascular section for repair of the vessels, and musculoskeletal for repair or tendons. The wound repair is included in these other codes for repair of the vessels, nerves, or tendons and so it should not be coded separately. These codes will be discussed later in those sections.

SELECTION OF CODES: Repair codes are differentiated by anatomic site, type of repair, and size of repair. Wound repair within code groups are added together to determine the correct code. Code groups would be 12001 and 12011 for simple repairs, 12031, 12041, and 12051 for intermediate repairs, and 13100, 13120, 13131, and 13151 for complex. It is helpful in selecting the proper codes to write down the code group and the measurement once you have determined which code group is correct. A code group is based first on the type of repair and secondly on the anatomic site which will be discussed below.

1. The first step is to determine what anatomic site is being repaired. If it is a tendon, vessel or nerve that requires the repair then no wound repair code is listed because it is contained within the repair code for the tendon, vessel, or nerve.
2. The second step is to determine the code group for type of repair, i.e., simple, intermediate, or complex.
3. The third step is to determine if there is extensive debridement or decontamination. Remember, if it is then simple repairs are upgraded to intermediate repair for coding purposes. With intermediate and complex, extensive debridement or contamination would be coded as a separate code in addition to the wound repair code.
4. The fourth step is to select the code group for the anatomic site that is involved. Notice that the codes vary in which anatomic sites are included in the codes. Note that the anatomic sites contained with a level of wound repair is not the same as the anatomic sites contained in other levels of wound repair, so read them carefully.
5. The fifth step is that since you now know which code group the wound repair is in, the length of the repair should be written under the code group. Notice that the codes differ by how the length is coded with some codes specifically listing each group of sizes (simple and intermediate) whereas the complex codes provide a first code for size, then add-on codes per additional specified additional amounts which would be coded then as the first code and then the add-on code with a multiplier for each additional amounts. For example, if the wound repair was a total of 15.5 cm for codes within the 13101 group, then it would be coded as 13101 and 13102 x 2 because the first code (13101) covers the first 7.5 cm, the second code (13102) covers the next 5 cm, but there is still leaves 3 cm so an additional 13102 is needed to provide code coverage for the entire lengths. Notice that the second use of 13102 is only for 3 cm but the code can cover up to an additional 5 cm, but we do not need to have the full 5 cm to list the code a second time.
6. The sixth step is to continue selection of proper repair code for any other wounds by repeating steps described above.
7. The seventh step is to add the lengths of the wounds within each code group. This will determine which code within the code group is the proper code.

While the repair of various anatomic sites will each be coded per their coding group, the most serious injury should always be listed first, which is true of any procedure.

Section 39.11: GRAFTS/FLAPS

Grafting is the transplantation of skin or other tissues to another part of the body to act as a replacement. A flap is a type of graft in which tissue is moved from one area of the body to another either through a free graft or adjacent graft. A free graft is the transplantation of tissue with complete removal of the tissue from the donor site and movement to the recipient site. Adjacent graft is the transplantation of tissue in which a portion of the tissue remains attached and is not completely severed but rather rotated to cover the defect area. A pinch graft is when a piece of skin is elevated and the skin cut to provide a graft.

Split-thickness graft (STSG) includes the epidermis and part of the dermis and is also known as partial thickness. Full-thickness graft (FTSG) includes all layers of the epidermis and all of the dermis which includes collagen, elastic fibers, and extrafibrillar matrix.

Autograft is a graft that comes from the person themselves and also known as an autologous graft. Allograft is a graft that comes from a donor of the same species, but not from the person themselves. Xenograft is a graft that comes from something other than the same species. This includes pigskin and Gortex. Acellular grafts are composed of cadaver skin that is chemically treated. Tissue-cultured graft is created when the patient's skin is used to grow more skin in a laboratory.

The site where the graft is taken from is known as the donor site. The site where the graft is transferred to is known as the recipient site. Graft codes are selected based on the size of the recipient site in addition to type of graft and material used except for children infants and children younger than age 10 which are measured in percentages.

ADJACENT TISSUE TRANSFERS: Adjacent tissue transfers (14000-14350) are when one side of the graft remains intact which is known as the base. Instead of the graft being cut away completely (as in a free graft) and then transferred to another site, with adjacent grafts only part of the graft is cut away; then the graft is manipulated so that the graft can cover the defect area. Only the graft is coded and not any other procedure to treat the defect, such as excision because the excision is included in the services to create the adjacent graft.

This type of graft is optimal because it allows the graft to retain a source of blood and tissues and so it does not have the problems of failure.

Types of adjacent grafts include Z-plasty, V-Y-plasty, W-plasty, island flap, advancement flap, double pedicle flap, and rotational flaps. These grafts obtain their name from the description of the procedure in which a Z, Y or W cut is used to excise the defect and then manipulate the skin over the defect area. Rotational flaps are usually curved or semicircular. Advancement flaps are the partial release of tissue at one area and the movement of it to another point further away. An island flap consists of skin and subcutaneous tissue as a pedicle that contains only the nutrient vessels. A double pedicle flap has pedicles at each end.

When coding for adjacent grafts, if a defect is being treated at the same time that an adjacent graft is performed to cover the defect area, then only the adjacent graft is coded because the defect is excised with the graft procedure. For example, if a lesion is removed and an adjacent graft is used to cover it, then only the graft is coded because the lesion was removed by the cuts for the grafts, then the tissue was rearranged to cover the defect area.

If incisions that resemble adjacent grafts are used to repair defects from lacerations but the procedure is not truly an adjacent graft, they are not coded as grafts but as wound repair because the appearance of it being a graft is only incidental and does not truly reflect the procedure being performed which would be only a repair.

FREE GRAFTS: In contrast to adjacent grafts, in free grafts (15002-15278) the entire tissue area is removed from the donor site and then transferred to the recipient site. The codes are based on the type of graft and recipient site only, i.e. anatomic site and size of defect area which is the recipient site. Type of graft refers to autograft, allograft, xenograft or other types as previously described in the terminology section.

There are two types of coding scenarios for free grafts. First, a defect occurred sometime before and now presents for grafting, so during this waiting time scar tissue has grown over the defect area. This means that whatever caused the defect in the first place, such as a burn, was treated before the visit for the graft and is not a part of the coding scenario. However, this means that the defect site will need to be prepared since it has scar tissue now. This is known as preparation of the site and is coded by anatomic site and size with codes 15002 to 15005. Notice that there are add-on codes which are to be used in conjunction with the primary code for the initial size and anatomic site. The primary codes are based on 100 sq. cm for adults and percentages for children under the age of 10; therefore, any additional area must be coded with the add-on code with the code being multiplied for each additional 100 sq. cm. For example, if the patient is receiving a 250 cm graft from the back and legs today due to burns suffered six months ago on her chest, the preparation codes would be 15002 and 15003 x 3 because we are coding for the recipient site, the chest. Remember that the code for the 100 sq. cm is still used even if the defect is not 100 sq.cm. Note that the add-on codes describe the use of the code as "each additional 100 sq. cm" which means the code is based on 100 sq. cm increments, even if the last code is only for a portion of the 100 sq. cm. After preparation of the recipient site, then the graft is performed which will be discussed in more details in the specific graft type below.

Second, if a defect is being treated at the same time that a graft (other than an adjacent graft) is performed, then the procedure to treat the defect is coded, such as an excision to remove a lesion and the code for the graft is also coded. There is no need for preparation codes because there was no preparation since the procedure to treat the defect has already provided preparation of the recipient site.

Usually the donor site is treated with simple closure; however, if the donor site also needs extensive repair (e.g. grafting for itself), then this procedure will also need to be coded.

FLAPS: Types of flaps include pedicle (graft which retains it blood supply and is not cut away completely from the defect site but rather is manipulated to cover another part of the body), muscle, myocutaneous (composed of skin and muscle), delayed (flap detached from its donor area in two or more stages), and fasciocutaneous (graft composed of deep muscle fascia with its overlying skin). The recipient site is used to determine the code, but if a tube is formed by attachment at another site of the body for later use, then the donor site is used to determine the code (15570-15738). If there is immobilization, e.g. plaster cast, of the site required, then this can be coded as an additional code because immobilization is not included in the graft code.

OTHER FLAPS AND GRAFTS: Other flaps and grafts (15740-15777) include neurovascular grafts, free muscle flaps, flaps with microvascular anastomosis, graft composites, derma-fat fascia graft, and punch grafts for hair transplants. Other procedures (15780-15879) include dermabrasion, abrasion, chemical peel, cervicoplasty, blepharoplasty, rhytidectomy, excision of excessive skin, grafting for nerve paralysis, removal of sutures, dressing changes, injection of agent to test vascular flow in grafts, and lipectomy.

Section 39.12: PRESSURE ULCERS

Pressure ulcers are also known as decubitus ulcers and develop over time when a portion of the body has been exposed to prolonged pressure. Treatment (15920-15999) consists of excision with possible flap closure or ostectomy which, in addition to anatomic site, is how the codes are differentiated.

Section 39.13: BURN TREATMENT

Burn treatment in this section (16000-16036) refers to local treatment of burns, including application of dressings and cleaning but are not related to any grafting procedures for coding purposes. For the purpose of using these codes, the TBSA (total body surface area) must be known to calculate the percentage of body burned as well as the depth of burn. The Lund and Browder chart (provided in the ICD-10 course) can be used to determine this if the physician does not provide the percentage but does describe the anatomic sites.

Section 39.14: DESTRUCTION

Destruction is differentiated from excisions and biopsies in that the tissue or specimen is destroyed and, therefore, cannot be biopsied. Means of destruction include electrocautery, electrodesiccation, use of chemicals, cryosurgery and laser. Codes 17000-17250 are used to code for means of removing lesions by destructive methods rather than excision which were described earlier. Methods includes electrosurgery, cryosurgery, surgical curettement, laser and chemical. Closure is usually not required but would need to be coded separately if necessary.

These codes vary on the criteria for differentiation. Destruction of premalignant lesions (17000-17004) are based on the number of lesions. Read the CPT notes in this section carefully to be sure you use the right criteria for differentiating the codes.

Destruction of premalignant lesions are based on the first lesion being coded as 17000, but the next 2 to 14 lesions are coded with the use of code 17003 in addition to 17000 for the first lesion. Notice that the notes under code 17003 describe that each lesion can be coded separately, so if a patient has 12 pre-malignant lesions removed, the codes would be 17000 and 17003 x 11.

Destruction of cutaneous vascular proliferative lesions is coded by size in sq. cm with codes 17106 to 17108.

Destruction of benign lesions is coded by number of lesions but differs from the coding criteria for premalignant lesions. With benign lesions, the first 14 lesions are coded as 17110, but they are not coded separately, 17110 includes all of the lesions up to 14. Code 17111 is for destruction of 15 or more lesions, so codes 17110 and 17111 cannot be listed together because either there are 14 or less lesions destroyed or there are 15 or more. In addition, there is no statement that these lesions can be coded separately or each. For example, if a patient has 12 benign lesions destroyed, then just 17110 should be listed.

Destruction of malignant lesions (17260-17286) are differentiated by anatomic site and lesion size, so each lesion is coded separately.

Section 39.15: MOHS SURGERY

Moh's surgery (17311-17315) is a microscopic procedure in which skin cancer is removed in stages with histological exam occurring in between excisions. The purpose of this type of procedure is so that as little tissue may be removed as possible yet to ensure that all of the malignancy has been removed.

The procedure begins with an initial excision of the malignant lesion, which is then examined by the same surgeon who removed it. The purpose of this examination is so the surgeon can be sure if all of the malignancy has been removed. If all of the malignancy has not been removed, then the surgeon returns to excise more with all of this occurring during the same operative session.

In order to code Moh's Surgery, the surgeon must perform both the excision and the tissue examination. If he does not, then only the portion of the procedure that he performed would be coded, i.e. the excision. The excised lesion would then be sent to the pathology department for examination by a pathologist and not by the surgeon, so the pathology department would be coding for the examination. However, there is not the timely provision of findings that is available in Moh's surgery which provides immediate findings and allows the surgeon to continue the procedure at the same visit rather than the patient having to return multiple times to have excisions performed.

These codes are differentiated based on anatomic site, number of stages, and number of tissue blocks. The first code for groups of anatomic sites is for the first stage and there is an add-on code for each additional stage thereafter. Note that the word "each" is used, so each time the surgeon must return to perform excisions is a new stage and each stage is coded. For example, if the surgeon had to return three times before removal of all malignancy on the chest, the codes would be 17313 and 17314 x 2. There is also another add-on code for additional tissue blocks beyond five (the first five tissue blocks are included in the first codes, 17311-17314). Tissue blocks are the divisions of the lesion site into parts which are to be removed and examined.

If additional repair is required to close the defect area (other than simple suturing), then this procedure should also be coded, such as a graft.

If non-routine stains are used, these should be coded additionally (88311-88314, 88342). See notes in the CPT book for Moh's Surgery for further information.

If a prior biopsy was never performed to confirm malignancy but a biopsy is performed during Moh's surgery and sent for confirmation then this biopsy can be coded (11100-11101 or 88331 for frozen) but modifier 59 will need to be attached to the procedural code.

Section 39.16: BREAST

Breast procedures can be performed on both males and females with some differences.

MODIFIERS: All of the procedures are performed as unilateral, so if the procedure is performed on both breasts, then modifier 50 would need to be attached to indicate that the procedure is bilateral. To use modifier 50, the two sides must be mirror images of each other anatomically so 50 can be applied to codes for ears, eyes, and breasts; however, modifier 50 cannot be used with the lungs or heart since the two halves are not the same. Modifiers LT and RT should be used, particularly if only a procedure is performed on only one side.

INCISIONS/PUNCTURES: Punctures (19000-19001) may be performed on breasts to remove fluid which is known as aspiration and is performed for cysts. Incisions (19020) can be used for exploration. Injection procedures for reporting purposes are coded as 19020-19030. If reporting is also performed (supervision and interpretation), then these should be coded additionally.

BIOPSIES: Types of biopsies include:

1. Incisional biopsy is when only a portion of a specimen is removed for pathological examination.
2. Excisional biopsy is when the entire specimen is removed for pathological examination.
3. Core needle biopsy is when a core of a specimen is taken for pathological examination.
4. Fine needle aspiration biopsy is when a needle is used to withdraw fluid or specimen for pathological examination, such as from a cyst.
5. Wire localization biopsy is when a wire is used to mark the location for the biopsy.

Biopsies of breasts without image guidance are coded with 19100-19101. Biopsies of the breast using placement of localization devices such as clips are coded per each lesion (19081-19086). Placement of image-guided devices without biopsies are coded as 19281-19298.

Remember that excisional biopsies (19120) are coded as excisions since the entire specimen is removed, and not a portion of it which are then sent to pathology for examination. If only a portion is removed, this is known as an incisional biopsy (19101) if it is sent to pathology for examination. A core needle biopsy (19100) is when core of tissue is removed. If fine needle aspiration biopsies are performed, then these are coded as 10021-10022, so all fine needle aspiration biopsies are code with these codes which are in another section. Wire localization biopsies in which a wire is used to locate and remove the biopsy are coded as 19125-19126 which are coded as each biopsy with the first code for the first biopsy and all additional biopsies coded with the add-on code. Placement of catheters in the breast for radiotherapy are coded as 19296-19298 depending on when they are placed, either during or after the mastectomy.

MASTECTOMY: Types of mastectomies include:

1. Partial mastectomy is the removal of part of the breast tissue. This includes lumpectomy and segmental mastectomy.
2. Complete simple mastectomy is the removal of the breast tissue but not the muscles and lymph nodes.
3. Subcutaneous mastectomy is the removal of subcutaneous tissue only of the breast with the skin and nipple remaining intact.
4. Radical mastectomy is the removal of the breast tissue, muscle and lymph nodes.
5. Modified radical mastectomy is the removal of breast tissue and the axillary lymph nodes and with or without removal of the pectoralis minor muscle but the pectoralis major muscle is not removed.

Mastectomies are coded based on what portions of the breast and surrounding area is removed as well as some codes reflect the reason the mastectomy was performed. A partial mastectomy is coded as 19300-19302. Simple complete mastectomy is coded as 19303. Subcutaneous mastectomy is coded as 19304. Radical mastectomy is coded as 19305-19306. Modified radical mastectomy is coded as 19307.

Biopsies or removals of lymph nodes can also be coded using codes 38500-38780. Repair and reconstruction of mastectomy sites are coded separately and are discussed below.

REPAIR/RECONSTRUCTION: There are various means of repair and reconstruction for mastectomies. This includes mastopexy (19316) and mammoplasty (19318-19325). Mastopexy is fixation of the breast whereas mammoplasty alters the shape of the breast either with reduction or augmentation with or without implants. These codes also include the removal of implants (19328-19330) or insertion of breast prosthesis (19340-19342). There can also be other reconstruction, such as with the nipple (19350-19355) or with tissue expanders (19357) or using flaps (19361-19364). A TRAM flap (Transverse Rectus Abdominis Myocutaneous) (19367-19369) is a surgical procedure most commonly employed for breast reconstruction.

Section 39.17: HCPCS

Some of the HCPCS used with integumentary and other surgical codes include:

1. A4550: Surgical tray (usually included in the surgical procedure and not coded separately).
2. G0127: Trimming of dystrophic nails, particularly for diabetic patients.
3. G0168: Closure of wound with adhesive only (band-aid type).
4. J7340: Dermal and epidermal tissue for graft (human).
5. J7341: Dermal tissue for graft (nonhuman).

INTEGUMENTARY QUIZ 28

1) In the ICU, after prepping with ChloraPrep, we used some 0.25% Marcaine with epinephrine. The patient is on the ventilator. The lower piercings were used first where a post went through and through. The area was localized with some 1% Xylocaine. The lower left side was removed first. We grasped the ball, screwed off the external cap, and then brought it into the oral cavity and removed the entire post and the inside cap. We then in a like manner, removed the lower cap on the right side, screwing off the external cap and grasping it internally and then reducing it through the internal cavity. Then the patient had 2 areas of the left cheek and the right cheek where there was a diamond-like cap that was attached to a plate that was beneath. I had to make a small incision and first the left side was done. It was anesthetized, ChloraPrep was used and we grasped it. Made a small incision with #11 blade, removed the plate that was holding it beneath, and the incision was small enough that it did not need a suture on the left side. On the right side, a like procedure was carried out. There was a small incision made. It was large enough that we removed the plate. We had to use a 4-0 nylon suture. This controlled the bleeding. He tolerated all this well and the procedure was ended.

2) What are the codes for an 8-year-old patient who had suffered second and third degrees burns over both fronts of her legs four months ago which totaled 15% of TBSA with 7% third degree? She is seen today for STSG from her back to cover the burned area.

3) What are the codes for a 32-year-old patient who had 17 skin tags removed electrosurgically?

4) What are the codes for a 23-year-old patient who cut her right index finger which was 3 cm while preparing dinner which required 8 stitches in the emergency room? History and exam were problem focused.

5) What are the codes for a 62-year-old diabetic patient who was treated for an infected right toe requiring extensive debridement and wound repair with single layer suturing?

6) What are the codes for a 47-year-old patient who had 3.5 cc of collagen injected into her chin to reduce wrinkles?

7) What are the codes for a 42-year-old patient who presents with an infection from her previous CABG for ASHD and MI two weeks ago? She is found to have MRSA and the site is prepared for drainage with continued monitoring with the patient remaining in the hospital for further observation. History and exam were detailed.

8) What are the codes for a 38-year-old female who had a mastectomy of both breasts which included removal of the axillary lymph nodes due to carcinoma of the breast with a TRAM?

9) What are the codes when a pathologist finds malignancy from a needle core biopsy of the left breast of a 32-year-old woman?

10) What are the codes for an 82-year-old nursing home patient who had excision of a sacral ulcer repaired with suturing and requiring an ostectomy?

11) What are the codes for a 49-year-old patient who was involved in a car accident and suffered extensive lacerations and broken collarbone? The patient had a BAC level of 1.0 as he has suffered for many years with alcoholism and went on a binge today. Lacerations were numerous including a 3.0 cm laceration of the right forearm which required layered closure, a 5.5 cm laceration of the right thigh which required retention sutures and ligation of arteries, 4.8 cm laceration of the chest which required simple closure but extensive debridement due to glass fragments, a 2.8 cm laceration of the right cheek which required layered closure, and a 3.0 cm laceration of the left thigh which required retention sutures.

12) What are the codes for a pathologist when a 2.5 cm malignant lesion of the left arm was destroyed?

13) What are the codes for a 22-year-old patient who had 5 corns removed by paring?

14) What are the codes for a 58-year-old patient who had excision of basal cell carcinoma of the back (2.2 cm) which was repaired with a Z-plasty?

15) The patient was brought to the operative suite, prepped and draped in the usual manner. A time-out was accomplished. Preop antibiotics were given and SCDs applied. The patient morbidly obese. The left chest wall mass, which was about 3.5 cm was removed first. An elliptical incision was made. Bleeding controlled with electrocautery. Mass was removed. Subcutaneous tissue was closed with 3-0 Vicryl. The skin was closed with interrupted 3-0 Prolene. This appeared to be a large inclusion cyst. Right breast mass was then removed. A circumareolar incision made in the outer quadrant. This mass was removed. All bleeding was controlled. The mass will be submitted to pathology for review. Rule out carcinoma. The subcutaneous tissue was closed with 3-0 Vicryl after hemostasis had been accomplished and then skin was closed with interrupted 3-0 Prolene. Following this, we turned his head slightly, removed the right posterior neck mass. An elliptical incision was made. Bleeding controlled with electrocautery. Mass was removed and we closed with some interrupted 3-0 Prolene. Sterile dressing applied to each of these incisions. We used 0.25% Marcaine with epinephrine and each one of them sent to recovery room in satisfactory condition.

16) What are the codes for a 44-year-old patient who is seen today for the first time with a history and exam that were expanded problem focused and who had a 3.2-cm mass of the back which was infected and required drainage which was found to be a sebaceous cyst?

17) What are the codes for a 15-year-old patient who was seen in the emergency room due to complaints of severe abdominal pain and hemoptysis? The patient was found to have Staph food poisoning and discharged with prescriptions. The history was expanded problem focused and the exam was problem focused.

18) What are the codes for a pathologist who performs the pathological review of the two biopsies of specimens from Moh's surgery for a 4.2 cm lesion on the back of a 48-year-old man?

19) What are the codes for a 38-year-old female who had a suspicious lump in her left breast with fine needle aspiration being completed and specimen sent to pathology?

20) What are the codes for a 17-year-old patient who is seen today for repair of burns sustained four months ago when hot water spilled on her? Her body had sustained second and third degree burns over 25% of her body (forearms and chest) with 13% of the burns being third degree. Repair at this time was a 50 sq. cm FTSG taken from her back and placed on the chest area which was 35 sq. cm in size.

CHAPTER 40
MUSCULOSKELETAL

You will learn the following objectives in this chapter:

A. Wound
   a. Open
   b. Closed
B. Incision/Excisions
   a. Excision
   b. Radical Resection
C. Introduction and Removal
   a. Aspiration
   b. Trigger Point Injections
   c. Carpal Tunnel Syndrome
   d. Arthrocentesis
D. Repairs
   1. Dislocations
   2. Fractures
   3. Spine
   4. Joint
E. General
   1. Wound Exploration
   2. Closed and Open Treatment
   3. Incision/Excision
   4. Introduction/Removal
   5. Replantation
   6. Grafts/Implants
   7. Other
   8. Amputation
F. Head
G. Neck/Thorax
H. Back/Flank
I. Spine
J. Abdomen
K. Shoulder
L. Humerus/Elbow
M. Forearm/Wrist
N. Hand/Fingers
O. Pelvis/ Hip Joint
P. Femur/Knee
Q. Leg/Ankle Joint
R. Foot/Toes
S. Casts/Strapping
T. Endoscopy/Arthroscopy

Section 40.1: MUSCULOSKELETAL

The musculoskeletal system includes the bones, tendons, muscles, and soft tissues. Notice that the musculoskeletal section is categorized by anatomic site with certain types of procedures listed in the same order within each anatomic site subheading, e.g. incision, excision, introduction, removal, repair, revision, reconstruction, fractures, dislocations, arthrodesis, and amputation.

INCISIONS/EXCISIONS: Incisions are indicated by the suffix "tomy" and excisions are indicated by the suffix "ectomy". Remember, "ec" means "out", to take out. Incisions are only cuts but excisions involve the removal of tissue. Excisions are also described as resections in the CPT book.

Types of excisions include:

1. Excision of subcutaneous soft tissue tumors involves the resection (excision) of tumors, usually benign, extending into the subcutaneous tissue but not into the deep fascia.
2. Excision of fascial or subfascial soft tissue tumors, usually benign, involves the resection (excision) of tumors extending into the deep tissue including tendons and muscles but not involving bone.
3. Radical resection of soft tissue involves the resection of the tumor, usually malignant, with wide margins and is not simple.
4. Radical resection of bone tumors involves the resection of bone tumors, usually malignant, with wide margins and is not simple. If tissue is also removed, then it is bundled into the code for the resection of the bone tumor.

INTRODUCTION AND REMOVAL: Introduction and removals include introduction as through injections of materials into the body as well as removal of materials such as foreign objects. These codes are limited and do not include all introductions and removals such as for prosthetics.

REPAIRS: Repairs can be primary which is the first repair of an anatomic site or secondary which is a repair after other treatments have been attempted but not successful resulting in a repair.

FRACTURE CARE: Types of fracture care are:

1. Closed treatment means the injury site was not opened for treatment (exposed to the outside) which can be achieved with or without manipulation and with or without out traction.
2. Open treatment means the injury site was open and exposed to the outside as part of the treatment.
3. Percutaneous skeletal fixation is treatment for a fracture that is neither open or closed in which a fixation device, e.g. pins, are placed across the fracture site, usually with x-ray imaging.
4. Manipulation is also known as reduction. It is the attempted reduction or restoration of fracture or dislocation to its original position by the use of force.

5. Skeletal traction is the application of a force to an injury site such as a pin, screw, wire or clamp. Skin traction is the application of the force to the injury site through the skin, e.g. strapping.
6. Fixation is immobilization and stabilization of the injury site usually utilizing some type of hardware, such as pins, rods, plates, or screws. A cast is not a fixation device.
7. External fixation involves the use of pins in addition to a device which holds the pins in place.

To code fractures, the following must be determined: anatomic site, open or closed treatment, is manipulation involved and is there any type of internal or external fixation applied such as pins, screws or plates. ORIF means open reduction internal fixation and is a procedure used to repair a fracture.

Other than fixation devices, application and removal of casts or traction devices are included in the main procedural code for the fracture care, known as a fracture package. However, if a different physician performs the removal they are allowed to code it separately.

JOINT: A joint is where two or more bones come together. There are three types of joints:

1. Synovial Joints: Synovial Joint is also known as diarthrosis. It is the most movable type of joint which occurs where two bones come together.
   a. Capsule: Synovial joints have capsules that surround the space where the bones come together and where movement occurs.
   b. Synovial Fluid: Synovial fluid is contained within the capsule and allows for the smooth movement of the joint.
2. Cartilaginous Joints: Bones are joined by cartilage.
3. Fibrous joint – Bones are joined by fibrous connective tissue.

Section 40.2: WOUND EXPLORATION

Wound exploration codes (20100-20103) are for wounds such as caused by gunshots or stabbing and are determined by anatomic site. These codes include surgical exploration and wound enlargement with dissection if necessary to determine the extent of the damage and presence and removal of any foreign bodies. It also includes minor ligation or coagulation of vessels as well as repair or muscle and muscle fascia.

Similar to integumentary repair codes, if more extensive repair is required of vessels or other structures then the codes for repair of these structures should be used instead with the wound exploration services included in these other codes.

Remember, if there is no wound exploration as described, then the integumentary repair codes should be used.

INCISIONS/EXCISIONS: Biopsies are coded from this section and are differentiated by whether the biopsy is superficial or deep. If needle or trocar bone biopsies are performed, these are coded as 20220-20225. However, if the needle or trocar bone biopsy is of the bone marrow, then 38221 should be used instead which from the hemic and lymphatic codes.

Imaging guidance (77002, 77012, 77021) should be coded separately.

Remember, fine needle aspiration is coded with 10021-10022 and evaluation of the specimen would be coded also as 88172-88173.

INTRODUCTION/REMOVAL: These codes are used for aspiration and injections (20500-20696) in tendons or muscles which may occur at the same time at the same location in which case only one code is necessary because both are included in the codes. This includes trigger point injections into muscles (20552-20553) and carpal tunnel syndrome injections (20526). Trigger Point Injections: Trigger points are particular sites in skeletal muscle or fascia where there is pain which is accompanied usually by twitching and is known to not have originated from a disease process, such as trauma, inflammation, degeneration, neoplasm or infection. These sites can be treated in numerous ways including electrostimulation and pressure; however, injections of substances are usually very successful even when other treatments are not. Types of substances include saline, local anesthetics (Procaine and Novocain), steroids, and botulinum toxin. Carpal Tunnel Syndrome: Carpal tunnel syndrome is when the median nerve is compressed at the wrist which can cause paresthesias, numbness and muscle weakness in the hand. This is corrected by either splinting or carpal tunnel syndrome surgery.

Removal of a foreign body from a muscle or tendon is coded as 20520-20525.

If needles or catheters need to be placed into muscle or soft tissue for radiotherapy treatment of cancer (when radioelements are inserted into the tissue to attack the cancer), then this is coded as 20555. Placement of radioelements in some other tissues may be coded with other codes, such as for breast (19296-19298) and prostate (55875), so be sure to read the notes in the CPT book under these codes (20555).

Arthrocentesis, aspiration, and injection is also coded from this section of the CPT codes (20600-20610) and are based on if they are placed into a small, medium, or major joint or bursa. Aspiration is the removal of fluid. Arthrocentesis is the removal of fluid from a joint with a needle or syringe.

Similarly, aspiration or injection into cysts are coded as 20612. If multiple cysts are treated, then the code must be listed for each one with modifier 59 listed after the additional codes (but not the first one) to indicate that the there was injection of more than one cyst. Aspiration and injection of bone cysts are coded as 20615.

Application and removals of fixation devices (such as pins, wires, or halos) are coded as 20650-20692. Adjustment or revisions of fixation devices are coded as 20693-20697. Notice that code 20650 is described as a separate procedure which means it would be included in the major procedure if performed at the same time. However, the other fixation codes are listed in addition to other procedural codes.

If substances are injected, then J codes from the HCPCS should be used to code for them.

Usually local anesthetics are used prior to the actual injection which should not be coded separately because it is included in the main procedure.

As with any code, supervision and interpretation or radiological guidance should be coded additionally.

REPLANTATION: Replantation is the reattachment of body parts due to complete amputation and codes are distinguished by anatomic sites (20802-20838). If the amputation was not complete, then this is coded as surgical repair codes for any body part involved, such as bone, ligaments, tendons, vessels, and nerves.

GRAFTS/IMPLANTS: These graft codes are for grafts other than skin, such as bone, cartilage, and tendon (20900-20926). Obtaining the graft may or may not be coded in addition to the plantation of the graft if obtaining the graft is not included in the plantation code. For example, code 21127 states that the bone graft is included, so obtaining the graft is not coded separately but is included in 21127. Spinal surgeries are also coded here (20930-20938). Notice though that these are all add-on codes and should be coded in addition to the major procedure, such as 22532 for arthrodesis (fixation of a joint) and discectomy (removal of a disc). If the obtainment of the graft is not included in the repair code, then you need to code this separately so there would be two codes, the repair and obtaining the graft.

OTHER: Bone grafts requiring the use of the microscope to complete anastomosis (connection of two normally separate parts) are coded as 20955-20962. Similarly, microvascular surgery for osteocutaneous flap are coded as 20969-20973. The use of modalities to promote bone healing is coded as 20974-20979, such as electrical stimulation and ultrasound. Ablation (removal of bone) of bone tumors is coded as 20982. If a computer system is used during a procedure then the add-on code 20985 should be listed.

Section 40.3: HEAD

INCISION/EXCISION: Excisions (resections) involve the removal of tumors and are coded by the location and the greatest diameter of the specimen removed which includes a narrow margin. Remember, the size should be derived from the physician's report and not the pathology report, if possible because the size may change. The codes are also differentiated by whether an osteotomy is included and if the resection is radical or not as described earlier in this packet.

If there is extensive exploration of vessels or neuroplasty (surgical repair of a nerve), then this should be coded separately.

Simple and intermediate repair are bundled into the excision code, but a complex repair is not and should be coded separately.

Remember that removal of a foreign body is coded elsewhere (41805-41806).

Resection of a bone tumor is only coded by location and not by size and whether the tumor is benign or malignant.

Notice that meniscectomies (21060) (Surgical removal of the meniscus of the knee) and coronoidectmies (21070) (surgical removal of the mandibular coronoid process) can be coded but are described as separate procedures; therefore, these would not be coded in addition to a major procedure that includes them.

MANIPULATION: There is only one code in this section for therapeutic manipulation for TMJ with anesthesia (21073). Without anesthesia, codes 97140-98943 should be used from the Medicine Section.

PROSTHESIS: These codes (21076-21089) are used when the physician designs and prepares the prosthesis for treatment of oral, facial or other head site involving the use of prostheses. This includes artificial eyes, nose, and ears.

INTRODUCTION/REMOVAL: The introduction (or application) of a fixation device applied to the head is coded from 21100-21110 codes. There is also a code for injection procedures for arthrography (211116).

REPAIR/REVISION/RECONSTRUCTION: Many of these codes which involve reshaping of the face are described as plasties. Genioplasties are included in this section (21120-21123. Genioplasties are reconstruction of the chin. A sliding genioplasty is the removal of a horseshoe-shaped piece of the chin bone and then the sliding it backwards or forwards and once corrected, it is fixed in place with screws.

Augmentation of the mandibular bone is coded as 21125-21127 as distinguished by with or without bone graft so the bone graft does not need to be coded extra.

Surgery to reduce the forehead are coded as 21137-21139 and are distinguished as occurring with or without a bone graft so the bone graft does not need to be coded extra.

Reconstruction of the face are coded as 21141-21235 and are distinguished by specific anatomic site, how many pieces are moved, and if bone grafts are included or not so, again, none of these would be coded extra. Some codes are differentiated by area size. Arthroplasties are also coded from these codes (arthroplasty is surgical repair of a joint) (21240-21243).

Canthopexies are coded as 21280-21282 and are described as separate procedures so they are only coded if done separately and not as part of a larger procedure. Canthopexies involved the tightening of the canthal tendons of the eyes which allow in older age, for the eyelids to sag. Canthoplasty and canthopexy both tighten the lower lid and change their tilt. In canthopexy the lower canthal tendon is tightened but in canthoplasty (67950) the tendon is divided, moved and tightened. There is a greater freedom to move the tendon in canthoplasty.

FRACTURES/DISLOCATIONS: For open (operative) repair of a skull fracture, then use codes 62000-62010 instead of these codes. However, closed treatment of a skull fracture as simply coded as an E/M visit since there is nothing else that is done at that time.

These codes (21310-21497) include anatomic sites, such as nose, jaw bones, cheekbones, forehead, sinuses, and eye orbits.

LeForts refer to fractures and types of repairs to the front of the face.

The lower red line is a LeFort I fracture; the middle blue line is a LeFort II, and the topmost green line is a fracture III (Wikipedia.org).

Section 40.4: NECK/THORAX

INCISION/EXCISION: These codes (21501-21632) include the soft tissues of the neck and down into the thorax and ribs. Notice that code 21502 includes a rib ostectomy (excision of rib bones). Excisions include tumors by size and depth of tissue involved as well as radical resections. There are also excisions of ribs and sternum.

REPAIR/REVISION/RECONSTRUCTION: These codes (21685-21750) include repair of the hyoid, scalenus anticus, sternocleidomastoid, pectus excavatum and sternum.

FRACTURE/DISLOCATIONS: These codes include fracture and/or dislocation repair of the ribs and sternum.

Section 40.5: BACK/FLANK

Excision: The only codes for back and flank (21920-21936) include biopsy of the back or flank and excision or radical resection of tumors by size and depth of tissue involved.

Section 40.6: SPINE

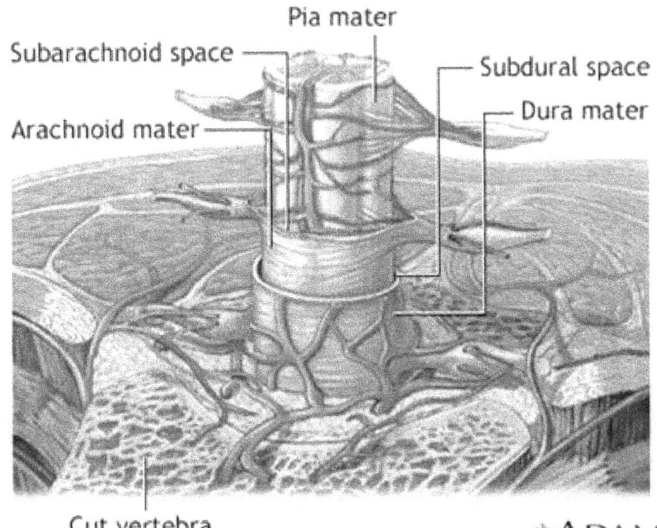

The spine is composed of the following:

1. Vertebral segment is the basic part of the spine composed of a single vertebral bone with articular process and laminae. Segments are sometimes referred to as body. (nih.gov)

2. Vertebral Interspace: Vertebral Interspace is the nonbony space between two vertebral segments which includes the disk.
3. Vertebral Processes: Protruding portions of the vertebral segment to which muscles and ligaments attach.

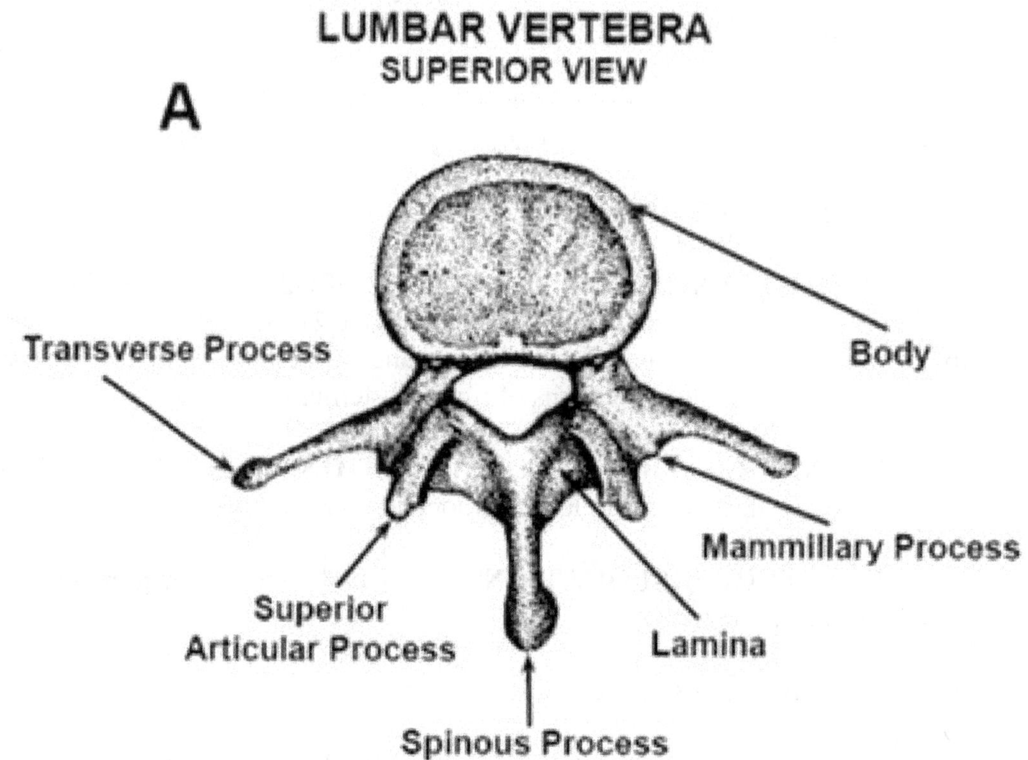

Nih.gov

INCISION/EXCISION: There are codes for incision and drainage as determined by anatomic site of the spine, cervical, thoracic, lumbar, or sacral (22010-22015). Excision codes (22100-22116) are used to code for excisions of components of the vertebral segments and not for other purposes.

Biopsies use codes from other sections as appropriate, such as 20220-20251 for bone biopsies, 21920-21925 for soft tissue biopsy of back. Removal of tumors is coded as 21930.

Excision codes are based on anatomic site of the spine and what portion of the vertebral segment or if the purpose if the excision is due to a lesion.

Notice that there are add-on codes for additional excisions of segments, so if more than one segment is involved in the procedure, then the add-on code would need to be listed. Notice too that this says that it is for each additional segment, so these add-on codes would need to be listed for each segment that is involved.

Also notice that if the nerves are involved in the removal of the segment, then 63081-63091 codes would be used instead which are from the Nervous Section. If spinal reconstruction is involved these would also be coded from the nervous section (e.g. 63085). You do not need to remember all of this, however, because it is impossible to understand everything in the medical field; however, you do need to be diligent about examining the code's description of the procedure and checking other nearby codes or codes referred to in the notes for that section to see if perhaps another code is more descriptive of the procedure.

OSTEOTOMY: Spinal osteotomy codes used when a portion of the vertebral segment is cut or removed. These codes do not include removal of a lesion (22100-22116).

If decompression is conducted, then it should be coded from the Nervous Section (63001-63305) as this involves the nerves.

The codes (22206-22226) are differentiated by columns involved, anatomic portion of the spine, approach, and number of vertebral segments. There are also add-on codes for each additional segment involved. Approach is the direction from which the procedure begins and proceeds, such as posterior or anterior. Columns refer to anterior, middle and posterior. Anterior includes two-thirds of the front portion of the segment. Middle refers to the posterior third of the vertebral segment. Posterior refers to the articular facets, lamina, and spinous process.

FRACTURE/DISLOCATIONS: Fracture/dislocation codes for the spine (22305-22328) include closed and open treatments as distinguished by anatomic site of the spine, such as processes and body with or without manipulation, casting, bracing, traction, anesthesia, internal fixation, grafting, and approach. Notice in the notes that if the approach is anterior or if decompression of the nerves are involved, then these codes are selected from the Nervous Section codes (63081-63091). There are also add-on codes for each additional vertebra for some procedures.

MANIPULATION: There is only one code for manipulation of the spine with anesthesia (22505). If no anesthesia is involved, then 97140 should be used instead.

EMBOLIZATION/INJECTION: Embolization is a procedure used to shrink a tumor or aneurysm by limiting the blood flow to that area by introducing an emboli which will occlude the blood vessel to that aneurysm or tumor. These codes (22520-22527) are for surgical repair (plasties). These codes are differentiated by anatomic site of the spine involved with add-on codes for each additional body involved.

Augmentation of vertebral body involves the injection of material, such as bone cement.

In intradiscal electrothermal annuloplasty (22526-22527), a hollow needle is inserted into the disc and then a heating wire placed with the purpose to seal any ruptures in the disc wall and possible burning of the nerves to lessen pain.

ARTHRODESIS: Arthrodesis is fixation which means fusion of vertebral segments of the spine. These codes (22532-22819) should be coded in addition to other spinal procedures.

These codes are differentiated by anatomic site of the spine, approach,

There are add-on codes for additional interspaces. Interspaces contain the disc and are described as the two segments on either side of the interspace, e.g., S1-S2. If additional interspaces are involved, then it would be described as S1-S3 which means there are two interspaces involved (S1-S2 and S2-S3), so two codes would be necessary to describe this procedure.

Codes for arthrodesis procedures to correct spinal deformities, such as scoliosis and kyphosis, are coded as 22800-22819. In these codes, many segments may be involved in the procedures so the codes are differentiated by number of segments involved. Kyphectomy (22818) is a specialized procedure for patients suffering from kyphosis in which the kyphotic portion of the spine is removed and then spinal fixation provided.

EXPLORATION: There is only one code (22830) used to describe exploration of spinal fusion.

SPINAL INSTRUMENTATION: Spinal instrumentation is also coded (22840-22865) in addition to any other spinal procedure. Many of these codes are add-on codes. Notice that some of the codes are differentiated by number of vertebral segments involved, direction of placement (anterior/posterior), and if segmental or nonsegmental.

There are two types of spinal instrumentation: segmental (fixation at each end and one bony attachment) and nonsegmental (fixation at each end possibly spanning several vertebral segments without additional attachments).

Removal of instrumentation codes are also coded from this section, as well as application of devices (e.g. bone dowels).

Surgical repair of discs with insertion of artificial discs (arthroplasties) are coded as 22856-22865 and based on anatomic site of spine and number of interspaces involved. Notice that arthroplasties of additional interspaces are coded with Level III codes, such as 0163T which can be found at the back of your CPT book.

BONE GRAFTS: Bone grafts are coded in addition to other spinal procedures. Bone grafts are coded from 20930-29038.

Section 40.7: ABDOMEN

EXCISION: The only procedures listed under Abdomen are excisions (22900-22999). These include excision of a tumor by size, what layer of skin is involved, and if it is radical or not.

Section 40.8: SHOULDER

INCISION/EXCISION: The shoulder is made up of the scapula clavicle, humerus head and neck, sternoclavicular joint, acromioclavicular joint and shoulder joint. Incisions codes

(23000-23044) are for various reasons, such as removal of calcaneous deposits, capsular contracture, incision and drainage, or joint incisions which includes exploration, drainage and/or removal of foreign body.

Excision codes (23065-23220) include biopsies, excision of tumors by size and depth of excision, radical resection of malignant tumor by size, joint incision, excision of part of the clavicle (23120), surgical repair of the acromion (23130), excision of bone cyst or tumor with or without graft by type of graft (which includes obtaining the graft also so this would not need to be coded additionally), and sequestrectomy (removal of a piece of dead bone which has separated from the healthy bone due to disease or injury.)

INTRODUCTION/REMOVAL: Introduction and removal codes (23330-23350) are used to code for removal of foreign bodies by type (subcutaneous, deep, or complicated as determined and described by physician) and injection procedures for shoulder x-rays. The injection procedures include fluoroscopy which is used to enhance the picture; however, enhanced CT or MR arthrography should be coded as an extra code. Removal of prosthesis is coded as 23334-23335.

REPAIR/REVISION/RECONSTRUCTION: These codes (23395-23491)muscle transfer, fixation of the scapula (scapulopexy), incision of the tendon (tenotomy), repairs, ligament release, reconstruction, tenodesis (suture of a tendon to a bone), resections (excisions), transplantations, capsulorrhaphy (suture of a tear in a joint capsule), arthroplasty (surgical repair of a joint), osteotomy (incision in a bone), and prophylactic treatment.

Notice that these codes are for procedures involving incisions and do not include the use of a scope during the procedure. There is a reference note with some of the codes which provides the code to be used if the procedure was performed with a scope, e.g. 23415 which would be coded as 29826 if a scope was used during the procedure.

FRACTURE/DISLOCATIONS: Other than fixation devices, application and removal of casts or traction devices are included in the main procedural code for the fracture care, known as a fracture package. However, if a different physician performs the removal they are allowed to code it separately.

There is one code for manipulation (23700) of the shoulder joint.

Arthrodesis is fixation of a joint and this section includes glenohumeral joint only (23800-23802) (with or without graft.) Amputation codes (23900-23921) include amputation or disarticulation (separation of two bones at the joint) of the shoulder.

Section 40.9: HUMERUS/ELBOW

INCISION/EXCISION: The elbow includes the head and neck of the radius and olecranon process. Incision codes (23930-24006) include incision and drainage and arthrotomy of the elbow. It is important to understand the physiology of a joint because some codes differentiate by the inclusion of the capsule in the procedure. Excision codes (24065-24155) include biopsies, excisions of tumors by size, radical resection of tumor, arthrotomy, excisions of burs and bone cysts, sequestrectomy, and partial excisions.

INTRODUCTION/REMOVAL: Introduction and removal codes (24160-24220) include removal of implants or foreign bodies, and injection procedures for x-rays (arthrography). Remember there are codes for implants and removals, such as K-wires and pins, which are coded from another section (20650-20680). Injections procedures for tennis elbow are coded as 20550, not from this section either.

REPAIR/REVISION/RECONSTRUCTION: These codes (24300-24498) include manipulation of the elbow under anesthesia, muscle or tendon transfers, tendon lengthening, tenotomy, tenoplasty, flexorplasty, tenodesis (fixation of a tendon), repair or tendons or muscles, reinsertion of ruptured tendons, repairs and reconstruction of ligaments, arthroplasty, osteotomies, osteoplasties, repairs of nonunion (bones did not heal together) or malunions (bones did not heal together properly) of bones, decompression, and prophylactic treatment.

FRACTURE/DISLOCATIONS: These fracture and dislocation codes (24500-24685) are for the humerus, and elbow as distinguished by the portion of the bone involved, open or closed treatment, with or without manipulation, and a wide variety of other procedural services.

Arthrodesis is fixation of the elbow joint with or without a graft (24800-24802). Amputation codes (24900-24940) is of the humerus with various procedures included such as implant or scar revision as well as stump elongation and cineplasty (surgical fitting of a lever to a muscle so an artificial hand can be attached).

Section 40.10: FOREARM/WRIST

INCISION/EXCISION: The forearm includes the radius, ulna, carpal bones and joints. Notice that the elbow is not included in these codes but is included in the upper arm section.

Incision codes (25000-25040) include incisions of tendon sheaths, decompression fasciotomy, incision and drainage and arthrotomy. Fasciotomy is when the fascia is cut to relieve tension or pressure and the subsequent loss of circulation to that area. This procedure is used to treat compartment syndrome which may result from stress or pressure-causing events such as application of a cast due to a fracture which causes compression of the nerves and vessels. A compartment is a closed space within the body, such as the lower leg.

Excision codes (25065-25240) include biopsies, excision of tumors by size, radical resection of tumors by size, capsulotomy, arthrotomy, excision of tendons, excisions of lesions, excision of bursa, synovectomy (removal of the synovial membrane of a joint), excision of bone cysts, sequestrectomy, carpectomy (excision of a carpal bone – bones of the wrist), and styloidectomy (excision of the part of the bone protruding at the end of the lower arm bones (ulna and radius) which attach to the wrist bones).

INTRODUCTION/REMOVAL: Introduction and removal codes (25246-25259) include injection procedures for wrist arthrography, exploration with removal of deep foreign body, removal of wrist prosthesis, and manipulation of wrist under anesthesia.

REPAIR/REVISION/RECONSTRUCTION: These codes (25260-25492) include repair or tendons and muscles, lengthening or shortening of tendons, tenotomy, tenolysis (release of tendon from adhesions), tenodesis (anchoring of tendons to stabilize (fixate) a joint), tendon transplantation, flexor origin slide (releasing at the origin of a flexor so it alters the length and tone which allows them to slide and provides flexion), capsulorrhaphy, reconstruction arthroplasty, osteotomy, osteoplasty, repair of nonunion or malunion from previous fracture repair, repair of defect with graft, and prophylactic treatment.

FRACTURE/DISLOCATIONS: Fracture/dislocation codes (25500-25695) are for the radius, ulna, carpals, ulnar, and lunate.

Arthrodesis: Arthrodesis codes (25800-25830) are of the wrist with or without bone graft and either complete or limited as described by the physician. Amputation: Amputation codes (25900-25931) include amputation of the forearm and wrist.

Section 40.11: HAND/FINGERS

INCISION/EXCISION: Incision codes (26010-26080) include drainage of simple or complicated abscesses, tendon sheaths, and bursa, incision of bone of the finger or hand, decompression of the fingers or hand, fasciotomy, tenotomy, and arthrotomy.

DIP is the distal interphalangeal joint (between distal and intermediate phalanges); PIP is proximal interphalangeal joint (between proximal and intermediate phalanges).

Excisions (26100-26262) include arthrotomy, excision of tumor by size, radical resection of tumor, fasciectomy with or without graft, synovectomy, excision of tendon, sesamoidectomy (excision of a sesamoid bone which are located where a tendon passes over a joint, such as the hand, knee, and foot), excision or curettage of bone cyst, excision of bone, and radical resection of malignant tumor.

INTRODUCTION/REMOVAL: Introduction and removal has one code (26320) for removal of implant from finger or hand.

REPAIR/REVISION/RECONSTRUCTION: These codes include manipulation of a finger joint so that it is put back into place (26340-26341). Repair or advancement of tendons is coded with or without graft as primary or secondary and in what area of the hand by zones for each tendon (26350-26434) and includes codes for excision and implantation of prosthesis (rod). (Tendons are the tissues that attach the muscle to the bones.) Primary repair is the first repair procedure and if the patient must return for an additional repair that is considered secondary.

No man's land is located on both sides at the base of the fingers as shown in the highlighted area. This area is prone to injuries and continued stiffness after surgery.

Tenolysis is coded as (26445-26449) and is the freeing of tendons from adhesions. These codes are differentiated by each tendon. Tenotomies (26450-26460) are differentiated by each tendon and is the incision or cutting of a tendon and are also known as releases. Tenodesis (26471-26474) are differentiated by each joint and is the fixation of a tendon, such as to a bone.

Lengthening and shortening of tendons (26476-26479) are differentiated by each tendon.

Transfer or transplants of tendons (26480-26498) are differentiated by each tendon and with or without graft. An opponensplasty is a tendon transfer procedure involving the thumb used to provide relief for severe carpal tunnel syndrome.

Other codes (26499-26510) include correction of a claw hand and release of thenar muscles.

Capsule procedures (26516-26525) include capsulodesis by number of digits and capsulectomy by each joint. Capsulodesis is fixation of the capsule of a joint in the hand and capsulectomy is an excision (resection or removal).

Arthroplasties (26530-26536) are surgical repair of joints of the hands and are differentiated by each joint and implantation of prosthesis.

FRACTURE/DISLOCATIONS: Fracture codes (26600-26785) are for the fingers by joints of the hand.

Arthrodesis (26820-26863) includes arthrodesis by joint, with or without fixation or graft. Notice that there are add-on codes for additional joints. Also notice that obtaining the graft is also included in the code and would not be coded separately. There is also fusion in opposition of the thumb (26820) which involves the fusing of the bones of the joint to alleviate pain.

Amputation (26910-26952) are differentiated by joint and can include interosseous transfer (between bone transfers which can involve nerves and tendons), neurectomies (excision of nerves) and advancement flaps (where skin is moved over to cover defect). An amputation is primary if it is used to treat an acute injury and it is secondary if it used to treat an injury that had received other medical care but which failed and now requires amputation.

Section 40.12: PELVIS/HIP JOINT

INCISION/EXCISION: Incision codes (26990-27036) include I&D of the pelvis and hip areas that are deep and not superficial, such as for hematomas, bursa, or abscess. Incisions into the cortex of the bone are also coded as 26992. Surgical division of a tendon to correct a deformity (tenotomy) are coded as 27000-27006 and can be open or percutaneous. Incision of the fascia is coded as 27025 or 27027 with decompression. Incision into a joint (arthrotomy) is coded as 27030-27033 with drainage or removal of loose or foreign bodies. Incision or excisions into the capsule of the joint are coded as 27035-27036.

Excision codes (27040-27080) include biopsies, excision or radical resection of tumors by size, arthrotomies with biopsy or synovectomy (excision of the synovial membrane surrounding the joint), decompression fasciotomy, excision of bursa or cyst or excision of the coccyx.

INTRODUCTION/REMOVAL: Introduction and removal codes (27086-27096) include removal of foreign bodies from within subcutaneous tissue, or deeper into the subfascial or intramuscular tissues. It also includes removal of an artificial hip joint (prosthesis), and injections of materials for arthrographies with or without anesthesia.

REPAIR/REVISION/RECONSTRUCTION: Repair, revision and reconstructions codes (27097-27187) include release of the hamstring, transfers of muscles, acetabulopasty (repair of the cavity of the acetabulum), hemiarthroplasty of the hip (surgical repair of part of the hip utilizing a prosthesis) or total hip replacement (arthroplasty 27130), hip arthroplasty conversions and revisions, osteotomies of hip and femur, bone graft, treatment of a slipped femoral epiphysis with or without pins, traction, and reduction. Slipped femoral epiphysis is slippage of the proximal femoral epiphysis on the neck of the femur, most often occurring during puberty and in obese children.

FRACTURE/DISLOCATIONS: Fractures and dislocation codes (27193-27269) include the pelvis, coccyx, acetabulum (hip socket), femur, and hip. Other than fixation devices, application and removal of casts or traction devices are included in the main procedural code for the fracture care, known as a fracture package. However, if a different physician performs the removal they are allowed to code it separately.

Manipulation: There is one manipulation code (27275) for manipulation of the hip joint with anesthesia. Arthrodesis codes (27280-27286) include fixation of sacroiliac joint, symphysis pubis, and hip joint. Amputation codes (27290-27295) include amputation of the hindquarter and hip.

Section 39.12: FEMUR/KNEE

INCISION/EXCISION: Incision codes (27301-27310) include I&D of abscess, bursa, hematoma as well as deep incision into the bone cortex of the femur or knee. It also includes fasciotomies, tenotomies, and arthrotomies.

Excision codes (27323-27365) include biopsy, neurectomy, excision of tumors by size and if radical, arthrotomy with or without meniscectomy or synovectomy which should not be coded additionally if performed since they are included in the code. These codes also include excision of bursa, cysts with or without a graft, and lesions. Patellectomies are removal of the patella of the knee.

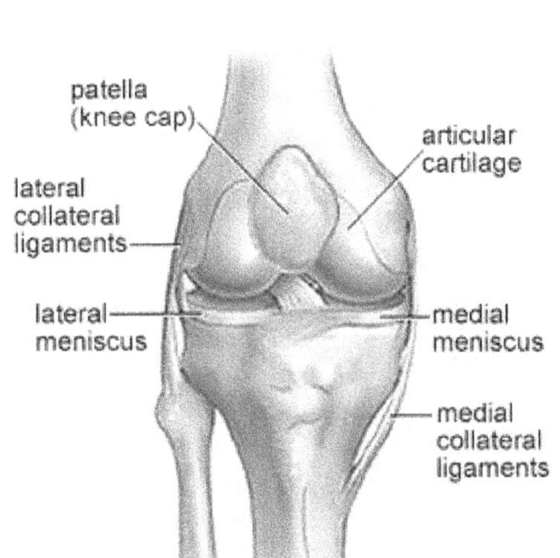

http://www.ithaca.edu/depts/img/17550_photo.jpg

INTRODUCTION/REMOVAL: Introduction and removal codes (27370-27372) include injections for arthrography (remember that the S&I must also be coded in addition using 73580) and removal of foreign bodies.

REPAIR/REVISION/RECONSTRUCTION: Repair, revision and reconstruction codes (27380-

27499) include primary or secondary suturing of tendons and tenotomies, lengthening transplanting, and transferring of tendons by number of tendons involved. These codes also include arthrotomy with meniscus repair of the knee, primary repair of a torn ligament of the knee, osteochondral grafts (bone and cartilage), and reconstruction of the patella with or without realignment, muscle advancement and patellectomy. Included also in these codes are open releases but note that an arthroscopic release is coded with a different code (29873) which you will find to be true of open versus arthroscopic procedures which will not be coded with the same codes. Reconstruction of ligaments of the knee either as within or outside of the joint (intra-articular and extra-articular respectively) are coded with these codes. Primary repair of the ligaments should be coded additionally as noted in these codes as 27405-27429. Surgical repair of the quadriceps to restore knee flexion caused by fractures is coded as 27430. Surgical repair of the joint (athroplasties) are coded for patella, knee, and femur as differentiated by specific sites within those areas. Osteotomies are also coded for femur and proximal tibia, which includes repair of bowlegs or knock-knees (27455-27457). Repair of the bone (osteoplasty) are performed on the femur as either or both shortening and lengthening. Repair of a nonunion or malunion of a fracture is coded as 27470-27472 either with or without a graft. Fixation or arresting of the epiphyseal by any method of the femur is coded as 27475-27479 as differentiated by femur, tibia or fibula and if it is partial or total. Revision of a total knee arthroplasty is coded as 27486-27487 and extent of body components involved. Removal of a prosthesis is coded as 27488. Decompression or release of the fascia to relieve stress is coded also with respect to extent of body components involved.

FRACTURE/DISLOCATIONS: Fracture and dislocation codes (27500-27566) include femur, patella, knee, tibia and fibula.

There is one manipulation code (27570) for the knee joint under general anesthesia. There is one arthrodesis code (27580) for the knee. The amputation codes (27590-27598) are for the thigh through the femur by method or at the knee.

Section 39.13: LEG/ANKLE JOINT

INCISION/EXCISION: Incision codes (27600-27612) include decompression fasciotomy of the leg by compartments (anterior, lateral, or posterior). I&D is also coded for the leg or ankle for deep abscess, hematoma or bursa. Tenotomies are coded for the Achilles tendon with local or general anesthesia. Arthrotomies for the ankle include exploration, drainage, removal of foreign body, and capsular release.

Excision codes (27613-27647) include biopsies, excision or radical resection of tumors by size, arthrotomies of the ankle which may include a synovectomy (excision of the synovial membrane), excision of lesion of the tendon or surrounding tissue, excision or curettage of bone cyst with or without graft, and partial excision of the bone (craterization or saucerization which is the removal of tissue which leaves a shallow depression with the purpose to allow for drainage of infected areas).

INTRODUCTION/REMOVAL: There is only one code for introduction and removal (27648) which is for injection procedures for arthrographies. Remember that the S&I codes will also need to be coded with 73615).

REPAIR/REVISION/RECONSTRUCTION: Repair, revision and reconstruction codes (27650-27745) include primary or secondary repair of the Achilles tendon with or without graft, and repair of a fascial defect of the leg. There are also numerous procedures performed on tendons, including primary or secondary repair, tenolysis per each tendon, lengthening or shortening, and transfer or transplant per each tendon with add-on codes for involvement of additional tendons. There are also codes for repair of ligaments and arthroplasties of the ankle including with implant or revision. Osteotomies and osteoplasties are performed on the tibia and fibula, but there is a code that includes both if both are involved so only this code would be coded and the tibia and fibular would not be coded separately then. Repair of malunions or nonunions are also coded as 27720-27726 and can include grafts and synotosis (when two bones have formed together as dysfunctional). Arrest of the epiphysis (fusion of the epiphysis and diaphysis which interrupts growth of the bones) of tibia or fibula, or both, or the femur is coded as 27730-27742.

FRACTURE/DISLOCATIONS: Fracture/dislocation codes (27750-27848) include treatment of the tibia, fibular, malleolus (bony prominence on each side of the ankle), and ankle.

There is one code for manipulation (27860) of the ankle. There are two codes for arthrodesis (27870-27871) for the ankle and tibiofibular joint. Amputation codes (27880-27889) are of the tibia, fibula, and ankle and include with fitting with cast, guillotine procedure, with secondary closure (such as grafting) and re-amputation.

Section 40.13: FOOT/TOES

INCISION/EXCISION: Incision codes (28001-28035) include I&D of bursa or abscess, fasciotomies, tenotomies, arthrotomies, and nerve decompression for entrapments.

Excision codes (28043-28175) include excisions and radical resections of tumors by size, arthrotomies, neurectomies, fasciectomies, synovectomies, curettage of bone cyst or tumor, ostectomies (complete or partial), craterization, resections of phalanges, metatarsectomy (removal of a metatarsal), and partial and complete phalangectomies (removal of phalanges).

The first joint, or the metatarsophalangeal (MTP) joint connects the toe to the foot. The second joint is the proximal interphalangeal (PIP) joint, and the third is the distal interphalangeal (DIP) joint.

INTRODUCTION/REMOVAL: Introduction and removal codes (28190-28193) include removal of foreign bodies from the foot as either subcutaneous, deep or complicated. If no incision is required and the foreign body is removed with an instrument such as tweezers, then removal of the foreign body should not be coded as this would be included in the E/M visit code. If the removal goes below the fascia then this would be considered complicated.

REPAIR/REVISION/RECONSTRUCTION: Repair, revision and reconstruction codes of the foot (28200-28360) are more complicated and detailed than for most other anatomic sites primarily because this section contains codes for bunionectomies (hallux valgus correction). Terminology is important in understanding these codes.

Hallux valgus is better known as a bunion in which the big toe turns inward towards the second toe and the joint at the base thereby becomes pronounced producing a deformity. Medically, it is the enlargement of bone and tissue at the joint at the base of the big toe, otherwise known as the metatarsophalangeal joint.

There are various methods used to correct bunions although the procedures are similar and vary more according to the severity of the deformity. The main procedure of all of the procedures is the removal of the bump (medial eminence) from the first metatarsal head of the great toe. Additional procedures include additional resections, fusions, transfer of tendons, osteotomies and insertion of wires which are identified by different names for the procedures.

The types of bunionectomies are:

Silver bunionectomy (28290) which is a simple excision of the medial eminence.

Keller bunionectomy (28292) which is excision of the medial eminence and a resection of the base of the proximal phalanx of the great toe which is just above the medical eminence site.

McBride bunionectomy (28292) is the same as Keller with excision of the medial eminence, resection of the base of the proximal phalanx, but also includes removal or release of the lateral sesamoid bone which is on the opposite side of the medial imminence, so on the inside of the big toe, so both sides are removed and the same code is used.

Keller-Mayo bunionectomy (28293) is the same as the Keller but includes the implantation of a double-stem implant such as a Kirschner wire.

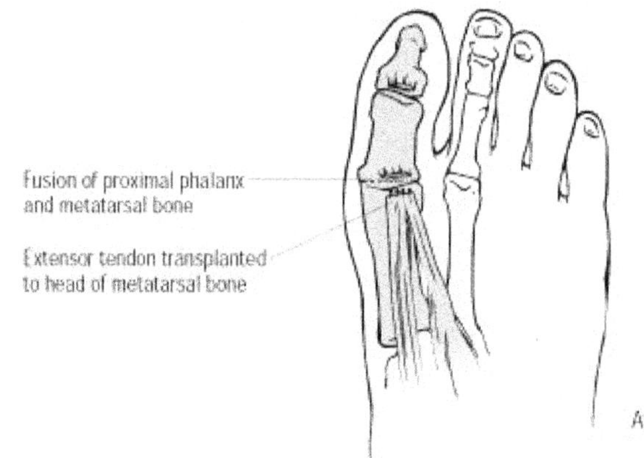

Joplin bunionectomy procedure (28294) includes excision of the medial eminence and fusion of the hallux interphalangeal joint of the great toe in addition to the extensor tendon being transferred to the head of the first metatarsal.

http://libweb.allencc.edu/images/28294.jpg

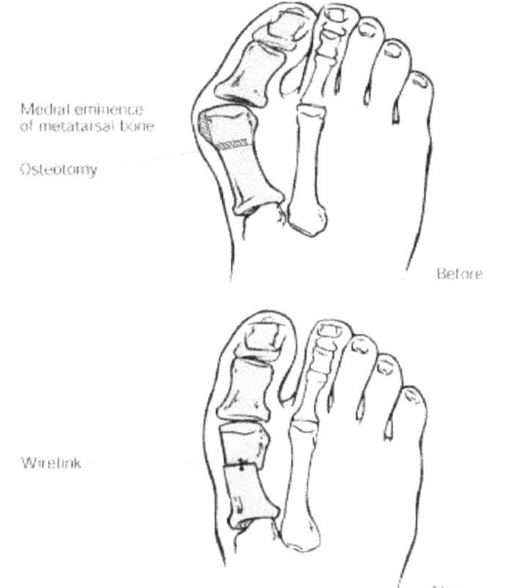

Mitchell Chevron bunionectomy (28296) includes the excision of the medial eminence and an osteotomy of the first metatarsal neck and repositioning of the metatarsal head.

http://libweb.allencc.edu/images/28296.jpg

Phalanx osteotomy procedure (28298) is the excision of the medial eminence and an Akin osteotomy in which a bony wedge is removed from the base of the proximal phalanx and a Kirschner wire may be implanted. If a double osteotomy is performed where the bone is cut in both the metatarsal bone and the proximal phalanx this is coded as 28299.

Other osteotomy codes (28300-28312) are performed on the calcaneus, talus, and tarsals, metatarsals and include shortening and grafts.

Other repair codes include repair of tendons with or without graft for each tendon and primary or secondary. They also include tenolysis, tenotomy, reconstruction, lengthening, and release for each tendon. Division of fascia and muscle is coded as 28250 and capsulotomy as 28260-28272 as specified by including medial release, tendon lengthening, and extensiveness by joint.

Syndactylization of the toes (28260) is used to correct deformities of the toes such as claw toe and results in an artificially produced webbing (syndactyl of the toes). Syndactylization is usually performed if more conservative procedures, such as arthroplasty and removal of bone from the affected toe, are not effective in correcting the deformities of the toes involved. Correction of deformities of the fifth toe, such as hammertoe, are coded as 28285-28288, such as correction of hammertoe.

There are also codes (28313-28360) for reconstruction of deformities of the toes, sesamoidectomies, repair of nonunions and malunions, and reconstruction of feet and toes for macrodactyly (when toes are larger than normal), polydactyly (when there are more than five toes per foot) and cleft foot.

FRACTURE/DISLOCATIONS: Fracture and dislocation codes (28400-28675) include the foot and toes.

Arthrodesis codes (28705-28760) for the toes and foot include osteotomies, and tendon lengthening and advancement. However, hammertoe operations are coded as 28285 and are not coded from these codes. Amputation codes for the toe and foot (28800-28825) are by site and joints.

Section 40.14: CASTS/STRAPPING

There are several scenarios in which coding for casting and strapping can occur. The reason for these scenarios is because typically casting and strapping are not coded because they are considered part of the procedure for fracture care (global postop), such as ORIF, but there are times when casting and strapping can be charged.

First, if the casting or strapping is a replacement it can be coded even if it occurs during the global postop period or after.

Second, if the casting or strapping was performed without the provision of any other major procedure of which the strapping or casting would have been included.

Third, if the casting or strapping is performed by a physician other than the one who provided the initial fracture care package or other major procedure in which the casting and strapping would otherwise have been included. In this scenarios, modifier 79 should be attached if the casting or strapping was provided during the postop global period which indicate that another physician provided the service rather than the physician who performed the initial procedure.

BODY/UPPER EXTREMITY: These codes (29000-29280) include the application of a halo body cast (used to immobilize the body and the spine after spinal procedures and fits onto the shoulders and circles the head), Risser jacket (extending from the patient's hips to the neck and sometimes including part of the head used to treat deformities of the spine such as scoliosis), turnbucket jacket (uses metal turnbuckles to twist two halves of the cast), body cast, figure-of-eight cast, splints (long or short arm or finger), and strapping by anatomic site.

LOWER EXTREMITY: These codes (29305-29584) include spica cast (cast which includes the trunk of the body and one or more limbs), long leg cast (thigh to toes) either as walking or ambulatory, brace, cylinder leg cast (thigh to ankle), short leg cast (below knee to toes), patellar tendon bearing cast, walker to assist with mobility when cast applied, rigid total contact leg cast, clubfoot cast, splints, and strapping.

REMOVAL/REPAIR: These codes (29700-29750) can only be used by a physician other than the physician who applied the cast. They include removal, repair, wedging, and windowing of casts.

Section 40.15: ENDOSCOPY/ARTHROSCOPY

Endoscopies and arthroscopies are performed with a scope (obviously) and are not considered open procedures. In fact, a procedure can be either scopic or open but not both. If a procedure begins as a scopic procedure and is converted to an open procedure, then ICD-10 code V64.41 should be used which indicates this.

There are different codes for a procedure performed with a scope and an open procedure. The CPT codes will usually provide a note under the code for each directing the use of the other code, so under endoscopic codes there is a note that an open procedure should be coded with other codes which are usually then provided in the note.

If a diagnostic scopic procedure is performed but continues into a surgical scopic procedure, then only the surgical scopic procedure is coded. The CPT codes make frequent mention of this requirement.

Multiple procedures can be performed through the scope and can be coded separately but they must be separate procedures and not related as part of each other. For example, arthroplasty of the knee with partial synovectomy are included in one code, 27443, and so they cannot be coded separately.

Section 40.16: HCPCS

Some frequently used HCPCS codes used with musculoskeletal codes are A4565 for slings, A4570 for splints, A4580 for cast supplies like plaster, A4590 for special casting materials such as fiberglass, Q4049 for finger splint. Sometimes Medicare will not accept CPT codes and HCPCS codes should be used instead, such as G0259 for injection procedures into the sacroiliac joint for arthrography and G0289 for arthroscopy of the knee for removal of loose material. Also, S2350 for anterior diskectomy and S2360 for percutaneous vertebroplasty.

MUSCULOSKELETAL QUIZ 29

1) What are the codes for a 62-year-old patient who experienced blunt trauma to the left orbit with a hematoma on the forehead which resulted in neuropathy and blindness in the left eye. The patient was found to have an extensive blowout fracture of the left orbital floor which was treated with a periorbital open procedure.

2) What are the codes for a 23-year-old patient who had removal of screws in the right knee due to fracture repair 5 months ago?

3) What are the codes for a 15-year-old patient who received arthroscopy of the left knee. There was exploration of the knee in the suprapatellar and patellofemoral region, and a partial medial meniscectomy was completed to repair a tear. There was no evidence of remaining loose body or other abnormality. A posterior horn tear of the medial meniscus was debrided back to a stable margins. The chondromalacia of the patella were noted and chondroplasty was performed.

4) What are the codes for a 17-year-old patient who was involved in a car accident and suffered skull fracture which required closed treatment of skull fracture in the emergency room with a history and exam that were both detailed?

5) What are the codes for a 42-year-old patient who had repair of an artificial fracture at a former pin site from a previous fracture of the right upper ulna which did not heal together properly and was repaired with external fixation?

6) What are the codes for a 13-year-old patient who had removal of glass from a wound of the right forearm into the dermis and fascia?

7) What are the codes for a 48-year-old patient who had repair of a bunion on the left foot with removal of the medial eminence with resection of part of the proximal phalanx and osteotomy with implantation of screw in addition to arthroplasty to repair the hammertoe of the second toe?

8) What are the codes for a 28-year-old patient who had received craniofacial reconstruction in the past and was now experiencing loosening of plate and screws. There were some irregularity in the temporal parietal bones. Old scar was excised and revised of both coronal sides. The plates, screws and wires were all removed from the area. Attention was directed to the craniofacial orbital region where some of the excess bone was reduced.

9) What are the codes for a 64-year-old patient who had a comminuted displaced distal fracture of the shaft of right radius and ulna which was repaired with ORIF?

10) What are the codes for a 62-year-old patient who had resection of the base of the DIP of the second toe on the left side with hemiphalengectomy and syndactylization due to Freiberg's?

11) What are the codes for the secondary procedure for a patient who had repair of a cranial deformity defect with a piece of titanium mesh as the primary procedure. Once this was complete, the secondary procedure was begun where a vertical incision was made transversely to the left side in order to allow exposure of the prominent right parietal bone with a contouring bur and reduced in size. Due to extensive tension on the wound repair, the old scar was removed. This was trimmed appropriately and hemostasis was achieved with electrocautery and closure with 2-0 Vicryl interrupted sutures and 3-0 nylon.

12) What are the codes for a 64-year-old patient with a history of insulin-dependent diabetes mellitus, coronary artery disease, chronic renal failure and heart failure who was initially admitted for congestive heart failure and nonhealing bilateral mid-foot ulcers treated for years with debridement and whirlpool. The patient was readmitted for acute diabetic right foot to be treated with incision and drainage of his right foot and first ray amputation but the infection had spread so right below-knee amputation was performed.

13) What are the codes for a 71-year-old patient who has osteoarthritis of the left thumb which required fusion?

14) What are the codes for a 77-year-old patient who received some traction with some manipulation and reduction for intertrochanteric fracture of the left hip in addition to A 6-inch incision was made beginning at the tip of the greater trochanter and going distally along the lateral thigh. The fascia was incised in line with the incision, and the vastus lateralis muscle was split by sharp resection down to the underlying femur and a Bennett retractor placed. A guide wire was placed and a 90-mm compression hip screw was then placed over the guidewire. Next, the 135° angle, four-hole sideplate was slipped over the shaft of the screw and fixed to the femoral shaft. Four screws were then placed by drilling, measuring, and putting in four tap screws.

15) What are the codes for a 32-year-old female who had a neoplasm removed from her left posterior shoulder in addition to a biopsy of the left axillary sentinel lymph node?

CHAPTER 41
RESPIRATORY

You will learn the following objectives in this chapter:

A. Respiratory System
   1. Paranasal Sinuses
   2. Endoscopy
   3. Endotracheal Intubation
   4. Tracheostomy
   5. Decortication
   6. Wedge Resection
   7. Fluoroscopic Guidance
B. Nose
C. Accessory Sinuses
D. Larynx
E. Trachea and Bronchi
F. Lungs and Pleura
   1. Lung Transplantation
   2. Surgical Collapse Therapy: Thoracoplasty

Section 41.1: RESPIRATORY SYSTEM

The respiratory system begins with the nose and mouth, then into the pharynx, larynx, trachea, bronchi and lungs. All of the codes in the respiratory section of the codes are by anatomic sites within this system and it is the same order of procedures within each anatomic site.

ENDOSCOPY

An endoscope is a lighted optical instrument which can be inserted into the body to view various anatomic structures. Endoscopes can be rigid or flexible. They are usually named after the anatomic structure that they are used to view, such as arthroscope and laryngoscope.

Fluoroscopic guidance is the use of radiologic imaging to assist in the placement of instrumentation for testing and procedures which involves the introduction of contrast materials into the body.

Section 41.2: NOSE

Although the nose is considered one anatomic site, if a procedure is performed on a part of the nose that lies on both sides, then that would be considered to be a bilateral procedure. If the procedure code does not describe that it includes both bilateral sides and the procedure was performed on both sides, then a modifier 50 needs to be applied to the procedure code which indicates this is a bilateral procedure (modifiers will be discussed more extensively later.), for example removal of polyps from both sides of the nose (30110).

INCISION: Most incisions are included in other surgical packages and, therefore, are not coded; however, incisions for drainage of abscesses or hematomas are using 30000-30020.

EXCISION: Biopsy is coded as 30100. Excisions of polyps (polypectomy) (30110-30115) are differentiated in the codes by being either a simple or complex procedure which must be defined by the physician; if not, query him. A complex polypectomy is usually done in a hospital setting.

Other procedures include excision/destruction of lesions through either an internal or external surgical approach (30117-30118) and removal of skin from the nose (rhinophyma) (30120). Excision of cysts can be either simple (subcutaneous) or complex (under the bone or cartilage) (30124-30125).

Excision of the inferior turbinates of the nose are coded as 30130-30140, but unlisted procedure is used for superior or middle turbinates (30999). In addition, ablation codes (e.g. 30801) should not be coded in conjunction with these excision codes since they would be included in the procedure.

A rhinectomy (excision of the nose) is coded as either partial or total (30150-30160).

INTRODUCTION/REMOVALS: Introductions are injections (30200), displacement therapy (30210) and insertion of prosthesis (30220). Removal of foreign bodies (30300-30320) are differentiated by requiring anesthesia, occurring in the office or requiring a lateral rhinotomy (incision into the nose).

REPAIR: Rhinoplasty codes (surgical repair) (30400-30462) are differentiated as primary or secondary; primary being the first surgery and the secondary a revision. The primary surgery codes are differentiated by what anatomical parts are included and if there is major septal repair. Revisions are differentiated by extent of revision: simple includes a small amount of nasal tip; intermediate includes bony work with osteotomies; and major includes nasal tip and osteotomies. If grafts are needed they need to be coded from their appropriate sections, such as musculoskeletal (20900-20926).

Repair of vestibular stenosis (30465) involves the spreading of the nose cartilage with insertion of a graft, known as a spreader graft. Septoplasty (repair of the septum) is coded as 30520. Repair of a fistula is coded as 30580. Repair of nasal septal perforations is coded as 30630.

DESTRUCTION: Destruction includes ablation (30801-30802) which is the removal of the top layer of tissue by electrocautery, radiofrequency, or tissue reduction. These codes are differentiated as to depth, either superficial or deeper (submucosal). Ablation codes should not be coded if they are performed during a more significant procedure.

OTHER: Other procedures for the nose include control of a nose bleed (hemorrhage) (30901-30906) which are differentiated as either anterior or posterior part of the nose and if they are simple or complex as described by the physician. Ligation of arteries is coded as 30915-30920 by artery. If the turbinates need to be fractured for treatment, this would be coded as 30930.

Section 41.3: ACCESSORY SINUSES

The accessory sinuses are the paranasal sinuses: frontal, maxillary, ethmoid and sphenoid. These sinuses exist on each side of the face so they are bilateral but the codes are unilateral so you will need to append a 50 modifier to your procedure code.

INCISION: Incision codes include a wide variety of services. Lavage (31000-31002) is differentiated by which sinus is involved. Sinusotomy (31020-31090) is differentiated several ways. For the maxillary it is as either accessed through the nose (intranasally) or if it is radical with or without removal of polyps. A radical sinusotomy is known as a Caldwell-Luc in which access is gained through the upper gum and into the sinus to allow drainage. Sinusotomy of the sphenoid is differentiated as with or without removal of polyps or mucosal stripping. Sinusotomy of the frontal sinuses is differentiated with or without obliterative or flap. If there is sinusotomy of 3 or more paranasal sinuses, code 31090 should be used.

EXCISION: Excision codes (31200-31230) includes ethmoidectomy which can be either anterior or total.

ENDOSCOPY: If a patient receives a diagnostic scopic procedure but it results in surgery, then we do not code the diagnostic scope because it is included in the surgical scopic procedure.

Codes for the use of scopes (31231-31297) are differentiated by which sinuses are involved and if it is diagnostic or surgical. Note that the first code for diagnostic nasal endoscopy (31231) is a separate procedure which means that it can only be coded separately with this code when it is not part of a more significant procedure. Surgical procedures via the scope that are coded in this section include polypectomy, control of hemorrhage, dacryocystorhinostomy, ethmoidectomy, maxillary antrostomy, sphenoidectomy, repair of cerebrospinal fluid leak, and orbital wall decompression.

Section 41.4: LARYNX

EXCISION: Excision codes (31300-31420) include laryngotomy with removal of tumor or laryngocele, larynectomy, pharyngolaryngectomy, adenoidectomy, and epiglottidectomy. These codes are all removal codes for the structures that lie within the larynx. They can be total or partial, with or without radical neck dissection, and/or with reconstruction. For partial excisions, the codes indicate which portion of the structure was excised.

INTRODUCTION: The Introduction codes (31500-31502) include an emergency endotracheal intubation. Endotracheal intubation is a procedure by which a tube is inserted through the mouth down into the trachea, such as before surgery or in emergency situations. A tracheostomy is a procedure in which a tube is inserted into the trachea to maintain an open airway. A tracheotomy is the incision into the trachea. It may be performed to open the airway if it becomes occluded and jeopardizing a person's ability to breathe. This procedure is sometimes performed on an emergency basis.

ENDOSCOPY: Endoscopic codes (31505-31579) are differentiated by several terms including anatomic site, direct or indirect, diagnostic or operative, with biopsy or removal of tumors, lesions or foreign body, as initial or subsequent, with grafts, and with or without injections. The code for diagnostic laryngoscopy using flexible fiberoptic scope (31575-31578) is for insertion of the scope, not the testing that may be conducted. Testing codes would be selected from 92612-92617 codes in addition.

Scopes can be either direct or indirect. With a direct scope there is direct visualization but with indirect scope mirrors are used.

If multiple procedures are performed, note that only one of those codes can be described as including the use of a microscope or telescope. The description of the code should indicate that a microscope or telescope was used with terms such as microscopic or telescopic. If the use of a microscope was described but the code does describe it, then code 69990 should be used to include the use of the microscope.

REPAIR: Repair codes (31580-31590) include laryngoplasty differentiated by the purpose and specific area of the larynx involved.

DESTRUCTION: Destruction code 31595 is for therapeutic sectioning of the laryngeal nerve and is a separate procedure.

Section 41.5: TRACHEA AND BRONCHI

INCISION: Incisions codes (31600-31614) include tracheostomy differentiated as planned or emergency, age, insertion of speech prosthesis (voice button), puncture, and revision with or without flap.

ENDOSCOPY: Endoscopy codes (31615-31649) are described by the anatomic structures that are involved. Remember that if a diagnostic scope is performed at the same time as a surgical scope, then only the surgical scopic procedure is coded.

This section codes for procedures in which injections or placements are performed so that other procedures can be done. For example, contrast material may need to be introduced in order for a test to be performed although the test code will come from the radiology or medicine codes. Catheters, indwelling tubes, or stents may be placed to assist with further treatment such as infusions.

Code 31615 is for a tracheobronchoscopy performed through an established tracheostomy incision.

Code 31620 is an add-on code for endobronchial ultrasound during a bronchoscopy and can be used with codes 31622-31646 as noted in the CPT book.

Bronchoscopies are performed for many purposes including to obtain cell washings, brushings, lavage, biopsy, placement of markers, treatment of fracture, placement of stents, removal of foreign body, excision of tumor, placement of catheter, therapeutic aspiration, and injection of contrast material for bronchography.

Some of these procedures may be computer-assisted and would then be coded additionally as 31627 which is marked as an add-on code for certain codes.

Note that the biopsies should only be coded once no matter how many biopsies of that area are taken.

INTRODUCTION: Introduction codes (31717-31730) include injection procedures for a bronchography, catheterization with biopsy, catheter aspiration, and introduction of needle wire dilator/stent or indwelling tube.

EXCISION, REPAIR: Excision/Repair codes (31750-31830) include tracheoplasty and bronchoplasty which are differentiated by either specific anatomic area or with graft or excision. Other codes include excision of tracheal stenosis with anastomosis, excision of tumor, suture of wound, closure of tracheostomy or fistula with or without plastic repair, and revision of tracheostomy scar.

Section 41.6: LUNGS AND PLEURA

INCISION: Incision codes (32035-32225) include thoracostomy with rib resection or open flap drainage. Thoracotomies can be for limited or major biopsies, control of traumatic hemorrhaging, repair of lung postoperative complications and massage. They can include pneumonolysis, removal of cysts, excision of bullae, and removal of foreign body. Pneumonostomies provide a tube to the outside of the body which allows for drainage of abscess or cyst.

EXCISION: Excision codes (32310-32405) include pleurectomy (excision of the pleura) of the parietal lobe which is a separate procedure and, therefore, would not be coded if included as part of a more significant procedure. They also include biopsies, either as open or percutaneously with a needle. If a fine needle aspiration is performed for the biopsy then codes 10021 or 10022 should be used. Radiological codes for the supervision and interpretation of these biopsy results should be coded separately.

Decortication is the removal of the surface layer, membrane, or fibrous cover of an anatomic structure, such as the lungs.

REMOVAL: Removal codes (32440-32540) include pneumocentesis (puncture to remove fluid or air) and thoracentesis (puncture of the pleural cavity to remove fluid or air). Pneumonectomy (removal of the lungs) can be total, resection of a segment, such as lobes (lobectomy), or a wedge resection. WEDGE RESECTION: Biopsy procedure in which a wedge-shaped piece of tissue is removed.

Other removal codes include resection of lung tumor with or without chest wall reconstruction and empyemectomy.

Notice that many of these procedures may be performed in conjunction with other procedures and may require additional coding as they may not be included in the global package; see CPT book notes. These additional codes include bronchplasties, decortications and tumor resection.

INTRODUCTION AND REMOVAL: Introduction and removal codes (32550-32553) include insertion of indwelling catheter, tube thoracostomy (insertion of chest tube), removal of indwelling catheter, and placement of interstitial devices for radiation therapy. These are very important codes that are used frequently today. The catheters and tube are used to support the ability to provide other treatments and services. If imaging guidance is used to place these radiology codes should be used (76942, 77002, 77012, 77021). Thoracentesis is the placement of a temporary chest tube into the lung to alleviate conditions such as pneumothorax. Thoracostomy is a more permanent placement of a chest tube into the lung, such as for drainage of the pleural space. Thoracentesis codes include 32554-32555.

DESTRUCTION: Destruction codes (32560-32562) include codes for instillation of agents to cause pleurodesis (obliteration of the pleural space to prevent recurrence of pneumothorax or pleural effusion) and fibrinolysis (breaking down of blood clots). There is an add-on code for the fibrinolysis codes for subsequent days; both this code and the code for initial day can only be coded once per day even if additional treatments are provided during the day.

ENDOSCOPY: Endoscopic codes (32601-32674) of the lungs are known as thoracoscopies and are differentiated by anatomic site with or without biopsy. They may also include pleurodesis, decortication, pneumonolysis, removal of foreign body or fibrin deposit, control of hemorrhage, excision of bullae, pleurectomy, wedge resection, removal of clot, creation of window or sac for drainage, pericardiectomy, excision of cysts or tumors, lobectomy, thoracic sympathectomy and esophagomyotomy.

Remember that surgical scope codes always include diagnostic scopes.

REPAIR: Repair codes (32800-32820) include repair of hernia in the lung, closure of chest wall following a flap opening for drainage, closure of fistula, and major reconstruction of chest wall due to injury.

LUNG TRANSPLANTATION: Lung transplantation codes (32850-32856) include three components which includes removal of cadaver organs, backbench work to prepare the organ for transplant, and the actual transplantation with or without cardiopulmonary bypass and differentiated as to single or double lobes.

SURGICAL COLLAPSE THERAPY/THORACOPLASTY: These codes (32900-32960) include resection of the ribs, thoracoplasty with or without closure of fistula, pneumonlysis, and therapeutic pneumothorax (surgical collapse therapy).

OTHER: Other procedures (32997-32999) include total lung lavage and ablation therapy to reduce or eradicate tumors (include radiology codes for guidance and monitoring, 76940, 77013, 77022).

RESPIRATORY QUIZ 30

1) Insertion of a tube into the mouth and down into the trachea is known as what?

2) What are the codes for a 52-year-old patient with metastatic cancer of the pleura from breast cancer a year ago which was excised at that time and is being seen today for tube thoracostomy and chest tube insertion?

3) What are the codes for a 67-year-old patient who is seen today for pleural effusion secondary to small cell carcinoma of the upper left lung with tube thoracostomy including indwelling cathether?

4) What are the codes for this 52-year-old patient who has a history of pulmonary nodule in the left lung? She was seen today for a CT of the Chest and Adrenals with oral and intravenous contrast. Today there is a 2-cm area of parenchymal density which has the appearance of interstitial changes without findings of significant nodule or mass. This finding can relate to scarring. There is no other nodule, mass, or effusion. No evidence of adenopathy in the mediastinum. The heart and great vessels are normal in appearance. No findings with the liver, spleen, kidneys, adrenals, or pancreas.

5) What are the codes for a 14-year-old patient who had cauterization and packing of both sides of nose posteriorly to control epistaxis?

6) Excision of polyps is known as what?

7) What are the codes for a 5-year-old patient who received a tracheobronchoscopy performed through an established tracheostomy incision when he swallowed part of a plastic toy and had stopped breathing at the scene?

8) What are the codes for a 16-year-old who had an emergency left thoracostomy with ligation of the eighth intercostal artery and partial upper lobectomy with placement of arterial femoral catheter due to severe lacerations of the left artery and lung due to a car accident?

9) What are the codes for a 3-year-old patient who had a computer-assisted bronchoscopy for biopsy of right lung which revealed upon physician's review that there were three coins.

10) What are the codes for a 71-year-old patient who has a long history of lung disease due to being a lifelong smoker. History of hypertension. The patient also had COPD and asthma with bullous emphysema. A PET scan was reviewed by the physician and revealed that she has a 3.5-cm nodule in the upper left lobe which is malignant. A lobectomy was performed.

11) What are the codes for an 18-year-old patient who has trouble breathing due to airway obstruction. It was found that this is due to turbinate hypertrophy and deviated septum

protruding into the left nasal airway for which a septoplasty and bilateral turbinectomy was performed.

12) What are the codes for a 38-year-old patient who presents with the complaint of SOB and dyspnea with wheezing that began approximately four hours ago and has worsened? She is seen in the emergency room today. Her medical history showed a history of asthma. The patient states that she had a cough for the past day but she denies any other problems. She denies any fever or chills. She denies any chest pain or palpitations. The patient had an asthma attack a month ago which required hospitalization and treatment. The patient has no other past surgical history. The patient does have HTN and hypercholesterolemia. The patient lives alone and she works at a local school. She has smoked for more than 20 years. Her father is deceased due to emphysema. ROS shows that the patient has no problems in any system including no abdominal pain, chest pain, or edema other than previously mentioned. Physical exam showed the patient to be tachypneic. She is well developed and well nourished with respiratory rate of 20 and blood pressure of 124/86. HEENT is normocephalic and atraumatic. Pupils equal and round, regular, reactive to light. Extraocular muscles intact. Nares and oropharynx negative. Neck is supple; no JVD, no lymphadenopathy, no carotid bruits, no thyromegaly. Lungs reveal bilateral wheeze diffusely. There are some decreased breath sounds bilaterally. No rhonchi. Cardiovascular: Regular rate and rhythm, without murmurs, gallops, or rubs. Normal S1 and S2. No S3, S4. Abdomen: Normal active bowel sounds, soft, nontender, nondistended. No hepatosplenomegaly. Extremities: No cyanosis, clubbing or edema. Today in the emergency room the patient received 4 nebulization treatments for her acute exacerbation of her asthma but continued to be hypoxic with room air oxygen saturation of 84%. She had some slight improvement in her wheeze with the nebulization treatments but without further improvement she was admitted to the hospital to be continued on Solu-Medrol 125 mg IV and supplemental O2.

13) What are the codes for this 41-year-old patient who had an esophagoscopy and microlaryngoscopy of the neck to determine if there was cancer secondary to lung cancer. The scope was advanced into the cervical esophagus which was found to be normal. It was noticed that there was tumor involving the anterior wall of the right portion of the neck extending approximately 1 cm below the pharyngeal epiglottic fold and into the hypopharyngeal wall of which a sample was obtained. The specimen was found to be malignant.

14) What are the codes for a 2-year-old patient who had a tracheobronchoscopy to remove a toy that he swallowed. The scope was established through a tracheostomy incision.

CHAPTER 42
CARDIOVASCULAR

You will learn the following objectives in this chapter:

A. Cardiovascular System
B. General
C. Heart and Pericardium
   1. Cardiopulmonary Bypass
   2. Coronary Artery Bypass Graft
D. Arteries and Veins
   1. Angioplasty
   2. Atherectomy
E. Spleen
F. General
G. Lymph Nodes and Lymphatic Channels
H. Mediastinum
I. Diaphragm
J. Definitions

Section 42.1: CARDIOVASCULAR SYSTEM

The blood, heart, and blood vessels form the cardiovascular system. (library.thinkquest.org)

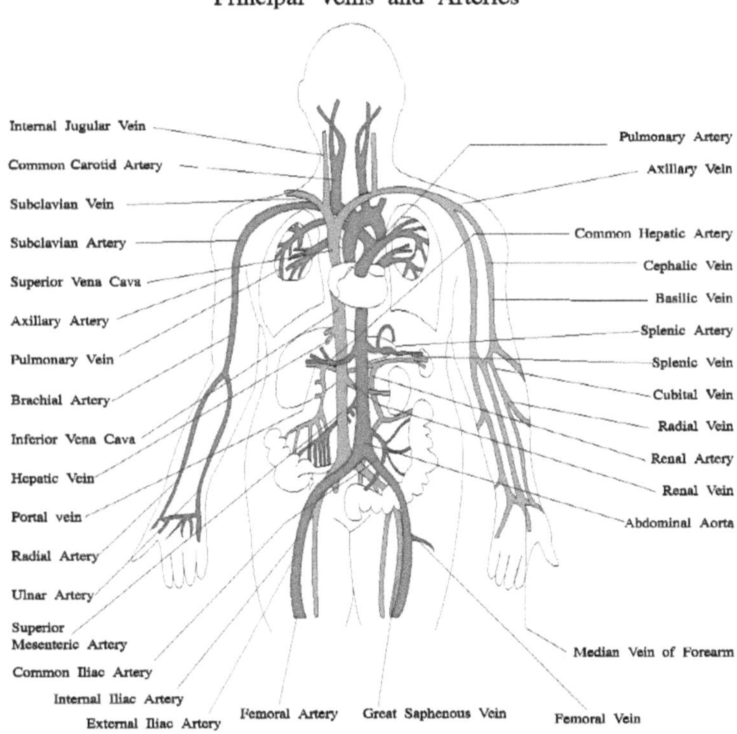

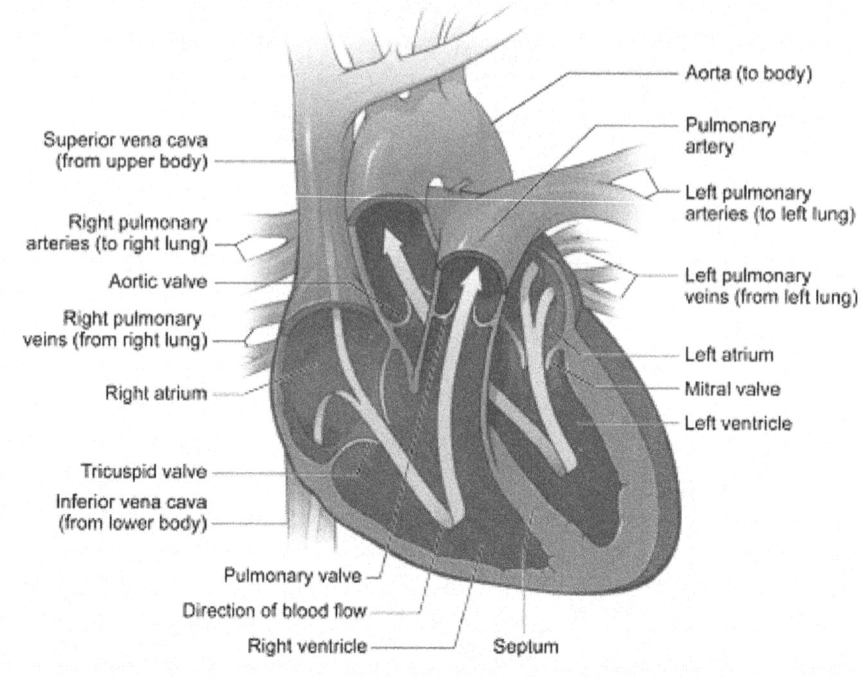

(nih.gov)

The lymph, lymph nodes, and lymph vessels form the lymphatic system.

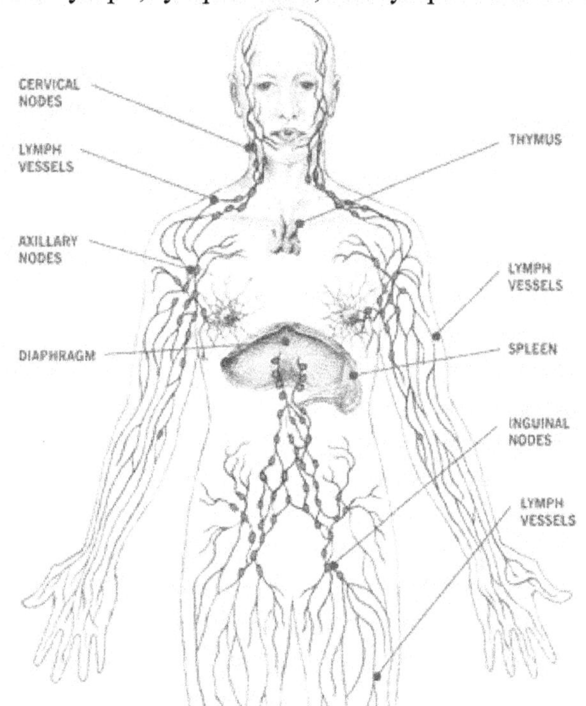

Nevgp.org

The cardiovascular system and the lymphatic system collectively make up the circulatory system.

AORTIC SINUS: There are three sinuses that originate from the ascending aorta and give rise to arteries. These are sinus of Valsalva which gives rise to the left coronary artery, sinus of Morgagni which gives rise to the right coronary artery, and Petit's sinus which comes from the posterior aortic sinus but no vessels arise from this.

Section 42.2: GENERAL

The codes in this section include procedures performed on the heart, pericardium, valves, veins, and arteries in addition to insertion of hyperalimentation (administration of nutrients by intravenous feeding,) or hemodialysis catheter and infusion pumps. These codes are differentiated by anatomic site and then by procedures which are listed in the same order within each anatomic section.

This section includes codes for procedures in which injections or placements are performed so that other procedures can be done. For example, contrast material may need to be introduced in order for a test to be performed although the test code will come from the radiology or medicine codes. Catheters, indwelling tubes, or stents may be placed to assist with further treatment such as infusions.

If any test is performed and the physician reviews the results, then codes for radiological and interpretation should also be coded as 75600-75978.

SECTION 42.3: PERICARDIUM

Pericardium codes (33010-33050) include pericardiocentesis (puncture to remove fluid from the pericardium) differentiated as initial or subsequent. This procedure is usually done with ultrasound guidance and so radiological supervision and interpretation codes should also be listed.

Also included in these codes is a tube pericardiostomy (creation of an opening of the pericardium leading to the outside), pericardiotomy for removal of clot or foreign body, creation of window or partial resection for drainage, pericardiectomy, (excision of the pericardium) and excision of cyst or tumor.

Section 42.4: CARDIAC TUMOR & REVASCULARIZATION

Cardiac tumor codes (33120-33130) include excision or resection of intracardiac or external tumor. Transymocardial revascularization codes (33140-33141) are for laser revascularization and can be either a separate code when not combined with a more significant procedure (33140) or as part of a significant procedure requiring the use of the 33141 code. This procedure involves the creation of holes in the heart surgical to help alleviate the pain of severe angina.

Section 42.5: PACEMAKER OR PACING CARDIOVERTER-DEFIBRILLATOR

Pacemaker and Pacing Cardioverter-Defibrillator codes (33202-33249) include the insertion or replacement of these devices.

A pacemaker is a battery –powered electrical system used to treat arrhythmias by ensuring normal heart rate. The pacemaker ensures normal heart rate by issuing a small electrical charge when the pace is too slow. A pacemaker consists of a pulse generator, a battery and one or more electrodes (leads). The pulse generator is placed in a devised pocket on the person in the abdominal or clavicular area. The electrode(s) lead(s) from the generator and are placed either on top of the heart (epicardial) or through a vein (transvenous). In a single chamber pacemaker, there is only one lead which is placed into either a ventricle or atrium. In a dual chamber pacemaker, there are two leads with one placed in the right atrium and the other in the right ventricle. On occasion a third lead may be placed into the left ventricle known as biventricle pacing.

A pacing cardioverter-defibrillator (known as implantable cardioverter-defibrillator, ICD) is a battery-powered electrical system which provides an electrical impulse to convert an improper heart rhythms to a proper one similar to an AED (automated external defibrillators) used by EMTs and paramedics. A pacing cardioverter-defibrillator is similar to the pacemaker and includes a pulse generator and electrodes although there may be multiple leads even if only inserted into a single chamber, but it can be either single or dual chambered. The generators are also placed into pockets and the electrodes are placed into the heart through the venous system (transvenously). If biventricular pacing is performed which is insertion of an additional lead into the left ventricle, then another code (33224 or 33225) should be coded in addition to the main procedure.

To select the proper code, you must know (1) if this is the initial insertion or replacement; (2) single or dual chamber; (3) surgical approach to place electrodes, and (4) if the pacemaker is temporary or permanent.

If a pacemaker or defibrillator is replaced, then two codes must be used – one for removal and one for insertion of the replacement. Sometimes only one part of the system may be replaced, so be sure to use the correct codes for what is replaced.

Repositioning of leads is reported with codes 33215 or 33226. Replacement is coded as 33206-33208, 33210-33123 or 33224.

If guidance is used to place the systems, use radiological supervision and interpretation codes.

Section 42.6: ELECTROPHYSIOLOGIC OPERATIVE PROCEDURES

Electrophysiologic procedures (33250-33266) include ablations and reconstruction which treat dysrhythmias by making a vessel nonfunctional. Ablation can be achieved by incision, radiofrequency, cryotherapy, microwave, ultrasound, or laser.

These codes are differentiated by the use of cardiopulmonary bypass during surgery, limited or extensive, and with or without the use of a scope, ablation described as extensive is the same procedure as the limited but includes additional ablations of atrial tissue involving the right atrium, atrial septum or left atrium.

Patient activated event recorder codes (33282-33284) include implantation of a recorder to monitor patient's cardiac activity or the removal of it.

Section 42.7: WOUNDS OF THE HEART AND GREAT VESSELS

Wounds of the heart and great vessels codes (33300-33335) include repair of cardiac wound, cardiotomy with removal of thrombus or foreign body, suture repair of a great vessel, insertion of graft into greater vessels. Most of these codes are differentiated by occurring with or without the use of cardiopulmonary bypass and with or without shunt.

Section 42.8: CARDIAC VALVES

Cardiac valve codes (33361-33478) are differentiated by aortic valve, mitral valve, tricuspid valve and pulmonary valve.

Procedures for aortic valve include valvuloplasty, construction of apical aortic conduit, replacement of an aortic valve, repair of obstruction by patch enlargement, resection for stenosis, ventriculomyotomy, and aortoplasty. Most of these codes are differentiated by occurring with or without the use of cardiopulmonary bypass and with or without graft, with or without enlargement.

Procedures for mitral valve include valvotomy either as open or closed, valvuloplasty with or without a prosthetic ring, and replacement.

Procedures for tricuspid valve include valvectomy, valvuloplasty with or without ring insertion, replacement, and valve respositioning and placation for Ebstain anomaly.

Procedures for pulmonary valve include valvotomy either as open or closed, replacement, resection for stenosis and outflow tract augmentation.

Other valvular procedure code is 33496 for repair of prosthetic valve dysfunction and is a separate procedure so it would be no coded if part of a more significant procedure.

Section 42.9: CORONARY ARTERY ANOMALIES

Coronary artery anomalies codes (33500-33507) include endarterectomy (removal of plaque from the wall of an artery) or angioplasties (surgical repair of vessels) so these procedures would not be listed as extra codes.

These codes include repair of a fistula and repair of an artery with an anomaly by means of a graft, construction of intrapulmonary artery tunnel, translocation from pulmonary artery to aorta, or unroofing.

Endoscopy code 33508 is an add-on code and is for harvesting of veins for coronary artery bypass procedure so it is listed in addition to codes for the other procedures.

Section 42.10: CORONARY ARTERY BYPASS GRAFTING

These codes (33510-33516) are for CABG procedures in which grafts come only from the venous system, such as the saphenous vein from the leg. These codes are differentiated by number of grafts.

Coronary Artery Bypass Graft (CABG) is a surgical procedure in which arteries or veins from elsewhere are grafted to the coronary arteries to bypass atherosclerotic narrowing and is usually performed with the use of cardiopulmonary bypass.

CORONARY ARTERY BYPASS GRAFT WITH VEIN: The procurement of the vein is included in these codes and is not coded separately from the CABG; however, procurement (harvesting) of an upper extremity vein (35500) or artery (35600), as well as a femoropopliteal vein (35572), is not included in the CABG code and would be coded additionally.

COMBINED ARTERIAL VENOUS GRAFTING FOR CORONARY ARTERY BYPASS: A CABG that includes both arterial and venous grafting requires the use of two codes: one for the arterial grafts (33533-33548) and one for the combined arterial-venous graft (33517-33530). These are distinguished by number of arterial grafts and the other for number of venous grafts. For this reason, notice that all of the combined codes are add-on codes. These codes are differentiated by number of grafts.

Procurement of the graft, such as the saphenous vein graft is included in these codes; however, procurement (harvesting) of an upper extremity vein (35500) or artery (e.g. radial artery) (35600), as well as a femoropopliteal vein (35572), is not included in the CABG code and would be coded additionally.

ARTERIAL GRAFTING FOR CORONARY ARTERY BYPASS: These codes (33533-33548) are used when the grafts are from arteries, such as the mammary artery, gastroepiploic artery, epigastric artery, radial artery and arterial conduits. They are also used when a combined arterial and venous grafting is performed as previously mentioned.

Procurement (harvesting) of an upper extremity artery (e.g. radial artery) (35600) is not included in the CABG code and would be coded additionally.

CORONARY ENDARTERECTOMY: Coronary endarterectomy (33572) (removal of plaque or blockage from artery) is an add-on code and should be listed in addition to other procedures including CABGs.

Section 42.11: CARDIAC ANOMALIES & PROCEDURES

SINGLE VENTRICLE AND OTHER COMPLEX CARDIAC ANOMALIES: Cardiac anomaly codes (33600-33622) include closure of heart valves, anastomosis of pulmonary artery to aorta, repair of cardiac anomaly, and repair of ventricles.

SEPTAL DEFECT: Septal defect codes (33641-33697) include repair and closures of septal defect with or without patch closure or venous drainage, and bending of pulmonary artery. Notice that repair of tetralogy of Fallot (congenital heart defect with four conditions: pulmonary stenosis, over-riding aorta, ventricular septal defect, and right ventricular hypertrophy) is included here (33692-33697).

SINUS OF VALSALVA: Repair of sinus of Valsalva fistula or aneurysm is coded (33702-33722) with cardiopulmonary bypass, repair of septal defect, or closure of ventricular tunnel.

VENOUS ANOMALIES: Venous anomalies codes (33724-33732) include repair or repair of stenosis, venous return, and repair of cor triatriatum (congenital defect in which one of the atriums is split into two parts) or mitral ring.

SHUNTING PROCEDURES: Shunting procedure codes (33735-33768) include atrial septectomy or septostomy (septum is the wall of tissue that separates the right and left atria of the heart) either as closed or open procedure, insertion of shunt by artery or with or without graft, and anastomosis of vena cava.

TRANSPOSITION OF THE GREAT VESSELS: Transposition (arteries improperly connected) of the great vessels codes (33770-33783) include repair of transposition of the great arteries with or without enlargement,

TRUNCUS ARTERIOSUS: Truncus arteriosis codes (33786-33788) are for repair or reimplantation of the pulmonary artery which did not properly close and form in the embryo.

AORTIC ANOMALIES: Aortic anomalies codes (33800-33853) include suspension for tracheomalacia, division of aberrant vessel with or without reanastomosis, obliteration of septal defect, repair of patent ductus arteriosis by ligation or division by age, excision of coarctation of aorta and repair of aortic arch.

THORACIC AORTIC ANEURYSM: Thoracic aortic aneurysm codes (33860-33877) include graft of the ascending aorta with valve suspension, reconstruction or replacement, as well as grafts of the transverse arch, descending thoracic aorta, or thoracoabdominal aortic aneurysm.

ENDOVASCULAR REPAIR OF DESCENDING THORACIC AORTA: Endovascular repair of descending thoracic aorta codes (33880-33891) include grafts for repair of descending thoracic aorta. All portions of these procedure are included in these codes, e.g. introduction, manipulation, positioning, angioplasty, and stent deployment.

However, introduction of guidewires to assist in placement, catheters, open arterial exposure and associated closures are coded separately and are not included in the codes. Transposition of some arteries, as described in the CPT book, are also coded separately. As usual, use of fluoroscopic guidance should also be coded as an additional code. Services for other arteries at the same time should also be coded separately.

PULMONARY ARTERY: Pulmonary artery codes (33910-33926) include embolectomy, endarterectomy, repair for stenosis and atresia (abnormal closure), transection of pulmonary artery, ligation and takedown of shunt, and repair of arborization (branching of arteries) anomalies.

HEART/LUNG TRANSPLANTATION: Heart/Lung transplantation codes (33930-33945) consist of three sets of components: (1) harvesting of the organ (cadaver donor cardiectomy with or without pneumonectomy of lungs); (2) backbench work (preparation of heart and lung), and (3) transplantation of the heart with or without lung). This does not include an artificial heart transplant.

CARDIAC ASSIST: Cardiac assist codes (33960-33993) include insertion of VAD (ventricular assist device) either as extracorporeal (outside of the body) or intracorporeal (within the body), as well as removal and replacement of either system or a portion of it, such as replacement of the pump only. These codes also include extracorporeal circulation of the heart (33960-33961) which is based on time.

Section 42.12: ARTERIES AND VEINS

While the previous section dealt with the heart, this section deals with arteries and veins, many of which are similar procedures to those performed on the heart. Sympathetectomies (surgical procedures that destroy nerves in the sympathetic nervous system to increase blood flow or decrease pain) are included in the codes as well as arteriograms by the surgeon.

ANGIOPLASTY: Angioplasty involves the use of a balloon catheter which is placed into a vessel using a guide wire. The balloon is then used to open up the vessel which is obstructed.

ATHERECTOMY: A surgical procedure in which a thin catheter with a scraping blade is inserted into the artery to remove plaque and obstructions.

EMBOLECTOMY/THROMBECTOMY: EMBOLECTOMY (removal of blood clot that is moving through the circulatory system) and thrombectomy (removal of blood clot) codes (34001-34490) codes are used to remove embolus or thrombus as specified by artery or vein involved.

VENOUS RECONSTRUCTION: Venous reconstruction codes (34501-34530) codes include valvuloplasty, reconstruction, transposition, cross-over graft, and anastomosis for specified veins.

ENDOVASCULAR REPAIR OF ABDOMINAL AORTIC ANEURYSM: Endovascular repair of abdominal aortic aneurysm codes (34800-34834) include graft for repair of an aneurysm in the abdominal aorta. These codes include angioplasty and stent placement.

Similar to other codes, placement of guidewires and catheters should be coded additionally as separate codes (36200, 36245-36248, 36140). If repair is more extensive than expected this should also be coded additionally (35226 or 35286). Fluoroscopic guidance is also coded additionally as a separate code. Notice that some of these codes are add-on codes and they direct you to code them as additional codes if performed. There are also codes (34841-34848) for endovascular repair of visceral and infrarenal aorta.

ENDOVASCULAR REPAIR OF ILIAC ANEURYSM; Endovascular repair of iliac aneurysm codes (34900) are similarly coded as previous arteries and veins in that angioplasties and stent placements are included in the code, but fluoroscopic guidance, guidewires and catheters are coded as separate additional codes.

DIRECT REPAIR OF ANEURYSM OR EXCISION (PARTIAL OR TOTAL) AND GRAFT INSERTION FOR ANEURYSM, PSEUDOANEURYSM, RUPTURED ANEURYSM AND ASSOCIATED OCCLUSIVE DISEASE: Direct repair of aneurysm codes (35001-35152) include preparation of artery for anastomosis and includes endarterectomy and are differentiated by artery.

REPAIR ARTERIOVENOUS FISTULA: Repair of arteriovenous fistula (abnormal passageway between two anatomic structures) codes (35180-35190) include repair of fistula by anatomic site and as either congenital or acquired.

REPAIR BLOOD VESSEL OTHER THAN FOR FISTULA, WITH OR WITHOUT PATCH ANGIOPLASTY: Repair of blood vessel codes (35201-35286) include repair of blood vessel by anatomic site and with or without graft.

THROMBOENDARTERECTOMY: Thromboendarterectomy codes (35301-35390) include thromboendarterectomies by artery and has an add-on code for any additional arteries involved. If grafts are involved, harvesting of the graft from the saphenous or upper extremity are included and are not coded separately.

ANGIOSCOPY: Angioscopy (use of a scope to view the lumen of a vessel) code (35400) is an add-on code and is for non-coronary vessels or grafts.

TRANSLUMINAL ANGIOPLASTY: Transluminal angioplasty codes (35450-35476) can be open or percutaneous. These include transluminal balloon angioplasty by artery or vein. For the percutaneous codes, catheter placement and for both open and percutaneous radiological supervision and interpretation should be coded separately as additional codes. Balloon angioplasties are also known as percutaneous transluminal coronary angioplasty (PTCA).

Bypass Graft: Bypass graft codes (35500-35671) refer to the vein and is then further differentiated by the vessel where the graft is going. Use of an artery (other than vein) is coded as 35600-35671 by artery used and where it is transferred to.

Harvesting of multiple vein segments from distant site are coded as composite grafts (35681-35683) and are coded as add-on codes (see below). Codes 35681-35683 are for grafts which include vein and a prosthetic material by number of vein segments involved in the graft.

Harvesting of a saphenous vein graft is included in the graft codes. Harvesting an upper extremity vein or artery is coded separately as an additional code (35500, 35600). Other veins harvested are included in the code for the graft.

Use of in-situ vein is coded as 35583-35587 and is coded as an additional code if used in combination with a vein graft. In situ vein graft uses the proximal and distal ends of the vein (e.g. saphenous) with most of the vein left in its original place which can promote greater success and recovery.

COMPOSITE GRAFT: These codes (35681-35683) are add-on codes and coded as additional codes to procedures for the graft. These are for

ADJUVANT TECHNIQUES: Adjuvant technique codes (35685-35686) are add-on codes for vein patch or cuff or creation of fistula that are used during a bypass graft to improve patency of the graft.

ARTERIAL TRANSPOSITION: Arterial transposition codes (35691-35697) include transposition or reimplantation of arteries and are differentiated by both the artery moved and to what artery it is moved to.

EXCISION, EXPLORATION, REPAIR, REVISION: Excision, exploration, repair and revision codes (35700-35907) include a code for reoperation which is an add-on code to be used with the major procedure but it needs to be noted that it is a reoperation. Other codes include exploration of a vessel with or without lysis or for postoperative hemorrhage, thrombosis or infection by anatomic site. Repair of fistula is also coded as well as thrombectomy, revision of stenosis in areas of grafts and excision of infected grafts.

VASCULAR INJECTION PROCEDURES: These codes do include the arteries, but they are complex. Vascular injection procedure codes (36000-36598) are similar to the codes used for left or right heart catheterization, except with these codes no left or right heart catheterization occurs although a catheter or device is inserted. If a left or right heart catheterization accompanied vascular injection procedures, then these are coded from the medicine codes (93541-93545).

Vascular injection procedures are used to examine and study the vascular system either to determine or assist in treatment. Vascular injection procedures involve the insertion of a catheter or device. These codes include introduction of the catheter, injection of contrast material;

however, the material injected is not included such as the contrast materials and would be coded separately.

With catheter codes, you must know where the catheter was inserted, where it went, and where it ended. Some of these codes are selected according to where the catheter was introduced (inserted) in the vascular system. For these purposes the vascular system is divided into families in which the primary or first order vessel is the beginning and then the remaining vessels branch from that and are categorized by how they branch. Again, I begins with the first order and then branches into a second, then third, and so on (Table 7-1). Appendix L provides a hierarchial classification of these order. First order are the main arteries which include innominate, left common carotid, left subclavian and axillary, celiac trunk and superior mesenteric and common iliac. The second and third order and beyond are also listed. Code only for the greatest level of division within a family, that is, if the catheter goes into a third order vessel, then code only for that third order in addition to placement. However, if the physician additionally goes into a different order, you must code for each separately distinct order. For example, if the physician goes into a third order, but then additionally goes into another third order of the same first and second order family, the must code for each third order. There are two codes, one for each third order, plus placement, but not first or second order, as described earlier.

Selective catheterization means the catheter is manipulated into areas other than where placed (e.g., 36012), which includes placement and introduction. Nonselective catheterization means the catheter remains within the vessel where originally placed without further manipulation, so this is an introduction only of catheter/needle (36000).

A tunneled catheter (e.g. Hickman or Broviac) is inserted through tissue, such as skin. A non-tunneled catheter is placed directly into the vessel.

The materials and supplies (catheters, drugs, and contrast media) are sometimes not included in these codes and can then be coded separately, as will be stated in the notes in the CPT book. If cardiovascular radiology codes state that they include contrast material, then do not code for injection and contrast material because they are a part of the radiological code.

These codes also include insertion of central venous access devices (CVD) which are used to create a means to provide ongoing treatment, such as administration of drugs, IV fluids, and other materials or to obtain blood samples, known as Port-a-Cath, PICC, and Hickman. There are two types: completely implanted or partially implanted. Insertion can be either central or peripheral. For central lines, access is usually through the subclavian or jugular veins of the neck. One type of central, known as a peripheral venous catheters (PICC), are placed peripherally in the veins of the arms, legs, feet or head. CVDs are known as implantable CVDs and allow for vascular access without repeated needle sticks, such as for total parenteral nutrition (TPN), chemotherapy, dialysis, etc. Ports are implanted VADs which supply medication or materials and is composed of an injection port (placed in a pocket) and a catheter which is tunneled from the vein into the subcutaneous tissue to the port.

Central venous access procedures are coded separately as insertion, repair, partial replacement, complete replacement or removal.

ARTERIAL: Arterial codes (36600-36660) include arterial puncture for withdrawal of blood, catheterization for sampling or infusion therapy, or of the umbilical artery in newborns.

INTRAOSSEOUS: The interosseous code (36680) is for placement of a needle for intraosseous infusion therapy.

HEMODIALYSIS ACCESS: Intervascular Cannulation for Extracorporeal Circulation or Shunt Insertion: Hemodialysis access codes (36800-36870) are to create access for hemodialysis through shunts, cannulas, arteriovenous fistulas, and anastomosis which allows for blood to pass directly from an artery or vein to another one, thereby bypassing the normal vascular network. Insertion of a cannula for hemodialysis through prolonged extracorporeal circulation membrane oxygenation is known as ECMO.

There are new codes for the creation of a dialysis circuit (36901-36909). These allow for the creation of a circuit so treatment can be easily rendered

PORTAL DECOMPRESSION PROCEDURES: Portal decompression procedural codes (37140-37183) include portal decompression procedures with anastomosis for treatment of blockages and hemorrhaging varices in the liver due to cirrhosis or cancer.

TRANSCATHETER PROCEDURES: Transcatheter procedural codes (37184-37217) are for mechanical thrombectomy, arterial mechanical thrombectomy and venous mechanical thrombectomy. Injection of the thrombolytic agent during the procedure is included and should be not coded separately. These codes are differentiated by vascular families by orders, e.g. first, second, etc as previously described with vascular injection procedures so additional thrombectomies of other families are coded as additional codes.

Codes for catheter placement, stent placement, balloon angioplasty and radiological supervision and interpretation should be coded as separate additional codes. However, note that fluoroscopic guidance is mentioned, so this is included in the codes and should not be coded separately. Transcatheter placement of a stent in either a vein or an artery is coded as 37236-37239.

These codes also include thrombolysis, transcatheter biopsy, retrieval, occlusions, embolization, therapy and placement of stents.

INTRAVASCULAR ULTRASOUND SERVICES/VASCULAR EMBOLIZATION: Vascular emobolization and occlusion procedures are coded as 37241-37253.

Intravascular ultrasound service codes (37252-37253) are add-on codes for use of ultrasound during any procedure or service.

ENDOSCOPY: Endoscopy codes (37500-37501) are for surgical vascular endoscopy which, as always, includes diagnostic scope.

LIGATION: Ligation codes (37565-37785) include ligations of veins and arteries as differentiated by vessel involved and anatomic site.

Section 42.13: SPLEEN

EXCISION: Excision codes (38100-38102) include splenectomy total or partial.

REPAIR: The repair code (38115) includes repair of ruptured spleen (splenorrhaphy) with or without splenectomy.

LAPAROSCOPY: Surgical laparoscopy codes (38120-38129) include the use of the scope during a splenectomy.

INTRODUCTION: The introduction code (38200) is for injection procedures for splenoportography.

Section 42.14: GENERAL

BONE MARROW OR STEM CELL SERVICES/PROCEDURES: Bone marrow or stem cell services and procedural codes (38204-38243) describe the various steps for preservation, preparation and purifying of bone marrow/stem cells prior to transplantation or reinfusion. Preparation includes thawing and cell depletion and removal. There are also codes for aspiration and harvesting of the bone marrow.

Section 42.15: LYMPH NODE AND LYMPHATIC CHANNELS

INCISION: Incision codes (38300-38382) include drainage of abscesses or for lymphadenitis of the lymph nodes. It also includes lymphangiotomy of the lymph channels or suture/ligation of the thoracic duct.

EXCISION: Excision codes (38500-38555) include biopsy or excision of lymph nodes either as an open procedure or by needle although fine needle aspiration is coded with a different code (10021-10022) and are differentiated by lymph node. Dissection and excision of cystic hygroma are also included in these codes.

LIMITED LYMPHADENECTOMY FOR STAGING: Limited lymphadenectomy for staging codes (38562-38564) is oftentimes included in combination with other procedures which requires the use of another code.

LAPAROSCOPY: Laparoscopy codes (38570-38589) are for surgical scope which includes diagnostic scope procedures. Surgical scopic procedures include biopsy (sampling) with lymphadenectomy.

RADICAL LYMPHADENECTOMY: Radical lymphadenectomy codes (387000-38780) are also known as radical resection of lymph nodes.

INTRODUCTION: Introduction codes (38790-38794) include injection procedures for lymphangiography, also for identification of sentinel nodes. Cannulation of the thoracic duct is also included in these codes.

Section 42.16: MEDIASTINUM

INCISION: Incision codes (39000-39010) include mediastinotomy for exploration, drainage, removal of foreign body and are differentiated by approach.

EXCISION: Excision codes (39200-39220) include excision of cyst or tumor of the mediastinum.

ENDOSCOPY: Endoscopy code 39400 includes mediastinoscopy with or without biopsy.

Section 42.17: DIAPHRAGM

REPAIR: Repair of the diaphragm codes (39501-39561) include repair of a laceration, hernia, resection of the diaphragm with simple or complex repair and imbrications (overlapping of muscles) of diaphragm. Complex repair involves the use of prosthetic material or flaps.

CPT CARDIOVASCULAR QUIZ 31

1) What are the codes for a 49-year-old male with insulin-dependent diabetes mellitus has been admitted with diabetic ketoacidosis and not having peripheral vein access. Through a percutaneous puncture, the subclavian vein was located, and using the Seldinger technique, a triple-lumen catheter was inserted without difficulty. There was observed a good blood return from all three ports, and then the port was irrigated. One single stitch was used to secure the catheter in place.

2) What are the codes for a 61-year-old right-handed patient with history of hypertension, CKD, and schizophrenia with OCD symptoms who presents to the ER as having dysphasia and numbness/weakness on the right side that she noticed yesterday and has not resolved since. She explained that she had a similar incident a month before but it resolved. The patient's parents are both alive and well. She does not smoke or drink. Her ROS was negative for all other systems. Exam revealed temp of 98.7, blood pressure of 168/92. HEENT is clear. Lungs clear. Heart regular rate and rhythm. Abdomen shows surgical scar. Normal bowel sounds. Extremities show no clubbing, cyanosis or edema. She was alert and oriented times 3. She had difficulty with speech, mostly lingual sounds. No aphasic symptoms. Normal flow, normal rate and normal content. No breathlessness noted. Cranial nerves showed right fundi with sharp discs, pupils reactive 3 to 2 bilaterally, full extraocular movements and full visual fields. Corneal reflexes were present bilaterally. Decreased V1 through V3 pinprick on the face. Masticatory muscles were normal. Face was symmetric. Eye closure, puffed cheeks and smile were symmetric. Uvula and tongue were midline. Her gag was present bilaterally, left greater than right. Motor examination showed increased tone in the left arm. Strength was 4/4 in the right upper and lower extremities and 5/5 in the left upper and lower extremities. Reflexes were 2+ throughout with downgoing toes. Sensory examination showed decreased pinprick on the right side. The patient was given an EKG which revealed that the patient had experienced an MI previously and a CVA within the past several days.

3) Where are the two ways that electrodes can be placed for a pacemaker?

4) What are the codes for a 49-year-old patient who has a history of ASHD. Left femoral artery was chosen for access because of recent cardiac catheterization from the right side. A diagnostic left coronary angiogram was performed which was advanced over a wire to the left coronary ostium. It revealed no change in the mid-LAD lesion. The wire was advanced across the lesion without difficulty, and initial PTCA was accomplished. Angiogram revealed less than 10% residual lesion, but in the left anterior oblique cranial view a nonocclusive dissection limited to the lesion was noted, therefore, stenting was performed.

5) What are the codes for an alcoholic 57-year-old patient who presents with compensated biliary cirrhosis and is suffering from recurrent variceal hemorrhage for which renal portal decompression with anastomosis was provided?

6) What are the codes for a 58-year-old patient who had a triple coronary artery bypass with

sequential left internal mammary artery anastomosis on the second diagonal of the left anterior descending, saphenous vein graft to the second obtuse marginal and the same to the posterior descending coronary artery due to ST elevated MI?

7) What is a PTCA?

8) The improper connection of the great arteries is known as what?

9) What are the codes for a 73-year-old patient with a history of aortic valve replacement and severe cardiomyopathy, chronic left bundle-branch block and diabetes who presents after having experience arrest early this morning characterized earlier by difficulty breathing and chest pain. The patient was cardioverted multiple times by EMTs and placed in ICU where he was seen several times from 8:00 am to 9:00 am, 11:30 to 12:45, and 4:15 pm to 5:30 pm but remained mostly unresponsive. Subsequent rhythm was sinus tachycardiac with a left bundle-branch block. He had a cardiac catheterization at the time of aortic valve replacement which showed normal coronary vessels three years ago. The patient does drink and smoke occasionally. His father died of a heart attack at age 75. ROS was unobtainable as the patient was not responsive. Exam showed blood pressure of 145/87, Pulse was 108 and respirations are 12 on ventilator. The patient is afebrile. HEENT show PERRLA. Neck is supple. Carotids have diminished upstroke without bruits. Lungs are clear. Anteriorly heart is tachycardiac . There is a prosthetic S2. The abdomen is soft and nontender without masses. Extremities have trace edema. Distal pulses are present. Neurologic exam: The patient is unresponsive. EKG shows sinus tachycardia with left bundle-branch block. Neurological and pulmonary evals are recommends. EKG should be repeated. Possible catheterization should be performed.

10) What codes are used if a procedure is changed from a laparoscopic procedure to an open procedure?

11) What are the codes for a 49-year-old patient who had a permanent pacemaker implanted with leads placed into the right ventricle and right atrium due to bradycardia. A pocket was made in the left anterior chest wall into which the pulse generator was inserted.

12) What are the codes for a 12-month-old baby with ventricular septal defect who had patch closure?

13) What are the codes for a 53-year-old male who was brought to the operating room and pulmonary artery catheter was inserted into the right internal jugular vein. The distal right saphenous vein was harvested from the medial malleolus to just above the knee. A midline sternotomy was performed and it was found that the ascending aorta was extremely calcified with diffuse atherosclerosis. Coronaries were marked for bypass, including posterior descending artery and a posterolateral branch One liter of cardioplegia was given antegrade to arrest the heart. Bypasses were accomplished, first using the reverse saphenous vein in an end-to-side fashion to the PDA. The second bypass was to the posterolateral branch. A bolus of cold cardioplegia was given, and the patient was rewarmed. With the crossclamp still in place, a single aortotomy was made in

the ascending aorta. The area was thickened and calcified, but had a decent lumen to allow suture of the proximal end of the PDA up to the ascending aorta. The remaining proximal anastomosis of the posterolateral branch was brought onto the hood of the PDA graft. The PDA was isolated with bulldog clamps. Venotomy was made, and the end-to-side anastomosis of the posterior left ventricle to the PDA was accomplished. The lungs were inflated. The patient was ventilated and weaned off bypass successfully without the aid of inotropic support.

14) What are the codes for a 55-year-old patient who had an acute MI with edema and received an intracorporeal left ventricular assist device as a bridge to cardiac transplantation several months ago. Now, after 100 days of support, the left ventricular assist device malfunctioned and the pump had to be replaced.

15) What are the codes for a 47-year-old patient with renal failure requiring hemodialysis so an AV cannula was placed for access?

CHAPTER 43
DIGESTIVE

You will learn the following objectives in this chapter:

A. Digestive System
B. General
C. Lips
D. Vestibule of Mouth
E. Tongue and Floor of Mouth
F. Dentoalveolar Structures
G. Palate and Uvula
H. Salivary Gland and Ducts
I. Pharynx, Adenoids, and Tonsils
J. Esophagus
K. Stomach
L. Intestines
M. Meckel's Diverticulum and the Mesentery
N. Appendix
O. Rectum
P. Anus
Q. Liver
R. Biliary Tract
S. Pancreas
T. Abdomen, Peritoneum and Omentum

Section 43.1: ANATOMY

DIGESTIVE SYSTEM
Nih.gov

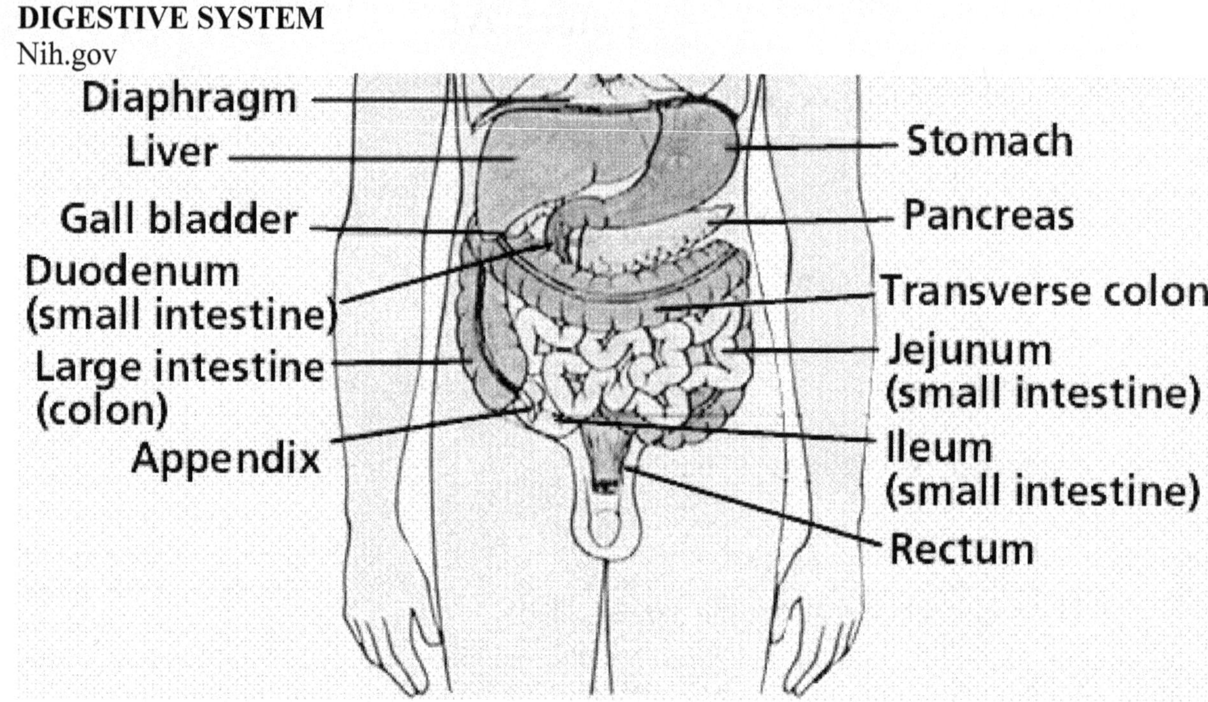

SALIVARY GLANDS: Salivary glands include the parotid gland, submandibular gland and sublingual gland.

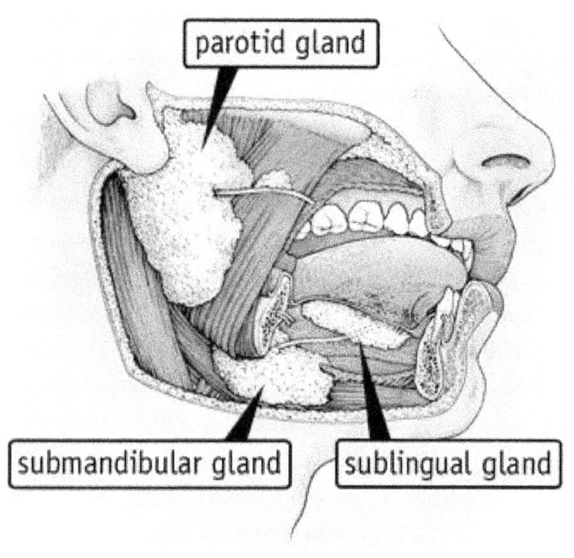

Fda.gov

INTESTINES: Food enters the intestines (also referred to as the bowels) from the stomach into the small intestine (duodenum, to the jejunum, to the ileum), then into the large intestine (cecum, to ascending colon, to transverse colon, to descending colon, to sigmoid colon and rectum).

Section 43.2: GENERAL

The basis to coding digestive is to know the combining forms for the different anatomic sites as these are usually included in most procedural descriptions, similar to the previous packets where some terms are combinations of combining forms, but particularly pronounced in this section.

A procedure can be performed as an open procedure, percutaneous, laparoscopic or endoscopic which are coded differently from each other. Endoscopic procedure involves the use of a tube which is inserted into the body for the purposes of viewing and without incisions. With laparoscopic, small incisions are made and the scope inserted although this procedure is minimally invasive.

If multiple procedures are performed through an endoscope, separate codes should be listed for each procedure. This includes removal or biopsy of lesions – each lesion is coded separately.

If a procedure starts with the scope and must be changed to an open procedure, then the open procedure code is used and a V code listed to indicate this.

A diagnostic scope is always included in a surgical scope if performed and the diagnostic scope is not coded separately.

Drains cannot be coded as additional code to major procedures but is included in the global packaging of a major procedure.

Section 43.3: LIPS

EXCISION: Excision codes (40490-40530) include biopsy, vermillionectomy (lip shave), excision of lip with or without reconstruction.

REPAIR: Repair codes (40650-40761) for the lips are known as cheiloplasties (lip reduction) and are based on if the codes are repair or plastic surgery. These codes are differentiated by height of lip repair and if the procedure is primary or secondary and one- or two-staged procedure and with or without flap.

Section 43.4: VESTIBULE OF MOUTH

INCISION: Incision codes (40800-40806) include the part of the oral cavity outside of the teeth and includes the mucosal and submucosal tissue of lips and cheeks. Incision codes include drainage of abscess, cyst, and hematoma differentiated as simple or complicated. These codes also include removal of foreign body and a frenotomy. (There are several frenulum sites in the mouth as these are membranes that attach tissues to other sites such as the mouth so you will find these codes listed throughout the sections of the digestive codes. One of the most common is the membrane that attaches the tongue to the base of the mouth).

EXCISION, DESTRUCTION: Excision and destruction codes (40808-40820) include biopsy, excision of lesion (with none, simple or complex repair), frenumectomy, frenulectomy, frenectomy, and destruction of lesion or scar.

REPAIR: Repair codes (40830-40845) include closure of laceration by size and vestibuloplasty (procedure designed to restore alveolar ridge height in the areas between the teeth and the cheek) by specific site. Vestibuloplasty is the surgical reconstruction of the alveolar ridge to restore it by lowering muscles of the buccal, labial and lingual areas.

Section 43.5: TONGUE AND FLOOR OF MOUTH

INCISION: Incision codes (41000-41019) include I&D of abscess, cyst or hematoma by specific site, frenotomy, and placement of devices for interstitial radioelement applications.

EXCISION: Excision codes (41100-41155) include biopsy by specific site, excision of lesion by specific site and with or without closure, frenectomy, glossectomy as complete or partial.

REPAIR: Repair codes (41250-41252) include repair of laceration by specific site and size.

OTHER PROCEDURES: Other procedures (41500-41599) include fixation, suturing, and suspension of tongue, as well as frenoplasty and ablation of the tongue base.

Section 43.6: DENTOALVEOLAR STRUCTURE

INCISION: Incision codes (41800-41806) include drainage of abscess, cyst or hematoma and removal of foreign body from tissues or bone.

EXCISION, DESTRUCTION: Excision and destruction codes (41820-41850) include gingivectomy, excision of tuberosities and lesion with no repair or simple or complex repair. Excision of hyperplastic alveolar mucosa and alveolectomy are also coded here.

There are no codes for tooth extraction because this is considered to be a dental procedure and would use dental codes from the Current Dental Terminology (CDT) code book.

OTHER PROCEDURES: Other procedures (41870-41899) include grafting, gingivoplasty and alveoloplasty by quadrant.

Section 43.7: PALATE AND UVULA

INCISION: The incision code (42000) is for drainage of abscess.

EXCISION, DESTRUCTION: Excision and destruction codes (42100-42160) include biopsy, excision or destruction of lesion (with no closure, simple or flap closure), resections, uvulectomy, and palatopharyngoplasty.

REPAIR: Repair codes (42180-42281) include repair of laceration by size, palatoplasty of cleft palate with or without bone graft or major revision, lengthening of palate, repair of palate or services for creation of prosthesis, such as impression and insertion.

Section 43.8: SALIVARY GLAND AND DUCTS

INCISION: Incision codes (42300-42340) include drainage of abscess by anatomic site and as either simple or complicated. It also includes sialolithotomy (excision of calculus from salivary gland) by anatomic site.

EXCISION: Excision codes (42400-42450) include biopsy of salivary gland by needle or incision, excision or marsupialization (procedure in which a slit is cut into a cyst and the edges sutured to form a continuous surface) of cyst, tumor or gland.

REPAIR: Repair codes (42500-42510) include plastic surgery of the salivary duct as primary or secondary procedure and diversion of the parotid duct with excision of glands.

OTHER PROCEDURES: Other procedure codes (42550-42699) include injection for sialography, closure of fistula, dilation of salivary duct, and ligation of salivary duct.

Section 43.9: PHARYNX, ADENOIDS, AND TONSILS

INCISION: Incision codes (42700-42725) include I&D of abscess by specific site and approach.

EXCISION, DESTRUCTION: Excision and destruction codes (42800-42894) include biopsy by anatomic site, limited or resection of pharynx and its wall (pharyngectomy), excision or destruction of lesions and cysts and removal of foreign body.

Tonsillectomy and adenoidectomy codes are based on the procedure being primary or secondary, specific anatomic site, age of patient and if they are performed alone or together. These codes are described as bilateral so a 50 modifier should not be attached to them but if a procedure involves only one side then a modifier 52 should be attached to indicate that the bilateral procedure was reduced to a unilateral procedure.

REPAIR: Repair codes (42900-42953) include repair and suturing of pharynx due to injury and pharyngoplasty.

OTHER PROCEDURES: Other procedure codes (42955-42999) include pharyngostomy to provide a means of feeding, and control of hemorrhage as simple, complicated or with secondary surgical intervention.

Section 43.10: ESOPHAGUS

INCISION: Incision codes 43020-43045) include esophagotomy to remove a foreign body and cricopharyngeal myotomy. If a laparotomy is performed for intubation this would be coded as 43510. (Cricoid is the ring-shaped cartilage at the end of the larynx.)

EXCISION: Excision codes (43100-43135) includes excision of lesions by approach, partial or total esophagectomy and diverticulectomy (excision of pouch or protrusion) of hypopharynx or esophagus.

ENDOSCOPY: Endoscopy codes (43191-43273) are many and are described by anatomic sites included in the procedure. Endoscopy involves the insertion of an endoscope through the mouth into the throat to the esophagus, stomach and into the duodenum and/or jejunum of the small intestine.

The scope can be rigid or flexible. The procedures can involve brushings and washings to collect specimens. Biopsies and treatment of varices are coded by type of treatment. Removal or destruction of foreign body, polyps, lesions or tumors are differentiated by technique and with or without placement of stent or use of guide wire. .

Esophagoscopies are coded as 43191-43233 and can include biopsies, removal of foreign body, and insertion of guide wires, with dilation by balloon or dilator, ablation of tumor or more.

Upper endoscopies are referred to as EGD (esophagogastroduodenoscopy) (43235-43259). These codes are differentiated by anatomic sites, with or without collection of specimen by brushing or washing, injections, ultra sound, fine needle aspiration, biopsy, drainage of pseudocyst, ablation of tumors, dilation with balloon, catheter placement, injections, band ligation, gastrostomy tube, removal of foreign body, use of guide wires, balloon dilation, removal or ablation of tumors and polyps, control of bleeding, stent placement, and use of thermal energy for treatment.

Endoscopic retrograde cholangiopancreatography (ERCP) are coded as 43260-43278. ERCP involves the use of the endoscope and fluoroscopy to diagnose and treat certain problems, such as gallstones. These codes are differentiated with or without brushings and washings to collect specimens, biopsy, incisions into specific anatomic sites, pressure measurements, removal or destruction of calculi, insertion of drainage tubes or stents, and removal or destruction of foreign body, cysts, tumors and lesion.

A surgical endoscopy includes a diagnostic endoscope if performed during the same surgery.

LAPAROSCOPY: Laparoscopy codes (43279-43289) involve incisions into the GI system and, therefore, differ from endoscopes although scopes are used in both procedures. The codes are differentiated by anatomic site involved and repair of hernia.

REPAIR: Repair codes (43300-43425) include esophagoplasty (surgical repair of esophagus), esophagostomy, esophagomyotomy, and fundoplasty with or without repair of fistula and by anatomic site or approach. Other codes include ligation of varices, closure of fistula or esophagostomy, suture of injury. Fundoplasties (e.g. Nissen fundoplication) involve the recreation of the valve at the lower end of the esophagus by wrapping part of the stomach around it which provides treatment for reflux disease (GERD) by preventing the backflow of stomach acid and foods from the stomach to the esophagus.

MANIPULATION: Manipulation codes (43450-43460) include dilation of esophagus differentiated by method (guide wires, bougie, balloon, or sound) and tamponade (constriction to stop blood flow).

OTHER PROCEDURES: Other procedures include free jejunum transfer which does involve the use of a microscope for anastomosis so the microscope is not coded separately.

Section 43.11: STOMACH

INCISION: Incision codes (43500-43520) include gastrotomy for removal of foreign body from the stomach, suture repair of bleeding ulcer or laceration and pyloromyotomy.

EXCISION: Excision codes (43605-43641) include gastrectomies which are partial or total removal of the stomach with Roux-en-Y reconstruction (anastomosis of the small bowel, oftentimes due to gastrectomy), creation of stoma, or formation of intestinal pouch. Biopsies are also included as well as vagotomy. Roux-en-Y reconstruction in this category is used for reconstruction of the excised portions and are used as treatments for cancers, infections, or damage.

LAPAROSCOPY: Laparoscopy codes (43644-43659) include the use of a scope to perform surgical gastric bypass (Roux-en-Y). Other codes include implantation, revisions, or replacement of gastric neurostimulator and electrodes and transection of vagus nerves. .

Note that if the procedure is open or begins with the use of a scope but is converted to an open procedure, then these codes should not be used; instead, the book directs you to use open procedure codes. Remember, there is a V code which describes the conversion to an open procedure (V64.41).

INTRODUCTION: Introduction codes (43752-43761) include placement, change or repositioning of gastrotomy tubes, such as the PEG (percutaneous endoscopic gastrostomy which is also known as the feeding tube). These also include nasogastric or orogastric tubes.

BARIATRIC SURGERY: Bariatric surgery codes (43770-43775) involves the placement, revision or replacement of a band on the stomach in addition to a subcutaneous port with additional codes for revision of the band (e.g. gastric banding procedures for weight control).

OTHER PROCEDURES: Other procedure codes (43800-43846) include pyloroplasty, gastroduodenostomy, gastrojejunostmy, gastrostomy, gastrorrhaphy, anastomosis, closure of fistula and gastrostomy, revision or removal of gastric neurostimulator electrodes and restrictive procedures. Restrictive procedures include the Roux-en-Y procedures for control of obesity that are known typically as gastric bypass surgery (43846).

Section 43.12: INTESTINES

INCISION: Incision codes (44005-44055) include enterolysis (freeing of intestinal adhesions) but this oftentimes is included in other major procedures and would usually not be coded as a separate code. However, sometimes adhesions can be extensive and/or require additional services for various reasons and should be coded separately with modifier 22 attached in addition to the major procedure. Other codes include duodenotomy or colotomy for exploration and/or biopsy and jejunostomy for enteral alimentation,

EXCISION: Excision codes (44100-44160) include allotransplantation, which like lung transplantation, is composed of three components: donor enterectomy, backbench work, and allotransplantation. These codes include biopsy, excision of lesions, enterectomy/resection by sections, anastomosis, enteroenterostomy, donor enterectomy from cadaver or living donor, allotransplantation, colectomy, colostomy, coloproctostomy, and colectomy.

LAPAROSCOPY: Laparascopy codes (44180-44238) include all of the following which are performed with the use of a scope and are not open procedures: enterolysis (freeing of adhesions), jejunostomy, ileostomy, colostomy, enterectomy, colectomy (either as partial or total and closure of enterostomy.

ENTEROSTOMY: Enterostomy codes (44300-44346) with or without placement of a tube for enterostomy or cecostomy although percutaneous of these tubes is coded elsewhere (49441-49442). Revision of ileostomy either as simple or complicated is also coded here. Colostomy or cecostomy are coded with or without biopsies in addition to revision of colostomy. Side to side anastomosis can be coded as an additional code to a major procedure, but an end to end (EEA) cannot be coded as an additional code.

ENDOSCOPY, SMALL INTESTINE AND STOMAL: Endoscopy codes for the small intestine (44360-44397) include enteroscopy with or without occurring through a stoma. These codes are differentiated by anatomic site for biopsy, stent placement, placement of jejunostomy tube, control of bleeding, removal of foreign body, removal or ablation of tumors, polyps, or lesions. Lower GI endoscopies include proctosigmoidoscopy which is examination of the rectum and sigmoid colon. Sigmoidoscopy is examination of the rectum, sigmoid colon, and part of descending colon.

Colonoscopy is examination of entire colon from rectum to cecum and possible examination of terminal ileum which can be via colostomy, colostomy, or rectum. Colonoscopies are coded according to how far anatomically the scope is advanced.

Procedures performed during a colonoscopy include removal of polyps via hot forceps, bipolar cautery, snare technique, cold biopsy forceps, and laser.

INTRODUCTION: Introduction code (44500) is for introduction of long gastrointestinal tube.

REPAIR: Repair codes (44602-44680) include suturing of small or large intestine due to perforated ulcer, diverticulum, wound, rupture, perforation or injury and with or without colostomy. Other codes include stricturoplasty, closure of enterostomy or fistula.

OTHER PROCEDURES: Other procedure codes (44700-44799) include exclusion of small intestine from the pelvis, colonic lavage, backbench work for preparation and reconstruction for transplantation.

Section 43.13: MECKEL'S DIVERTICULUM AND THE MESENTRY

EXCISION: Excision of Meckel's diverticulum is coded as 44800-44820.

SUTURE: Suture of mesentery is coded as 44850.

Section 43.14: APPENDIX

INCISION: Incision codes for the appendix (44900) include I&D of abscess either as an open procedure or percutaneously.

EXCISION: Excision codes for appendix (44950-44960) include appendectomy as the major procedure or at time of other procedure and for ruptured appendix or not.

LAPAROSCOPY: Laparoscopy procedures for appendix (44970-44979) include appendectomy or other procedure. Notice that these codes, just as with all of the codes, can be done either laparoscopically or as an open procedure and that these procedures use different codes though they have the same purpose.

Section 43.15: RECTUM

INCISION: Incision codes for rectum (45000-45020) include drainage of abscess or I&D of abscess.

EXCISION: Excision codes for rectum (45100-45172) can differ by approach and anatomic site. They include biopsies, myomectomy, protectomy either complete or partial, exenteration (removal of all organs) for malignancy, excision of tumor and anastomosis.

DESTRUCTION: Destruction code for rectum (45190) includes destruction of tumor.

ENDOSCOPY: Endoscopy codes for the rectum (45300-45392) include proctosigmoidoscopy (rectum and sigmoid colon), sigmoidoscopy (entire rectum, sigmoid colon and part of descending colon), and colonoscopy (entire colon from rectum to the cecum and may include terminal ileum). The scope can be rigid or flexible.

Endoscopies are performed for collection of specimens by brushing or washing, dilation, biopsy, control of bleeding, removal of foreign body, tumor, polyp or cyst.

LAPAROSCOPY: Laparoscopic procedures of the rectum (45395-45499) include protectomy with or without colostomy or repair such as proctopexy (fixation of rectum) for prolapse.

REPAIR: Repair codes for rectum (45500-45825) include proctoplasty for stenosis or prolapsed, injections for prolapsed, repair or rectocele (prolapsed of rectum into vaginal area), repair of injury, and closure of fistula.

MANIPULATION: Manipulation codes for the rectum (45900-45915) include reduction of procidentia (prolapse of rectum, extending even beyond the anus), dilation of anal sphincter, dilation of rectal stricture and removal of impacted feces.

OTHER PROCEDURES: Other procedures (45990-45999) codes include anorectal exam.

Section 43.16: ANUS

INCISION: Incision codes for the anus (46020-46083) include placement or removal of a seton (ligature which is inserted into the fistula and tied, so that it can be tightened over time to eliminate the fistula), I&D of abscess, sphincterotomy, and incision of thrombosed hemorrhoid.

EXCISION: Excision codes for the anus (46200-46320) include fissurectomy, sphincterotomy, hemorhoidectomy by ligation or band, excision of papilla or tag, surgical treatment of fistula, and hemorrhoidectomy.

Hemorrhoidectomy code are differentiated by internal or external or both, and if fissurectomy was also performed. Each different procedure to remove hemorrhoids should be coded. A simple hemorrhoidectomy involves simple removal such as by ligature. A complex hemorrhoidectomy involves plastic surgery. For a thrombosed external hemorrhoid, code 46083 should be used; for ligation codes 46221-46945 are used, 46946; for excision codes 46250-46262 and 46320 are used; for injection 46500 is used; for destruction 46930 is used; and for cryosurgery code 46999 is used. A column or band hemorrhoid is the hemorrhoid appearing as a pillar or column due to the rectal vein being swollen.

For fistulectomies, a submuscular involves the division of the sphincter muscle but a subcutaneous does not. A complex fistulectomy involves the excision of multiple fistulas.

INTRODUCTION: Introduction codes for the anus (46500-46505) include injection of sclerosing agent for treatment of hemorrhoid and chemodenervation of internal anal sphincter.

ENDOSCOPY: Endoscopy codes for the anus (46600-46615) include anoscopy with brushings and washing, dilation, biopsy, removal or destruction of foreign body, cyst, tumor, or polyp.

REPAIR: Repair codes for the anus (46700-46947) include anoplasty, repair of fistula or pouch, repair of anus or anomalies, sphincteroplasty, graft for rectal incontinence or prolapse, and hemorrhoidopexy (fixation of hemorrhoid).

DESTRUCTION: Destruction codes for anus (46900-46947) include destruction of lesions and hemorrhoids by electrodessicaton, cryosurgery, laser, chemical, radiofrequency, infrared coagulation, or excision, and curettage or cautery of fissures.

Section 43.17: LIVER

INCISION: Incision codes for liver (47000-47015) include biopsy by itself or as part of another procedure, hepatotomy for drainage of abscess or cyst and laparotomy with aspiration or injection.

EXCISION: Excision codes for the liver (47100-47130) include wedge biopsy, hepatectomy for resection and lobectomies varying by parts of liver excised.

LIVER TRANSPLANTATION: Liver transplantation codes for the liver (47133-47147) include allotransplantations which are composed of donor hepatectomy, backbench work, and recipient liver allotransplantation, as with any other transplantation as previously mentioned. These codes vary by portion of the liver transplanted.

REPAIR: Repair codes for the liver (47300-47362) include marsupialization (creation of a pouch with the lining of a cyst on the liver and then suturing the edges) of cyst or abscess, management of hemorrhage differentiated as simple, complex, exploration, or re-exploration.

LAPAROSCOPY: Laparoscopy codes for the liver (47370-47379) include ablation of tumor by radiofrequency or cryosurgery.

OTHER PROCEDURES: Other procedures codes for the liver (47380-47399) include ablation of tumor as an open procedure by radiofrequency or cryosurgery.

Section 43.18: BILIARY TRACT

INCISION: Incision codes for the biliary tract (47400-47480) include procedures for removal of calculus including hepaticotomy, hepaticostomy (formation of an opening into a hepatic duct), choledochotomy (incision into the common bile duct), choledochostomy (creation of an opening into the common bile duct), sphincterotomy, sphincteroplasty (surgical repair of rectal sphincter), cholecystotomy (creation of an opening the gall bladder), or cholecystostomy. Notice again the importance of the terms as the pattern continues to repeat itself based upon combining forms and anatomic sites.

INTRODUCTION: Introduction codes for the biliary tract (47490-47530) include injection procedures for cholangiography percutaneously or through an existing catheter, introduction or change of catheter or stent, and revision or reinsertion of transhepatic tube.

ENDOSCOPY: Endoscopy codes for the biliary tract (47550-47556) include an add-on code for biliary endoscopy and other codes for biopsy, removal of calculi, and dilation of biliary duct with or without stent.

LAPAROSCOPY: Laparoscopy codes for the biliary ducts (47560-47579) include laparoscopy with or without guided cholangiography with or without biopsy. Other procedures include cholecystectomy with cholangiography, exploration, or cholecystoenterostomy (.surgical anastomosis of the gallbladder and intestinal tract).

EXCISION: Excision codes for the biliary duct (47600-47715) include cholecystectomy with or without cholangiography, exploration, choledochoenterostomy (anastomosis of the bile duct to the intestine), sphincteroplasty, or sphincterotomy. Other codes include extraction of biliary duct stones, exploration of atresia of bile ducts, portoenterostomy (anastomosis of the jejunum to a certain area of the liver), excision of tumor or choledochal (bile ducts) cyst.

REPAIR: Repair codes for the biliary tract (47720-47999) include cholecystoenterostomy (surgical anastomosis of the gallbladder and intestinal tract) as direct, with gastroenterostomy, and Roux-en-Y. Other codes include anastomosis of certain anatomic sites, reconstruction, hepaticoenterostomy (surgical anastomosis between ducts and intestines), and suture for injury.

Section 43.19: PANCREAS

INCISION: Incision codes for the pancreas (48000-48020) include removal of calculus.

EXCISION: Excision codes for the pancreas (48100-48160) include biopsy open or percutaneous, resection, debridement, excision of lesion, and pancreatectomy as total, subtotal, or near total.

INTRODUCTION: Introduction code for the pancreas is 48400 and is an add-on code for injection procedure for pancreatography and is coded in addition to the primary procedure.

REPAIR: Repair codes for the pancreas (48500-48548) include marsupializtion of cyst, drainage of pseudocyst either as open or percutaneous, anastomosis for cyst, Roux-en-Y, duodenal exclusion with gastrojejunostomy for injury and pancreaticojejunostomy (anastomosis of the pancreatic duct to the jejunum) with anastomosis.

PANCREAS TRANSPLANTATION: Pancreas transplantation codes (48550-48556) include the three components that are present in other transplantation: donor pancreatectomy, backbench work and recipient pancreas allotransplantation.

Section 43.20: ABDOMEN, PERITONEUM AND OMENTUM

INCISION: Incision codes (49000-49084) include exploratory laparotomy, re-opening of laparotomy, drainage of abscess or lymphocele as either open or percutaneous by anatomic site, and centesis procedures. Notice that the terminology for the anatomic sites are included in the descriptions, such as peritoneocentesis (surgical puncture of the peritoneal cavity to obtain fluid.)

EXCISION, DESTRUCTION: Excision and destruction codes (49180-49255) include biopsy, excision or destruction of tumors, cysts or enometriomas by size, staging laparotomy for Hodgkins disease, umbilectomy, omphalectomy (excision of the umbilicus) and omentectomy (remove part or all of the omentum, a fold of the peritoneum).

LAPAROSCOPY: Laparoscopy codes (49320-49329) include diagnostic with brushings and washings to collect specimen, biopsy, aspiration of cyst, drainage of lymphocele, and insertion or replacement of cannula or catheter.

INTRODUCTION, REVISION, REMOVAL: Introduction, revision and removal codes (49400-49465) include injection of contrast material, removal of foreign body, placement of interstitial (between tissues or directly into, such as radioactive material placed directly into a tumor) devices for radiation therapy, and insertion of removal or cannula, shunt, or catheter for drainage or dialysis either as temporary or permanent.

There are specific codes for several other procedures. Initial placement codes are for insertion, conversion and replacement of tubes for gastrostomy, duodenostomy, jejunostomy, and cecostomy. If the replacement occurs through a different site than the removal of the original tube, then these two procedures must be coded separately. Notice that these codes include the use of fluoroscopic guidance so this would not be coded as an additional separate code. Also, NG (nasogastric) and OG (orogastric) tube placements are included in these codes and are not coded separately. There is an important other code for cleaning of any of these tubes (49460). Usually the contrast injection is included in these codes; however, if only a radiological evaluation is performed with contrast injection then this would be coded alone as 49465.

REPAIR: Hernias are protrusions of an organ or the fascia of an organ through the wall of the cavity Hernia codes are based on type of hernia. Types of hernias include inguinal (groin area), lumbar (back area), incisional (at site of previous incision), femoral (groin area), epigastric (above the navel), ventral (midline of the abdomen, usually at an incisional site oftentimes ventral hernias are considered incisional hernias), umbilical (navel area), hiatal (protrusion of a hernia of the stomach up into the thorax and can involve the esophagus), and Spigelian (rectus area above the epigastric vessel).

Hernias can be repaired by manipulation and stitches, use of mesh (e.g. Marlex and Prolene), or laparoscopically. When mesh is used to repair a hernia it is usually not coded as an additional code but is included; however, in repair of incisional or ventral hernias the use of mesh is coded as an additional separate code (49568).

Repair codes (49491-49659) include repair of hernias, i.e. hernioplasty, herniorrhaphy, and herniotomy. Hernia repairs (herniorrhaphies) are common procedures. Hernia codes are differentiated by (1) type or site of hernia, (2) age of patient, (3) history of hernia (initial or recurrent), and (4) clinical presentation. Clinical presentation includes reducible (protrusion can be returned to original position by manipulation), sliding (includes colon, cecum and/or urinary bladder), incarcerated (cannot be reduced or manipulated back into place), and strangulated (incarcerated hernia in which blood supply is compromised or reduced which presents as a medical emergency). If a hernia is strangulated, then the repair of the strangulated organ should be coded separately. Diaphragmatic and hiatal hernias are not coded from this section as they are not part of this anatomic site and should be coded from 43332-43337 codes.

CPT DIGESTIVE QUIZ 32

1) The patient was brought to the operative suite, prepped and draped in the usual manner. A right paramedian incision was made basically just above the umbilicus. Bleeding controlled with electrocautery. The rectus muscle was split and the peritoneal cavity was entered. We used 0.25% Marcaine with epinephrine prior to making the incision. We had to lengthen it to get some exposure. I had problems finding the appendix, as the appendix with generalized peritonitis came off and was tethered into the retroperitoneal area. I asked Dr. Vaughan to assist for exposure. We were able to basically mobilize the right colon and then we dissected the appendix from the cecum but once we found it, it was coming out fairly high off of the cecum. We tied it twice, divided it, cauterized the tip, then dissected, used the LigaSure for the mesentery and dissected it off of the duodenum. All bleeding was controlled. We irrigated thoroughly with saline, made certain that the bowel was properly placed back into the abdomen. Omentum was placed over it. We used a sheet of Seprafilm over the cecum and the right colon and another one over the omentum. The sponge, instrument, and needle count was correct and then we closed with double looped Maxon for the fascia, subcutaneous tissue closed with 2-0 Vicryl and skin was closed with V-Loc. Steri-Strip was applied. Sterile dressing was applied. Sent to recovery room in satisfactory condition. Tolerated the procedure well.

2) What are the codes for a 54-year-old patient who had a Roux-en-Y reconstruction following a complete gastrectomy for stomach cancer?

3) What are the codes for a 57-year-old patient who had a diverting colostomy with Hartmann pouch with sepsis and excision and debridement of a stage 3 sacral decubitus ulcer with ostectomy which had become necrotic.

4) What are the codes for a 62-year-old hypertensive patient who had a colostomy placed 9 days ago after resection of colonic carcinoma. Earlier today, he felt nauseated and stated that his colostomy stopped filling. He also had a sensation of "heartburn." He denies vomiting but has been nauseated. He denies diarrhea. He denies hematochezia, hematemesis, or melena. He denies abdominal pain or fever. Bowel obstruction was found and the colostomy had to be repaired.

5) What are the codes for a 41-year-old patient who had an ERCP for identification and removal of gallstones?

6) What are the codes for a 44-year-old patient in whom a videoendoscope was inserted under direct vision. The patient was found to have a meat bolus in the distal esophagus with diffuse inflammation causing compression. The bolus was displaced into the stomach. The stomach itself had an inflamed gastric mucosa as well as the first segment of the duodenum. Biopsies were obtained of the stomach and duodenum which were negative and esophageal dilatation which did not find anything.

7) What are the codes for a 41-year-old patient who was complaining of a bulging mass in the right side of the abdomen which correlated with a ventral hernia of the right abdominal wall. At this point, plication of the rectus abdominis muscle was done and Marlex mesh was applied.

8) What are the codes for a 52-year-old patient who was placed in the supine position and the F2 focus of the MSL 5000 lithotriptor, shock wave lithotripsy was started at 17 kV and went up to 23, where a total of 3000 shocks were given to the stone with fragmentation of this left renal calculi.

9) The patient brought to the operative suite, prepped and draped in the usual manner. Timeout was accomplished. Preoperative antibiotics were given and SCDs applied. Low midline incision was made, bleeding controlled with electrocautery. Fascia divided and peritoneal cavity was entered. Bookwalter retractor was placed. We able to see the area where India ink had been injected in the sigmoid colon. We used the GIA proximally and distally, divided the mesentery using the ligature. One vessel was stick-tied with 3-0 silk. We then opened the specimen and there was no polyp in it, so we then opened the bowel proximally thinking that the polyp might be just above where we had resected and, indeed, we found the polyp on a very long stalk. Resected another portion of the colon, then used a pursestringer. Placed a pursestring proximally. Used the dilators. A 29 EEA was selected. We tied the pursestring and then brought the EEA in from below, made the anastomosis. We then tested it, and there were some air bubbles, and so we had to use 3-0 silk. There was a small rent in the anastomosis on the right lateral side. This was sutured. We then tested it again. Put the anastomosis under water and produced air from below using an Asepto syringe. There were no leaks. After making sure we had a good tight anastomosis, I also brought some surrounding fat over the area where we had reinforced and put a couple more silks anteriorly. Left a 19 Blake drain through a separate stab incision through the right side, sutured in place with a 2-0 Prolene. Then used 2 sheets of Seprafilm by the omentum over the small bowel. Had a correct sponge, instrument, and needle count. Closure was a double loop of Maxon along with some interrupted #1 Vicryl, subcutaneous tissue closed with 2-0 Vicryl, and skin was closed with V-Loc subcuticular. Steri-Strip applied. Sterile dressing applied. Sent to recovery room in satisfactory condition. Tolerated the procedure well.

10) What are the codes for a 78-year-old patient who has had profound microcytic, hyperchromic anemia, initially presenting with a hemoglobin of 6.5. A few weeks ago, she was transfused, discharged, and then returned with a hemoglobin of 6.4 with recurrent anginal pectoris and marked fatigue. She reports having black tarry stool immediately prior to admission. The scope was passed through the oropharynx into the stomach. The esophagus was well seen and was normal. There was a small hiatal hernia but no evidence of erosions in the gastric mucosa. The body of the stomach distended. The instrument was withdrawn into the stomach at this point. The enteroscope was then passed into the descending duodenum and down to the jejunum. The patient was given oral contrast to facilitate visualization of the small bowel. No abnormalities or neoplasia.

CHAPTER 44
GENITOURINARY/ENDOCRINE

You will learn the following objectives in this chapter:

A. Kidney
B. Ureter
C. Bladder
D. Urethra
E. Male Genital System
F. Reproductive System Procedures
G. Intersex Surgery
H. Female Genitalia
   1. Gynecology
   2. Obstetrics
I. Oviduct/ovary
J. Ovary
K. In Vitro Fertilization
L. Maternity Care and Delivery
M. Endocrine System

Section 44.1: URINARY SYSTEM

The urinary system produces, stores, and eliminates urine consisting of two kidneys, two ureters, the bladder, the urethra, and two sphincter muscles. (cancer.gov)

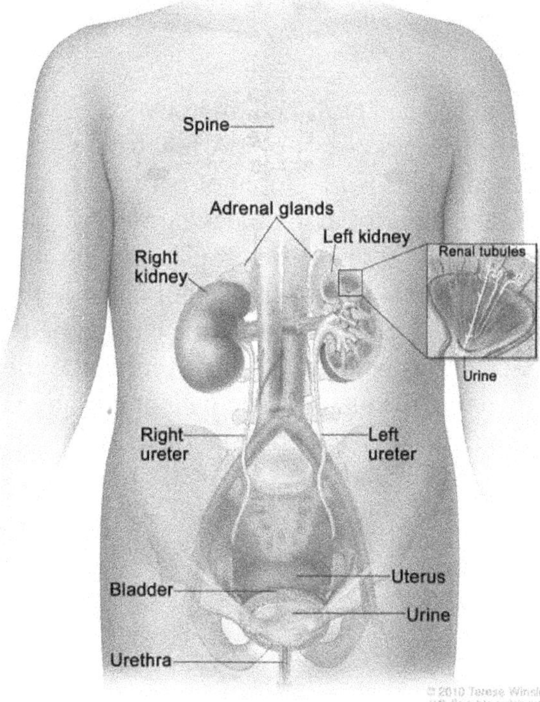

Section 44.2: KIDNEY

INCISION: Incision codes for the kidneys (50010-50135) include exploration, drainage of abscess either as open or percutaneous, nephrostomy (artificial opening created between the kidney and the skin which allows for the drainage of urine), nephrotomy with drainage of exploration, nephrolithotomy (incision for removal of calculi/stones), nephrostolithotomy (removal of medium-sized or larger renal calculi /kidney stones from the patient's urinary tract), pyelostolithotomy (removal of a calculus (stone) through an incision into the renal pelvis), stenting, lithotripsy (crushing of stones/calculi), transection or repositioning of renal vessels, pyelotomy, pyelolithotomy (incision of the renal pelvis for removal of calculi), and pyelostomy (forming an artificial opening in the renal pelvis of a kidney in order to provide a drainage route for urine) which can be differentiated as a secondary procedure or as complicated.

EXCISION: Excision codes for the kidney (50200-50290) include biopsy by needle or surgical exposure and nephrectomy in conjunction with other procedures and which can also be differentiated as complicated or radical or partial or total. Other codes include ablation of lesions and excision of cysts.

RENAL TRANSPLANTATION: Renal allotransplantation codes (50300-50380) include the three components of all transplantation: donor nephrectomy, back bench work, and recipient renal allotransplantation. There are also codes for autotransplanation (50380).

INTRODUCTION: Introduction code for the kidneys (50382-50398) include procedures on stents and catheters defined as internally dwelling or externally accessible. Procedures include removal and replacement of ureteral stents or catheters and are differentiated by approach, such as percutaneous or transurethral. Other introduction procedures include aspiration and injection of cyst and instillation of therapeutic agent through a stoma, such as nephrostomy or pyelostomy. Introduction of catheter into the renal pelvis for drainage or injection is also coded here as well as change of tubes, such as nephrostomy.

REPAIR: Repair codes for the kidney (50400-50540) include pyeloplasty as simple or complicated,). Notice that the symphsiotomy code is listed as being either unilateral or bilateral which means that this code is used once even if it is performed on both sides and it is not reduced if the procedure is performed on only one side.

LAPAROSCOPY: Laparoscopy codes for the kidneys (50541-50549) include the use of a scope to perform the following procedures: ablation of cyst or mass, partial or radical nephrectomy, pyeloplasty, and donor nephrectomy.

ENDOSCOPY: Endoscopy codes for the kidneys (50551-50580) include endoscopy through a previously created stoma (i.e. nephrostomy or pyelostomy) for biopsy, fulguration, removal of foreign body, and resection of tumor. Other codes includes endoscopy through an incision for ureteral catheterization, biopsy, endopyelotomy, fulguration and removal of foreign body.

OTHER PROCEDURES: An important and common procedure, lithotripsy is coded as 50590 which uses extracorporeal shock waves to break up calculi. Other codes in this section (50592-50593) include ablation of tumors either through radiofrequency or cryotherapy. This procedure is described as unilateral, so if this procedure is performed on both sides, a modifier 50 for bilateral procedure would need to be attached to the procedure.

Section 44.3: URETER

INCISION: Incision codes for the ureters (50600-50630) include ureterotomy for exploration or drainage, insertion of indwelling stents, (Remember that the insertion of temporary stents is usually included in a procedure but indwelling permanent stents are not and should be coded in addition to any other procedure. Remember too that a stent is a thin tube inserted into a part of the body, such as vessels or tubes, such as ureters, which then maintain an opening within the area.) Other codes include ureterolithotomy (removal of stone by incision) by portion of the ureter involved.

EXCISION: Excision codes for the ureters (50650-50660) include ureterectomy (excision of ureters).

INTRODUCTION: Introduction codes for the ureters (50684-50690) include injection procedure for ureterography (x-ray of ureters) or ureteroplyelography (x-ray of ureter and renal pelvis), manometric (measures strength of muscles) studies, and change of ureterostomy tube or stent.

REPAIR: Repair codes for the ureters (50700-50940) include ureteroplasty, ureterolysis (freeing ureters of adhesions), revision of anastomosis, ureteropyelostomy (surgical creation connecting ureter and the renal pelvis), ureteroocalycostomy (anastomosis of ureter to the calyceal system), ureteroureterostomy (end-to-end anastomosis of the two portions of a transected ureter), transureteroureterostomy (joining of one ureter to the other across the midline), ureteroneocytostomy (transplantation of a ureter to a different site in the bladder), ureteroenterostomy (anastomosis of one or both ureters to the wall of the intestine), ureterosigmoidostomy (ureters are diverted into the sigmoid colon), creation of ureterocolon or ureteroileal conduits, continent diversion (surgical procedure to provide an alternate pathway to release urine from the body), ureterostomy, ureterorrhaphy, closure of fistula, and deligation of ureter (removal of a ligature (e.g. thread) that was placed in a previous surgery).

LAPAROSCOPY: Laparoscopy procedures for the ureters (50945-50949) include the use of a scope for ureterolithotomy and ureteroneocystostomy.

ENDOSCOPY: Endoscopy procedures for the ureters (50951-50980) can be performed through an ureterostomy or ureterotomy for procedures such as catheterization, biopsy, fulguration, and removal of foreign bodies or calculus.

Section 44.4: BLADDER

Incision: Incision codes for the bladder (51020-51080) include cystotomy and cystostomy for insertion of radioactive material, cryosurgical removal of lesions, drainage, placement of catheter or stent, cystolithotomy (incision of bladder to remove calculus/stones), and ureterolithotomy.

REMOVAL: Removal codes for the bladder (51100-51102) include aspiration or insertion into bladder by needle, trocar, or catheter.

EXCISION: Excision codes for the bladder (51500-51597) include excision of cyst with or without hernia repair, cystotomy for excision of part of the bladder, cystotomy for repair of ureterocele, simple or complicated cystectomy which can be partial or total, and pelvic exenteration.

INTRODUCTION: Introduction codes for the bladder (51600-51720) include injection procedures for cystography or urethrocystography, bladder irrigation, insertion of temporary or non-indwelling bladder catheter, change of cystostomy tube as simple or complicated, bladder instillation, and injection of implant material.

URODYNAMICS: Urodynamic codes for the bladder (51725-51798) involve the flow of urine and include simple or complex cystometrograms (measuring the amount of fluid present in bladder upon first need to urinate), voiding pressure studies, simple or complex uroflowmetry (measuring volume of urine released), electromyography studies (EMG) (measuring electrical activity of muscles) by needle or other means, stimulus evoked response, and measurement of post-void residual urine by ultrasound.

REPAIR: Repair codes for the bladder (51800-51980) include cystoplasty, cystourethroplasty (surgical revision of the urinary bladder and urethra), vesicourethropexy (suspension of the bladder involving the bladder and urethra), urethropexy as simple or complicated, suspension, cystorrhaphy (suturing to repair bladder), closure of cystostomy or fistula, closure of exstrophy (congenital anomaly in which part of the bladder is outside of the body) and enterocystoplasty (using part of the intestines to provide a graft to the bladder).

LAPAROSCOPY: Laparscopic codes for the bladder (51990-51999) include the use of a scope for surgical suspension of the bladder with or without sling operation (which creates a hammock type of suspension by suturing) due to stress incontinence.

ENDOSCOPY: Endoscopy codes for the bladder (52000-52010) include cystoscopy, urethroscopy and cystourethroscopy.

TRANSURETHRAL SURGERY: Transurethral surgery codes (52204-52356) are classified as either urethra and bladder or ureters and pelvis. Therapeutic cystourethroscopy always includes diagnostic cystourethroscopy.

Procedures for the urethra and bladder include cystourethroscopy with biopsy and fulguration of lesions, or tumors by size (small, medium or large). Other cystourethroscopies include insertion of radioactive substance, biopsy, fulguration, urethrotomy, sphincterotomy, calibration of stenosis, insertion of permanent stent, steroid injections, ureteral meatotomy, fulguration of ureterocele or resection of diverticulum, removal of foreign body, and litholapaxy (crushing of a stone in the bladder and washing out the fragments through a catheter) which is differentiated as simple or complicated and removal of small or large fragments. Some of these codes are described as including both unilateral and bilateral procedures, so no additional codes or modifiers are necessary whether the procedure is bilateral or not.

Procedures for ureter and pelvis include cystourethroscopy for elimination of calculus by removal, fragmentation, lithotripsy, fulguration, injection of implant material, and manipulation. Other codes include cystourethroscopy with insertion of guide wire to establish a nephrostomy, treatment of stricture, ureteroscopy, pyeloscopy and resection of tumor.

For insertion and removal of temporary stent, these procedures are included in the primary procedure and are not coded separately. For permanent indwelling stent, code 52332 should also be coded in addition to the primary procedure. For removal of the permanent indwelling stent, codes 52310 and 52315 should be coded and modifier 58 attached.

VESICAL NECK AND PROSTATE: Vesical Neck and Prostate codes (52400-52700) include cystourethroscopy with transurethral resection, fulguration, resection of urethral valves, transurethral incision or resection of the prostate, laser coagulation or vaporization of prostate, including TURP (52630) (transurethral resection of the prostate).

Section 44.5: URETHRA

INCISION: Incision codes for the urethra (53000-53085) include urethrotomy, urethrostomy, meatotomy (incisional enlargement of the external urethral), drainage of abscess, drainage of extravasation (leakage of urine from urethra into other parts of the body) and drainage of Skene's gland (located on each side of the urethra) abscess or cyst.

EXCISION: Excision codes for the urethra (53200-53275) include biopsy, urethrectomy for female or male, excision or fulguration of cancer, excision or marsupialization of diverticulum for female or male, excision of bulbourethral (Cowper) gland, and excision or fulguration of polyps, caruncle, Skene's glands, or prolapse.

REPAIR: Repair codes for the urethra (53400-53520) include urethroplasty as either first or second stage of the procedure for treatment of a fistula or diverticulum, reconstruction, tubularization for incontinence, sling operation for incontinence, insertion, repair and removal codes for inflatable sphincter, urethromeatoplasty, urethrolysis, urethrorrhaphy, or closure of fistula.

MANIPULATION: Manipulation codes for the urethra (53600-53665) include dilation of stricture either as initial or subsequent procedure.

OTHER PROCEDURES: Other procedures codes for the urethra (53850-53899) include transurethral destruction of prostate tissue by microwave or radiofrequency and insertion of temporary stent.

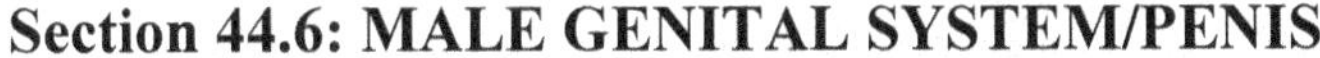

Section 44.6: MALE GENITAL SYSTEM/PENIS

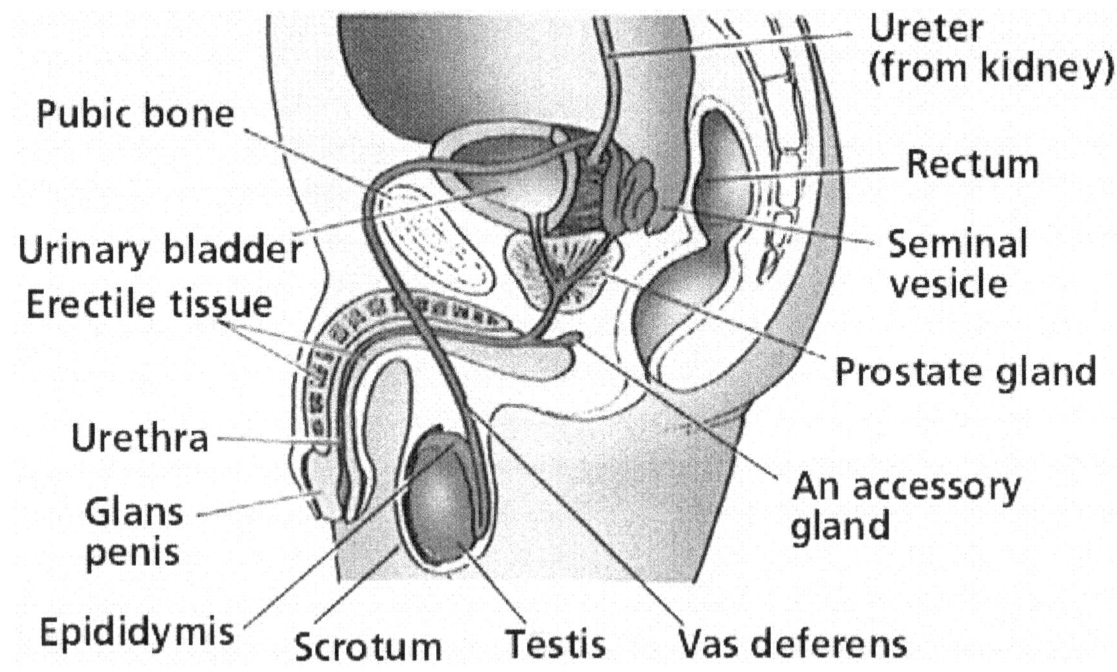

www.emc.maricopa.edu

INCISION/DESTRUCTION: Incision codes are 54000-54015. Destruction codes for the penis (54050-54065) include destruction of lesions by chemical, electrodesiccation, cryosurgery, laser or excision and as simple or extensive.

EXCISION: Excision codes for the penis (54100-54164) include circumcision which are differentiated by use of clamp or other device and if the patient is newborn or not. If the circumcision is performed on a newborn (28 days or younger) then a code for the anesthetic should also be coded (64450-47) unless it is a clamp circumcision in which case the anesthesia is included in the primary code.

OTHER CODES: Other codes include biopsy, excision of plaque with or without graft, removal of foreign body, amputation as partial or complete, lysis of excision of adhesions and frenulotomy of penis.

INTRODUCTION: Introduction codes for the penis (54200-54250) include injection for Peyronie disease (fibrosis in the penis causing hardening and other difficulties), irrigation for priapism (persistent, usually painful, erection that lasts for more than four hours) or for cavernosography (radiographic visualization of the corpus cavernosum of the penis used in conjunction oftentimes with cavernosometry in which fluid is pumped into the penis and then the vascular pressure is measured), plethysmography (process of measuring changes in volume within an organ) and test for tumescence or rigidity.

REPAIR: Repair codes for the penis (54300-54440) include straightening, urethroplasty for correction of hypospadias (congenital opening of the urethra is on the underside of the penis) by stages and associated complications, correction of angulation, correction of epispadias (congenital malformation of the penis in which the urethra ends in an opening on the upper aspect of the penis), insertion or removal of prosthesis, insertion of shunts, fistulization and treatment of an injury.

MANIPULATION: Manipulation code for the penis (54450) is for foreskin manipulation.

Section 44.7: TESTIS

EXCISION: Excision codes for the testis (54500-54535) include biopsy by needle or incision, excision of lesion, and orchiectomy (removal of the testicles) as simple, partial or radical.

EXPLORATION: Exploration codes for the testis (54550-54560) include exploration for undescended testicles by area.

REPAIR: Repair codes for the testis (54600-54680) include reduction of torsion of testicles, fixation, orchiopexy (moving an undescended testicle into the scrotum and permanently fixing it there), insertion of prosthesis, suture or repair of injury and transplantation of testicles to thigh.

LAPAROSCOPY: Laparoscopy codes for the testis (54690-54699) include the use of a scope to perform an orchiectomy or orchiopexy.

Section 44.8: EPIDIDYMIS

INCISION: Incision code for the epididymis (54700) is for I&D of abscess or hematoma.

EXCISION: Excision codes for the epididymis (54800-54861) include biopsy by needle, excision of lesion or spermatocele, and epididymectomy (surgical removal of the epididymis).

EXPLORATION: Exploration code for the epididymis (54865) is for exploration with or without biopsy.

REPAIR: Repair codes for the epididymis (54900-54901) include epididymovasostomy (severing of the vas deferens with anastomosis to the epididymis) with different codes for either unilateral or bilateral.

Section 44.9: TUNICA VAGINALIS

INCISION: Incision code for tunica vaginalis (55000) is for puncture aspiration of hydrocele.

EXCISION: Excision codes for tunica vaginalis (55040-55041) include excision of hydrocele with different codes if unilateral or bilateral.

REPAIR: Repair code for tunica vaginalis (55060) is for repair of hydrocele.

Section 44.10: SCROTUM

INCISION: Incision codes for scrotum (55100-55120) includes drainage of abscess, scrotal exploration and removal of foreign body.

EXCISION: Excision code for scrotum (55150) is for resection of scrotum.

REPAIR: Repair codes for scrotum (55175-55180) includes scrotoplasty as either simple or complicated.

Section 44.11: VAS DEFERENS

INCISION: Incision code for vas deferens (55200) is for vasotomy for cannulization.

EXCISION: Excision code for vas deferens (55250) is for a vasectomy and is described as unilateral or bilateral so no additional codes or modifiers are necessary if the procedure is performed either way. This procedure does include postoperative semen examination to determine if the semen contains sperm.

INTRODUCTION: Introduction code for vas deferens (55300) is for vasotomy for vasograms, vesiculograms or epididymograms with both bilateral and unilateral coded with the same one code.

REPAIR: Repair code for vas deferens (55400) is for vasovastostomy or vasovarsorrhaphy.

SUTURE: Suture code for vas deferens (55450) is for ligation of the vas deferens.

Section 44.12: SPERMATIC CORD

EXCISION: Excision codes for spermatic cord (55500-55540) include excision of hydrocele, lesion, or varicocele by approach including as abdominal or with hernia repair.

LAPAROSCOPY: Laparoscopy codes for spermatic cord (55550-55559) include the use of scope for ligation for varicocele.

Section 44.13: SEMINAL VESICLES

INCISION: Incision codes for seminal vesicles (55600-55605) include vesiculotomy (surgical incision of a seminal vesicle).

EXCISION: Excision codes for seminal vesicles (55650-55680) include vesiculectomy or excision of Mullerian duct cyst.

Section 44.14: PROSTATE

INCISION: Incision codes for prostate (55700-55725) include biopsy by needle, punch, or incision and prostatotomy for drainage of abscess either as simple or complicated.

EXCISION: Excision codes for prostate (55801-55865) include prostatectomy for bleeding, vasectomy, meatotomy, dilation, urethrotomy, prostatectomy with or without lymphadenectomy, exposure for insertion of radioactive material with lymph node biopsy or lymphadenectomy.

LAPAROSCOPY: Laparoscopy code for prostate (55866) is for prostatectomy using a scope.

OTHER PROCEDURES: Other procedure codes for prostate (55870-55899) include electroejaculation, ablation, and insertion of needles or catheters for placement of interstitial radioelements.

Section 44.15: REPRODUCTIVE SYSTEM PROCEDURES

The code for reproductive system procedure (55920) is for placement of needles or catheters into pelvic organs and/or genitalia for interstitial radioelement application for therapy.

Section 44.16: INTERSEX SURGERY

The codes for intersex surgery (55970-55980) are differentiated as male to female or female to male, respectively.

Section 44.17: FEMALE GENITALIA

Gynecology is the study of female reproduction. Obstetrics is the specialty dealing with the care of women and their children during pregnancy.

Section 44.18: VULVA, PERINEUM, AND INTROITUS

The first sections of these codes are for women who are not pregnant (nonobstetrical); there is a separate section for pregnancy codes to be discussed later. Also, some services and procedures related to the female genitalia are located in other coding sections, such as destruction of endiometriomas is coded from the digestive section.

INCISION: Incision codes (56405-56442) include I&D for abscess, marsupialization, lysis of adhesions, and hymenotomy.

DESTRUCTION: Destruction codes (56501-56515) include destruction of lesions which are differentiated as simple or extensive and the code can only be listed once as it includes all lesions (notice that the code is described as "lesion(s)" and is not described as being for each separate lesion.

EXCISION: Excision codes (56605-56740) include vulvectomy which are differentiated as simple, radical, partial or complete. Simple involves the removal of skin and superficial subcutaneous tissues. Radical involves the removal of skin and deep subcutaneous tissue. Partial involves the removal of less than 80% of the vulvar area. Complete involves the removal of greater than 80% of the vulvar area.

Codes also include biopsies per lesion with an add-on code for additional lesions biopsied, excision of cyst and partial hymenectomy or revision of hymenal ring.

REPAIR: Repair codes (56800-56810) include repair of introitus, perineoplasty (repair of perineum), and clitoroplasty for intersex surgery.

ENDOSCOPY: Endoscopy codes (56820-56821) include colposcopy with or without biopsy.

Section 44.19: VAGINA

INCISION: Incision codes for vagina (57000-57023) include colpotomy for exploration or drainage for abscess, colpocentesis (surgical puncture of vagina) and I&D of hematoma.

DESTRUCTION: Destruction code for vagina (57061-57065) include destruction of lesions as either simple or extensive using laser, electrosurgery, cryosurgery or chemosurgery.

EXCISION: Excision code for vagina (57100-57135) include biopsy of mucosa as either simple or extensive, vaginectomy as either partial or complete with removal of other tissues as described in the codes. Other excision codes include colpoclesis (surgical closure of the vaginal canal), excision of vaginal septum, or excision of tumor or cyst.

INTRODUCTION: Introduction codes for vagina (57150-57180) include irrigation with medication to treat infection, insertion for clinical brachytherapy (internal radiotherapy), fitting and insertion of pessary or other support device, fitting of diaphragms, and introduction of hemostatic agent to control bleeding.

Insertion of a suprapubic catheter is not coded here but is coded as 51102. Procedures for interstitial radioelement application are coded as 55920 and for insertion of radioelements such as sources and ribbons from 77761-77787 codes.

REPAIR: Repair codes for vagina (57200-57335) include colporrhaphy (suturing of vagina) for repair of injury or repair or cystocele or rectocele, colpoperineorrhaphy (suturing of vagina and perineum), plastic surgery on urethral sphincter, repair of urethrocele, repair or enterocele, colpopexy, closure of fistulas, sling operation, construction of artificial vagina with or without graft, and repair of defects. Many of these repair code differ by approach, such as vaginal, abdominal, transperineal, transvesical or intra-peritoneal.

Notice that there is a code for the use of mesh or other prosthesis used to repair a defect. This code (57267) is an add-on code and should be added to the primary procedure.

MANIPULATION: Manipulation codes for vagina (57400-57415) include dilation of vagina, pelvic examination, and removal of foreign body with anesthesia. If removal of the foreign body is performed without anesthesia, an E/M code should be used instead.

ENDOSCOPY/LAPAROSCOPY: Endoscopy/Laparoscopy codes for vagina (57420-57426) include colposcopy with or without biopsy, repair of defect, colpopexy, and revision of prosthetic graft.

Section 44.20: CERVIX UTERI

ENDOSCOPY: Endoscopy codes for cervix uteri (57452-57461) include colposcopy which include biopsies and LEEP or LOOP procedures (excision of tissue with electrosurgical device) with or without colposcopy or vaginoscopy.

EXCISION: Excision codes for cervix uteri (57500-57558) include biopsies, curettage, cautery of cervix, conization (removal of cone-shaped portion of tissue performed by cold knife or laser), excision of cervical stump by abdominal or vaginal approach and D&C.

REPAIR: Repair codes for cervix uteri (57700-57720) include cerclage (placement of stitches in the cervix to hold it closed; also known as tracheloplasty) and trachelorrhaphy (sutures of the cevix uteri).

MANIPULATION: Manipulation code for cervix uteri (57800) is for dilation of cervical canal.

Section 44.21: CORPUS UTERI

EXCISION: Excision codes for corpus uteri (58100-58294) include D&C (dilatation and curettage) for nonobstetrical patients and should not be used for a patient who is pregnant, in delivery, or postpartum. If the D&C is part of a primary procedure, then it would not be coded but is included as part of the primary procedure. These codes also include endometrial sampling (biopsy) either alone (58100) or as part of another primary procedure (58110; add-on code). Myomectomies (excision of tumors) are differentiated by number and weight of the tumors as well as by approach.

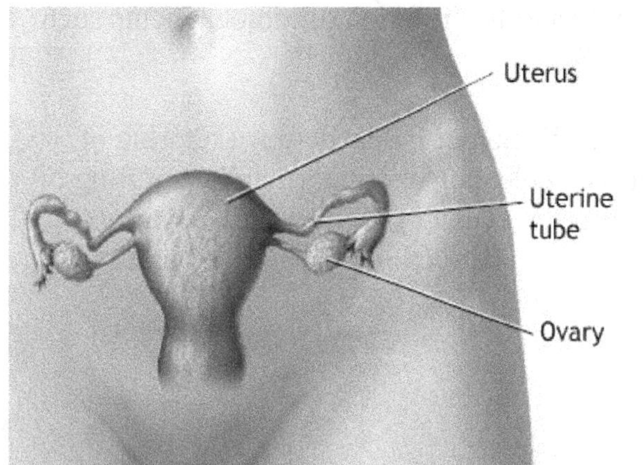

When codes describe procedures on tube(s), then the procedure is unilateral or bilateral and so no additional codes or modifiers are necessary if the procedure is performed on one or two tubes.

Nih.gov
Hysterectomies are coded as 58150-58294. They are distinguished as total, subtotal or radical as described earlier and by weight of the uterus. Complete or total hysterectomy involves the removal of the uterus and cervix. Partial or subtotal hysterectomy (supracervical) involves the removal of upper two-thirds of the uterus and leaves the cervix intact. Radical hysterectomy involves the removal of the uterus, cervix, part of the vagina, and supporting tissues.

INTRODUCTION: Introduction codes for corpus uteri (58300-58356) include insertion of IUD (intrauterine device for contraception), artificial insemination, sperm washing, catheterization of saline or contrast material for testing purposes, capsules for brachytherapy, introduction of catheter into tubes, and ablation.

REPAIR: Repair codes for corpus uteri (58400-58540) include uterine suspension with or without sympathectomy (destruction of nerves to increase blood flow), hysterorrhaphy and hysteroplasty.

LAPAROSCOPY/HYSTEROSCOPY: Laparoscopy/Hysteroscopy codes for corpus uteri (58541-58579) include the use of a scope for hysterectomy by size of uterus and type as previously discussed, myomectomy (removal of uterine leiomyomas), hysteroscopy (hysteroscope is a thin telescopic instrument that is inserted into the uterus to allow direct visualization), as diagnostic or surgical for lysis, polypectomy, removal of leiomyomata, removal of foreign body, and ablation.

Section 44.22: OVIDUCT/OVARY

INCISION: Incision codes (58600-58615) include procedures performed on the oviduct (fallopian tubes) and ovaries. Tubal ligations are performed by ligation, transaction or other means. Tubal ligations are performed during the delivery visit then code 58605; when it is performed without delivery but during another procedure of C-section, then code 58611 should be used.

LAPAROSCOPY: Laparoscopy codes (58660-58679) include fulguraton of any tissue using a scope. Note that uterine adnexae includes fallopian tubes, ovaries, pelvic viscera and peritoneal surfaces so all of these are included in the code and are not coded separately. Codes also include the use of a scope for lysis of adhesions, oophorectomy, salpingectomy, fulguration of oviducts, fimbrioplasty (surgery to repair the fimbria of a damaged or blocked fallopian tube), and salpingostomy.

EXCISION: Excision codes (58700-58720) include removal of fallopian tubes and ovaries (salpingectomy and/or oophorectomy as an open procedure) which are described as separate procedures and so should not be coed in addition to a primary procedure as they would be included in the primary procedure code.

REPAIR: Repair codes (58740-58770) include lysis of adhesions which is a separate procedure and would not be coded in addition to a primary procedure performed at the same time. Codes also include anastomosis, implantation, fimbrioplasty, and salpingostomy.

Section 44.23: OVARY

INCISION: Incision codes for ovary (58800-58825) include drainage of cysts or abscesses (both unilateral and bilateral included in the one code) and differentiated by approach, either vaginal or abdominal.

EXCISION: Excision codes for ovary (58900-58960) include oophorectomy (ovariectomy; removal of ovaries) and bilateral salpingo-oophorectomy (removal of both fallopian tubes and ovaries). Codes also include biopsy, wedge resection, ovarian cystectomy, resection of tumor or malignancy.

Section 44.24: IN VITRO FERTILIZATION

In vitro fertilization codes (58970-58976) include follicle puncture for oocyte retrieval, embryo transfer and transfer of gamete, zygote or embryo.

Section 44.25: MATERNITY CARE AND DELIVERY

Pregnancy is the state of carrying a developing baby within the female body. The three divisions of a pregnancy are:

1. ANTEPARTUM: Period prior to delivery/birth in a pregnant woman.
2. LABOR/DELIVERY: Labor begins with contractions and dilation of the cervix in preparation for delivery following which the placenta and membranes (afterbirth) are expelled from the body.
3. POSTPARTUM/PUERPERIUM: Six-week period following delivery.

One important issue with coding maternity care and delivery is that multiple codes must be listed if there are multiple births, such as twins (multiple gestations). A code must be listed for each birth; however, only one of those codes can include the antepartum and postpartum care so as to not duplicate coding for the provision of one service since the mother will not have double the antepartum or postpartum care. If one of the babies is born via C-section, then this code should include the antepartum and postpartum care as the care is more involved typically with a C-section. If both babies are born vaginally, then a second code for the vaginal delivery only would be coded in addition to the vaginal delivery code including all services. However, if both babies are born via C-section, then only one code is listed, i.e. a C-section code including antepartum and postpartum care since the C-section only occurs once.

ANTEPARTUM AND FETAL INVASIVE SERVICES: Antepartum and Fetal Invasive Services codes (59000-59076) include amniocentesis as diagnostic or therapeutic, cordocentesis, chorionic villus sampling, fetal contraction stress test, fetal scalp blood sampling, fetal monitoring, amnion fusion fetal fluid drainage, and fetal shunt placement.

EXCISION: Excision codes (59100-59160) include hysterotomy, treatment of ectopic pregnancy. Ectopic pregnancy codes are differentiated by inclusion or not of salpingectomy and/or oophorectomy and where located (ovarian, abdominal, interstitial, or cervical).

INTRODUCTION: Introduction code (59200) is for insertion of cervical dilator to enable other treatment.

REPAIR: Repair codes (59300-59350) include episiotomy or vaginal repair, cerclage of cervix, and hysterorrhaphy of ruptured uterus.

VAGINAL DELIVERY, Antepartum and Postpartum Care: Vaginal Delivery codes (59400-59430) are usually packaged with all services included. The most common code is 59400 for vaginal delivery or 59510 for C-section which includes all of the following services:

Antepartum care includes monthly visits up to 28 weeks gestation, then biweekly visits to 36 weeks, and weekly visits until delivery. Any additional complications or services beyond this are billed separately including additional complications during delivery, antepartum or postpartum.

Delivery services include admission to hospital, exams, management of uncomplicated labor, vaginal delivery and episiotomy.

Postpartum (pueripeum) care includes visits up to six weeks after delivery.

If a woman has multiple births, then a code for delivery with antepartum and postpartum services, if provided, would be coded in addition to the code for a vaginal birth with no extra services for each additional baby.

If the patient had a previous C-section and is scheduled for a vaginal delivery (VBAC – vaginal birth after Cesarean), then code 59610 would be listed which includes all antepartum, delivery, and postpartum care as described above. If only the VBAC was performed by the physician, then code 59612 would be listed. If postpartum care was included in the VBAC, then code 59614 would be listed. If the VBAC failed and a C-section was performed, then code 59618 would be listed which includes antepartum, delivery, and postpartum care. If only the C-section was performed after failed VBAC then code 59620 would be listed. If the C-section after failed VBAC and postpartum care was provided, then code 59622 would be listed.

Sometimes a patient may not receive full service (antepartum, delivery, and postpartum care) from one physician. In this case there are codes based on the number of visits or services the patient did complete with the one physician. If only delivery was provided then the code for vaginal delivery only is 59409 but if there was also postpartum care included with the vaginal delivery then it would be coded as 59410. If the delivery was Cesarean and no antepartum or postpartum care was provided, then code 59514 would be used. If postpartum services were provided after the C-section then code 59515 would be coded. If only antepartum visits were provided, then codes 59425-59426 would be listed depending on number of visits that did occur.

However, if the number of visits were less than 4 (1-3 visits), then the visits would be coded as office visits using E/M codes. If only postpartum care was provided then code 59430 would be listed.

If the baby presented breech and needed to be turned so the head was first, code 59412 would be listed which is described as external cephalic version.

If a hysterectomy was performed after C-section, then code 59525 should be listed an additional code as it is an add-on code.

CESAREAN DELIVERY: Cesarean Delivery codes (59510-59525) were previously described.

DELIVERY AFTER PREVIOUS CESAREAN DELIVERY: Delivery After Previous Cesarean Delivery codes (59610-59622) (VBAC) were previously described.

ABORTION: Abortion codes (59812-59857) include D&C for obstetric/pregnant patient. If the D&C is part of a primary procedure, then it would not be coded but is included as part of the primary procedure.

Abortions can be incomplete, missed or induced. A missed abortion must be described by the physician, which involves fetal death before 20 weeks yet retention of the fetus in the uterus during that time. Induced abortions are differentiated by method, such as D&C, injections, evacuation, suppositories and hysterotomy.

OTHER PROCEDURES: Other procedure codes (59866-59899) include procedures to reduce (eliminate one or more of multiple fetuses), uterine evacuation and curettage for mole and removal of cerclage suture.

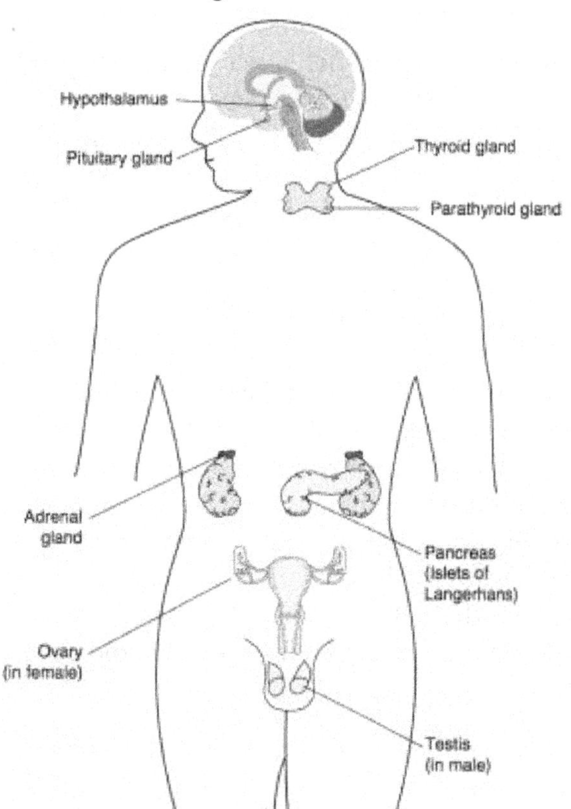

Section 44.26: ENDOCRINE SYSTEM

THYROID GLAND: Incision code for the thyroid gland (60000) is for I&D of infected cyst. Excision codes for the thyroid gland (60100-60281) include biopsy, excision of cyst or adenoma, partial or total lobectomy of the thyroid, thyroidectomy (total, subtotal, or complete), and excision of cyst. The removal code for thyroid (60300) is for aspiration and/or injection into a cyst.

PARATHYROID, THYMUS, ADRENAL GLANDS, PANCREAS, AND CAROTID BODY: Excision codes (60500-60605) include parathyroidectomy, exploration, autotransplantation, thymectomy as differentiated by approach and inclusion of radical mediastinal dissection, adrenalectomy with or without removal of tumor and excision of tumor with or without excision of carotid artery.

Laparoscopy code (60650) is for adrenalectomy (removal of adrenals) with the use of a scope.

php.med.unsw.edu.au

CPT GENITOURINARY QUIZ 33

1) What are the codes for a 37-year-old ESRD patient who is seen for insertion of dialysis catheter. Attention was directed to the right neck and with direct puncture the right internal jugular vein was cannulated with a guidewire. Advanced over the guidewire were two-vessel dilators, then the Schon temporary dialysis catheter advanced.

2) What are the codes for this 41-year-old with urodynamically documented intrinsic sphincter deficiency. Attention was turned to the anterior vaginal wall. The sling material was then prepared with packing on either side of the dissection. A strip of cadaveric fascia was incised for its width and tacked at each of the corners. A series of four interrupted sutures of 2-0 PDS were then used to tack the sling at the UVJ and down the urethra to minimize the risk of the sling rolling under the urethra. The sling was under minimal tension under the urethra. Generous purchases of the cadaveric fascia were taken and tacked.

3) What are the codes for a 38-year-old patient who had a percutaneous nephrostomy due to hydronephrosis with right ureteral obstruction?

4) What are the codes for a 32-year-old patient who had a scar in the right upper quadrant, and through that same scar the abdominal cavity was entered. Upon entering the abdominal cavity, the gallbladder was evaluated and was noted to be full of stones and phlegm. The operative cholangiogram showed some stenotic area along the common bile duct and the hepatic duct with some dilatation, but there was no obstruction. At this point the gallbladder was removed.

5) What are the codes for this 23-year-old patient who has volunteered to be a living, related kidney donor to her brother, who suffers from end-stage renal disease?

6) What are the codes for a 42-year-old patient who had fulguration of cancerous tumors in the urethra?

7) What are the codes for a 42-year-old patient who had calculus of the right kidney which was removed with ESWL?

8) What are the codes for 35-year-old unmarried patient who has 7 children. After obtaining informed consent and also discussing with the patient the alternatives, including natural family planning, birth control pills, tubal ligation, barrier methods of birth control, and vasectomy; the patient chose to continue with a vasectomy. In the operating room, the left vas deferens was identified and isolated adjacent to the scrotal skin. A 2.5-cm segment of vas deferens was then excised between hemostats. The ends of the vasa were then cauterized with Bovie electrocautery. The distal end was suture-ligated and folded back upon itself with 3-0 chromic. The proximal end was suture-ligated and then, using a second suture of 2-0 chromic, ligated and folded back upon itself. Next, attention was directed to the right side where the procedure was performed, done in identical mirror-

image fashion.

9) What are the codes for this 38-year-old man with carcinoma of the prostate who is seen today for lymphadenectomy which was done by mobilizing pelvic tissue on both sides. Frozen section revealed these to be negative. The posterior urethra was now incised and there was retropubic resection of the prostate off the rectum. A portion of this ejaculatory duct was removed with the seminal vesicles, and the bladder neck was mobilized against some mild traction of the Foley, sparing about a 1-cm section of prostatic urethra. This was everted with 3-0 chromic sutures on the seromuscular layer and anastomosed to the urethra using the Greenfield suture guide.

10) What are the codes for a 41-year-old patient who had repair of an inguinal hernia and hydrocelectomy on both sides as well as orchiopexy on the right for undescended testis?

11) What are the codes for a 28-year-old patient with excessive bleeding due to menorrhagia. The patient was then placed in Trendelenburg. Endocervical D&C was then done. A hysteroscope was placed through the cervix into the uterus. The uterine cavity was examined. There was a questionable polyp versus just a tear of the superficial endometrium noted anteriorly. The remainder of the cavity seemed normal, with normal ostia. Sharp curettage was done, and a small amount of tissue was obtained. The cervix was examined, and the hysteroscope was removed. There was no evidence of any abnormalities in the cervical canal. Specimens were submitted to pathology.

12) What are the codes for a 25-year-old patient who had TAH-BSO for uterine fibroids, endometriosis stage 4 and menometrorrhagia?

13) What are the codes for a 34-year-old patient who had surgery in which peritoneal biopsies were obtained scopically. Cul-de-sac biopsy and peritoneal omental biopsies were obtained. Uterosacral ligaments were clamped, cut, and ligated bilaterally. Uterine vessels were clamped, cut, and ligated bilaterally. Vessels in the broad ligament were clamped, cut, and ligated. There was visualization of uterine fibroids and the uterus and left ovary were then removed.

14) What are the codes for a 23-year-old patient who had a LEEP procedure today due to abnormal PAP which showed cervical dysplasia?

15) What are the codes for a 23-year-old patient who progressed to delivery; however, there was shoulder dystocia. Epsiotomy was performed. Forceps were used but did not work but shortly after with additional push, the baby was delivered. The baby was 10 pounds 3 ounces.

16) What are the codes for a 21-year-old patient who received a repeat low-abdominal Pfannenstiel incision from previous c-section due to obstructed labor. The rectus muscles were divided in the midline by sharp dissection. The lower uterine segment was carefully incised with a scalpel and extended laterally. A living female infant was delivered from the vertex right occipitotransverse position. The head was noted to be wedged into the

pelvis but was easily elevated with a hand. The baby was suctioned and cried immediately. There was marked bleeding coming from the laceration of the left uterine artery which was sutured. The first layer of uterine closure was with running-locking #1 chromic catgut suture. The second layer was with imbricating #1 chromic catgut suture.

17) What are the codes for a 31-year-old patient who is seen in ER this morning complaining of intense pelvic pain with vaginal bleeding. The patient is 8 weeks pregnant. She denies any dizziness or shoulder pain. The patient had a c-section previously and 2 normal vaginal births prior to that. She had one miscarriage. The patient smokes and does drink regularly and is diabetic. The patient's mother was also positive for diabetes and COPD with asthma. ROS negative for all systems other than previously stated. Exam revealed a well-developed, well-nourished female in no acute distress with stable vital signs and afebrile. HENT WNL. Neck is supple without masses. Lungs clear. Heart shows regular rate and rhythm without murmur or gallop. Bowel sounds are present. Pelvic shows normal external genitalia. Cervix shows some bleeding. Slightly tender to motion. Uterus: Tender. Ectopic pregnancy cannot be ruled out. Patient had an ultrasound which demonstrated ruptured tubal ectopic pregnancy which was removed laparoscopically.

18) What are the codes for this 42-year-old patient who has been having trouble sleeping. It Using the laryngeal mirror, the adenoid tissue was found to be very enlarged and totally obstructing the back of the nose which was excised and sent to pathology for diagnosis. Using the electrocautery, the hypertrophic right tonsil was amputated and sent to pathology for diagnosis. The left tonsil was then seen to have purulent material and also hypertrophic; therefore it was also excised.

19) What are the codes for a 45-year-old patient who had a total thyroidectomy with modified radical neck dissection on the right due to carcinoma metastatic to cervical lymph nodes?

20) What are the codes for a 39-year-old patient who noticed a large lump in the left side of their neck. The large left thyroid lobe was dissected from its loose attachments laterally. This was sent for pathologic examination and found to be carcinoma. It was elected to proceed with a total thyroidectomy. The superior parathyroid gland was found, dissected off the thyroid gland, and left intact.

CHAPTER 45
NERVOUS/SENSES

You will learn the following objectives in this chapter:

A. Nervous System
   1. Central Nervous System
   2. Peripheral Nervous System
   3. Sympathetic Nerves
   4. Parasympathetic Nerves
B. Skull, Meninges, and Brain
C. Spine and Spinal Cord
D. Eye Anatomy
E. Ear Anatomy
F. Operating Microscope

Section 45.1: NERVOUS SYSTEM

The nervous system is a network of neurons that carry electrical signals between the brain and the rest of the body to effect action. The central nervous system which contains the brain, spinal cord, and retina. The peripheral nervous system extends throughout the rest of the body, including 12 cranial nerves, 31 spinal nerves, and autonomic nervous system.

NERVES: Sympathetic nerves are autonomic nerves which stimulate the body, such as increasing heart rate, sweating, dilation of airways, increase blood pressure, secretion of adrenaline and inhibit digestion. Parasympathetic nerves are also autonomic nerves which slow down the body, such as contracting the pupils of the eye, lowering blood pressure, and slow down heart rate.

BRAIN: The brain is surrounded by the meninges (connective tissue membranes) which are the pia mater which is the closet to the brain, the arachnoid mater which is the middle and the dura mater which is on the outside There is a space below the arachnoid mater which contains cerebrospinal fluid (CSF) circulating in the spaces in between known as ventricles which protects and nourishes the brain.

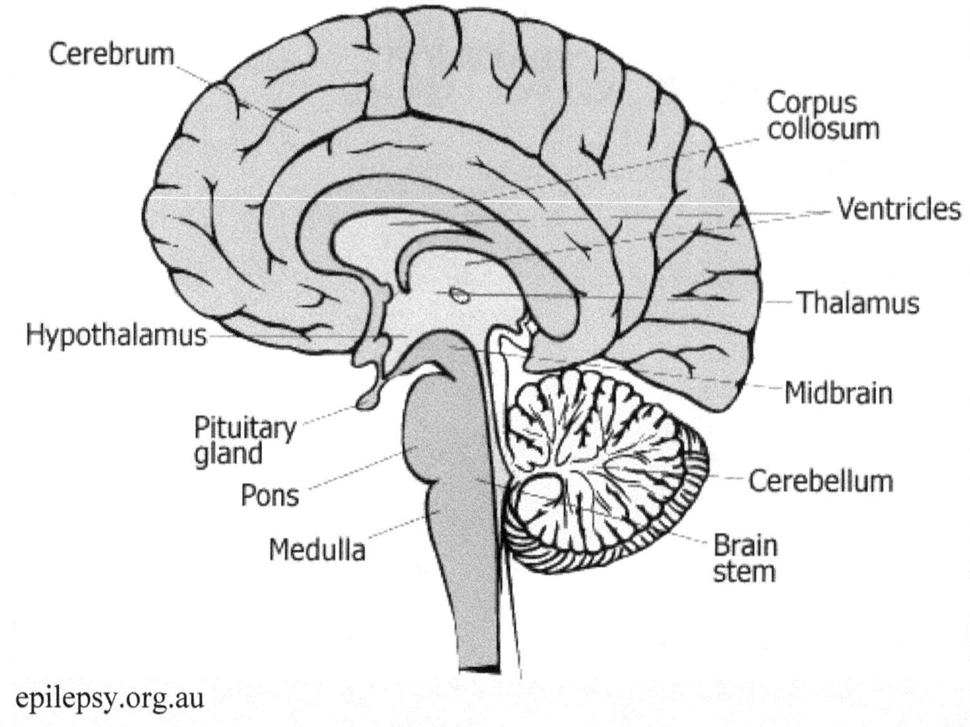

epilepsy.org.au

SPINE: Also known as backbone or vertebral column; it contains 33 vertebrae which surround and protect the spinal cord which is the collection of nerves which extend throughout the body.

VERTEBRAE: Each vertebrae consists of two parts: vertebral body in the front and vertebral arch on the posterior side which contains the vertebral foramen. The vertebral arch is formed by a pair of pedicles and a pair of laminae, and supports seven processes (4 articular, 2 transverse, and 1spinous).

LAMINAE: The two plates extending from the pedicles inwards to the spine.

Section 45.2: SKULL, MENINGES, AND BRAIN

INJECTION, DRAINAGE OR ASPIRATION: Injection procedures for graphies should be coded with other codes (36100-36218; 61026, 61120, 61055). Injection, drainage, or aspiration codes (61000-61070) include taps into the skull, punctures through burr holes with or without injection of medication, punctures into the C1-C2 of the spine and puncture of shunt tubing. For S&I of radiological tests, codes from radiology should be used in addition.

TWIST DRILL, BURR HOLES OR TREPHINE (surgical tool used to cut out bone): Twist drill hole or burr holes into the skull (61105-61253) codes are differentiated on procedure and location. These are usually used to gain access so a procedure can then be accomplished. This includes drainage, aspiration, biopsy, implantation of catheters, and insertion of reservoirs or pump for infusion systems. Some procedural codes include the holes but some do not, so if the code does not include the holes but holes were created then these codes would need to be coded in addition to the procedure.

CRANIECTOMY OR CRANIOTOMY: Craniectomy and craniotomy codes (61304-61576) are differentiated on procedure and area of the brain involved with add-on codes for grafts. Procedures include exploratory, evacuation of hematoma, drainage of abscess, lobectomy, decompression, removal of lesion, tumor or foreign body, implantation of electrodes, and repair of craniosynotosis (congenital defect in which sutures of a baby's head close too early).

SURGERY OF SKULL BASE: Skull base surgery is composed of three parts: (1) approach (61580-61598), (2) definitive procedure (61600-61616), and (3) repair/reconstruction (61618-61619). The repair and reconstruction is only coded if it is extensive, such as grafting, flaps, grafts or cranioplasty required.

ENDOVASCULAR THERAPY: Endovascular therapy codes (61623-61642) include balloon occlusion of arteries accompanying neurological monitoring and S&I of angiography, use of a catheter to create permanent occlusion or embolization such as for destruction of tumors, balloon angioplasty within the brain, placement of stents in the brain, and balloon dilatation of vessel.

SURGERY FOR ANEURYSM, ARTERIOVENOUS MALFORMATION OR VASCULAR DISEASE: Surgeries (61680-61711) include surgery of arteriovenous malformations by locations and as simple or complex. There are also surgeries of aneurysms and anastomosis. These codes include craniotomies as means of accessing the skull.

STEREOTAXIS: Stereotaxis codes (61720-61791) are for surgical techniques in which 3D medical imaging is used to find a specific site where a surgical procedure will be focused. This can be performed for biopsy, aspiration, excision, burr holes, implantation of electrodes and insertion of catheters. S&I codes from radiology should also be coded. The application of the head frame for stereotaxis is included in the procedure unless it is done at a different time at which time it can be coded as 20660.

STEREOTACTIC RADIOSURGERY: Stereotactic radiosurgery (61796-61800) is the same as stereotaxis but for the purposes of administering radiation to remove lesions. Each additional lesion removal should be coded with the add-on codes. Code 61793 must be coded only once no matter how many times this procedure is performed because the code includes "one or more sessions".

NEUROSTIMULATORS: Neurostimulators are used to treat disorders such as Parkinsons or intractable pain. These codes (61850-61888) are for simple and complex neurostimulators in the brain, and not in the spine. These codes are for placement of the neurostimulators, known as arrays, and do not include reprogramming, S&I, or testing. Recordings are included, however, and should not be coded separately. Additional arrays should be coded with add-on codes.

REPAIR: Repair codes (62000-62148) include elevation of depressed skull fracture as simple or compound, reduction of craniomegalic skull (when hydrocephalus was treated and now needs to be restored to original condition; hydrocephalus is CSF builds up in the ventricles of the brain) with cranioplasty, graft and/or reconstruction, repair of encephalocele, cranioplasty for skull defect, and removal of bone flap.

NEUROENDOSCOPY: Neuroendoscopy codes (62160-62165) include scopic procedures using a scope for placement or replacement of catheters, dissection of adhesions, retrieval of foreign body, and excision of brain or pituitary tumor.

CEREBROSPINAL FLUID SHUNT: Cerebrospinal fluid shunt codes (62180-62258) are for various systems used to remove excess CSF fluid from the brain including ventriculocisternostomy (surgical formation of opening between the ventricles of the brain and the cerebellomedullary cistern), creation of shunt, replacement of catheter, replacement of irrigation catheter, and removal of shunt system.

Section 45.3: SPINE AND SPINAL CORD

INJECTION, DRAINAGE OR ASPIRATION: Injections and punctures codes (62263-62319) are differentiated by anatomic site, whether the procedure is diagnostic or therapeutic, injection material, and single or continuous injection/infusion.

Types of spinal injections are epidural, subarachnoid, caudal, or subdural.

Injection of contrast material is included in these codes so do not code them separately (this is specified in the codes). Fluoroscopic guidance to determine the exact location for treatment is not and should be coded with 77003 but not coded for formal contrast studies (myelography, epidurography or arthrography) as it is included in those codes.

Code 62263 for catheter-based treatment can include lysis of multiple adhesions or scars by injections so these should not be coded separately. This code is also coded by multiple over a period of 2 days or more. Only one day of injections would be coded as 62264.

Other codes include aspiration, biopsy, spinal puncture (diagnostic or therapeutic), epidural injection, injection or infusion of neurolytic substance, injections for myelography/tomography, decompression (procedures performed to relieve pressure on disks of the spine), discography (record of the discs) by each level of the spine, treatment of occlusions, and chemonucleolysis (procedure to dissolve the nucleus puplosus (NP) which is the cushioning material between vertebrae which prevents them from rubbing against each other and absorbs shock; however, sometimes this material can bulge or tear which causes pain and is known as a herniated NP or better known as a herniated disk.)

Catheter Implantation: Catheter implantation codes (62350-62355) implantation, revision, removal or repositioning of catheters for long term medication administration.

Reservoir/Pump Implantation: Reservoir/pump implantation codes (62360-62370) include implantation, replacement, removal and electronic analysis of programmable pump for drug infusion.

Posterior Extradural Laminotomy or Laminectomy for Exploration/Decompression of Neural Elements or Excision of Herniated Intervertebral Discs: The codes for laminotomy or laminectomy (63001-63051) include excision (laminectomy), incisions, (laminotomies) and surgical repair (laminoplasty) of intervertebral disks by portion of the spine involved as treatment for herniated discs.

Intervertebral disks are described the spaces between disks, so one space would be designated as S1-S2. Two disks could be designated as S1-S3 which are two intervertebral disks at the beginning of the sacral area.

A laminotomy is a hemi-laminectomy. These codes are differentiated as to if facetectomy (excision of the articular facet of a vertebra), discectomy, or foraminotomy (procedure used to enlarge the space through which the spinal nerves pass in order to alleviate pressure on the nerves) also was performed.

TRANSPEDICULAR OR COSTOVERTEBRAL APPROACH FOR POSTEROLATERAL EXTRADURAL EXPLORATION/DECOMPRESSION: These exploration/decompression codes (63055-63066) are differentiated by approach, either transpedicular or costovertebral, which spinal segment, and how many segments involved.

ANTERIOR OR ANTEROLATERAL APPROACH FOR EXTRADURAL EXPLORATION/DECOMPRESSION: These codes (63075-63091) are also for exploration and decompression but the approach is by anterior or anterolateral. These codes are differentiated by specific and number of segments. These codes also include vertebral corpectomy (removal of the body of the vertebra).

LATERAL EXTRACAVITARY APPROACH FOR EXTRADURAL EXPLORATION/DECOMPRESSION: These codes (63101-63103) are also for exploration and decompression but the approach is by lateral extracavitary. These codes are differentiated by specific and number of segments. These codes also include vertebral corpectomy (removal of the body of the vertebra).

INCISION: Incision codes (63170-63200) include laminectomies with various additional services, such as myelotomy (severing of the fibers in the spinal cord), drainage of cyst, rhizotomy (selective severing of nerve roots in the spinal cord), excision of nerves or ligaments, cordotomy (cutting of the spinal cord in a specified area) and release of tethered (tissue attachments which limit flexibility) spinal cord.

EXCISION BY LAMINECTOMY OF LESION OTHER THAN HERNIATED DISC: Laminectomy of lesion codes (63250-63295) are differentiated by specific area of the spine and if it the lesion is a neoplasm or not. If reconstruction is required, then this is coded as 63295 as an add-on code.

EXCISION, ANTERIOR OR ANTEROLATERAL APPROACH, INTRASPINAL LESION: Excision of lesion of the spine in these codes (63300-63308) are differentiated by approach as either anterior or anterolateral, if it was intradural (within the subarachnoid area) or extradural (outside the thecal sac) and by specific area of the spine.

STEREOTAXIS: Stereotaxis codes (63600-63615) are for stereotactic creation of lesion, stimulation of the spinal cord, biopsy, aspiration or excision of lesion.

STEREOTACTIC RADIOSURGERY: Stereotactic radiosurgery codes (63620-63621) is used to define a target to administer radiation to the tumor. There is an add-on code for each additional lesion that is treated.

NEUROSTIMULATORS: Neurostimulator codes (63650-63688) are for both simple and complex neurostimulators. These codes include placement, revision, replacement or removal of the catheter electrodes as the neurostimulators. Arrays are collection of electrode contacts that are on one catheter that is implanted.

REPAIR: Repair codes (63700-63710) are for repair of meningocele (protrusion of membranes covering the spine) by size, repair of CSF (cerebrospinal fluid) leak or pseudomeningocele (collection of CSF fluid), and spinal dural graft.

SHUNT, SPINAL: Shunt codes (63740-63746) include creation, removal or replacement of shunt.

Section 45.4: EXTRACRANIAL NERVES, PERIPHERAL NERVES, AND AUTONOMIC NERVES

INTRODUCTION/INJECTION OF ANESTHETIC AGENT, DIAGNOSTIC OR THERAPEUTIC: Introduction and injection codes (64400-64530) include injection of anesthetic, steroid, and therapeutic agent by nerve into extracranial nerves (those outside of the brain) which include somatic, paravertebral and autonomic nerves.

NEUROSTIMULATORS: Neurostimulator codes (64550-64595) for the extracranial nerves include implantation and revisions of electrodes as neurostimulators.

DESTRUCTION BY NEUROLYTIC AGENT: Destruction by neurolytic agent codes (64600-64681) include injections for destruction, chemodenervation and therapy.

NEUROPLASTY: Neuroplasty codes (64702-64727) is the decompression or freeing of nerves from scar tissue by specific nerve.

TRANSECTION OR AVULSION: Transection or avulsion codes (64732-64772) are reported by specific nerve.

EXCISION: Excision codes (64774-64823) are differentiated by nerve (somatic or sympathetic).

NEURORRHAPHY Neurorrphaphy codes (64831-64876) involve suturing of nerves for repair and is differentiated by specific nerve and if suturing was delayed.

NEURORRHAPHY WITH NERVE GRAFT, VEIN GRAFT OR CONDUIT: Neurorrhaphy with nerve grafts codes (64885-64911) are for suturing that involves a graft.

Section 45.5: EYE

The anterior segment is the front third of the eye that includes the structures in front of the vitreous humor: the cornea, iris, ciliary body, and lens. The anterior segment is composed of the anterior and posterior chambers. The anterior chamber is located directly between the cornea and iris. The posterior chamber is located between the iris and the lens.

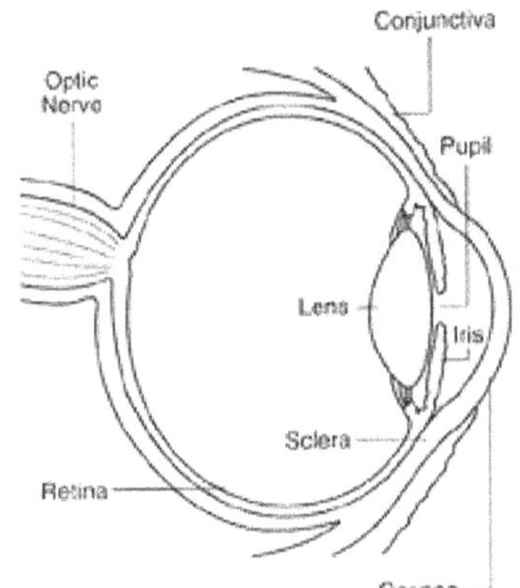

The posterior segment is the back two-thirds of the eye that includes the anterior hyaloid membrane and all of the optical structures behind it: the vitreous humor, retina, choroid, and optic nerve.

For most procedures, laterality needs to be indicated as left or right eye using RT and LT attached to the end of the procedure code.

Nih.gov

REMOVAL OF EYE: Removal of eyeball codes (65091-65114) include evisceration (surgical removal of contents of eye) with or without implant, enucleation (removal of entire eye) of eye with or without implant and exenteration (removal of all contents) with removal of orbital contents or bone and use of flap for repair.

SECONDARY IMPLANT PROCEDURES: Secondary implant procedures (65125-65175) include insertion, removal or modification of implant.

REMOVAL OF FOREIGN BODY: Removal of foreign body codes (65205-65265) are based on location of the foreign body (external or intraocular), if embedded, and use of a slit lamp to perform the procedure.

REPAIR OF LACERATION: Repair of laceration codes (65270-65290) include direct closure, mobilization, and rearrangement by anatomic site and with or without hospitalization.

ANTERIOR SEGMENT: Cornea codes (65400-65782) include excision of lesion, biopsy, scraping of cornea, destruction of lesion, and keratoplasty (corneal transplant using grafts and donor material) and are distinguished as lamellar (outermost layers of the cornea) and penetrating (full-thickness corneal tissue).

Other procedures include keratomileusis, keratophakia, keratoprosthesis, radial keratotomy, corneal wedge resection, and ocular surface reconstruction.

Anterior chamber codes (65800-66030) include treatment of glaucoma by several methods, including goniotomy (use of knife to open the trabecular meshwork and increase flow of fluids), trabeculoplasty (use of trabecultome to open the trabecular meshwork and increase flow of fluids), trabeculoplasty with laser (laser creates holes in the trabecular meshwork), fistulization of sclera (extra holes are created in the sclera to allow flow of fluids), trabeculectomy ab externo (flap is created to provide additional reservoir for fluids), and aqueous shunt to an extraocular reservoir for fluid.

Anterior sclera codes (66130-66250) include excision of lesion, fistulization of sclera for glaucoma, aqueous shunt, and trabeculotomy as mentioned above for treatment of glaucoma.

Iris, Ciliary body codes (66500-66770) include iridotomy, iridectomy, repairs, sutures, and destruction by diathermy, cyclophotocoagulation (use of laser surgery to reduce the amount of fluid entering the eye), cryotherapy, and cylodialysis, iridoplasty and destruction of lesions.

LENS: Lens codes (66820-66986) include procedural codes for treatment of cataracts. These procedures include many other procedures which are included in the code and not coded separately, such as capsulotomy, canthotomy and insertion of intraocular lens if performed at same time.

There are two types of lens extraction for cataract surgery: ECCE (extracapsular cataract extraction) and ICCE (intracapsular cataract extraction). With ECCE, the posterior capsule is not removed but with ICCE the posterior capsule is removed. The lens is also removed in these procedures.

Ocular implants are also part of the cataract surgery and if not performed at the same time as the extraction of the cataract, then they can be coded. These implants are known as IOL, intraocular lens.

Other codes include phacoemulsification which is a cataract extraction procedure using ultrasound waves to break up the lens. Phacofragmentation is a technique in which the lens is broken into pieces by mechanical means. Intraocular lens procedure codes (66982-66986) are described above.

Other procedure codes (66990-66999) include use of ophthalmic endoscope in addition to other procedures and is an add-on code.

POSTERIOR SEGMENT: Vitreous codes (67005-67043) include vitrectomy (removal of vitreous fluid) and implantation or replacement of intravitreal drug delivery system. Vitrectomy involves the removal of the vitreous humor and replacement with another solution.

Retina or choroid codes (67101-67229) include repair of retinal detachment by diathermy, cryotherapy or photocoagulation. Only one of these codes can be listed even if several of these modalities were used; the primary modality would be the only listed code.

Retinal detachment (when layers of retina separate) is corrected with surgical reattachment by one of several procedures including sclera buckling or vitrectomy.

Destruction codes include destruction of lesions by diathermy, photocoagulation, photodynamic, cryotherapy, or radiation as well as treatment of diabetic retinopathy.

Posterior sclera codes (67250-67255) include scleral reinforcement with or without graft.

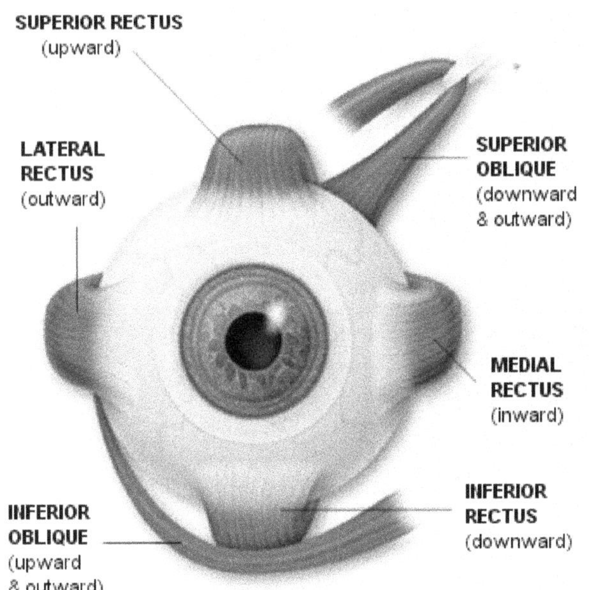

OCULAR ADNEXA: Extraocular muscle codes (67311-67399) include correction of strabismus. These codes are based on the muscles of the eye which are composed of "six extraocular eye muscles, two horizontal (lateral rectus and medial rectus) and four vertical (inferior rectus, superior rectus, inferior oblique, and superior oblique). There is a separate code if the strabismus surgery is for the superior oblique muscle.

www.cs.txstate.edu

There are additional add-on codes if this procedure is not the first strabismus surgery because there are additional services required if there has been a previous surgery. If adjustable sutures are also provided, these should also be coded as an additional code (67335).

Orbit codes (67400-67599) include orbitotomy with drainage, removal of lesion, bone flap, or removal of foreign body. Other codes include fine needle aspiration of orbital contents, injections of medication, orbital implant, optic nerve decompression.

Eyelid codes (67700-67999) include blepharotomy for drainage of abscess, severing of tarshorrhaphy (procedure to temporarily close the eyes), canthotomy, excision of chalazion differentiated by lids involved, biopsy, correction of trichiasis (when eye lashes grow in towards the eyes), excision or destruction of lesions.

Other codes include repair of brow ptosis or blepharoptosis as differentiated by muscles, correction of lid retraction, repair of ectropion (lower eyelid turns outward) or entropion (eyelids turn inwards) by suture, thermocauterization, excision wedge, or as extensive. Reconstruction includes suture of wound as partial thickness or full thickness, removal of embedded foreign body, canthoplasty, and reconstruction of eyelid.

CONJUNCTIVA: Incision and Drainage codes (68020-68040) include I&D of conjunctiva and expression of follicles.

Excision and destruction codes (68100-68135) include biopsy and excision or destruction of lesions. Injection code (68200) is for subconjunctival injections. Conjunctivoplasty codes (68320-68340) include conjunctivoplasty with grafts or reconstruction and repair of symblepharon (adhesion of eyelids to eyeball) with or without graft.

Other procedure codes (68360-68399) include conjunctival flap and harvesting of allograft.

Lacrimal System codes (68400-68899) include I&D of lacrimal gland or sac, excision of lacrimal sac or gland as total or partial, biopsy, removal of foreign body, and excision of tumor. Other codes include plastic surgery of canaliculi, dacryocystorhinostomy (fistulization of lacrimal sac to nasal cavity), conjunctivorhinoplasty (fistulization of conjunctiva to nasal cavity), closure of lacrimal punctum, dilation of lacrimal punctum, and probing of nasolacrimal duct as differentiated by insertion of stent, catheter, or anesthesia.

Section 45.6: EAR

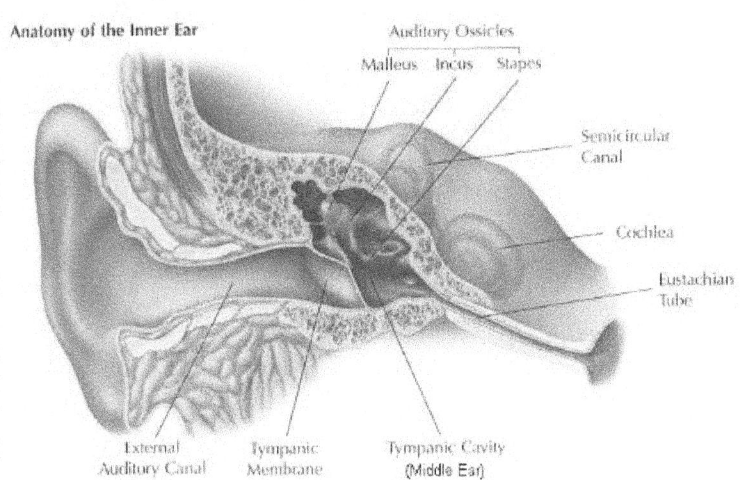

EXTERNAL EAR: Incision codes for external ear (69000-69090) include ear piercing and drainage of abscess or hematoma as simple or complicated. Excision codes for external ear (69100-69155) include biopsy, excision or amputation of external ear with or without neck dissection.

www.ent.uci.edu

Removal codes for external ear (69200-69222) include removal of foreign body with or without anesthesia, removal of impacted cerumen (ear wax), and debridement and mastoidectomy as simple or complex.

Repair codes for external ear (69300-69320) include otoplasty and reconstruction of external ear or canal.

MIDDLE EAR: Introduction codes for middle ear (69400-69405) include inflation of Eustachian tube with or without catheterization. Incision codes for middle ear (69420-69450) include myringotomy, tympanostomy (insertion of ventilating tubes, usually for infections), and removal of ventilating tubes. Other codes include middle ear exploration and tympanolysis.

Excision codes for middle ear (69501-69554) include antrotomy, resection of temporal bone, excision of polyp or tumor and mastoidectomy (surgery to remove cells in the hollow, air-filled spaces in the skull behind the ear due to infection; these codes are differentiated as complete, modified radical or radical),

Repair codes for middle ear (69601-69676) include revision of mastoidectomy so more comprehensive, tympanic membrane repair, repair of fistula and tympanic neurectomy, myringoplasty (surgical procedure to close a hole in the ear drum), tympanoplasty with or without prosthesis and dependent upon structures involved, stapes mobilization, stapedectomy (,removal of innermost bone (stapes) of the middle ear with replacement a prosthesis). Other procedures (69700-69799) include suturing, replacement of a graft, and closure of a fistula.

INNER EAR: Incision and Drainage codes for inner ear (69801-69840) include fenestration and labyrinthotomy (incision into the labyrinth of the ear) with or without mastoidectomy. Excision codes for inner ear (69905-69915) include labyrinthectomy with or without mastoidectomy. Introduction code for inner ear (69930) is for cochlear device implantation.

TEMPORAL BONE, MIDDLE FOSSA APPROACH: Codes 69950-69970 include vestibular nerve section, total facial nerve decompression, decompression of internal auditory canal and removal of tumor.

Section 45.7: OPERATING MICROSCOPE

Code 69990 is for the use of a microscope which can only be coded if surgery involves the use of a microscope but the microscope is not already included in the primary procedural code. Terms such as microvascular or microscopic within a code's description indicates that the microscope is already included in the primary procedure's code and so this code should not be coded additionally.

CPT NERVOUS/SENSES QUIZ 34

1) What are the codes for a 44-year-old patient who had epidural blocks to treat herniated discs at L4-S1?

2) What are the codes for a 61-year-old patient who has left lower extremity footdrop and received an EMG which was abnormal and confirmed peroneal nerve dysfunction on the left side at the fibular head and does not seem to suggest a problem regarding the L5 nerve root.

3) What are the codes for a 37-year-old patient with chronic low back pain which is sympathetic. I have suggested to the patient that we go ahead and perform a rhizotomy. A line was drawn to mark the sacral ala and the medial and superior aspects of each transverse process. There was radiofrequency facet denervation from L1-S1. A total of 10 lesioning denervation rhizotomies sites were performed.

4) What are the codes for a 69-year-old patient who had excision of intervertebral discs C4-6 with arthrodesis using an anterior approach for spondylosis and displacement with myelopathy?

5) What are the codes for a 33-year-old patient who had release of right carpal tunnel?

6) What are the codes for a 22-year-old patient who had left frontal burr hole for placement of ventriculostomy due to brain swelling suffered after falling from a roof?

7) What are the codes for a 42-year-old patient who had decompression at the L4-S1 levels due to severe back pain. The fusion was done using the posterior lumbar interbody technique with BAK instrumentation. X-rays were taken throughout the procedures with fluoroscopy. There was an abundant quantity of bone from the laminectomy, so no bone graft was needed from elsewhere. This bone graft was packed into the cage at the distal end and then the cage was inserted. The proximal end of the cage was then packed with bone as well. The same technique was then done on the right-hand side and the same technique was done at the L5-S1 level, for a total of four cages. Because this was a two-level cage procedure, the pedicle screw instrumentation was used to augment the stabilization.

8) What are the codes for a patient whose right eye was prepared and draped in the usual sterile fashion. Conjunctival incisions were made nasally and temporally, and a 4-mm infusion cannula was sutured into the inferotemporal quadrant 4 mm posterior to the limbus using a 4-0 Vicryl suture. After cannula tip placement in the vitreous cavity had been verified, infusion was begun. Supranasal and superotemporal sclerotomies were performed, and the trocar and cannula system was introduced to correct primary open-angle glaucoma, severe stage. The vitrectomy was performed. The posterior vitreous was not detached. It was elevated from the posterior pole and trimmed back into the far periphery. We then selected a biopsy site inferiorly and cut out a 2 x 2-mm piece of retina at 6 o'clock at the border of infected and noninfected retina. There was no significant

bleeding. We then performed a fluid-gas exchange, flatting the retina through the biopsy site. Laser was placed around the biopsy for 360 degrees to demarcate the peripheral retinitis. We then filled the eye with silicone oil. The sclerotomies were sutured shut with 7-0 Vicryl, and the conjunctiva was closed with 6-0 plain. Sub-Tenon's Ancef and Decadron were injected. The patient tolerated the procedure well and was returned to the recovery room in stable condition.

9) What are the codes for this 48-year-old patient whose right eye was prepped and draped for the procedure. Chalazion forceps were used to grasp the upper right eyelid. The pretarsal conjunctival surface of the chalazion was incised. The contents of the chalazion were curetted.

10) What are the codes for a 68-year-old patient who was seen for pseudophakic bullous keratopathy of left eye. Blepharostat was inserted and sutured to the episclera. A 7.5-mm trephine was then used for the recipient until penetration occurred. Curved corneal scissors to the right and left were used to completely excise the recipient button. The pupil was enlarged and small amounts of capsule and cortical material were also excised. The donor corneal button was transferred to the operative field, where it was secured. The intraocular Healon was evacuated and replaced with balanced salt solution. The blepharostat was removed and subconjunctival injections of gentamicin, Ancef and Celestone were given and a drop of Betagan 0.5% was instilled.

11) What are the codes for this 47-year-old patient who had a amyloid pterygium marked and subconjunctival injection of 1% lidocaine with epinephrine. The pterygium of the left eye was then resected. The head of the pterygium was dissected off the cornea. A conjunctival graft measuring 10 × 8 mm was harvested from the superior bulbar conjunctiva and replanted.

12) What are the codes for this 63-year-old patient who had the excess skin of upper lid of both eyes crease demarcated to repair paralytic ptosis. Utilizing sharp dissection, the eyelid skin and orbicularis were removed.

13) What are the codes for a 42-year-old patient who had a MSICS and capsulotomy of the nucleus, due to diabetic cataracts. A phacoemulsification tip was introduced and a large bowl sculpted. The remaining nucleus was brought into the anterior chamber, and with the pulse mode and phacoemulsification with high vacuum, the remaining nucleus was prolapsed and removed without complication. A posterior chamber lens implant of the appropriate power was placed.

14) What are the codes for this 47-year-old patient who had strabismus surgery two years ago and is seen today for the same which was for correction of monocular pattern esotropia of the left eye?

15) What are the codes for this 64-year-old patient who had repair of retinal detachment with single break of the right eye by cryothermy and photocoagulation?

16) What are the codes for a 61-year-old patient who has been experiencing slow, decreasing vision in the right eye secondary to punctate cataract formation. A fornix-based conjunctival flap was formed with Westcott scissors. Clear-cornea paracentesis wound was made. A crescent blade was used to fashion a scleral tunnel through which the anterior chamber was entered and anterior capsulotomy performed with a capsulorrhexis technique. The nucleus was hydrodissected with balanced salt solution and emulsified with the phacoemulsification device. The remaining cortex was removed using irrigation and aspiration. Using a smooth lens forceps, we introduced the lens into the eye.

17) What are the codes for this 8-year-old patient seen today for chronic suppurative otitis media of both ears. Using the Zeiss operating microscope, the left tympanic membrane was visualized. The canal was cleaned of cerumen. A radial incision was made in the anteroinferior quadrant. "Glue" was found behind this ear, and this was suctioned. A 0.40 Shepard tube was put into place. Cortisporin Otic suspension drops were instilled, and a cotton ball was placed at the meatus. The right tympanic membrane was then visualized using the same Zeiss operating microscope. The canal was cleaned of cerumen. Using the laryngeal mirror, the adenoid tissue was found to be moderately enlarged but was not removed.

18) What are the codes for a 6-year-old patient who had bilateral myringotomy and tubes for chronic Eustachian tube dysfunction and recurrent acute serous otitis media?

19) What are the codes for patient in whom a scope was used to visualize and inspect. There was a small retention cyst noted arising from the anterior medial wall of the left maxillary sinus which was filled full of a whitish glue-type material and inflamed, although it was nonpurulent and so an antrostomy was performed to remove it in addition to ethmoidectomy.

20) What are the codes for this 12-year-old patient who has continued to have problems with acute serous otitis media so an anterior inferior myringotomy was performed on the left tympanic membrane. An Armstrong tube was placed and ear drops following into the canal. With the use of an operating microscope, an anterior inferior myringotomy was performed on the right tympanic membrane, and through it no effusion was suctioned. An Armstrong tube was placed and ear drops following into the canal.

TEST 4
ICD-10 AND CPT CHAPTERS 1 - 46

1. What are the codes for this 8-year-old patient seen today for chronic suppurative otitis media of both ears. Using the Zeiss operating microscope, the left tympanic membrane was visualized. The canal was cleaned of cerumen. A radial incision was made in the anteroinferior quadrant. "Glue" was found behind this ear, and this was suctioned. A 0.40 Shepard tube was put into place. Cortisporin Otic suspension drops were instilled, and a cotton ball was placed at the meatus. The right tympanic membrane was then visualized using the same Zeiss operating microscope. The canal was cleaned of cerumen. Using the laryngeal mirror, the adenoid tissue was found to be moderately enlarged but was not removed.

2. What are the codes for a 6-year-old patient who had bilateral myringotomy and tubes for chronic Eustachian tube dysfunction and recurrent acute serous otitis media?

3. What are the codes for a patient whose right eye was prepared and draped in the usual sterile fashion. Conjunctival incisions were made nasally and temporally, and a 4-mm infusion cannula was sutured into the inferotemporal quadrant 4 mm posterior to the limbus using a 4-0 Vicryl suture. After cannula tip placement in the vitreous cavity had been verified, infusion was begun. Supranasal and superotemporal sclerotomies were performed, and the trocar and cannula system was introduced to correct primary open-angle glaucoma, severe stage. The vitrectomy was performed. The posterior vitreous was not detached. It was elevated from the posterior pole and trimmed back into the far periphery. We then selected a biopsy site inferiorly and cut out a 2 x 2-mm piece of retina at 6 o'clock at the border of infected and noninfected retina. There was no significant bleeding. We then performed a fluid-gas exchange, flatting the retina through the biopsy site. Laser was placed around the biopsy for 360 degrees to demarcate the peripheral retinitis. We then filled the eye with silicone oil. The sclerotomies were sutured shut with 7-0 Vicryl, and the conjunctiva was closed with 6-0 plain. Sub-Tenon's Ancef and Decadron were injected. The patient tolerated the procedure well and was returned to the recovery room in stable condition.

4. An incision was made supertemporally to expose the right medial rectus muscle which was disinserted from the globe and reattached to the glob for treatment of esotropia. The right superior rectus muscle was then hooked to the muscle, disinserted and reattached to the globe. The left medial rectus muscle was then recessed in a similar manner.

5. What are the codes for a 68-year-old patient who was seen for pseudophakic bullous keratopathy of left eye. Blepharostat was inserted and sutured to the episclera. A 7.5-mm trephine was then used for the recipient until penetration occurred. Curved corneal scissors to the right and left were used to completely excise the recipient button. The pupil was enlarged and small amounts of capsule and cortical material were also excised. The donor corneal button was transferred to the operative field, where it was secured. The intraocular Healon was evacuated and replaced with balanced salt solution. The

blepharostat was removed and subconjunctival injections of gentamicin, Ancef and Celestone were given and a drop of Betagan 0.5% was instilled.

6. What are the codes for this 47-year-old patient who had a conjunctival pterygium marked and subconjunctival injection of 1% lidocaine with epinephrine. The pterygium was then resected. The head of the pterygium was dissected off the cornea. A conjunctival graft measuring 10 × 8 mm was harvested from the superior bulbar conjunctiva and replanted.

7. What are the codes for this 63-year-old patient who had the excess skin of upper lid of both eyes crease demarcated to repair paralytic ptosis. Utilizing sharp dissection, the eyelid skin and orbicularis were removed.

8. What are the codes for a 61-year-old patient who has been experiencing slow, decreasing vision in the right eye secondary to punctate cataract formation. A fornix-based conjunctival flap was formed with Westcott scissors. Clear-cornea paracentesis wound was made. A crescent blade was used to fashion a scleral tunnel through which the anterior chamber was entered and anterior capsulotomy performed with a capsulorrhexis technique. The nucleus was hydrodissected with balanced salt solution and emulsified with the phacoemulsification device. The remaining cortex was removed using irrigation and aspiration. Using a smooth lens forceps, we introduced the lens into the eye.

9. What are the codes for a 61-year-old patient who has left lower extremity footdrop and received an EMG which was abnormal and confirmed peroneal nerve dysfunction on the left side at the fibular head and does not seem to suggest a problem regarding the L5 nerve root.

10. What are the codes for a 37-year-old patient with chronic low back pain which is sympathetic. I have suggested to the patient that we go ahead and perform a rhizotomy. A line was drawn to mark the sacral ala and the medial and superior aspects of each transverse process. There was radiofrequency facet denervation from L1-S1. A total of 10 lesioning denervation rhizotomies sites were performed.

11. What are the codes for a 42-year-old patient who had decompression at the L4-S1 levels due to severe back pain. The fusion was done using the posterior lumbar interbody technique with BAK instrumentation. X-rays were taken throughout the procedures with fluoroscopy. There was an abundant quantity of bone from the laminectomy, so no bone graft was needed from elsewhere. This bone graft was packed into the cage at the distal end and then the cage was inserted. The proximal end of the cage was then packed with bone as well. The same technique was then done on the right-hand side and the same technique was done at the L5-S1 level, for a total of four cages. Because this was a two-level cage procedure, the pedicle screw instrumentation was used to augment the stabilization.

12. What are the codes for this 42-year-old patient who has been having trouble sleeping. It Using the laryngeal mirror, the adenoid tissue was found to be very enlarged and totally

obstructing the back of the nose which was excised and sent to pathology for diagnosis. Using the electrocautery, the hypertrophic right tonsil was amputated and sent to pathology for diagnosis. The left tonsil was then seen to have purulent material and also hypertrophic; therefore it was also excised.

13. What are the codes for a 45-year-old patient who had a total thyroidectomy with modified radical neck dissection on the right due to carcinoma metastatic to cervical lymph nodes?

14. What are the codes for a 47-year-old patient with ESRD. The patient had no superficial veins large enough on the distal forearm that would suffice for bypass and AV fistula creation. An incision was made in the antecubital fossa, dissection carried down to identify the brachial artery and the basilic vein . Second small incision was made on the volar aspect of the forearm distally and graft was sutured in the vein in end-to-side fashion with running 6-0 Prolene suture. Attention was directed to the brachial artery, vascular clamp was applied, arteriotomy made and a 4-mm end of the graft was sutured end-to-side to the artery. Attention was directed to the right neck and by direct puncture the right internal jugular vein was cannulated with a guidewire and two-vessel dilators advanced, then the temporary dialysis catheter advanced over the guidewire and superior cava.

15. What are the codes for a 23-year-old patient who progressed to delivery; however, there was shoulder dystocia. Epsiotomy was performed. Forceps were used but did not work but shortly after with additional push, the baby was delivered. The baby was 10 pounds 3 ounces.

16. What are the codes for a 21-year-old patient who received a repeat low-abdominal Pfannenstiel incision from previous c-section due to obstructed labor. The rectus muscles were divided in the midline by sharp dissection. The lower uterine segment was carefully incised with a scalpel and extended laterally. A living female infant was delivered from the vertex right occipitotransverse position. The head was noted to be wedged into the pelvis but was easily elevated with a hand. The baby was suctioned and cried immediately. There was marked bleeding coming from the laceration of the left uterine artery which was sutured. The first layer of uterine closure was with running-locking #1 chromic catgut suture. The second layer was with imbricating #1 chromic catgut suture.

17. What are the codes for a 31-year-old patient who is seen in ER this morning complaining of intense pelvic pain with vaginal bleeding. The patient is 8 weeks pregnant. She denies any dizziness or shoulder pain. The patient had a c-section previously and 2 normal vaginal births prior to that. She had one miscarriage. The patient smokes and does drink regularly and is diabetic. The patient's mother was also positive for diabetes and COPD with asthma. ROS negative for all systems other than previously stated. Exam revealed a well-developed, well-nourished female in no acute distress with stable vital signs and afebrile. HENT WNL. Neck is supple without masses. Lungs clear. Heart shows regular rate and rhythm without murmur or gallop.Bowel sounds are present. Pelvic shows normal external genitalia. Cervix shows some bleeding. Slightly tender to

motion. Uterus: Tender. Ectopic pregnancy cannot be ruled out. Patient had an ultrasound which demonstrated ruptured tubal ectopic pregnancy which was removed laparoscopically.

18. What are the codes for a 25-year-old patient who had cerclage due to cervical incompetence?

19. What are the codes for this 47-year-old patient who had an exploratory laparotomy. revealed a large left 15-cm ovarian mass in the right adnexa.. To facilitate dissection of the large left ovarian mass, we dissected the left ureter which was occluded and adherent to the mass. We were eventually able to completely perform extrafascial hysterectomy, and the uterus (filled with fibroids), large left adnexal mass, right ovarian endometrioma, and tubes were removed as a single specimen.

20. What are the codes for a 29-year-old patient who had scopic removal of a polyp with D&C on the vaginal wall due to postmenopausal bleeding with glandular dilatation and proliferative endometrium?

21. What are the codes for a 27-year-old patient with ectopic pregnancy which required a salpingectomy on the left?

22. What are the codes for a 31-year-old patient with incompetent cervix at 8 weeks which required a McDonald cerclage placement?

23. What are the codes for this 38-year-old man with carcinoma of the prostate who is seen today for lymphadenectomy which was done by mobilizing pelvic tissue on both sides. Frozen section revealed these to be negative. The posterior urethra was now incised and there was retropubic resection of the prostate off the rectum. A portion of this ejaculatory duct was removed with the seminal vesicles, and the bladder neck was mobilized against some mild traction of the Foley, sparing about a 1-cm section of prostatic urethra. This was everted with 3-0 chromic sutures on the seromuscular layer and anastomosed to the urethra using the Greenfield suture guide.

24. What are the codes for a 59-year-old who was found to have prostate cancer. Routine bilateral pelvic lymph node dissections were performed. The lymph node packets were sent for final histopathologic diagnosis. Retropubic dissection of the prostate was then performed rectopubically.

25. What are the codes for a 41-year-old patient who had repair of an inguinal hernia and

26. What are the codes for a 48-year-old patient who had cystoscopy and ureteroscopy which revealed ureteral calculus in the left which was treated with lithotripsy and basket extraction with bilateral retrograde pyelograms?

27. What are the codes for a 53-year-old male who has BPH and also has recurrent UTIs now. Today he had TURP and removal of prostatic chips which were occluding the

bladder vault using a resectoscope. A 22-French Foley catheter 30-cc balloon was inserted. The balloon was inflated to 55 cc. The catheter was irrigated. The return was blood tinged. The catheter was connected to straight drainage.

28. What are the codes for a 37-year-old ESRD patient who is seen for insertion of dialysis catheter. Attention was directed to the right neck and with direct puncture the right internal jugular vein was cannulated with a guidewire. Advanced over the guidewire were two-vessel dilators, then the Schon temporary dialysis catheter advanced.

29. Crushing of a stone in the bladder and washing out the fragments through a catheter is known as what?

30. What are the codes for this 41-year-old with urodynamically documented intrinsic sphincter deficiency. Attention was turned to the anterior vaginal wall. The sling material was then prepared with packing on either side of the dissection. A strip of cadaveric fascia was incised for its width and tacked at each of the corners. A series of four interrupted sutures of 2-0 PDS were then used to tack the sling at the UVJ and down the urethra to minimize the risk of the sling rolling under the urethra. The sling was under minimal tension under the urethra. Generous purchases of the cadaveric fascia were taken and tacked. The sling was well positioned but not under any tension from the urethra. The bladder was then inspected with a cystoscope. The urethra was normal. There was no evidence of any trauma to the urethra or bladder. The urine was clear.

31. What are the codes for this 78-year-old patient status post multiple colon resections for carcinoma. She has received radiation chemotherapy and was recently noted on CT scan to have bilateral hydronephrosis, right worse than left, and therefore for further evaluation underwent the above procedure. Findings were Retroperitoneal fibrosis. The cystoscope was introduced per urethra without any difficulty. Under vision it was placed into the bladder. There was no evidence of stone or tumor. Retrograde pyelogram was undertaken. Cystoscope was removed and the ureteroscope was inserted under direct vision and with hydrostatic dilatation it was advanced up to the point of obstruction where complete obstruction was visualized secondary to extrinsic compression likely from mild retroperitoneal fibrosis. A guidewire was inserted through the working port of the ureteroscope and advanced up the collecting system as confirmed under fluoroscopic control. Retrograde pyelogram demonstrated the guidewire to be in the renal collecting system. The ureteroscope was then removed and the cystoscope was reintroduced over the guidewire. A 6-French, 24-cm double-J stent was inserted over the guidewire and advanced up the collecting system as confirmed under fluoroscopic control. The string was cut from the stent and then the guidewire was removed.

32. What are the codes for a 42-year-old patient who had calculus of the right kidney which was removed with ESWL?

33. What are the codes for a 45-year-old patient who was diagnosed with carcinoma of the bladder. Resectoscope was placed and cystopanendoscopy was performed. The urethra was within normal limits. There was a large fungating bladder carcinoma which was

obviously necrotic. The tumor extended to the entire surface of the left lateral wall and was resected using the resectoscope. No other lesions were identified. A separate biopsy of the prostatic urethra was obtained. The chips were removed and the bladder was once again inspected and found to be free of evidence of injury, and the ureteral orifices were intact at the conclusion of the procedure.

34. The patient was brought to the operative suite, prepped and draped in the usual manner. A right paramedian incision was made basically just above the umbilicus. Bleeding controlled with electrocautery. The rectus muscle was split and the peritoneal cavity was entered. We used 0.25% Marcaine with epinephrine prior to making the incision. We had to lengthen it to get some exposure. I had problems finding the appendix, as the appendix came off and was tethered into the retroperitoneal area. I asked Dr. Vaughan to assist for exposure. We were able to basically mobilize the right colon and then we dissected it from the cecum but once we found it, it was coming out fairly high off of the cecum. We tied it twice, divided it, cauterized the tip, then dissected, used the LigaSure for the mesentery and dissected it off of the duodenum. All bleeding was controlled. We irrigated thoroughly with saline, made certain that the bowel was properly placed back into the abdomen. Omentum was placed over it. We used a sheet of Seprafilm over the cecum and the right colon and another one over the omentum. The sponge, instrument, and needle count was correct and then we closed with double looped Maxon for the fascia, subcutaneous tissue closed with 2-0 Vicryl and skin was closed with V-Loc. Steri-Strip was applied. Sterile dressing was applied. Sent to recovery room in satisfactory condition. Tolerated the procedure well.

35. What are the codes for a 54-year-old patient who had a Roux-en-Y reconstruction following a complete gastrectomy for stomach cancer?

36. What are the codes for a 57-year-old patient who had a diverting colostomy with Hartmann pouch with sepsis and excision and debridement of a sacral decubitus ulcer stage 3 with ostectomy which had become necrotic .

37. What are the codes for a 41-year-old patient who was complaining of a bulging mass in the right side of the abdomen which correlated with a ventral hernia of the right abdominal wall. At this point, plication of the rectus abdominis muscle was done and Marlex mesh was applied.

38. What are the codes for a 52-year-old patient who was placed in the supine position and the F2 focus of the MSL 5000 lithotriptor, shock wave lithotripsy was started at 17 kV and went up to 23, where a total of 3000 shocks were given to the stone with fragmentation of this left renal calculi.

39. The patient brought to the operative suite, prepped and draped in the usual manner. Timeout was accomplished. Preoperative antibiotics were given and SCDs applied. Low midline incision was made, bleeding controlled with electrocautery. Fascia divided and peritoneal cavity was entered. Bookwalter retractor was placed. We able to see the area where India ink had been injected in the sigmoid colon. We used the GIA proximally and

distally, divided the mesentery using the ligature. One vessel was stick-tied with 3-0 silk. We then opened the specimen and there was no polyp in it, so we then opened the bowel proximally thinking that the polyp might be just above where we had resected and, indeed, we found the polyp on a very long stalk. Resected another portion of the colon, then used a pursestringer. Placed a pursestring proximally. Used the dilators. A 29 EEA was selected. We tied the pursestring and then brought the EEA in from below, made the anastomosis. We then tested it, and there were some air bubbles, and so we had to use 3-0 silk. There was a small rent in the anastomosis on the right lateral side. This was sutured. We then tested it again. Put the anastomosis under water and produced air from below using an Asepto syringe. There were no leaks. After making sure we had a good tight anastomosis, I also brought some surrounding fat over the area where we had reinforced and put a couple more silks anteriorly. Left a 19 Blake drain through a separate stab incision through the right side, sutured in place with a 2-0 Prolene. Then used 2 sheets of Seprafilm by the omentum over the small bowel. Had a correct sponge, instrument, and needle count. Closure was a double loop of Maxon along with some interrupted #1 Vicryl, subcutaneous tissue closed with 2-0 Vicryl, and skin was closed with V-Loc subcuticular. Steri-Strip applied. Sterile dressing applied. Sent to recovery room in satisfactory condition. Tolerated the procedure well.

40. What are the codes for an 8-year-old patient who had suffered second and third degrees burns over both fronts of her legs four months ago which totaled 15% of TBSA with 7% third degree? She is seen today for STSG from her back to cover the burned area.

41. What is an I&D?

42. What are the codes for a 32-year-old patient who had 17 skin tags removed electrosurgically?

43. What are the codes for a 38-year-old female who had a mastectomy of both breasts which included removal of the axillary lymph nodes due to carcinoma of the breast with a TRAM?

44. What are the codes when a pathologist finds malignancy from a needle core biopsy of the left breast of a 32-year-old woman?

45. What are the codes for an 82-year-old nursing home patient who had excision of a sacral pressure ulcer stage 2 repaired with suturing and requiring an ostectomy?

46. What are the codes for a 49-year-old patient who was involved in a car accident and suffered extensive lacerations and broken collarbone? The patient had a BAC level of 1.0 as he has suffered for many years with alcoholism and went on a binge today. Lacerations were numerous including a 3.0 cm laceration of the right forearm which required layered closure, a 5.5 cm laceration of the right thigh which required retention sutures and ligation of arteries, 4.8 cm laceration of the chest which required simple closure but extensive debridement due to glass fragments, a 2.8 cm laceration of the right cheek which required layered closure, and a 3.0 cm laceration of the left thigh which

required retention sutures.

47. What are the codes for a 44-year-old patient who is seen today for the first time with a history and exam that were expanded problem focused and who had a 3.2-cm mass of the back which was infected and required drainage which was found to be a sebaceous cyst?

48. What are the codes for a 15-year-old patient who was seen in the emergency room due to complaints of severe abdominal pain and hemoptysis? The patient was found to have Staph food poisoning and discharged with prescriptions. The history was expanded problem focused and the exam was problem focused.

49. What are the codes for a pathologist who performs the pathological review of the two biopsies of specimens from Moh's surgery for a 4.2 cm lesion on the back of a 48-year-old man?

50. What are the codes for a 64-year-old patient with a history of insulin-dependent diabetes mellitus, coronary artery disease, chronic renal failure and heart failure who was initially admitted for congestive heart failure and nonhealing bilateral mid-foot ulcers treated for years with debridement and whirlpool. The patient was readmitted for acute diabetic right foot to be treated with incision and drainage of his right foot and first ray amputation but the infection had spread so right below-knee amputation was performed.

51. What are the codes for a 67-year-old patient who is seen today for pleural effusion secondary to small cell carcinoma of the upper left lung with tube thoracostomy including indwelling catheter?

52. What are the codes for this 52-year-old patient who has a history of pulmonary nodule in the left lung? She was seen today for a CT of the Chest and Adrenals with oral and intravenous contrast. Today there is a 2-cm area of parenchymal density which has the appearance of interstitial changes without findings of significant nodule or mass. This finding can relate to scarring. There is no other nodule, mass, or effusion. No evidence of adenopathy in the mediastinum. The heart and great vessels are normal in appearance. No findings with the liver, spleen, kidneys, adrenals, or pancreas.

53. What are the codes for a 71-year-old patient who has a long history of lung disease due to being a lifelong smoker. History of hypertension. The patient also had COPD and asthma with bullous emphysema. A PET scan was reviewed by the physician and revealed that she has a 3.5-cm nodule in the upper left lobe which is malignant. A lobectomy was performed.

54. What are the codes for an 18-year-old patient who has trouble breathing due to airway obstruction. It was found that this is due to turbinate hypertrophy and deviated septum protruding into the left nasal airway for which a septoplasty and bilateral turbinectomy was performed.

55. What are the codes for a 38-year-old patient who presents with the complaint of SOB and dyspnea with wheezing that began approximately four hours ago and has worsened? She is seen in the emergency room today. Her medical history showed a history of asthma. The patient states that she had a cough for the past day but she denies any other problems. She denies any fever or chills. She denies any chest pain or palpitations. The patient had an asthma attack a month ago which required hospitalization and treatment. The patient has no other past surgical history. The patient does have HTN and hypercholesterolemia. The patient lives alone and she works at a local school. She has smoked for more than 20 years. Her father is deceased due to emphysema. ROS shows that the patient has no problems in any system including no abdominal pain, chest pain, or edema other than previously mentioned. Physical exam showed the patient to be tachypneic. She is well developed and well nourished with respiratory rate of 20 and blood pressure of 124/86. HEENT is normocephalic and atraumatic. Pupils equal and round, regular, reactive to light. Extraocular muscles intact. Nares and oropharynx negative. Neck is supple; no JVD, no lymphadenopathy, no carotid bruits, no thyromegaly. Lungs reveal bilateral wheeze diffusely. There are some decreased breath sounds bilaterally. No rhonchi. Cardiovascular: Regular rate and rhythm, without murmurs, gallops, or rubs. Normal S1 and S2. No S3, S4. Abdomen: Normal active bowel sounds, soft, nontender, nondistended. No hepatosplenomegaly. Extremities: No cyanosis, clubbing or edema. Today in the emergency room the patient received 4 nebulization treatments for her acute exacerbation of her asthma but continued to be hypoxic with room air oxygen saturation of 84%. She had some slight improvement in her wheeze with the nebulization treatments but without further improvement she was admitted to the hospital to be continued on Solu-Medrol 125 mg IV and supplemental O2.

56. What are the codes for this 41-year-old patient who had an esophagoscopy and microlaryngoscopy of the neck to determine if there was cancer secondary to lung cancer. The scope was advanced into the cervical esophagus which was found to be normal. It was noticed that there was tumor involving the anterior wall of the right portion of the neck extending approximately 1 cm below the pharyngeal epiglottic fold and into the hypopharyngeal wall of which a sample was obtained. The specimen was found to be malignant.

57. What are the codes for a 73-year-old patient with a history of aortic valve replacement and severe cardiomyopathy, chronic left bundle-branch block and diabetes who presents after having experience arrest early this morning characterized earlier by difficulty breathing and chest pain. The patient was cardioverted multiple times by EMTs and placed in ICU where he was seen several times from 8:00 am to 9:00 am, 11:30 to 12:45, and 4:15 pm to 5:30 pm but remained mostly unresponsive. Subsequent rhythm was sinus tachycardiac with a left bundle-branch block. He had a cardiac catheterization at the time of aortic valve replacement which showed normal coronary vessels three years ago. The patient does drink and smoke occasionally. His father died of a heart attack at age 75. ROS was unobtainable as the patient was not responsive. Exam showed blood pressure of 145/87, Pulse was 108 and respirations are 12 on ventilator. The patient is afebrile. HEENT show PERRLA. Neck is supple. Carotids have diminished upstroke without bruits. Lungs are clear. Anteriorly heart is tachycardiac . There is a prosthetic S2.

The abdomen is soft and nontender without masses. Extremities have trace edema. Distal pulses are present. Neurologic exam: The patient is unresponsive. EKG shows sinus tachycardia with left bundle-branch block. Neurological and pulmonary evals are recommends. EKG should be repeated. Possible catheterization should be performed.

58. What are the codes for a 49-year-old patient who had a permanent pacemaker implanted with leads placed into the right ventricle and right atrium due to bradycardia. A pocket was made in the left anterior chest wall into which the pulse generator was inserted.

59. What are the codes for a 55-year-old patient who had an acute MI with edema and received an intracorporeal left ventricular assist device as a bridge to cardiac transplantation several months ago. Now, after 100 days of support, the left ventricular assist device malfunctioned and the pump had to be replaced.

60. What are the codes for a 47-year-old patient with renal failure requiring hemodialysis so an AV cannula was placed for access?

CHAPTER 46
REIMBURSEMENT

You will learn the following objectives in this chapter:

A. Overview of Coding and Reimbursement
B. Medical Terms
C. Claims
D. Reports
E. Insurances
F. Payments
G. Encoder
H. Federal Register
I. Coverage Determinations
J. Billing Forms
    a. CMS-1500
    b. CMS-1450
    c. Explanation of Benefits
    d. Medicare Summary Notice
    e. Advance Beneficiary Notice
K. Medicare
    a. Beneficiaries
    b. Part A
    c. Part B
    d. Part C
    e. Part D
    f. Medigap
    g. Medicare as Secondary Payer
    h. Medicare Administrative Contractors
L. Medicaid
M. SCHIP
N. Tricare
O. Medi-Medi
P. Private Payers
    a. HMOs
    b. PPOs
    c. IPAs
Q. Professional Courtesy
D. Possible Reimbursement Errors

Section 46.1: RESOURCE BASED RELATIVE VALUE SCALE

Resource Based Relative Value Scale (RBRVS) was implemented in 1992 as a means of establishing predetermined values for reimbursement for physician services for Medicare. RBRVS calculates the amount to be paid for a code using the relative value unit of the service, geographical location, and a conversion factor. The basis, relative value units, is determined by the healthcare provider's work, overhead, and malpractice costs which is then adjusted for geographic practice cost indices (GPCIs) and multiplied by a conversion factor.

The formula used by the government for reimbursement is:
non-Facility Pricing Amount = [(Work RVU * Work GPCI) +
(RB Non-Facility PE RVU * PE GPCI) + (MP RVU * MP GPCI)] * Conversion Factor

Relative values used to determine the amount paid for services or materials can be found at CMS's website: http://www.cms.hhs.gov/PhysicianFeeSched/PFSRVF/list.asp#TopOfPage.

	A	B	C	D	E	F
1 2	Carrier Number	Locality Number	Locality Name	[1]Work GPCI	PE GPCI	MP GPCI
3	00510	00	Alabama	1.000	0.858	0.752
4	00831	01	[2]Alaska	1.670	1.670	1.670
5	00832	00	Arizona	1.000	0.985	1.069
6	00520	13	Arkansas	1.000	0.839	0.438
7	31146	26	Anaheim/Santa Ana, CA	1.036	1.210	0.954
8	31146	18	Los Angeles, CA	1.049	1.147	0.954
9	31140	03	Marin/Napa/Solano, CA	1.025	1.294	0.651
10	31140	07	Oakland/Berkley, CA	1.048	1.303	0.651
11	31146	99	Rest of California*	1.007	1.043	0.733
12	31140	99	Rest of California*	1.007	1.043	0.733
13	31140	05	San Francisco, CA	1.064	1.501	0.651
14	31140	06	San Mateo, CA	1.061	1.484	0.639
15	31140	09	Santa Clara, CA	1.073	1.460	0.604
16	31146	17	Ventura, CA	1.028	1.152	0.744
17	00824	01	Colorado	1.000	1.003	0.803
18	00591	00	Connecticut	1.044	1.163	0.900
19	00902	01	Delaware	1.016	1.026	0.892
20	00903	01	DC + MD/VA Suburbs	1.049	1.208	0.926
21	00590	03	Fort Lauderdale, FL	1.000	1.003	1.703
22	00590	04	Miami, FL	1.008	1.049	2.269
23	00590	99	Rest of Florida	1.000	0.940	1.272
24	00511	01	Atlanta, GA	1.008	1.074	0.966
25	00511	99	Rest of Georgia	1.000	0.882	0.966
26	00833	01	Hawaii/Guam	1.001	1.118	0.800
27	05130	00	Idaho	1.000	0.874	0.459

Section 46.2: BILLING TERMS

ACCEPT ASSIGNMENT: A physician may choose to accept assignment which means they will accept what Medicare pays as payment in full per the Medicare Physician Fee Schedule (MPFS) which is based on Resource-Based Relative Value Scale (see below) and they cannot bill the beneficiary for any additional amounts beyond the traditional copayments and deductibles. Copayments for Part B typically are 20 percent which the patient pays and Medicare then pays 80 percent. Healthcare providers who accept assignment are known as participating (PAR) and those who do not accept assignment are known as non-PAR. When a physician accepts assignment it also means that CMS will pay the healthcare provider directly, not the patient. In addition, the healthcare provider is paid at 5 percent higher than non-PAR providers, claims are processed faster, and they are listed as a Medicare provider for marketing purposes. A non-PAR provider can charge the beneficiary more than PARs who cannot charge the beneficiary at all, but non-PARs are limited to 15 percent above Medicare's allowable amount per the MFS; however, the Medicare allowable amount is 5% less than the PAR's allowable charge of which Medicare pays 80% and the patient pays for the copay and additional allowable 15% amount. For example, if a PAR is allowed $100 he will be reimbursed for $80; however, the non-PAR's allowable amount is $95 of which he will receive $76 from Medicare and he will then charge the additional $15 to the patient in addition to any other charges such as the patient's 20% copay.

AGING REPORT: A report that shows the status of claims as to payment and the length of time for claims that have not been paid.

BENEFICIARY: The person eligible to receive care.

CAPITATION: A payment method in which the healthcare provider is paid a fixed amount by the insurance company per month per patient for the provision of services, even if the patient does not receive services.

CLEAN CLAIM: A clean claim is a claim that has been found to be error-free, usually by a software program which checks claims for errors.

CLEARINGHOUSE: A company that provides centralized claims processing.

COINSURANCE: The portion of the cost of services which the beneficiary must pay and is not paid by the insurance company. Coinsurance is usually 20% for the insured and 80% for the insurance company for most government plans, HMOs and PPOs.

COORDINATION OF BENEFITS (COB): When a person has multiple insurance coverages, there is an order to payment; in other words, certain insurances would be billed first (primary payer) and other insurances would follow after that (secondary payer) with the last insurance to be billed known as payer of last resort, which is known as coordination of benefits. Medicare is considered the payer of last resort after private insurances. Medicaid is the payer of last resort after Medicare.

If a patient has multiple private insurances, such as a child with both parents providing health insurance coverage, then the insurance company of the parent whose birthday occurs first in the year will be the first payer. This is known as the Birthday Rule.

Once a claim has been sent to the first payer, if it is denied then the claim would be sent to the secondary payer, such as Medicare to see if they will pay.

COPAYMENTS: Copayments are standard charges which the patient must pay for each visit, i.e. $10 or $20.

DEDUCTIBLES: The amount of money that must be paid by the beneficiary for healthcare services before the insurance company will begin payments.

ENCODER: Software which automates the coding process by providing codes based upon entries.

FEDERAL REGISTER: The Federal Register is a publication which lists the rules and regulations of the federal government and is a good source for locating information concerning governmental healthcare regulations.

GUARANTOR: Guarantor is the person responsible for payment, i.e. it is usually the person who is the carrier of the insurance policy.

LOCAL COVERAGE DETERMINATONS (LCD): LCDs provide guidance on what services are covered by Medicare and under what circumstances which are known as edits for the national coverage determination rules (NCD).

NATIONAL CORRECT CODING INITIATIVES (NCCI): A listing of edits which are the coding rules upon which reimbursement is determined by Medicare. These edits are issued quarterly.

NATIONAL COVERAGE DETERMINATIOIN (NCD): Rules developed by CMS that specify the circumstances under which services are paid which are outlined in the Local Coverage Determination (LCD).

OUTPATIENT CODE EDITOR (OCE): An Outpatient Code Editor is a software program which edits claims to check for errors.

PREMIUMS: Premiums are the dollar amount monthly for insurance coverage by either the employer and/or the employee.

REMITTANCE ADVICE: A form sent to the healthcare provider which explains the current status of claims.

UNIFORM HOSPITAL DISCHARGE DATA SET (UHDDS): Uniform Hospital Discharge Data Set is a standard set of data for collecting patient information which, therefore, ensures consistent health care for patients since other healthcare providers will have the necessary and consistent information so that they can provide proper care. This includes age, sex, race, residence of patient, length of stay, diagnosis, physicians, procedures, disposition of the patient and sources of payment.

Section 46.3: BILLING FORMS

CMS-1500: Center for Medicare and Medicaid developed the billing form that is used for submission of claims to them, but which has also been adopted by private insurers as well. This is known as the 1500 form, and was formerly known as HCFA-1500 (CMS was formerly known as Health Care Financing and Administration). As you may be noticing, most private insurers follow the government's lead with coding and reimbursement.

The form can be submitted either by paper or electronically. A 1500 form is located at the end of this packet and will be discussed more thoroughly in the CPT course. Directions on proper completion of this form are described later in this chapter.

CMS-1450: The CMS-1500 form is used for billing physician services. A different form, CMS-1450 is used to bill for hospital inpatient services and is quite different from the CMS-1500 form.

EXPLANATION OF BENEFITS: This form is provided to the healthcare provider (e.g., physician) and the patient which explains the services provided, the cost, and payments.

MEDICARE SUMMARY NOTICE (MSN): The explanation of benefits form provided by Medicare which explains the services provided, the cost, and the payments.

ADVANCE BENEFICIARY NOTICE (ABN): If a service may not be reimbursed by Medicare, an Advance Beneficiary Notice needs to be signed by the patient to indicate that the patient has been informed that the services may not be reimbursed by Medicare and that the patient will be responsible for payment. It must be issued each time for services provided; one ABN does not provide coverage for more than one service and new ABNs must be obtained for other services provided. If an ABN is not obtained prior to the service being provided, then the patient cannot be charged for the service.

Section 46.4: MEDICARE

Medicare was established as part of the Social Security Act and is overseen by the Department of Health and Human Services.

BENEFICIARIES: Medicare benefits are provided to people over the age of 65, blind, disabled, and end-stage renal disease (ESRD) who are known as beneficiaries.

PART A: Part A is known as hospital insurance and pays for costs for hospitals, skilled nursing facilities (SNF), and hospice, and eligible home health care. There is no premium to be paid by beneficiaries.

PART B: Part B is known as supplemental insurance and pays for physician services, laboratory, therapies, outpatient mental health care, home health care not covered under Part A, outpatient hospital services, ambulance services, renal dialysis, chemotherapy, Pap smears every 24 months, mammograms, prostate screenings, and vaccines for pneumonia, hepatitis B and influenza, and durable medical equipment.

Medicare does not pay for routine preventive exams (except mammograms), routine dental and eye exams, most foot care, and cosmetic surgery.

Beneficiaries must pay a premium. There are deductibles and copayment costs associated with Part B benefits.

PART C: Private insurance that is obtained by a patient's selection of a private insurance company instead of the traditional medicare and whereby Medicare contracts with the private insurance company to provide Medicare Part A and Part B benefits, known as Medicare+Choice, also known as Medicare Advantage. Medicare Advantage Plans are HMOs, PPOs, or Private Fee-for-Service Plans.

PART D: Medicare Part D is insurance coverage to subsidize the costs of prescription drugs. It was enacted as part of the Medicare Prescription Drug, Improvement, and Modernization Act of 2003 (MMA) and went into effect on January 1, 2006.[1]

MEDIGAP: Beneficiaries may purchase additional insurance to supplement costs that are not paid by Medicare, such as Medicare Select.

MEDICARE FEE SCHEDULE (MFS); A schedule of how much Medicare pays for services (example listed below).

Physician fee schedules can be found at: http://www.cms.hhs.gov/PhysicianFeeSched/

	A	B	C	D	R	S	T	U	V	W	X	Y	Z	AA
1			**2005 National Physician Fee**											
2			*CPT codes and descriptions only are c*											
3			*Dental codes (D codes) are copyright 2*											
4			REVISED 2/9/2004											
5													PHYSICIAN	
6													SUPERVISION OF	
7				STATUS	POST	MULT	BILAT	ASST	CO-	TEAM	ENDO	CONV	DIAGNOSTIC	CALCULATION
8	HCPCS	MOD	DESCRIPTION	CODE	OP	PROC	SURG	SURG	SURG	SURG	BASE	FACTOR	PROCEDURES	FLAG
9														
10	A0021		Outside state ambulance serv	I	0.00	9	9	9	9	9		37.8975	9	0
11	A0080		Noninterest escort in non er	I	0.00	9	9	9	9	9		37.8975	9	0
12	A0090		Interest escort in non er	I	0.00	9	9	9	9	9		37.8975	9	0
13	A0100		Nonemergency transport taxi	I	0.00	9	9	9	9	9		37.8975	9	0
14	A0110		Nonemergency transport bus	I	0.00	9	9	9	9	9		37.8975	9	0
15	A0120		Noner transport mini-bus	I	0.00	9	9	9	9	9		37.8975	9	0
16	A0130		Noner transport wheelch van	I	0.00	9	9	9	9	9		37.8975	9	0
17	A0140		Nonemergency transport air	I	0.00	9	9	9	9	9		37.8975	9	0
18	A0160		Noner transport case worker	I	0.00	9	9	9	9	9		37.8975	9	0
19	A0170		Transport parking fees/tolls	I	0.00	9	9	9	9	9		37.8975	9	0
20	A0180		Noner transport lodgng recip	I	0.00	9	9	9	9	9		37.8975	9	0
21	A0190		Noner transport meals recip	I	0.00	9	9	9	9	9		37.8975	9	0
22	A0200		Noner transport lodgng escrt	I	0.00	9	9	9	9	9		37.8975	9	0
23	A0210		Noner transport meals escort	I	0.00	9	9	9	9	9		37.8975	9	0
24	A0225		Neonatal emergency transpor	I	0.00	9	9	9	9	9		37.8975	9	0
25	A0380		Basic life support mileage	I	0.00	9	9	9	9	9		37.8975	9	0
26	A0382		Basic support routine suppls	X	0.00	9	9	9	9	9		37.8975	9	0
27	A0384		Bls defibrillation supplies	X	0.00	9	9	9	9	9		37.8975	9	0
28	A0390		Advanced life support mileag	I	0.00	9	9	9	9	9		37.8975	9	0
29	A0392		Als defibrillation supplies	X	0.00	9	9	9	9	9		37.8975	9	0
30	A0394		Als IV drug therapy supplies	X	0.00	9	9	9	9	9		37.8975	9	0
31	A0396		Als esophageal intub suppls	X	0.00	9	9	9	9	9		37.8975	9	0
32	A0398		Als routine disposble suppls	X	0.00	9	9	9	9	9		37.8975	9	0
33	A0420		Ambulance waiting 1/2 hr	X	0.00	9	9	9	9	9		37.8975	9	0
34	A0422		Ambulance 02 life sustaining	X	0.00	9	9	9	9	9		37.8975	9	0
35	A0424		Extra ambulance attendant	X	0.00	9	9	9	9	9		37.8975	9	0
36	A0425		Ground mileage	X	0.00	9	9	9	9	9		37.8975	9	0
37	A0426		Als 1	X	0.00	9	9	9	9	9		37.8975	9	0
38	A0427		ALS1-emergency	X	0.00	9	9	9	9	9		37.8975	9	0
39	A0428		bls	X	0.00	9	9	9	9	9		37.8975	9	0
40	A0429		BLS-emergency	X	0.00	9	9	9	9	9		37.8975	9	0
41	A0430		Fixed wing air transport	X	0.00	9	9	9	9	9		37.8975	9	0
42	A0431		Rotary wing air transport	X	0.00	9	9	9	9	9		37.8975	9	0
43	A0432		PI volunteer ambulance co	X	0.00	9	9	9	9	9		37.8975	9	0
44	A0433		als 2	X	0.00	9	9	9	9	9		37.8975	9	0
45	A0434		Specialty care transport	X	0.00	9	9	9	9	9		37.8975	9	0
46	A0435		Fixed wing air mileage	X	0.00	9	9	9	9	9		37.8975	9	0
47	A0436		Rotary wing air mileage	X	0.00	9	9	9	9	9		37.8975	9	0

PPRRVU05

MEDICARE ADMINISTRATIVE CONTRACTORS (MAC): CMS contracts with Medicare Administrative Contractors (private insurance companies) to provide services related to claims.

MEDICARE AS SECONDARY PAYER (MSP): Medicare is a secondary payer in certain circumstances, that is when (1) the patient has a primary employer insurance through themselves or their spouse; (2) this is a disability claim to be paid by the disability insurance; (3) when worker's compensation or an auto insurance company are responsible for patient's healthcare costs; (4) when the patient has black lung disease; (5) patient has end-stage renal disease and coverage is provided through employer, and (6) Veteran or enlisted.

When Medicare is the secondary insurance, it cannot be billed first; the other company must be billed first; then Medicare can be billed for what the primary insurance would not cover.

FISCAL INTERMEDIARIES: Insurance companies that process claims for the government programs.

Section 46.5: MEDICAID

Medicaid is also a government healthcare program originating in the Social Security Act which provides healthcare to the poor. Medicaid is administered jointly by the federal and state governments with states determining benefits and eligibility, so benefits can vary across states. In Arizona, Medicaid is known as AHCCCS.

By federal regulation, states must provide certain services in their Medicaid programs which include inpatient and outpatient hospital services, family planning services, home health, emergency room services, medically necessary physician services, prenatal care, home health and SNF services, and preventive health care for children known as Early and Periodic Screening, Diagnosis and Treatment (EPSDT).

Medicaid is always the payer of last resort; all other insurance plans should be billed before Medicaid.

Section 46.6: SCHIP

SCHIP is a new government program known as the State Children's Health Insurance Program, which pays for health care for children who are uninsured by any other program.

Section 46.7: TRICARE

Once formerly known as CHAMPUS (Civilian Health and Medical Program of the Uniformed Services), TRICARE provides health insurance coverage to the retired military personnel and their families.

There are three options to TRICARE: (1) TRICARE Prime; (2) TRICARE Extra, and (3)

TRICARE Standard. Prime offers the most coverage while Extra has lower costs and only healthcare providers who have agreed to participate can provide services and Standard provides selection of any provider with the insurance covering a percentage of the cost.

CHAMPVA (Civilian Health and Medical program of the Veterans Administration) provides health insurance coverage for spouses and children of veterans who are disabled or deceased due to duty-related service.

Section 46.8: MEDI-MEDI

Some patient may be covered by both Medicaid and Medicare, which is known as Medi-Medi. With Medi-Medi, Medicaid is considered the payer of last resort.

Section 46.9: PRIVATE PAYERS

There are several types of private payers with many companies offering a selection from the following: HMOs and PPOs.

HMOs: HMOs are health maintenance organizations in which subscribers (insurance carrier) pays a monthly premium and then can utilize the services with payment of copayments and deductibles from healthcare providers who have joined the HMO. HMOs can be staff model (healthcare provider is an employee); network model (HMO company contracts with a network of healthcare providers), group model (HMO provides services through a privately owned practice), or IPA in which independent physicians who provide services and the HMO reimburses them.

IPAs: Independent physician associations are a type of HMO in which physicians treat a predefined group of patients in their own offices and charge for their services on a predetermined rate.

PPOs: Preferred Provider Organizations in which a group of providers contract to provide services to an employer at a discounted rate.

FEE-FOR-SERVICE: In fee-for-service, the healthcare provider is paid directly for his services.

SECTION 46.10: PROPER COMPLETION OF THE CMS-1500 FORM

For auditing and coding purposes, we will examine only the bottom half of the -CMS-1500 form.

Blocks 17 and 17A must be filled out if a patient was referred by another physician. This can be used when a patient is simply referred by another physician for services offered by another physician. However, it is necessary when the patient is referred to another physician for a consultation. Be sure to include the referring physician's tax identification number (UPIN).

Block 18 must be filled out if the patient is in the hospital for the services charged. This box must link to Block 24B, which indicates the place of service. If a patient is in the hospital, block 24B must be 21 to indicate that services were provided in the hospital.

Block 21 is used to list ICD-10 codes with up to four codes allowed. If there are more diagnoses listed than four, you must select the four most important and relevant codes. Remember, too, that some codes will indicate that other codes must be coded in addition; this means that if you list the one code, you must list the other required code. This takes up two lines then, which can be limiting when you have many diagnoses but only four lines, but a required code must be listed in addition to the code that required it.

ICD-10 codes must then be properly linked to CPT/HCPCS codes as listed in block 24D. This **linkage** is crucial today in proving medical necessity and, thus, ensure reimbursement. Medical necessity is demonstrated through the linkage of ICD-10s and CPTs through blocks 21 through 24 by providing justification for the provision of services charged. Block 24E is used to denote this linkage. Line numbers from block 21 are used in block 24E to link the ICD-10s and CPTs. The line number of the relevant ICD-10 code is selected and then applied in block 24E, which corresponds with the service provided. Do not list the codes themselves in block 24E, only line numbers as indicated in block 21. Several line numbers may be used to demonstrate multiple links, such as a patient who has diabetes and a laceration that are both relative to the care of the wound; therefore, both diagnostical codes would be relative to the repair of that wound and so the line numbers for both codes can be listed in block 24E.

Block 24 includes several different blocks, that is, date(s) of services, place of service, type of service, CPT/HCPCS code, diagnosis code, charges, and units within block 24. Places of service are specifically designated numbers: 11 is used to indicate an office visit, 21 for inpatient hospital, 12 patient's home, 22 outpatient hospital, 23 emergency room, 31 skilled nursing facility, and 34 hospice. Not all carriers use type of service, which can include 1 for medical care, 2 for surgical care, 3 for consultation, 4 for x-rays, 5 for laboratory, 6 for radiation therapy, and 7 for anesthesia.

CPT/HCPCS codes as listed in block 24D are, of course, required. Up to six CPT/HCPCS codes may be included on this form. Remember, both -ICD-10s and CPT/HCPCS must be listed in order to be reimbursed. You cannot charge for services without some type of code, even when results are normal and there is no chief complaint. Modifiers must be included after the code, as indicated on the form. Multiple modifiers may be applied. Be sure to not unbundle CPT/HCPCS codes by listing codes that are included within the services of another code already listed. Check Correct Coding Initiative (CCI) edits.

Do not forget to include charges and units in blocks 24F and G. Charges are charged by the unit and then totaled in block 28. Be careful to not charge for additional units if a code does not permit coding for each unit separately and additionally. Some codes will include charges for a multitude of units, such as skin tag code 11200, which includes up to 15 tags.

The tax identification number, whether it is a social security number (SSN) or federal employer identifi-cation number (EIN), must be included in order to receive reimbursement. The SSN or EIN box must be checked.

In block 27, the Accept Assignment box should be checked.

Total charges, amount paid, and balance due should be completed as necessary.Signature and date must be included in block 31, as well as address and phone in block 33 for reimbursement.

Billing errors, whether purposeful or not, may be interpreted as fraud and/or abuse with accompanying fines and possible imprisonment. The coder is a good defense for a medical practice against such punishments with the proper application of their expertise and knowledge. The coder is also essential in ensuring prompt reimbursement, as well as -follow-up for claims that are not paid to investigate why the claims were rejected and not paid. The following lists provide some types of billing errors that may prevent proper and prompt reimbursement, which may be included in some form on the national coding exams. Many of the examples in this section are representative of the first part of the -CCS-P exam (multiple choice).

Section 46.11: POSSIBLE REIMBURSEMENT ERRORS

CODES

1. Overcoding. Undercoding.
2. **Upcoding. Downcoding.**
3. Wrong or improperly applied code, particularly in reference to number of required digits.
4. Improperly applied modifier.
5. Improper linkage of -ICD-10 and CPT/HCPCS codes.
6. Unbundling.
7. Failure to demonstrate medical necessity.
8. Lack of necessary information to validate codes.
9. Transposed or wrong codes.

BILLING

10. Billing for services not rendered.
11. Billing for services provided to another patient.
12. Billing of services provided by another provider.
13. Billing for services not covered or for patients who are not covered.
14. Billing for the provision of services by unauthorized personnel.
15. Duplication of charges.
16. Duplication of services.
17. Billing for more units of services than allowed or in improper increments.
18. Overcharging, particularly in regards to Medi-care patients.
19. Failure to bill payers in proper order, i.e., primary and secondary.
20. Improper mathematical determination of units and accompanying cost.
21. Wrong physician name, address, or ID number.

DOCUMENTATION

22. Alteration of report information to receive higher reimbursement, either before or after reports have been completed.

23. Missing or inadequate documentation.
24. Lack of proper signatures.
25. No referring physician with ID, particularly for consultations.
26. Wrong dates or locations.
27. Improper information, such as place of service.

Appendix A
Resources

A. CODING WEBSITES

http://www.ahima.org

http://www.aapc.com

You absolutely need to access these websites to be fully informed about the coding field and for testing information. Applications for national coding exams are completed online at these sites. Be sure to read the handbook thoroughly from these websites before taking the national exams as there is highly specific information provided.

In addition, these sites provide examples of the test, requirements for continuing education units to maintain your national certification, and additional information about certifications, such as the RHIT. In addition, these sites provide extensive information and research about the health administrative field and accredited schools.

Remember, the AHIMA coding certifications are known as Certified Coding Specialist (CCS) for inpatient and outpatient coding and Certified Coding Specialist – Physician for physician coding.

AAPC coding certifications include Certified Professional Coder Hospital (CPC-H) for outpatient hospital and Certified Professional Coder (CPC) for the physician.

B. GOVERNMENT WEBSITES

http://www.oig.hhss.gov (office of inspector general for health administration information.)
http://www.cdc.gov (Centers for Disease Control and Prevention)
http://www.gpoaccess.gov (Federal Register)
http://www.fedstats.gov (Federal Statistics)
http://www.hrs.gov (Health Resources and Services Administration
http://www.hhs.gov (US Department of Health and Human Services)
http://www.cms.gov (Centers for Medicare and Medicaid Services)
http://www.medicare.gov (Medicare)
http://www.cdc.gov/nchs (National Center for Health Statistics)
http://www.ncvhs.hhs.gov (National Committee on Vital and Health Statistics)
http://www.nih.gov (National Institutes of Health)
http://www.osha.gov (Occupational Safety and Health Administration)
http://www.ssa.gov (Social Security Administration)
http://www.tricare.osd.mil (TRICARE)
http://www.bls.gov (US Bureau of Labor Statistics)
http://www.va.gov (Veterans Administration)

C. ORGANIZATIONS WEBSITES

http://www.ama-assn.org (American Medical Association)
http://www.ahrq.gov (Agency for Healthcare Research and Quality)
http://www.achca.org (American College of Health Care Administrators)
http://www.ache.org (American College of Healthcare Executives)
http://www.aha.org (American Hospital Association)
http://www.asq.org (American Society for Quality)
http://www.bcbsa.com (Blue Cross/Blue Shield Association)
http://www.codingandreimbursement.net (Coding and Reimbursement Network)
http://www.himss.org (Healthcare Information and Management Systems Society)
http://www.jointcommission.org (Joint Commission)
http://www.nahq.org (National Association for Healthcare Quality)
http://www.ncqa.org (National Committee for Quality Assurance)
http://www.nubc.org (National Uniform Billing Committee)
http://www.nucc.org (National Uniform Claims Committee)
http://www.rbrvs.com (Resource-Based Relative Value System)

D. RESEARCH WEBSITES

http://www.ansi.org (American National Standards Institute)
http://www.advance .com (Advance Health Administration magazine)

HIPAA information can be found at:

http://www.aspe.hss.gov/adminsimp/ (Administrative Simplification Provisions of the Health Insurance Portability and Accountability Act.)
http://www.hhs.gov/ocr (HIPAA Privacy and Security Administration)

Annual ICD-10-CM-9-CM updates and revisions can be found at

http://www.cdc.gov/nchs/datawh/ftpserv/ftpICD-10-CM9/ftpICD-10-CM9.htm#guidelines
http://www.cms.hhs.gov/medlearn.ncci.asp (National Correct Coding Initiative)

APPENDIX B
SAMPLES OF REPORTS

HISTORY AND PHYSICAL REPORT

PATIENT'S NAME: REBECCA MILLER
PATIENT'S DOB: 10/02/89

ADMIT DIAGNOSES: Abdominal pain.

DETAILED HISTORY: This is an elderly 78-year-old female who has a history of atrial fibrillation, coronary artery disease and chronic A-Fib also. She was admitted with some abdominal pain, left upper quadrant radiating to the back, associated with some sharp pain. During admission she was found to have a drop in her blood counts and with her having a history of peptic ulcer disease and staying on anticoagulation she has been consulted for risk assessment and the presence of any ulcer disease, which may limit the use of anticoagulation on her. She at the moment is not having gross hematemesis or any hemotochezia.

PAST MEDICAL HISTORY: Coronary artery disease, A-Fib, hypertension, history of ulcer disease.

PAST SURGICAL HISTORY: Bypass grafting. She also has chronic hyponatremia and is being worked up at the moment.

MEDICATIONS: Consists of lisinopril, digoxin, metolazone, nitroglycerin, Coumadin, folic acid.
ALLERGIES: NKA.

FAMILY HISTORY: Noncontributory.

SOCIAL HISTORY: No alcohol. No tobacco abuse.

REVIEW OF SYSTEMS: All systems reviewed and negative and detailed on chart.

PHYSICAL EXAM: GENERAL: She was seen in the medical ward. Alert and oriented. HEENT: Atraumatic, normocephalic. CARDIOVASCULAR: S1, S2 irregular. RESPIRATORY: Clear bilaterally. ABDOMEN: Soft and nontender. NEUROLOGICAL: Nonfocal.

LAB WORKUP: Shows a white count of 4.7, hemoglobin of 10, has come down from 11, platelet count is normal, INR is 3.3, Chem 7 shows sodium of 120, potassium is 5, BUN is 20.

ASSESSMENT: This elderly 78-year-old female with chronic anticoagulation with slight drop in her blood counts with having a history of peptic ulcer disease and also presented initially with abdominal pain. Would want to do an upper endoscopy and I would do it diagnostically to see if there is any ulcers present. If they are then we will have to discuss with the physician regarding whether Coumadin is safe to continue in the immediate settings. For the moment continue on PPIs.

RE: David Jones
DATE: 12/01/10
DOB: 12/01/65

HISTORY OF PRESENT ILLNESS: This is a 43-year-old black man with no apparent past medical history who presented to the emergency room with the chief complaint of weakness, malaise and dyspnea on exertion for approximately one month. The patient also reports a 15-pound weight loss. He denies fever, chills, and sweats. He denies cough and diarrhea. He has mild anorexia. Past Medical History: Essentially unremarkable except for chest wall cysts which apparently have been biopsied by a dermatologist in the past, and he was given a benign diagnosis. He had a recent PPD which was negative in August 1994.

MEDICATIONS: Advil and Ibuprofen.

ALLERGIES: NO KNOWN DRUG ALLERGIES.

SOCIAL HISTORY: He occasionally drinks. He is a nonsmoker. The patient participated in homosexual activity in Haiti during 1982, which he described as "very active." He denies intravenous drug use. The patient is currently employed.

FAMILY HISTORY: Unremarkable.

PHYSICAL EXAMINATION:
General: This is a thin, black cachectic man speaking in full sentences with oxygen.
Vital Signs: Blood pressure 96/56, heart rate 120. No change with orthostatics. Temperature 101.6 degrees Fahrenheit. Respirations 30.
HEENT: Funduscopic examination normal. He has oral thrush.
Lymph: He has marked adenopathy including right bilateral epitrochlear and posterior cervical nodes.
Neck: No goiter, no jugular venous distention.
Chest: Bilateral basilar crackles, and egophony at the right and left middle lung fields.
Heart: Regular rate and rhythm, no murmur, rub or gallop.
Abdomen: Soft and nontender.
Genitourinary: Normal.
Rectal: Unremarkable.
Skin: The patient has multiple, subcutaneous mobile nodules on the chest wall that are nontender. He has very pale palms.

LABORATORY: Sodium 133, potassium 5.3, BUN 29, creatinine 1.8, hemoglobin 14, white count 7100, platelet count 515, total protein 10, albumin 3.1, AST 131, ALT 31, urinalysis shows 1+ protein, trace blood, total bilirubin 2.4, and direct bilirubin 0.1.

X-RAYS: Electrocardiogram shows normal sinus rhythm. Chest x-ray shows bilateral alveolar and interstitial infiltrates.

IMPRESSION:

1. Bilateral pneumonia; suspect atypical pneumonia, rule out Pneumocystis carinii pneumonia and tuberculosis.
2. Thrush.
3. Elevated unconjugated bilirubin.
4. Hepatitis.
5. Elevated globulin fraction.
6. Renal insufficiency.
7. Subcutaneous nodules.
8. Risky sexual behavior in 1982 in Haiti.

PLAN:

1. Induced sputum, rule out Pneumocystis carinii pneumonia and tuberculosis.
2. Begin intravenous Bactrim and erythromycin.
3. Begin prednisone.
4. Oxygen.
5. Nystatin swish and swallow.
6. Dermatologic biopsy of lesions.
7. Check HIV and RPR.
8. Administer Pneumovax, tetanus shot, and Heptavax if indicated.

APPENDIX C
CMS-1500 FORM

1500

HEALTH INSURANCE CLAIM FORM

APPROVED BY NATIONAL UNIFORM CLAIM COMMITTEE 08/05

PICA | PICA

CARRIER

1. MEDICARE (Medicare #) | MEDICAID (Medicaid #) | TRICARE CHAMPUS (Sponsor's SSN) | CHAMPVA (Member ID#) | GROUP HEALTH PLAN (SSN or ID) | FECA BLK LUNG (SSN) | OTHER (ID)

1a. INSURED'S I.D. NUMBER (For Program in Item 1)

2. PATIENT'S NAME (Last Name, First Name, Middle Initial)

3. PATIENT'S BIRTH DATE MM DD YY SEX M F

4. INSURED'S NAME (Last Name, First Name, Middle Initial)

5. PATIENT'S ADDRESS (No., Street)

6. PATIENT RELATIONSHIP TO INSURED Self Spouse Child Other

7. INSURED'S ADDRESS (No., Street)

CITY STATE

8. PATIENT STATUS Single Married Other

CITY STATE

ZIP CODE TELEPHONE (Include Area Code) ( )

Employed Full-Time Student Part-Time Student

ZIP CODE TELEPHONE (Include Area Code) ( )

9. OTHER INSURED'S NAME (Last Name, First Name, Middle Initial)

10. IS PATIENT'S CONDITION RELATED TO:

11. INSURED'S POLICY GROUP OR FECA NUMBER

a. OTHER INSURED'S POLICY OR GROUP NUMBER

a. EMPLOYMENT? (Current or Previous) YES NO

a. INSURED'S DATE OF BIRTH MM DD YY SEX M F

b. OTHER INSURED'S DATE OF BIRTH MM DD YY SEX M F

b. AUTO ACCIDENT? YES NO PLACE (State)

b. EMPLOYER'S NAME OR SCHOOL NAME

c. EMPLOYER'S NAME OR SCHOOL NAME

c. OTHER ACCIDENT? YES NO

c. INSURANCE PLAN NAME OR PROGRAM NAME

d. INSURANCE PLAN NAME OR PROGRAM NAME

10d. RESERVED FOR LOCAL USE

d. IS THERE ANOTHER HEALTH BENEFIT PLAN? YES NO *If yes*, return to and complete item 9 a-d.

READ BACK OF FORM BEFORE COMPLETING & SIGNING THIS FORM.

12. PATIENT'S OR AUTHORIZED PERSON'S SIGNATURE I authorize the release of any medical or other information necessary to process this claim. I also request payment of government benefits either to myself or to the party who accepts assignment below.

SIGNED ______ DATE ______

13. INSURED'S OR AUTHORIZED PERSON'S SIGNATURE I authorize payment of medical benefits to the undersigned physician or supplier for services described below.

SIGNED ______

PATIENT AND INSURED INFORMATION

14. DATE OF CURRENT: MM DD YY ILLNESS (First symptom) OR INJURY (Accident) OR PREGNANCY(LMP)

15. IF PATIENT HAS HAD SAME OR SIMILAR ILLNESS. GIVE FIRST DATE MM DD YY

16. DATES PATIENT UNABLE TO WORK IN CURRENT OCCUPATION FROM MM DD YY TO MM DD YY

17. NAME OF REFERRING PROVIDER OR OTHER SOURCE

17a. 17b. NPI

18. HOSPITALIZATION DATES RELATED TO CURRENT SERVICES FROM MM DD YY TO MM DD YY

19. RESERVED FOR LOCAL USE

20. OUTSIDE LAB? YES NO $ CHARGES

21. DIAGNOSIS OR NATURE OF ILLNESS OR INJURY (Relate Items 1, 2, 3 or 4 to Item 24E by Line)

1. ___ . ___ 3. ___ . ___

2. ___ . ___ 4. ___ . ___

22. MEDICAID RESUBMISSION CODE ORIGINAL REF. NO.

23. PRIOR AUTHORIZATION NUMBER

	24. A. DATE(S) OF SERVICE From MM DD YY To MM DD YY	B. PLACE OF SERVICE	C. EMG	D. PROCEDURES, SERVICES, OR SUPPLIES (Explain Unusual Circumstances) CPT/HCPCS MODIFIER	E. DIAGNOSIS POINTER	F. $ CHARGES	G. DAYS OR UNITS	H. EPSDT Family Plan	I. ID. QUAL.	J. RENDERING PROVIDER ID. #
1									NPI	
2									NPI	
3									NPI	
4									NPI	
5									NPI	
6									NPI	

25. FEDERAL TAX I.D. NUMBER SSN EIN

26. PATIENT'S ACCOUNT NO.

27. ACCEPT ASSIGNMENT? (For govt. claims, see back) YES NO

28. TOTAL CHARGE $

29. AMOUNT PAID $

30. BALANCE DUE $

31. SIGNATURE OF PHYSICIAN OR SUPPLIER INCLUDING DEGREES OR CREDENTIALS (I certify that the statements on the reverse apply to this bill and are made a part thereof.)

SIGNED DATE

32. SERVICE FACILITY LOCATION INFORMATION

a. NPI b.

33. BILLING PROVIDER INFO & PH # ( )

a. NPI b.

PHYSICIAN OR SUPPLIER INFORMATION

NUCC Instruction Manual available at: www.nucc.org *PLEASE PRINT OR TYPE* APPROVED OMB-0938-0999 FORM CMS-1500 (08-05)

APPENDIX D AUDIT FORM

CHIEF COMPLAINT:	Problem Focused	Exp. Prob. Focused	Detailed	Compre-hensive
HPI (history of present illness) elements: ☐ Location ☐ Severity ☐ Timing ☐ Modifying factors ☐ Quality ☐ Duration ☐ Context ☐ Associated signs and symptoms	Brief 1-3 Elements	Brief 1-3 Elements	Extended ≥ 4 elements or status of ≥ 3 chronic or inactive	Extended
ROS (review of systems): ☐ Constitutional (Wt. Loss, etc.) ☐ Ears, nose, mouth, throat ☐ GI ☐ GU ☐ Integumentary (skin, breast) ☐ Edno ☐ Eyes ☐ Card/Vasc ☐ Musculo ☐ Neuro ☐ Hem/Lymph ☐ All/Imm ☐ Resp ☐ Psych ☐ All others negative	None	Pertinent to problem 1 system	Extended 2-9 systems	Complete ≥ 10 systems, or some systems with statement "All Others Negative"
PFSH (past medical, family, social history) areas: ☐ Past history (the patient's past experiences with illnesses, operations, injuries and treatments) ☐ Family history (a review of medical events in the patient's family, including diseases which may be ☐ hereditary or place the patient at risk).	None	None	Pertinent 1 or 2 history areas	Complete 2 or 3 history areas

Circle history type within appropriate grid under Level of Service

If physician is unable to obtain history, the record should describe circumstances which preclude obtaining it.	**No PFSH required:** Subseq hospital care; Followup inpt consults; Subseq nursing facility care	**PFSH requirement:** Established patient (office/outpatient, dorms, home) and emergency department: pertinent - 1 history area; Complete history areas. New patient (office/outpatient, dorms, home). Consultations, initial hospital, hospital observation, comprehensive nursing facility assessments: Pertinent - 2 history areas; Complete - 3 history areas

GENERAL MULTI-SYSTEM EXAM		SINGLE ORGAN SYSTEM EXAMS
1-5 elements identified by bullet (*)	Problem Focused	1-5 elements identified by bullet (*)
≥ 6 elements identified by bullet (*)	Exp Problem Focused	≥ 6 elements identified by bullet (*)
≥ 2 elements identified by bullet (*) from 6 areas / systems <u>OR</u> ≥ 12 elements identified by bullet (*) from ≥ 2 areas / systems	Detailed	≥ 12 elements identified by bullet (*) <u>EXCEPT</u> ≥ 9 elements identified by bullet (*) for eye and psychiatric exams
Perform all elements identified by bullet (*) from ≥ 9 areas / systems <u>AND</u> document ≥ 2 elements identified by bullet (*) from 9 areas /	Comprehensive	Perform all elements identified by bullet (*); document all elements in shaded boxes; document ≥ 1 element in unshaded boxes

Circle exam type within appropriate grid under Level of Service

COMPLEXITY

A Number of Diagnoses of Treatment Options

Problems to Exam Physician	Number X Points = Results	
Self-limited or minor (Stable, improved or worsening)	1	Max = 2
Est. problem (to examiner): stable, improved	1	
Est. problem (to examiner): worsening	2	
New problem (to examiner): no additional workup planned	3	Max = 3
New prob. (to examiner): add, workup plannec	4	
	TOTAL	

Bring total to line A in Final Result for Complexity

C Amount and/or Complexity of Data to Be Reviewed

Data to Be Reviewed	Points
Review and/or order of clinical lab tests	1
Review and/or order of tests in the radiology section of CPT	1
Review and/or order of tests in the medicine section of CPT	1
Discussion of test results with performing physician	1
Decision to obtain old records and/or obtain history from someone other than patient	1
Review and summarization of old records and/or obtaining history from someone other than patient and/or discussion of case with another health care provider	2
Independent visualization of image, tracing or specimen itself (not simply review of report)	2
TOTAL	

Bring total to line C in Final Result for Complexity

Final Result for Complexity

A	Number diagnoses or treatment options	≤1 Minimal	2 Limited	3 Multiple	≥ 4 Extensive
B	Highest Risk	Minimal	Low	Moderate	High
C	Amount and/or complexity of data	≤ 1 Minimal or Low	Limited	Moderate	≥ 4 Extensive
	Type of decision making	Straight Forward	Low Complex	Moderate Complex	High Complex

B Risk of Complications and/or Morbidity or Mortality

Level of Risk	Presenting Problems(s)	Diagnostic Procedure(s) Ordered	Management Options Selected
MINIMAL	One self-limited or minor problem, e.g. cold, insect bite	Laboratory tests requiring venipuncture * Chest X-rays * EKG / EEG * Urinalysis * Ultrasound * KOH prep	* Rest * Gargles * Elastic bandages * Superficial dressings
LOW	* Two or more self-limited or minor problems * One stable chronic illness, e.g. well controlled hypertension, non-insulated dependent diabetes, contact, BPH * Acute uncomplicated illness or injury, e.g. cystitis	* Physiologic tests not under stress, e.g. function tests * Non-cardiovascular imaging studies with contrast, e.g. barium enema * Superficial needle biopsies * Clinical laboratory tests requiring arterial puncture * Skin biopsies	* Over-the -counter drugs * Minor surgery with no identified risk factors * Physical therapy * Occupational therapy * IV fluids without additives
MODERATE	* One or more chronic illnesses with mild exacerbation, progression, or side effects of treatment * Two or more stable chronic illnesses * Undiagnosed new problem with uncertain prognosis, e.g. lump on breast * Acute illness with systemic symptoms, e.g. pyelonephritis * Acute complicated injury, e.g. head injury with brief loss of consciousness	* Physiologic tests under stress, e.g. cardiac stress test, stress test * Diagnostic endoscopies with no identified risk factors * Deep needle or incisional biopsy * Cardiovascular imaging studies with contrast and no identified risk factors, e.g. arteriogram, cardiac cath * Obtain fluid from body cavity, e.g. lumbar punction, thoracemtesis,	* Minor surgery with identified risk factors * Elective major surgery (open percutaneous or endoscopic) with no identified risk factors * Prescription drug management * Therapeutic nuclear medicine * IV fluids with additives * Closed treatment of fracture or dislocation without manipulation
HIGH	* One or more chronic illnesses with severe exacerbation, progression * Acute or chronic illnesses or injuries that may pose a threat to life or badily function, e.g. trauma, acute MI, severe respiratory distress, progressive severe rheumatoid arthritis, psychitatiric illness with potential threat to self or others, acute renal failure * An abrupt change in neurologic status, e.g. seizure, TIA, weakness, or sensory loss	* Cardiovascular imaging studies with contrast with identified risk factors * Cardiac electrophysiological tests * Diagnostic endoscopies with identified risk factors * Discography	* Elective major surgery (open, percutanepus or endoscopic) with identified risk factors * Emergency major surgery (open, percutanepus or endoscopic) * Parenteral controlled substances * Drug therapy requiring intensive monitoring for toxicity * Decision not to resuscitate or to de-escalate care because of poor prognosis

APPENDIX E
AUDIT FORM/CLAIM DENIAL FOLLOWUP (resource aafp.org)

Plan/Payer name: ____ Date submitted: ____/____/____

Patient name: ____ Birth date: ____/____/____
FIRST M.I. LAST

Subscriber name: ____ Date of service: ____/____/____

Policy #: ________________ Group #: ________________ Original claim #: ______________

Initial Claim Submitted by: Employee: ______________________ Date: ________________

Deficiencies on the claim include (reason for denial):

- ❍ Policy number wrong. .
- ❍ Date of service incorrect; correct date is ____/____/____.
- ❍ CPT code incorrect. Correct CPT code is ______________ to replace ______________.
- ❍ Diagnosis code incorrect. Correct diagnosis code is ____________ to replace ____________.
- ❍ Not submitted to primary carrier first.
- ❍ Not medically necessary.
- ❍ Units incorrect
- ❍ Service was unbundled or part of global and should not have been billed.
- ❍ UPIN information was omitted.
- ❍ Date of service wrong: ______________________
- ❍ Place of service incorrect: ______________________.
- ❍ Duplicate billing: ______________________
- ❍ Services are not eligible for coverage: ______________________
- ❍ Records not legible ______________________
- ❍ Documents lack proper signatures ______________________
- ❍ Other reason for correction: ______________________

Patient ID	*Provider initials*	*Date of service*	*Procedure codes from superbill*	*Procedure codes from patient account*	*Procedures documented in medical record*	*Procedures provided but not billed*	*Allowed charges for all procedures*	*Date and amount paid by insurance*	*Lost revenue*	*Need explanation of benefits?*	*Notes*
1	BAN	5/8/08	99213	None	Office visit	99213	$85	None	$85	No	Charge never entered
2	JAL	5/8/08	Not found	None	New patient visit, quick strep test	99203 87880	$128	None	$128	No	Lost superbill
3	BAN	5/8/08	99396 82270 90718	Same	Same, plus vaccine administration	90471	$168	$143 on 5/28/08	$25	No	Service provided but not billed
4	BAN	5/8/08	99214 17000	Same	Same	None	$210	$125 on 5/24/08	$85	Yes	Two problems addressed, two diagnoses. E/M not paid

APPENDIX F
SAMPLE SUPERBILL

Date of service:	Waiver? yes / no	
Patient name:	Insurance:	
Address:	Subscriber name:	
	Group #:	Previous balance:
	Account #:	Today's charges:
Phone:	Copay:	Today's payment:
DOB: Age: Sex:	Physician name:	Balance due:

RA	Office visit	New	Est
	Minimal		99211
	Problem focused	99201	99212
	Exp problem focused	99202	99213
	Detailed	99203	99214
	Comp	99204	99215
	Comp (new patient)	99205	
	Significant, sep serv	-25	-25
	Well visit	**New**	**Est**
	< 1 y	99381	99391
	1-4 y	99382	99392
	5-11 y	99383	99393
	12-17 y	99384	99394
	18-39 y	99385	99395
	40-64 y	99386	99396
	65 y +	99387	99397
	Medicare preventive services		
	Pap		Q0091
	Pelvic & breast		G0101
	Prostate/PSA		G0103
	Tobacco couns/3-10 min		G0375
	Tobacco couns/>10 min		G0376
	Welcome to Medicare exam		G0344
	ECG w/Welcome to Medicare		G0366
	Flexible sigmoidoscopy		G0104
	Hemoccult, guaiac		G0107
	Flu shot		G0008
	Pneumonia shot		G0009
	Consultation/preop clearance		
	Exp problem focused		99242
	Detailed		99243
	Comp/mod complex		99244
	Comp/high complex		99245
	Other services		
	After posted hours		99050
	Evening/weekend appointment		99051
	Home health certification		G0180
	Home health recertification		G0179
	Post-op follow-up		99024
	Prolonged/30-74 min		99354
	Special reports/forms		99080
	Disability/Workers comp		99455
	Radiology		
Diagnoses			
1			
2			
3			
4			
Next office visit			
Recheck • Prev • PRN	____ D W M Y		
Instructions:			

RA	Office procedures		
	Anoscopy		46600
	Audiometry		92551
	Cerumen removal		69210
	Colposcopy		57452
	Colposcopy w/biopsy		57455
	ECG, w/interpretation		93000
	ECG, rhythm strip		93040
	Endometrial biopsy		58100
	Flexible sigmoidoscopy		45330
	Flexible sigmoidoscopy w/biopsy		45331
	Fracture care, cast/splint		29__
	Site: ________________		
	Nebulizer		94640
	Nebulizer demo		94664
	Spirometry		94010
	Spirometry, pre and post		94060
	Tympanometry		92567
	Vasectomy		55250
	Skin procedures		**Units**
	Burn care, initial	16000	
	Foreign body, skin, simple	10120	
	Foreign body, skin, complex	10121	
	I&D, abscess	10060	
	I&D, hematoma/seroma	10140	
	Laceration repair, simple	120__	
	Site: _______ Size: _____		
	Laceration repair, layered	120__	
	Site: _______ Size: _____		
	Lesion, biopsy, one	11100	
	Lesion, biopsy, each add'l	11101	
	Lesion, excision, benign	114__	
	Site: _______ Size: _____		
	Lesion, excision, malignant	116__	
	Site: _______ Size: _____		
	Lesion, paring/cutting, one	11055	
	Lesion, paring/cutting, 2-4	11056	
	Lesion, shave	113__	
	Site: _______ Size: _____		
	Nail removal, partial	11730	
	Nail removal, w/matrix	11750	
	Skin tag, 1-15	11200	
	Wart, flat, 1-14	17110	
	Wart, plantar, single	17000	
	Wart, plantar, each add'l	17003	
	Medications		**Units**
	Ampicillin, up to 500mg	J0290	
	B-12, up to 1,000 mcg	J3420	
	Epinephrine, up to 1ml	J0170	
	Kenalog, 10mg	J3301	
	Lidocaine, 10mg	J2001	
	Normal saline, 1000cc	J7030	
	Phenergan, up to 50mg	J2550	
	Progesterone, 150mg	J1055	

RA	Laboratory		
	Venipuncture		36415
	Blood glucose, monitoring device		82962
	Blood glucose, visual dipstick		82948
	CBC, w/ auto differential		85025
	CBC, w/o auto differential		85027
	Cholesterol		82465
	Hemoccult, guaiac		82270
	Hemoccult, immunoassay		82274
	Hemoglobin A1C		85018
	Lipid panel		80061
	Liver panel		80076
	KOH prep (skin, hair, nails)		87220
	Metabolic panel, basic		80048
	Metabolic panel, comprehensive		80053
	Mononucleosis		86308
	Pregnancy, blood		84703
	Pregnancy, urine		81025
	Renal panel		80069
	Sedimentation rate		85651
	Strep, rapid		86403
	Strep culture		87081
	Strep A		87880
	TB		86580
	UA, complete, non-automated		81000
	UA, w/o micro, non-automated		81002
	UA, w/ micro, non-automated		81003
	Urine colony count		87086
	Urine culture, presumptive		87088
	Wet mount/KOH		87210
	Vaccines		
	DT, <7 y		90702
	DTP		90701
	DtaP, <7 y		90700
	Flu, 6-35 months		90657
	Flu, 3 y +		90658
	Hep A, adult		90632
	Hep A, ped/adol, 2 dose		90633
	Hep B, adult		90746
	Hep B, ped/adol 3 dose		90744
	Hep B-Hib		90748
	Hib, 4 dose		90645
	HPV		90649
	IPV		90713
	MMR		90707
	Pneumonia, >2 y		90732
	Pneumonia conjugate, <5 y		90669
	Td, >7 y		90718
	Varicella		90716
	Immunizations & Injections		**Units**
	Allergen, one	95115	
	Allergen, multiple	95117	
	Imm admin, one	90471	
	Imm admin, each add'l	90472	

Aafp.org

APPENDIX G
COMBINING FORMS & ABBREVIATIONS

A

a, an	absence, without
ab	away from
abdomino	abdomen
ac	pertaining to
acous	hearing
acro	extremity
acusis	hearing
ad	toward
adeno	gland
adip	fatty
adren	adrenal glands
emia	blood condition
al	pertaining to
abl	white
algia	pain
allo	different
ambi	two
an	not, without
angio	blood vessel
ante	before
anti	against
arthro	joints
aur	ear
auto	self
axill	armpit

B

bi	two
bio	life
blepharo	eyelid
brachio	arm
brady	slow
bucco	cheek

C

capit	head
carcin	cancer
cardio	heart
carp	wrist
cele	hernia, pouch
centesis	surgical puncture
cephal	head
cerebr	brain
cervic	neck
cholecysto	gall bladder
chrondro	cartilage
circum	around
contra	against
costo	rib
crine	secrete
cryo	cold
cutan	skin
cyano	blue color
cyst	urinary bladder
cyt	cell

D

dactyl	finger, toe
de	away from
dermato	skin
dia	through
dis	take apart
dorso	back
dynia	pain
dys	bad

E

ec	out, away
ectasis	dilation
ectomy	excision
emesis	vomiting
emia	blood condition
endo	within
entero	intestine
eu	good
ex	out

G

gastro	stomach
gen	to form
genu	knee
gingiv	gums
gloss	tongue

gluco	sugar, glucose
glycol	sugar
gram	record, picture
graph	record, picture
graphy	process of recording

H

hemato	blood
hemi	one-half
hepato	liver
hetero	other
histo	tissue
hydro	water
hyper	above
hypo	below
hysteron	uterus

I

ia	condition
iatro	medicine, treatment
idio	self
infra	below
inter	between
intra	within
ism	condition
iso	equal
ist	one who specializes
it is	inflammation
ium	tissue, structure

K

kerato	cornea

L

labio	lip
lacrimo	tear
laparo	abdomen
lingu	tongue
lipo	fat
litho	stone, calculus
logo	knowledge
lysis	destruction

M

macro	large
malacia	softening
megaly	enlargement
melano	black
meso	middle
meta	change
micro	small
mono	single
morpho	form, shape
myo	muscle
myelo	bone marrow
myringo	eardrum
myxo	mucus

N

necro	death
neo	new
nephro	kidney
neuro	nerve

O

oculo	eye
odon	teeth
odyn	pain
oid	resembling
oligo	few, little
oma	tumor
omphalo	navel
onco	tumor
onycho	nail
ophthalmo	eye
oro	mouth
ortho	straight
ose	full
osis	abnormal condition
osteo	bone
oto	ear

P

palpebro	eyelid
pan	all
para	abnormal
paresis	paralysis
patho	disease
ped	foot
penia	deficiency
pepsia	digestion
per	through
peri	surrounding
pexy	fixation

phage	**eating**
pharmaco	**drug**
pharyng	**pharynx**
phlebo	**veins**
phobo	**fear**
phono	**sound**
photo	**light**
phren	**diaphragm**
plasia	**formation**
plasty	**surgical repair**
plegia	**paralysis**
pleura	**ribs**
pneumo	**lungs**
pod	**foot**
poiesis	**production**
poly	**many**
post	**after**
pre	**before**
presbyo	**old**
pro	**before**
procto	**rectum**
psycho	**mind**
ptosis	**drooping, falling**
ptysis	**spitting**
pulmon	**lungs**
pyo	**pus**
pyro	**fever**

R

rachio	**spine**
re	**back**
ren	**kidney**
retro	**back**
rhino	**nose**
rrhage	**burst forth**
rrhaphy	**suture**
rrhea	**flow, discharge**

S

sangui	**blood**
sarco	**flesh**
scope	**instrument for viewing**
semi	**half**
sialo	**saliva**
sinistro	**left**
sis	**condition**
somato	**body**
splen	**spleen**
spondylo	**vertebrae**
stasis	**stop**
steno	**narrowing**
stoma	**mouth**
stomy	**creation of an opening**
sub	**underneath**
super	**above, excess**
supra	**above**
syn	**together, with**

T

tachy	**fast**
thoraco	**chest**
thrombo	**blood clot**
toco	**childbirth**
tome	**cutting instrument**
tomy	**cutting**
trans	**across**
tripsy	**crushing**
trophy	**development**
tympano	**eardrum**

U

ule	**small**
ultra	**beyond, excessive**
ungui	**nail**
uni	**one**

ABBREVIATIONS

AB abortion
AD right ear
ADD attention deficit disorder
AIDS acquired immune Deficiency syndrome
ALS amyotrophic lateral Sclerosis
AMA against medical advice
AP anteroposterior
AS left ear
AU both ears

BBB bundle branch block
BKA below knee amputation
BPH benign prostatic hyperplasia
Bx biopsy

CA cancer
CABG coronary artery bypass graft
CAD coronary artery disease
CAPD continuous ambulatory Peritoneal dialysis
CAT computerized axial tomography
CBC complete blood count
CC chief complaint
CHD coronary heart disease
CHF congestive heart failure
CNS central nervous system
COPD chronic obstructive pulmonary disease
CRF chronic renal failure
C-section cesarean section
CSF cerebrospinal fluid
CT computed tomography
CVA cerebrovascular accident
CX chest x-ray

D&C dilation and curettage
DM diabetes mellitus
DNR do not resuscitate
DT delirium tremens
DTR deep tendon reflexes
Dx diagnosis

EEG electroencephalogram
EENT eyes, ears, nose and throat
EGD esophagogastroduodenoscopy
EKG electrocardiogram
ESRD end stage renal disease
ESWL extracorporeal shock wave Lithotripsy

Fx fracture

G gravid (pregnancy)
GERD gastroesophageal reflux Disease

HIPAA Health Insurance Portability& Accountability Act
HIV human immunodeficiency virus
HPI History of present illness
HTN hypertension

IBD irritable bowel disease
I&D incision and drainage
IHD ischemic heart disease
IOL intraocular lens
IPPB intermittent positive pressure Breathing
IVP intravenous pyelogram

KUB kidney, ureter & bladder x-ray

LA left atrium
LAD left anterior descending coronary Artery
Lat lateral
LBBB left bundle branch block
LFT liver function test
LLL left lower lobe (lung)
LP lumbar puncture

LVAD left ventricular assist device

MAC monitored anesthesia care
MMR measles, mumps, rubella
MRI magnetic resonance imaging

NB newborn
NICU neonatal intensive care unit
NSAID nonsteroidal anti-inflammatory Drug

OA osteoarthritis
OB/GYN obstetrics/gynecology
OD right eye
ORIF open reduction internal fixation

PA posteroanterior
PAC premature atrial contraction
Para number of viable births
PD peritoneal dialysis
PEEP positive end-expiratory pressure
PEG percutaneous endoscopic Gastrostomy (feeding tube)
PERRLA pupils equal, round and reactive To light and accommodation
PET positive emission tomography
PE tube ventilating tube for eardrum
PID pelvic inflammatory disease
PIP proximal interphalangeal joint
PKU phenylketonuria
PMH past medical history
PMS premenstrual syndrome
p.o. by mouth
prn as needed
PSA prostate specific antigen
PTCA percutaneous transluminal Coronary angioplasty
PTH parathyroid hormone
PTSD post traumatic stress disorder
PVC premature ventricular contraction

RA rheumatoid arthritis
RBBB right bundle branch block
RBC red blood count
RDS respiratory distress syndrome
R/O rule out

SC subcutaneous
SARS severe acute respiratory syndrome
SIDS sudden infant death syndrome
SLE systemic lupus erythematosus
SOAP subjective, objective, assessment, plan
SOB short of breath
SVC superior vena cava
SVD spontaneous vaginal delivery

T&A tonsillectomy and adenoidectomy
TAB therapeutic abortion
TAH total abdominal hysterectomy
TB tuberculosis
TIA transient ischemic attack
TM tympanic membrane
TNM tumor, nodes, metastases
TPN total parenteral nutrition
TVH total vaginal hysterectomy

UA urinalysis
URI upper respiratory infection
UTI urinary tract infection

APPENDIX H
RESOURCES

Medical Coding Specialist's Exam Review, Lyn Olsen, 2006, Cengage/Delmar Publishing Co.

CPT/HCPCS Coding and Reimbursement for Physician Service. Lynn Kuehn, AHIMA, 2008.

Correct Coding for Medicare, Compliance, and Reimbursement, Belinda Frisch, 2007, Cengage/Delmar Publishing.

Today's Health Information Management, Dana McWay, Thomson/Delmar, 2008.

International Classification of Diseases-10th Revision-Clinical Modification, 2015.

Current Procedural Terminology, American Medical Association, 2009.

Healthcare Common Procedure Coding System, CMS, 2009.

CPT: Beyond the Basics. Gail Smith. AHIMA, 2000.

Netter's Atlas of Human Anatomy for CPT Coding. Celeste Kirschner, AMA, 2005.

The Complete Procedure Coding Book. Shelley Safian, McGraw-Hill, 2009.

APPENDIX I: ANSWERS

REGULATIONS QUIZ 1

1. What does OIG stand for? Office of Inspector General

2. What does HIPAA stand for? Health Insurance Portability and Accountability Act

3. Explain the Stark Laws. Healthcare providers cannot recommend patient to other places for services if the provider has an affiliation with the other place and would benefit monetarily or otherwise.

4. What are the fines for healthcare fraud? $10,000 per incident plus triple amount of discrepancy.

5. What other prosecutory actions are levied besides fines for healthcare fraud? Prison time and loss of patients.

6. What is the three areas of healthcare offenses and describe them. Fraud is purposeful intent to gain funds illegally. Abuse is failure to perform fair and reasonable practices as would be performed in other similar practices. Acts of omissions and mistakes which have no intent to defraud and were not failure to perform reasonably.

7. Where can you find what areas OIG will be focusing on for fraud and abuse for that year? OIG work plan, oig.hhs.gov

8. Describe the components of a good compliance program. Written standards, compliance and security officer, proper training, established complaint process, enforcement policies for violations, audits and evaluations, and investigation/remediation of violations and problems.

9. What does Qui Tam mean? Private citizen files lawsuit in the name of the US Government for fraud on behalf of others.

10. Who is responsible for development of the ICD codes? WHO, World Health Organization.

REPORT FORMAT QUIZ 2

1. Name and describe the three types of health record formats. Source oriented based on department, specialty or other category. Integrated based on chronology (time). Problem oriented based on diagnosis or problem.

2. Describe the advantages and disadvantages of each type of health record format. Source oriented is easy to find and follow specific treatment plans by departments or specialties but may make it hard to find reports based on diagnosis or time. Integrated gives a congruent time line of services but hard to find specific reports for diagnosis or specialty. Problem oriented known as POMR (problem oriented medical record) gives entire picture of diagnosis treatment but does not provide coherent and consistent picture of overall healthcare which includes other diagnosis or problems.

3. Describe the two types of progress notes. SOAP (subjective, objective, assessment, plan) and SNOCAMP (subjective, nature of presenting problem, objective, counseling and coordination of care, assessment, medical decision making and plan.)

4. What are five types of medical reports? History and Physical, Discharge, Operative, Pathology, Radiology.

5. Describe the content of the history and physical report. Admitting diagnosis, history of present illness, past family social history, allergies, review of systems, exam, impression.

6. What are the two most important parts of medical reports for coding purposes? Headings such as admit discharge and description of procedure.

7. Describe abstracting. Reviewing a patient's record/report to determine codes (not superbills or other templates).

8. Describe two ways in which changes can be made to a medical report. Line drawn through error followed by date and initials of who made the changes and add an addendum.

9. Describe four criteria for proper completion of medical records. Handwriting must be legible, black ink, date and time for entries and changes, proper signatures.

10. What is the coder's motto concerning medical records? Not documented not done.

STRUCTURE QUIZ 3

1. What number most often represents an unspecified code? 9

2. What is the code for encephalopathy that is not specified? G93.40

3. Derangement of a previous ligament of the right knee is what code? M23.8X1

4. What are the codes for a perforation of the esophagus that was traumatic? S27.819A

5. What number most often represents a code in which more information is provided but there is no specific code for the condition? 8

6. What is the code for spina bifida occulta? Q76.0

7. What are the codes for otitis due to impetigo? L01.00

8. What are the codes for excessive vomiting in a pregnant woman? O21.9

9. What does NEC stand for? Not elsewhere classified

10. What is the code for postviral encephalitis? A86

11. What is the code for a patient who is seen today for crushing chest injury? S28.0XXA

12. A patient is seen today for a headache and polyneuropathy due to Type 1 diabetes. What are the codes? E10.40, R51

13. A patient is seen today to rule out a hernia due to abdominal pain. What are the codes? R51

14. A patient is seen today for arthropathy due to TB of the hip. What are the codes? A18.02

15. A patient is seen today for a stomach ache and headache and was found to be due to botulism. What are the codes? A05.1

INFECTIOUS DISEASES QUIZ 4

1. Is AIDS pandemic or epidemic? pandemic
2. What are the codes for septicemia due to anthrax? A22.7
3. What are the codes for a patient seen today for septic urinary tract infection due to E. coli? N39.0, B96.20,, A41.9
4. What are the codes for a patient seen with hepatitis D associated with Hepatitis B? B17.0
5. What are the codes for a patient with uveitis due to syphilis? A51.43
6. What are the codes for a patient who has H. influenza due to meningitis? B16.1
7. What are the codes for a patient who has infection of the colon due to Clostridium difficile? A04.7
8. What are the codes for a patient seen today for HIV and related Kaposi's sarcoma of the lymph nodes? B20, G46.3
9. What are the codes for a patient seen today with HIV? Z21
10. What are the codes for chronic spondylitis? M46.90
11. What are the codes for a patient seen today for bacteremia with septic shock? R78.81 R65.21
12. What are the codes for a patient with acute bronchitis due to Pseudomonas? J21.8, B96.5
13. What are the codes for a patient with pernicious complications of malaria with nephropathy? B52.0
14. What are the codes for a patient seen today for SIRS with septic shock? R65.21
15. What are the codes for a 23-year-old patient who is seen today for MRSA? B95.62

NEOPLASMS QUIZ 5

1. What are the codes for intramural leiomyoma of the uterus? D25.1

2. What are the codes for a patient who is seen today for nausea and vomiting due to chemotherapy two days ago of metastatic brain cancer? R11.2, C80.1, T45.1X5

3. What are the codes for traumatic asphyxiation? T71.9XXX

4. What are the codes for benign leiomyoma of the abdomen? D21.4

5. What are the codes for a patient who has metastatic brain cancer? C79.31

6. What are the codes for Paget's disease of the extramammary skin? C44.90

7. What are the codes for a patient with carcinoma of the body of the uterus and contiguous sites? C54.8

8. What are the codes for carcinoma of the rectum and colon metastatic from the anterior wall of the bladder? C67.3, C78.5

9. What are the codes for adenoma of the chief cell? D35.1

10. What are the codes for a patient who is seen today for prophylactic chemotherapy a year after having a mastectomy due to breast cancer with treatment completed three months ago? Z40.01 Z85.3

11. What are the codes for a patient who has Hodgkin's lymphoma of the lymph nodes of the neck and axilla and the spleen? C81.98, C81.97

12. What are the codes for patient with malignant schwannoma of the abdomen? C49.4

13. What are the codes for leiomyoblastoma (include the M code) of the chest? D48.1

14. What are the codes for osteochondroma of the coccyx? D16.8

15. What are the codes for patient with UTI due to E. coli? N39.0, B96.20

BLOOD DISORDERS QUIZ 6

1. What are the codes for a patient with senile dementia? F03.90

2. What are the codes for a patient experiencing septic shock due to UTI? N39.0, R65.21303

3. What are the codes for a patient suffering from dipsomania? F10.20

4. What are the codes for a patient with goat's milk anemia? D52.0

5. What are the codes for a patient who metastatic cancer of the uterus? C79.82

6. What are the codes for an anemic patient due to hemorrhaging of a lower leg wound caused by a car accident? S81.829A, D62, V49.9XXA

7. What are the codes for a patient who has sickle cell anemia Hb-SS with acute chest syndrome? D57.01

8. What are the codes for a patient who has vegan anemia? D51.3

9. What are the codes for a patient who has malignant schwannoma of the hip? C49.20

10. What are the codes for a patient experiencing a crisis with sickle cell anemia? D57.00

11. What are the codes for a patient who is diagnosed with anemia due to a chronic gastric ulcer? K25.7, D63.8

12. What are the codes for a patient with Hodgkins lymphoma of the spleen and axillary and neck lymph nodes who has neutropenia due to chemotherapy? C81.97, C81.98, D7.01

13. What are the codes for a patient with traumatic asphyxiation? T71.9XXX

14. What are the codes for a patient with a coagulation defect due to Vitamin K deficiency? D68.4

15. What are the codes for a patient who Pelger-Huet anomaly? D72.0

ENDOCRINE QUIZ 7

1. What are the codes for a patient with drug-induced Cushing's syndrome? E24.2
2. What are the codes for a patient with H. influenza with meningitis? G00.0
3. What are the codes for a patient with anemia and ALS? G12.21, D64.9
4. What are the codes for a patient with polyuria due to possible diabetes mellitus? R35.8
5. What are the codes for a Type I diabetic patient with cataracts? E10.9, H26.9
6. What are the codes for a patient with arthritis due to chronic gout? M1A.9XX0
7. What are the codes for a patient with Hodgkins lymphoma of the spleen and axillary and neck lymph nodes? C81.97, C81.98
8. What are the codes for a patient treated with insulin in the emergency room due to severe ketoacidosis due to their diabetes mellitus? E11.69
9. What are the codes for a patient who experienced hypovolemic shock due to trauma? T79.4XXA
10. What are the codes for a patient with goiter related to hyperthyroidism with storm? E05.01
11. What are the codes for a patient with diabetic retinal microangiopathy with edema? E11.311
12. What are the codes for a patient with a headache and possible concussion? R51
13. What are the codes for hypopituitarism due to the administration of radiotherapy? E23.1, T66.XXXA
14. What are the codes for a patient experiencing a thyrotoxic crisis due to Graves' Disease? E05.01
15. What are the codes for a patient who has amputation of two toes on the right foot due to gangrene related to Type 2 diabetic peripheral vascular disease? E11.52

MENTAL QUIZ 8

1. What are the codes for a patient with carcinoma of the lower outer quadrant of the breast metastatic to the left lung? C50.519, C78.02

2. What are the codes for patient experiencing panic attack with agoraphobia? F40.01

3. What are the codes for a patient who is experiencing combat fatigue? F430

4. What are the codes for a patient who has chronic alcoholism with cirrhosis? F10.20, K70.30

5. What are the codes for a patient with anorexia? R63.0

6. What are the codes for a patient suffering from depression due to the death of her husband? F43.21

7. What are the codes for a teenager who has been experiencing problems with significant school truancy? F91.2

8. What are the codes for a patient with subacute borderline schizophrenia? F21

9. What are the codes for a patient with a long history of alcoholism who was binge drinking over the superbowl weekend and seen for drunkenness? F10.229

10. What are the codes for a patient with dementia due to alcohol intoxication? F10.27

11. What are the codes for a 62-year-old patient with paranoid senile dementia? F03.90

12. What are the codes for a patient with bulima nervosa? F50.2

13. What are the codes for a patient with chronic PTSD? F43.12

14. What are the codes for a patient who has an IQ of 65? F70

15. What are the codes for a patient with acute exacerbation of chronic myeloid leukemia? C92.10

NERVOUS QUIZ 9

1. What are the codes for a patient with a classic migraine with aura? G43.109
2. What are the codes for a patient with an IQ of 45 who has ringworm? F71, B35.9
3. What are the codes for a patient who has MS? G35
4. What are the codes for a patient who has pars planitis? H30.23
5. What are the codes for a patient who has double vision? H53.2
6. What are the codes for a patient who has pigmentary open-angle glaucoma? H40.1390
7. What are the codes for a patient who has Fusarium keratitis? B48.8, H16.8
8. What are the codes for a patient who has tonic-clonic epilepsy? G40.309
9. What are the codes for a patient who has restless leg syndrome? G25.81
10. What are the codes for a patient who presents today because she has not been taking her insulin as prescribed for her for the past four years and she is now experiencing polyneuropathy due to Type 2 diabetes? E11.40, Z79.4
11. What are the codes for a patient who has presenile cortical cataract of the left eye and is Type I diabetic? H26.019, E109
12. What are the codes for a patient who has epilepsy marked by grand mal seizures which is not responding to treatment? G40.311
13. What are the codes for a patient who has tic douloureux? G50.0
14. What are the codes for a patient who has pseudocyesis? F45.8
15. What are the codes for a patient who has Huntington's dementia? G10, F02.80

TEST 1 ANSWERS

1. What is the code for a patient who is seen today for chest pains due to possible MI? R07.9
2. What is the code for a patient who is seen today for crushing chest injury? S27.9XXA
3. What are the codes for a patient who has metastatic brain cancer? C79.31
4. What are the codes for a patient seen today for chemotherapy for ongoing treatment of breast cancer which was excised two months ago? Z51.11, C50.919
5. An 8-year-old patient is seen today for enteritis due to Clostridium difficile. What are the codes? A04.7
6. What does HIPAA stand for? HEALTH INSURANCE PORTABILITY AND ACCOUNTABILITY ACT
7. What other prosecutory actions are levied besides fines for healthcare fraud? PRISON TIME AND CAN'T PROVIDE CARE TO GOVERNMENT PATIENTS
8. What number most often represents an unspecified code? 9
9. What is Volume 2 of the ICD book known as? ALPHABETICAL INDEX
10. Derangement of a previous ligament of the knee is what code? M23.8X9
11. What are the codes for a perforation of the esophagus that was traumatic? S27.819A
12. What is the code for postviral encephalitis? B97.89, G04.30
13. /3 indicates what in M codes? MALIGNANCY IN PRIMARY SITE
14. What are the two supplementary classifications in Volume 1? V AND E CODES
15. Name and describe the three types of health record formats. SOURCE-ORIENTED (BASED ON SPECIALTY OR DEPARTMENT), INTEGRATED (CHRONOLOGICALLY), PROBLEM-ORIENTED (DIAGNOSIS/PROBLEM)
16. Describe the two types of progress notes. SOAP (SUBJECTIVE, OBJECTIVE, ASSESSMENT, PLAN) AND SNOCAMP (SUBJECTIVE, NATURE OF PRESENTING PROBLEM, OBJECTIVE, COUNSELING/COORDINATION OF CARE, ASSESSMENT, MEDICAL DECISION MAKING AND PLAN
17. What does CPC mean? CERTIFIED PROFESSIONAL CODER
18. What types of coding does a CPC perform? PHYSICIAN
19. What types of coding does a CCS perform? INPATIENT AND OUTPATIENT HOSPITAL
20. Explain the Stark Laws. PROVIDERS CANNOT RECOMMEND PATIENTS TO RECEIVE SERVICES FROM AN ORGANIZATION IN WHICH THEY MAY RECEIVE MONETARY BENEFITS
21. What are the codes for traumatic asphyxiation? S27.9XXA
22. What are the codes for benign leiomyoma of the abdomen? D21.4
23. What are the codes for a patient who was binge drinking over the weekend and was seen in the emergency room who experienced alcoholic stupor? F10.10, R40.1

24. A patient is seen today for arthropathy due to TB. What are the codes? A18.02, M01.X0
25. ICD-10-CM stands for what? INTERNATIONAL CLASSIFICATION OF DISEASES – 9TH REVISION – CLINICAL MODIFICATION
26. What federal department is CMS a part of? HEALTH AND HUMAN SERVICES
27. How many volumes are there in the ICD today? 3
28. What are the codes for a patient seen today for septic urinary tract infection due to E. coli? N39.0, A41.9, B96.20
29. What are the codes for a patient seen with hepatitis D associated with inactive Hepatitis B? B17.0
30. What are the codes for a patient with uveitis due to syphilis? A51.43
31. What is the code for a patient with acute bronchitis due to Pseudomonas J21.8, B96.5
32. What are the codes for malaria with pernicious complications with hepatitis? B51.8, K77
33. What are the codes for a 23-year-old patient who is seen today for MRSA? B95.62
34. What are the codes for leiomyoma of the uterus? D25.9
35. What are the codes for a patient who is seen today for nausea and vomiting due to chemotherapy? R11.2, C80.1, T45.1X5
36. What are the codes for a patient with carcinoma of the breast metastatic to the left lung? C50.919, C78.02
37. AHIMA stands for what? AMERICAN HEALTH INFORMATION MANAGEMENT ASSOCIATION
38. What does CCS-P mean? CERTIFIED CODING SPECIALIST – PHYSICIAN
39. What are the codes for patient experiencing panic attack with agoraphobia? F40.01
40. What are the codes for a patient who has MS? G35
41. What are the codes for a patient who has pars planitis? H30.23
42. What are the codes for a patient who is experiencing combat fatigue? F43.0
43. A patient is seen today for a stomach ache and headache and was found to be due to E. coli food poisoning. What are the codes? B96.20, A058
44. Define presenile dementia. YOUNGER THAN 65
45. What are the codes for a patient with anorexia? R63.0
46. What are the codes for a patient suffering from depression due to the death of her husband? F43.21
47. Describe the CNS. BRAIN AND SPINAL CORD
48. What are the codes for a patient with a classic migraine with aura? G43.109
49. What are the codes for a patient who has meningitis due to Aerobacter aerogenes? G009
50. What are the codes for a patient who has double vision? H53.2
51. What is the difference between hemiplegia and hemiparesis? HEMIPLEGIA IS TOTALLY PARALYSIS ON ONE SIDE OF THE BODY, HEMIPARESIS IS WEAKNESS ON ONE SIDE OF THE BODY
52. Infantile cerebral palsy occurs when? DURING BIRTH

53. What are the codes for a patient who has Fusarium keratitis? B48.8, H16.8
54. What are the codes for a patient who has osteitis with chronic mastoiditis due to TB? A18.03, M90.80
55. What does idiopathic mean? NO KNOWN CAUSE
56. When two major changes were added in the ninth revision? EXPANDED FOR HOSPITAL PROCEDURES AND INTRODUCTION OF FIFTH DIGIT
57. What are the codes for septicemia due to anthrax? A22.7
58. What are the codes for a patient who has Huntington's dementia? G10, F02.80
59. What is the difference between a TIA and a CVA? CVA IS CEREBROVASCULAR DISEASE AND TIA IS TRANSIENT ISCHEMIC ATTACK SO TIA IS TEMPORARY INTERRUPTION OF BLOOD FLOW WITH NO DAMAGE IN CONTRAST TO CVA WHICH CAN BE LONG-LASTING AND DOES PRODUCE DAMAGE
60. What are the fines for healthcare fraud? $10,000 PLUS TIMES 3 PER INCIDENT

CIRCULATORY QUIZ 10

1. What are the codes for a patient with congestive heart failure and hypertension? I50.9, I10
2. What are the codes for a patient with elevated blood pressure? R03.0
3. What are the codes for a patient with malignant hypertensive stage IV CKD? I12.9, N18.4
4. What are the codes for a patient with benign CKD stage 4 and ASCVD due to hypertension? I13.10, N18.4, I50.9
5. What are the codes for a patient with acute and chronic pericarditis? I30.9, I31.8
6. What are the codes for a patient who has a complete AV heart block? I44.2
7. What are the codes for a patient who has strangulated internal hemorrhoids with bleeding? K64.8
8. What are the codes for a patient who has hemiplegia after experiencing a CVA 6 months ago? I69.959
9. What are the codes for a patient who was diagnosed nine weeks ago with chronic coronary insufficiency? I25.9
10. What are the codes for a patient who had an appendectomy due to appendicitis who has postoperative hypertension? I97.3
11. What are the codes for a patient who is not presenting with any symptoms but was diagnosed as having MI on an EKG reading? I25.2
12. What are the codes for a patient diagnosed with intermediate coronary syndrome? I20.0
13. What are the codes for a patient with chest pain due to acute MI of the inferoposterior wall as part of initial care? I21.11
14. What are the codes for a patient with RBBB? I45.10
15. What are the codes for a patient who has aplastic anemia due to radiation therapy? D61.1, Y84.2

RESPIRATORY 11

1. What are the codes for a patient with lower respiratory infection? J22
2. What are the codes for an asthmatic patient with status asthmaticus and COPD? J44.0
3. What are the codes for a patient with COPD and emphysema? J44, J43.9
4. What are the codes for a patient with chronic respiratory failure and chronic edema? J96.10, J81.1
5. What are the codes for a patient with ARDS? J80
6. What are the codes for a patient who is dehydrated and has pneumonia of the right lobe? J18.9
7. What are the codes for a patient with pleurisy due to TB? A15.6
8. What are the codes for a collapsed lung? J98.19
9. What are the codes for a patient with a sore throat? J02.9
10. What are the codes for a patient with tonsillitis and adenoiditis? J03.90
11. What are the codes for a patient who is seen today for a high fever and chest congestion due to the common cold? J00
12. What are the codes for a patient with COPD with pneumonia? J44.9, J18.9
13. What are the codes for a patient with acute and chronic bronchitis and COPD? J42, J44.1
14. What are the codes for a patient with chronic bronchitis and emphysema? J42, J43.0
15. What are the codes for a patient with asthma that was precipitated by exercise? J45.990

DIGESTIVE QUIZ 12

1. What is the code for a patient diagnosed with a peptic ulcer? K27.9
2. What are the codes for a patient with a perforated appendix with an abscess? K35.3
3. What are the codes for a patient with Crohn's disease? K50.90
4. What are the codes for a patient with gastritis and duodenitis? K29.90
5. What is the code for GERD? K21.9
6. What are the codes for a patient with hemorrhagic alcoholic gastritis? K29.21
7. What are the codes for a patient with dysentery and gastritis due to Salmonella? A02.0
8. What are the codes for a patient with Crohn's disease of large and small intestines? K50.80
9. What are the codes for a patient with acute cholecystitis with bile duct calculus and obstruction? K80.43
10. What are the codes for a patient with volvulus with hernia of the intestine with gangrene? K46.1
11. What are the codes for a patient with postoperative hernia? K43.2
12. What are the codes for a patient with acute gastric ulcer? K25.3
13. What are the codes for a patient with gastritis due to alcoholism? K29.20
14. What are the codes for a patient with retropharyngeal abscess? J39.0
15. What are the codes for a patient with incarcerated inguinal hernia? K40.30

INTEGUMENTARY QUIZ 13

1) What are the codes for a patient with severe dermatitis due to her use of pierced earrings? L24.81

2) What are the codes for a patient with infected corn on the right big toe with cellulitis with possible sepsis and COPD with diabetes? L84, J44.9, E11.9

3) What are the codes for a 2-month-old baby who presents with a diaper rash? L22

4) What are the codes for a patient with nonbullous erythema multiforme? L51.0

5) What are the codes for a patient with second degree sunburn? L55.1

6) What are the codes for a patient with exfoliation on 34% of their body due to erythema multiforme with arthropathy? L51.9, L49.3, M12.80

7) What are the codes for a patient with pilonidal cyst with abscess? L05.01

8) What are the codes for a patient with cheloid scar after an appendectomy? L91.0

9) What are the codes for a patient with impetiginous dermatitis? L01.00

10) What are the codes for a patient with impetigo simplex? L01.00

11) What are the codes for a patient with albinism? E70.30

12) What are the codes for a patient with winter's itch? L29.8

13) What are the codes for a patient with dermatitis due to allergy to dust? J30.89

14) What are the codes for a patient with a stage 2 ulcer that developed from a cast that was applied to their right lower leg for 3 months due to a fracture? L89.92

15) What are the codes for a patient with chronic lymphangitis due to staph? B95.8, I89.1

MUSCULOSKELETAL QUIZ 14

16) What are the codes for a patient who has traumatic asphyxiation? S27.9XXA

17) What are the codes for a patient who has pathological fracture of the vertebra due to osteoporosis? M81.0, M80.08XA

18) What are the codes for a patient who has SLE with chronic nephritis? M32.10, N08

19) What are the codes for a patient who has Achilles tenosynovitis? M66.369

20) What are the codes for a patient who has pyogenic arthritis of the hip due to staph? M00.059

21) What are the codes for a patient who has nonunion nondisplaced neck fracture of the left radius? S52.125K

22) What are the codes for a patient who has degenerative joint disease of the knee? M17.9

23) What are the codes for a patient who has chronic obstructive asthma and neuropathy due to Type 2 diabetes which required treatment with insulin because it was uncontrolled? E11.42, J44.9

24) What are the codes for a patient who has old bucket tear of the lateral meniscus of the right knee? M23.200

25) What are the codes for a patient who has a bone spur? M25.70

26) What are the codes for a patient who has acute osteomyelitis of the right ankle and foot? M86.271

27) What are the codes for a patient who has osteopathy due to typhoid fever? A01.00, M90.80

28) What are the codes for a patient who has rheumatic polyarthritis with myopathy? M06.9, G73.7

29) What are the codes for a patient who has carpal tunnel syndrome of the left arm? G56.02

30) What are the codes for a patient who has Sjogren's disease? M35.00

GENITOURINARY QUIZ 15

1. What are the codes for a patient with acute pyelonephritis due to E. coli? N10, B96.20
2. What are the codes for a patient with oophoritis and salpingitis? N70.93
3. What are the codes for a patient with chronic uremia with acute pericarditis? N18.9, N18.9
4. What are the codes for a patient with urinary incontinence and genital prolapse? N81.9, R32
5. What are the codes for a patient with orchitis and epididymitis due to diphtheria? A36.89, N51
6. What are the codes for a patient with menorrhagia? N92.0
7. What are the codes for a patient with post-hysterectomy vaginal prolapse? N99.3
8. What are the codes for a patient with acute cholecystitis with bile duct calculus with obstruction? K80.43
9. What are the codes for a patient with subacute nonsuppurative nephritis? N04.9
10. What are the codes for a patient with renal disease with membranous proliferative glomerulonephritis? N02.2
11. What are the codes for a patient with diverticulitis of the ileum with hemorrhage and peritonitis? K57.13, K65.9
12. What are the codes for a patient with vesicoureteral reflux with bilateral reflux nephropathy? N13.722
13. What are the codes for a patient with ureteral calculus and renal calculus? N20.0, N20.1
14. What are the codes for a patient with posttraumatic renal failure? T79.5XXA
15. What are the codes for a patient with septic UTI due to E. coli? N39.0, B96.20, A41.9

PREGNANCY QUIZ 16

1) What are the codes for a 36-year-old pregnant woman who has a C section due to fetal distress at 39 weeks? O68, Z37.0

2) What are the codes for a 25-year-old pregnant woman who is 33-weeks gestation, has gestational diabetes and is seen today for dehydration? O24.419, E86.0

3) What are the codes for an 18-year-old pregnant woman who has difficulty in labor due to the birth of a 12 pound baby boy? O65.4, O33.5XX0, Z37.0

4) What are the codes for a pregnant woman who delivered liveborn twins with one normal and the other breech at 32 weeks with both weighing 5 pounds? O30.003, O32.1XX0, O60.14X0, Z37.0

5) What are the codes for a pregnant woman who has had three previous miscarriages at approximately 18 weeks and presents today at 20 weeks gestation who is experiencing cramping? O26.22, R10.9

6) What are the codes for a 39-year-old pregnant woman whose baby at 32-weeks gestation is known to have Down's syndrome? O35.1XX0, O09.513

7) What are the codes for a pregnant 23-year-old woman who delivered by C-section a liveborn today at 35 weeks due to severe eclampsia and decreased fetal movement? O15.1, O36.8130, O60.14X0, Z37.0

8) What are the codes for a pregnant woman who delivered a liveborn girl which required an episiotomy to aid in delivery? O80, Z37.0

9) What are the codes for a pregnant woman who delivered twins with a normal delivery? O30.003, Z37.2

10) What are the codes for a 25-year-old pregnant woman who delivered a 10 pound baby boy but the mother's pelvic was too small and forceps had to be used but when these did not work a C-section was done? O65.4, O66.5, O33.4XX0, Z37.0

11) What are the codes for a 38-year-old pregnant woman, 37 weeks gestation, who is seen today for her checkup? O09.51

12) What are the codes for a pregnant 31-year-old woman who is seen today for deep thrombophlebitis which she developed four days after her delivery of liveborn at 42 weeks? O87.1

13) What are the codes for a pregnant woman who had an induced abortion two days ago and

is admitted for a severe infection? O071, Z37.0

14) What are the codes for a pregnant woman who was in a car accident and fractured her tibia? S82.201A, V22.2

15) What are the codes for a woman who delivered a liveborn vaginally at 39 weeks and who had a C-section for her previous pregnancy? O34.21, Z37.0

PERINATAL QUIZ 17

1) What is the code for a liveborn whose was delivered with the use of forceps at 34 weeks and weighing 1260 grams due to placentia previa? Z38.00, P03.2, P07.37, P07.15, P02.0

2) What are the codes for a newborn whose mother was addicted to cocaine and the newborn is experiencing withdrawal? Z38.00, P96.1, P04.41

3) What are the codes for a newborn at this visit who is diagnosed with neutropenia which is not transient? Z38.00, D70.0

4) What are the codes for a newborn with jaundice who was delivered at 34 weeks? Z38.00, P07.37, P59.0

5) What are the codes for a 1-year-old girl who was diagnosed with sepsis due to UTI due to E. coli? A41.50, N39.0

6) What are the neonatal codes for congenital TB? P37.0

7) What are the codes for a neonate who is diagnosed with diabetes? P70.2

8) What are the codes for a neonate with hyperbilirubinema who was premature at birth and so remained in the hospital with this her third day and weighed 2100 gm at birth? Z38.00, P590, J01.40

9) What are the codes for a baby born at 43 weeks who experienced asphyxia due to the cord wrapped around her neck? Z38.00, P84, P02.5, P08.22

10) What is the code for the newborn when her mother dies during childbirth? Z38.00, P01.6

11) What are the codes for a patient with a bunion on the right foot? M20.10

12) What are the codes for a 1-month old baby who has not gained any weight? R62.51

13) What are the codes for a patient with lower respiratory infection? J22

14) What are the codes for a fetus whose mother has been diagnosed with rubella? P00.2

15) What are the codes for a newborn whose mother received an anesthetic during delivery with a C-section performed because the newborn's heart rate slowed and was in fetal distress due to the cord being wrapped about her neck with newborn suffering hypoxia? Z38.1, P03.4, P04.0, P02.5, P19.1

CONGENITAL QUIZ 18

1) What are the codes for a newborn who was born with a hemangioma of the neck? Z38.00, D18.01

2) What are the codes for a patient with lateral epicondylitis due to crushing injury? S57.80XA, M77.10

3) What are the codes for a fetus at 35 weeks gestation who is diagnosed with a myelocele and spina bifida of C2-4 and hydrocephalus? Q05.0

4) What are the codes for a newborn during this visit with congenital toxoplasmosis with hydrocephalus? Z38.00, P37.1

5) What are the codes for a fetus who has been diagnosed with Tetralogy of Fallot? Q21.3

6) What are the codes for a missed abortion before 22 weeks for the mother? O02.1

7) What are the codes for an 8-year-old who is seen today for clubfoot that has developed over time? M21.549

8) What are the codes for a pregnant woman whose baby has been diagnosed with Down's Syndrome? O35.1XX0

9) What are the codes for a 3-day old baby who remains in the hospital after birth due to a diagnosis of Fallot's triad? Z38.00, Q22.2

10) What are the codes for a 30-week pregnant woman with aplastic anemia? O99.013, D61.9

11) What at the codes for a patient who has traumatic asphyxiation? S27.9XXA

12) What are the codes for a 44-year-old man who has arthritis of his shoulder due to Lyme disease? A69.20, M01.X19

13) What are the codes for a 2-year-old child who has been diagnosed with congential hypothyroidism? E00.9

14) What are the codes for a baby born on this visit via C-section with fetal alcohol syndrome due to her mother's alcoholism and occasional cocaine? Z38.01, Q86.0, P04.41

2. What are the codes when a 1750 gm baby at 28 weeks gestation is delivered due to hypertonic labor? Z38.00, , P03.6, P07.31

SYMPTOMS QUIZ 19

1) What are the codes for a 4-year-old patient with high fever, sore throat, and runny nose who is found to have acute right otitis media with rhinitis? J00, H66.90

2) What are the codes for a patient with pathological fracture of the distal radius and COPD with Type I diabetes? M84.439A, J44.9, E10.9

3) What are the codes for a patient who is 82-years-old and broke her right hip and has been severely depressed since? S72.009A, F43.21

4) What are the codes for a patient with second and third degree burns covering 25% of her body with 10% being third degree with infection? T31.21, T79.8XXA

5) What are the codes for a pregnant patient who ws seen for vaginal bleeding at 20 weeks gestation and she had three prior spontaneous abortions at this same time in the pregnancy? O20.9, O26.22

6) What are the codes for a patient who underwent chemotherapy today for small cell carcinoma lung cancer and is now experiencing vomiting without nausea? Z51.11, C34.90, R11.11

7. What are the codes for a patient who has old bucket tear of the lateral meniscus? M23.202

8. What are the codes for a patient with an infected wound of the right humerus which was greenstick fractured with a dislocation and laceration of the axillary nerves? S42.312D, T79.8XXA, S44.31XA

9. What are the codes for a patient with stage 5 renal disease and hypertension as well as arteriolar nephritis and chronic hypertensive uremia? I12.0, N18.5

10. What are the codes for a 45-year-old man with shortness of breath? R06.02

11. What are the codes for a patient with scar tissue of his chest from a third degree burn six months ago? L90.5, T21.31

12. What are the codes for a patient with complaints of dyspnea and tachycardia which the physician believes might be ARDS? R06.00, R00.0

13. What are the codes for a patient with acute and chronic bronchitis with COPD and ASHD? J42, J44, I25.10

14. What are the codes for a 72-year-old man who is seen for elevated liver function studies but hepatitis profile and sugar levels were normal? He is also diabetic Type 2 and has

cholelithiasis. E11.9, K80.20, R94.5, R79.89

15. What are the codes for a 57-year-old man who was admitted to the hospital for possible MI with complaints of chest pain with numbness of the left arm? EKG and stress tests were performed but were negative. R07.9, R20.1

INJURIES QUIZ 20

1) What are the codes for a patient who is diagnosed with pneumothorax due to gunshot wound? S27.0XXA

2) What are the codes for a patient who is diagnosed with a laceration of the right patella with dislocation? S83.091A

3) What are the codes for a patient who is diagnosed with a third degree burn of the chest area? T21.31XA

4) What are the codes for a patient who is diagnosed with comminuted fracture of the shaft of the left humerus with dislocation? S42.351A

5) What are the codes for a patient who is diagnosed with pneumothorax due to stab wound in the chest? S27.0XXA

6) What are the codes for a patient who is diagnosed with swelling of right thumb due to a non-venomous spider bite? S60.361A

7) What are the codes for a patient who is diagnosed with a sprain of the lateral medial collateral ligament of the right knee? S93.411A

8) What are the codes for a patient who is diagnosed with swelling and fever due to rattlesnake bite on her right ankle? T63011A

9) What are the codes for a patient who is diagnosed with second degree burns of the upper right arm? T22.211A

10) What are the codes for a patient who is diagnosed with a pathological fracture of the femur? M84.459A

11) What are the codes for a patient who is diagnosed with frostbite with necrosis of the right ear? T34.011

12) What are the codes for a patient who is diagnosed with a sprain of the posterior cruciate ligament of the left knee? S83.522

13) What are the codes for a patient who is diagnosed with crushing injury of the left lower leg and foot? S87.82XA, S97.82XA

14) What are the codes for a small child who was seen for a bean in his right ear? T16.1XXA

LATE EFFECTS/POISONINGS QUIZ 21

1) What is the code for a patient with an embolism due to their pacemaker? T82.817A

2) What is the code for a patient with gastritis after ingesting Percodan with alcohol and OTC antihistamines? K29.60, T40.2X1A, T5.191XA, T45.0X1A

3) What is the code for a patient with scar tissue due to a second and third degree burn on both legs six months ago? L90.5, T24.009S

4) What is the code for a patient with dislocation of an artificial hip joint? T84.029A

5) What is the code for a patient with CMV infection due to transplanted liver? B25.9, T86.40

6) What is the code for a patient with joint pain of the knees from rickets a year ago? M25.561, M25.562, E64.3

7) What is the code for a patient with a pressure ulcer with necrosis from her cast of the left lower leg due to a fractured upper tibia? L97.223, S89.002

8) What is the code for a patient with esophageal reflux due to ingestion of drain cleaner as an attempted suicide? K21.9, T54.3X2A

9) What is the code for a patient with failure of skin graft of the left upper arm sustained after a burn six months ago when boiling water fell on her? T86.821, T22.00XS

10) What is the code for a right-handed patient with hemiparesis of the left side due to a CVA four months ago? I69.954

11) What is the code for a patient with mental retardation due to viral encephalitis more than 5 years ago? F79, B94.1

12) What is the code for a patient with ataxia due to alcohol and carbamazepine? R27.0, T51.91XA, T42.1X1A

13) What is the code for a patient with an infection and pain due to his peritoneal dialysis catheter? T85.71XA, T82.848A, R52

14) What is the code for a patient with sequelae from a gunshot wound of the right leg a month ago? S81.809S

15) What is the code for a patient with dihescence of a mastectomy wound a week ago with infection? T81.32XA, T81.4XXA

SUPPLEMENTARY CODES QUIZ 22

1) What are the codes for a patient seen for follow-up exam of breast cancer which was removed a year ago and treated with chemotherapy? Z08, Z85.3

2) What are the codes for a patient seen who had a replacement of their colostomy? Z43.3

3) What are the codes for a patient seen today for prophylactic administration of Nolvadex for breast cancer which metastasized from skin cancer on the back which was removed a year ago with positive estrogen receptor status? Z79.810, C79.8, Z17.0

4) What are the codes for a woman who delivered a newborn who was 550 grams at 34 weeks with hyperbilirubinemia? O60.14X0, Z37.0

5) What are the codes for a patient who is leaving the country and needed a cholera vaccination? Z23

6) What are the codes for a patient seen today for counseling regarding instructions in the use of an insulin pump for her diabetes Type I and high blood pressure? E10.9, R03.0, Z46.81

7) What are the codes for a patient seen today for cataracts and diabetic neuropathy Type II with long term use of insulin and ASHD? H26.9, E11.40, I25.10, Z79.4

8) What are the codes for a 3-year-old child during a well check who was to receive DTP vaccination but was uncontrollable and so the vaccine was not administered? Z00.129, Z28.89

9) What are the codes for a patient who was seen today for laparoscopic resection of the small intestine with anastomosis which had to be changed to an open procedure for cancer? C17.9

10) What are the codes for a patient seen today for routine PAP test with no findings? Z01.419

11) What are the codes for a patient who is a bone marrow donor? Z52.3

12) What are the codes for a patient seen today for adjustment of peritoneal dialysis catheter during dialysis? Z49.02

13) What are the codes for a patient seen today for possible gout due to complaints of stomach pain but tests were negative? R10.9, Z13.0

14) What are the codes for a patient seen today for exercise therapy after suffering a severe crushing injury to the left lower leg four months ago? Z51.89, S87.80XS

15) What are the codes for a patient seen today for drug resistant pulmonary TB? A15.0, Z16.30

TEST 2 ANSWERS

1. What are the codes for a patient with senile dementia? Z16.30
2. What are the codes for a patient who has sickle cell anemia Hb-SS with acute chest syndrome? D57.00, J99
3. What is hemolysis? BREAKDOWN OF BLOOD
4. What are the codes for a patient who is diagnosed with anemia due to a chronic gastric ulcer? K25.7, D63.8
3. What are the codes for a patient with benign CKD stage 4 and ASCVD due to hypertension? I13.10, N18.4, I50.9
4. What are the codes for a pregnant woman who has had three previous miscarriages at approximately 18 weeks and presents today at 20 weeks gestation who is experiencing cramping? O26.22, R10.9
5. What are the codes for a patient with Crohn's disease? K50.90
6. What is the term for painful menstruation? DYSMENOHRRHEA
7. What are the codes for a patient with oophoritis and salpingitis? K50.90
8. What are the codes for a patient with cellulitis with possible sepsis and COPD with diabetes? L03.90, J44.9, E11.9
9. What are the codes for a 2-month-old baby who presents with a diaper rash? L22
10. What is the code for a patient with gastritis after ingesting Percodan with alcohol and OTC antihistamines? K29.60, T40.2X1A, T5.191XA, T45.0X1A
13. What is the code for a patient with scar tissue due to a second and third degree burn on both legs six months ago? L90.5, T24.009S
14. What are the codes for an anemic patient due to hemorrhaging of a lower leg wound caused by a car accident? S81.829A, D62, V49.9XXA
15. What are the codes for a patient with a stage 2 ulcer of the ankle that developed from a cast that was applied to their left lower tibia for 3 months due to a transverse fracture of the shaft? L89.522, S82.225
16. What are the codes for a patient who has pyogenic arthritis of the hip due to staph? M00.059
17. What are the codes for a patient with acute and chronic pericarditis? I30.9, I31.8
18. What are the codes for a patient with amebic carditis? I51.89, A06.89
19. What are the codes for a patient who has right heart failure? I50.9
20. What are dilated, swollen, painful veins in the anus or rectum known as? HEMORRHOID
21. What are the codes for a patient with COPD and emphysema? J44, J43.9
22. What are the codes for a Type II diabetic patient with neuropathy and pneumonia due to MRSA and a fever? J15.21, E11.40
23. What are the codes for a patient with asthma that was precipitated by exercise? J45.990
24. What are the codes for a patient with a perforated appendix with an abscess? K35.3
25. What are the codes for a patient with RAD? 493.90 REACTIVE AIRWAY DISEASE
26. What three things must occur for a woman to be diagnosed as having preeclampsia? ELEVATED BLOOD PRESSURE, EXCESSIVE PROTEIN IN THE BLOOD AND EDEMA

27. What are the codes for a 36-year-old pregnant woman who has a C section due to fetal distress at 39 weeks? O68, O09.513, Z37.0
28. What is another term for delivery? PARTURITION
29. What is considered a high blood pressure? 140/90
30. What are the codes for a patient who has mitral valve stenosis with aortic valve insufficiency? I08.0
31. What are the codes for a patient who was diagnosed nine weeks ago with chronic coronary insufficiency? I25.9
32. What are the codes for a 25-year-old pregnant woman who is 33-weeks gestation, has gestational diabetes and is seen today for dehydration? O24.419, E86.0
33. What are the codes for an 18-year-old pregnant woman who has difficulty in labor due to the birth of a 12 pound baby boy? O65.4, O33.5XX0, Z37.0
34. What are the codes for a pregnant woman who delivered liveborn twins with one normal and the other breech at 32 weeks with both weighing 5 pounds? O30.003, O32.1XX, O60.14X0, Z37.0
35. What are the codes for a patient with ASHD and chest pain due to an MI that was treated 10 weeks ago? I25.9
36. What are the codes for a patient with second degree sunburn? L5.51
37. What are the codes for a patient with pilonidal cyst with abscess? L05.01
38. What are the codes for a patient experiencing septic shock due to UTI? N39.0, R65.21303
39. What are the codes for a patient with goat's milk anemia? D52.0
40. What are the codes for a patient who metastatic cancer of the uterus? C79.82
41. What are the codes for a patient who has nonunion fracture of the left humerus? S49.002S
42. What are the codes for a patient who has degenerative joint disease of the knee? M17.9
43. What are the codes for a patient who is seen today for a high fever and chest congestion due to the common cold? J00
44. What are the codes for a patient who has right heart failure? I50.9
45. What are the codes for a patient who is diagnosed with pneumothorax due to gunshot wound? S27.0XXA
46. What are the codes for a patient who has old bucket tear of the lateral meniscus? M23.202
47. What are the codes for a newborn who was born with a hemangioma of the neck? Z38.00, D18.01
48. What are the codes when a 1750 gm baby at 28 weeks gestation is delivered due to hypertonic labor? Z38.00, , P03.6, P07.31
49. What are the codes for a neonate who is diagnosed with diabetes? P70.2
50. What are the codes for a baby born at 43 weeks who experienced asphyxia due to the cord wrapped around her neck? Z38.00, P84, P02.5, P08.22
51. What is the code for the newborn when her mother dies during childbirth? Z38.00, P01.6
52. What are the codes for a patient with second and third degree burns covering 25% of her body with 10% being third degree with infection? T31.21, T79.8XXA
53. What causes essential hypertension? CAUSE UNKNOWN
54. What is reactive airway disease? ASTHMA
55. What are the codes for a patient with lower respiratory infection? J22

56. What are the codes for an asthmatic patient with status asthmaticus and COPD? J44.0
57. What is the code for a patient with dislocation of an artificial hip joint? T84.029A
58. What is the code for a patient with CMV infection due to transplanted liver? B25.9, T86.40
59. What is the code for a patient with anoxic brain damage resulting from their bypass graft surgery for an MI? G97.81, G93.1
60. What is the code for a patient with failure of the battery of the pacemaker after two years requiring replacement? T82.111A

E/M CODES QUIZ 23

1) What are the codes for a patient who received IV infusion of non-chemotherapeutic drugs for 3 hours for septicemia? A41.9, 96365, 96366x2

2) What are the correct codes for a 32-year-old patient, well known to the physician, presents with complaints of fever, backache, and blood in urine. Patient states that the backache began a week ago, but the blood appeared last night with the pain worsening overnight. ROS is negative for all systems except for GI for which the patient has had ulcers in the past which were treated with prescriptions. Exam today found the patient to be malnourished as he has not been eating for several days now due to the pain. HEENT is negative and PERRLA. Head is normocephalic. Throat is clear. No adenopathy. Heart shows normal S1 and S2. No syncope or murmur. Lungs are clear to P&A. Extremities move well with no edema. Patient is ordered to get x-rays and blood labs were sent and patient was given a prescription. Patient is to return if pain continues after a week. R31.9, R50.9, M54.9, 99214

3) What would the codes be for a patient who was seen today at the doctor's office for their regular checkup for their diabetes Type I which is exacerbated with a high blood sugar so the history is PF and the exam is EPF. The physician conducts further testing and counseling including discussion with patient for further evaluation and treatment which was 50 more minutes? E10.65, 99215

4) What are the codes for a new patient who is having difficulty breathing and is seen today in the office? The patient's father had a history of asthma as does the patient. The patient does have COPD. The patient states that the breathing became more difficult after a long afternoon of playing basketball but has not been alleviated by his asthma medication and has only become more difficult overnight. The ROS is negative except for the history of breathing problems. During the exam, the patient's condition worsened and he was admitted to the hospital by the physician with the exam finding that GU, GI, skin, and HEENT normal. The patient does have hypertension which is treated with medication. Extremities move well with no edema. Cranial nerves are intact. J44.0, I10, 99221

5) What are the codes for a patient who was admitted to the hospital at 9 pm due to various trauma from a car accident with numerous facial lacerations as well as a possible concussion when they hit the windshield with the patient having lost consciousness in the ambulance? Patient was intoxicated so it was difficult to get a history and the exam was detailed. The patient then left AMA at 11:30 pm. S09.93XA, R40.1, F10.10, 99234

6) What are the codes for a patient who was admitted yesterday and seen today in the hospital for various testing due to difficulty breathing and pain to determine if the patient was a candidate for surgery to remove carcinoma of the left lung, but the patient is not a good candidate with history being detailed and exam detailed? C34.90, 99231

7) What are the codes for a 30-day old newborn who was admitted to the hospital for

complications due to withdrawal due to mother's use of cocaine during the pregnancy which included anoxia, failure to thrive, and seizures requiring critical care. The history is EPF and the exam is detailed. P96.1, 99471

8) What are the codes for a physician who was on standby for 45 minutes to assist with a C-section at which time he did assist for a successful C-section of a single liveborn male? O82, Z37.0, 59514-80

9) What are the codes for a 65-year-old patient who was referred to a cardiologist by their PCP due to possible CVA with hemiplegia on the left side with an EPF history and exam and Moderate MDM? G81.90, 99202

10) What are the codes for this new patient who is seen today in the office as referred by his PCP for possible AIDS with the patient's labs positive for HIV and tests are positive for Kaposi's sarcoma as was suspected with EPF History and Exam and moderate MDM so the physician spent 25 minutes counseling the patient and his family? B20, C46.9, Z71.7, 99204

11) What are the codes for a patient who is required by the insurance company for a consultation for a work-related injury when the patient fell from the roof and injured his back with a comprehensive History and Exam and Moderate MDM? S39.82XA, 99244-32

12) What are the codes for a 2-year-old who is seen today for a well check as part of continuing pediatric care with the office? Z00.129, 99392

13) What are the codes for an alcoholic patient who was admitted to the hospital at 9 pm due to possible concussion in a car accident with acute intoxication but who was transferred to another hospital at 11 pm for further treatment with a PF history and exam and moderate MDM? F10.229, 99234

14) What are the codes for a patient who was admitted to the hospital with a Detailed History and Exam and moderate MDM due to possible kidney failure, which was later diagnosed as kidney failure and the patient was provided critical care from 10:30 to 12:30 and 2:30 to 4:00? N19, 99291, 99292x5

15) What are the codes for a 3-year-old child who is seen in the emergency room after hitting their head on the fireplace that required sutures with PF History and EPF exam with SF MDM? S01.90XA, 99281, 12020

16) What are the codes for a premature baby born at 32 weeks who was in NICU an. received services from the physician from 9:30pm to 11:00 pm and then from 11:30 pm to 1:00 am? Z38.00, P07.3, 99468, 99469

17) What are the codes for a patient who is seen today in the office for follow-up after repair of a greenstick facture of the shaft of right radius with manipulation that occurred a week

ago with a PF history and exam with SF MDM? S52.311A, V67.4, 99024

18) What are the codes for a well-known patient who was seen in the office for checkup of COPD and asthma due possibly to pneumonia with the History PF history, EPF exam, and SF MDM, but the patient was found to be experiencing a severe headache and hemiparesis so the patient was admitted to the hospital for possible CVA with an EPF history and EPF exam and moderate MDM? Later that day another physician from the practice visited the patient on rounds and found that the patient's condition had deteriorated with neurological disturbances and further tests were ordered with a Detailed History and Exam and high complexity MDM. J44.9, 784.0, 342.90, 99221

19) What are the codes for a patient well known to this doctor who is seen today for a check of his diabetes Type I who cut his toe a week ago and which is now infected with a PF history, EPF exam, and moderate MDM and who had removal of a 1.5-cm lesion from her right hand? The patient was also examined for a suspicious neoplasm on his back which was removed and specimen sent to path. L08.9, E10.9, D48.5, 11100, 99213-25

20) What are the codes for a patient who was admitted to the hospital for observation for 24 hours due to complaints of chest pains after having undergone a CABG for ASHD and MI a month before but tests were negative? R07.9, 99218

ANESTHESIA QUIZ 24

11) What are the anesthesia codes for a patient who had a lobectomy of the right lung due to small cell carcinoma which metastasized to the kidney and who was admitted to the hospital with severe difficulty breathing which was also complicated by pneumoniae pneumonia? C79.00, C34.90, J13, 00546

12) What are the anesthesia codes for a patient who was given an epidural during her delivery due to prolonged delivery because of a large baby at 42 weeks? O63.9, O480, O33.5XX0, O65.4, Z370, 01960

13) What are the anesthesia codes for a 75-year-old patient who had emergency amputation of their left leg below the knee due to gangrene and sepsis after the patient was experiencing septic shock? R65.21, I96, 99100, 01482-P4

14) What are the anesthesia codes for a patient who has an esophagectomy performed due to esophageal cancer that has metastasized to the liver and brain? C15.9, C79.31, C78.7, 00320

15) What are the anesthesia codes for removal of an infected dental molar from a 3-year-old which required general anesthesia? K04.4, 00170-23

16) What are the anesthesia codes for a 1-year-old child who had tubes placed in her ears for suppurative otitis media?
H66.43, 00126

17) What are the anesthesia codes for a patient who required a C-section due to fetal distress at 34 weeks? O68, O6014X0, Z37.0, 01961

18) What are the anesthesia codes for a patient who had two left toes removed due to frostbite after the patient was lost in a snowstorm and experienced hypothermia? T34.832A, 01480, 99116

19) What are the anesthesia codes for a patient who had a rectal endoscopy with biopsy due to bleeding? K62.5, 00902

20) What are the anesthesia codes for a patient who had a pacemaker implanted due to ventricular fibrillation and hypertension? I10, I49.01, 00530

RADIOLOGY QUIZ 25

1) What are the codes for a 48-year-old patient who had a computed axial tomography of T1-T3 with contrast material for severe back pain and difficulty breathing? M549, R06.00, 72129

2) What are the codes for a 26-year-old patient who has gastroparesis and had a study for gastric emptying of the stomach? K31.84, 78264

3) What are the codes for a 66-year-old patient with ASHD who had angiography with noncardiac vascular flow imaging with cardiac stress test with treadmill with continuous monitoring and supervision by physician of the internal mammary artery? I25.10, 93015, 75756

4) What are the codes for a 37-year-old patient who is suspected of having lymphoma of the abdominal lymph nodes because of ongoing constipation and abdominal pain and today receives a whole body bone marrow imaging? R10.9, K59.00, 78104

5) What are the codes for a 48-year-old patient who had hysterosonography with color Doppler with introduction of saline and found to have septate uterus? Q51.2, 76831, 58340

6) How would you indicate that someone only did S&I? -26 modifier

7) What are the codes for a 48-year-old patient who had MRI of the ankle due to extreme pain and inflammation which demonstrated acute distal tibiofibular syndesmotic injury of the left ankle? S93.439A, 73721

8) What contrast materials are not coded as separate from the test? Oral & rectal

9) What are the codes for a 45-year-old patient who had imaging for carcinoma of the thyroid with urinary recovery which was found to be positive? C73, 78016

10) What are the codes for a 48-year-old patient who had CT of the head with oral contrast materials after falling from the roof and was unconscious for approximately 10 minutes but results were negative? R40.1, 70450

PATHOLOGY/LABORATORY QUIZ 26

1) What are the codes when a physician tests to determine how much Lithium an 8-year-old patient ingested? quantitative

2) What are the codes for a 42-year-old male who has a blood count smear with manual WBC count and bleeding time is also tested and the patient is found to be positive for von Willebrand's? D68.0, 85007, 85002

3) What are the codes for a path exam of a PAP smear that required physician interpretation due to patient complaints of erratic vaginal bleeding but there were no abnormal findings? Z01.419, Z13.21, 88141

4) What are the codes for the gross examination of a wedge from the liver of a 43-year-old patient which is found to be cancerous? C22.9, 88300

5) What are the codes for a semiquantitative immunoassay test for chlamydia with a reagent strip which is found to be negative? Z11.59, 86318

6) What are the codes for a 77-yo patient who had a blood draw and a finger stick on his office visit with complaints of fatigue? Z00.00, 36415, 36416

7) What are the codes for a 67-year-old patient who has tests for carbon dioxide, potassium, bilirubin, chloride, sodium, and glucose for a well check? 80051, 82247, 82947

8) What are the codes for when a physician tests a 17-year-old female to determine if she has taken barbiturates because of general fatigue? R53.83, 80101

9) What are the codes when a 37-year-old female is tested for histoplasm antibody which is found to be positive for histoplasmosis? B39.9, 86698

10) What are the codes for a hamster penetration test which was found to be negative for insterility? Z31.41, 89329

11) What are the codes for measurement of hemoglobin performed transcutaneously and is positive for polycythemia? 88738

12) What are the codes for microscopic and gross examination of a left breast of a 48-year-old woman which includes the lymph nodes which is found to be cancerous? C50.519, C49.9, 88309

13) If I was checking for the presence of antibodies, why type of test would I use? qualitative

14) The substance being chemically tested is known as what? analyte

15) What are the codes for testing for cocaine and meth? 80100

MEDICINE QUIZ 27

1) What are the codes for a patient who had training for the use of a TENS unit? 90901

2) What are the codes for a 52-year-old patient with ESRD who had monthly dialysis services with only 13 days of services this past month? N18.6, 90970x13

3) What are the codes for a 43-year-old patient with complaints of severe abdominal pain who has an IVP with KUB study for possible kidney stones? R10.9, 74400

4) What are the codes for a 3-year-old patient who is seen today for her well-check and received oral polio and DTP whole cell IM with flu vaccine which were administered by the nurse? Z00.129, V04.81, 90460, 90461, 99392, 90720, 90712

5) What are the codes for a 27-year-old patient who is hospitalized at this time for depression and suicide watch who was counseled by the psychiatrist concerning proper use of her prescriptions? F32.9, 90863

6) What are the codes for a 22-year-old patient who is seen today in the office for yellow fever vaccine before leaving the country? Z23, 90717, 90471

7) What are the codes for a 23-year-old OCD patient whose parents had a therapy session with her psychiatrist? F42, 90846

8) What are the codes for a 51-year-old patient who suffers from SSS and whose dual lead pacemaker is evaluated and programmed after implantation? I49.5, 93280

9) What are the codes for a 49-year-old patient who had a TEE for possible dysrhythmia due to fatigue and difficulty breathing? R53.83, R06.02, 93318

10) What are the codes for 48-year-old patient who had a lymphangiography of both legs due to restless leg syndrome? G25.81, 75803

11) What are the codes for 62-year-old patient who had an audiological screening of both ears due to tinnitus? H93.19, 92551

12) What are the codes for a 32-year-old patient who receives 45 minutes of electrical stimulation and acupuncture to help relieve chronic neck and back pain? M54.9, M54.2, 97813, 97814x2

13) What are the codes for a 34-year-old patient who was treated today for sepsis due to MRSA with an antibiotic injection of Avelox? A41.01, 96372

14) What are the codes for a 73-year-old diabetic patient with a history of COPD and emphysema who was admitted to the hospital due to her diabetes Type I being

uncontrolled at this time resulting in a diabetic coma? She was placed on a ventilator at this time and spirometry and testing of thoracic gas volume. E10.11, Z99.11, J44.9, J43.9, 94726, 94002, 94010, 99223

15) What are the codes for a 17-year-old patient who purposely overdosed on Xanax and Lithium and was treated in the ER with gastric intubation, aspiration, and lavage with history and exam being EPF? T42.4X2A, T56.892, 99283, 43753

16) What are the codes for a 48-year-old patient who is seen today for IM nonhormonal chemotherapy with Xolair due to small cell carcinoma of the left lung? Z51.11, C34.90, J2357, 96401

17) What are the codes for a 15-year-old patient who had three scratch allergy tests of which two are extracts and the other is drug which were negative? Z01.89, 95004x2

18) What are the codes for a 29-year-old patient of a sleep study with attendant which was staged with ventilation, respiratory effort, EEG, ECG and oxygen saturati for sleep apnea? G47.30, 95807

19) What are the codes for a 59-year-old patient seen today for electrical stimulation and hot packs due to rotator cuff syndrome? M75.100, 97010, 97014

TEST 3 ANSWERS

1. What are the seven components used to determine the E/M levels? HISTORY, EXAM, MEDICAL DECISION MAKING, COUNSELING, COORDINATION OF CARE, NATURE OF PRESENTING PROBLEM, TIME
2. What are the codes for a patient who is admitted to the hospital at 11 pm for a gunshot wound but leaves AMA at 12:30 am with a Detailed History, EPF exam, and moderate MDM? F10.229, E922.9, 99221, 99238
3. What are the codes for a 51-year-old patient who suffers from SSS and whose dual lead pacemaker is evaluated and programmed after implantation? I49.5, 93280
4. What are the codes for a 49-year-old patient who had a TEE for possible dysrhythmia due to fatigue and difficulty breathing? R53.83, R06.02, 93318
5. What are the codes for a computerized ophthalmic diagnostic imaging of the posterior segment that is computerized for both eyes which includes professional services? 92133
6. What are the codes for a patient who is required by the insurance company for a consultation for a work-related injury when the patient fell from the roof and injured his back with a comprehensive History and Exam and Moderate MDM? S39.82XA, 99244-32
7. If a report states that the patient is a smoker and his father died of lung cancer from smoking, what level of PFSH is this? PERTINENT
8. What are the correct codes for a patient who had an electromyography of two extremities in the paraspinal areas for paresis? G83.9, 95861
9. What type of HPI would the following be: The patient presents with complaints of chest pain with possible MI. The patient states that it began last night after eating and has not lessened over the night. BRIEF
10. What level of exam would the following be: The patient is a well-developed well-nourished white male whose GI and GU are negative. He has COPD but otherwise his respiratory is negative. He does present with complaints of chest pains today but otherwise his S1, S2 are normal. PEERLA and head is normocephalic. EOMs are intact. Neck is supple. Skin does present with some lesions which should be checked in the future. EXPANDED PROBLEM FOCUSED
11. What are the codes for a patient seen for COPD and chronic bronchitis who is new to this doctor and the history was EPF, Exam was PF and MDM was SF? J44.9, 99201
12. What are the codes for a patient who was admitted to the hospital at 9 pm due to various trauma from a car accident with numerous facial lacerations as well as a possible concussion when they hit the windshield with the patient having lost consciousness in the ambulance? Patient was intoxicated so it was difficult to get a history and the exam was detailed. The patient then left AMA at 11:30 pm. S09.93XA, R40.1, 99234
13. What are the codes for a physician who was on standby for 45 minutes to assist with a C-section at which time he did assist for a successful C-section of a single liveborn male? O82, Z37.0, 59514-80
14. What are the codes for a patient who is seen today for a second opinion consultation regarding possible renal cancer which was diagnosed by his PCP a week ago due to complaints of suspicious renal mass with an EPF history and exam and moderate complexity MDM? N28.9, 99202

15. What are the key components for determining a history portion of the office visit? HISTORY OF PRESENT ILLNESS, REVIEW OF SYSTEMS AND PAST FAMILY SOCIAL HISTORY
16. What are the codes for an established 78-year-old patient seen today for a well check and follow-up for her emphysema and diabetes Type I? E10.9, J43.9, Z00.00, 99397
17. What are the codes for a patient who was seen today by his regular PCP for fracture follow-up care of his left tibia a week ago when he was out of town visiting his ex-wife which was repaired with ORIF? S82.201A, 27535-55
18. What level of Exam would the following report constitute: General: Patient is well-developed, well-nourished. HEENT is normal with PERRLA. Respiratory, GI and GU are negative. Cardiovascular and skin are positive. DETAILED
19. What is the code for a new patient whose visit consisted of a PF history, Detailed Exam and moderate MDM? 99201
20. What are the codes for a new patient who is having difficulty breathing and is seen today in the office? The patient's father had a history of asthma as does the patient. The patient does have COPD. The patient states that the breathing became more difficult after a long afternoon of playing basketball but has not been alleviated by his asthma medication and has only become more difficult overnight. The ROS is negative except for the history of breathing problems. During the exam, the patient's condition worsened and he was admitted to the hospital by the physician with the exam finding that GU, GI, skin, and HEENT normal. The patient does have hypertension which is treated with medication. Extremities move well with no edema. Cranial nerves are intact. R06.9, J44.0, 401.9, 99221
21. What are the codes for a patient who received IV infusion of non-chemotherapeutic drugs for 3 hours for septicemia? A41.9, 96365, 96366X2
22. What is the code for a patient who is an established patient whose visit consisted of a PF History, EPF exam and SF MDM? 99212
23. What are the codes for a 3-year-old child who is seen in the emergency room after hitting their head on the fireplace that required sutures with PF History and EPF exam with SF MDM? S09.90XA, 99281, 12020
24. What are the codes for a patient well known to this doctor who is seen today for a check of his diabetes Type I who cut his toe a week ago and which is now infected with a PF history, EPF exam, and moderate MDM and who had removal of a 1.5-cm lesion from her right hand? The patient was also examined for a suspicious neoplasm on his back which was removed and specimen sent to path. L08.9, E10.9, D48.5, 11100, 99213-25
25. What is a DMERC? DURABLE MEDICAL EQUIPMENT REGIONAL CARRIER
26. If a patient is given 500 mcg of filgrastim by injection, what are the codes for this? J1440, J1441
27. What HCPCS codes are used for outpatient prospective payment system? C CODES
28. If a patient in the hospital after a procedure is given IV pain medication, what type of codes will the physician use to charge for this? J CODES
29. What does HCPCS mean? HEALTHCARE COMMON PROCEDURE CODING SYSTEM
30. If a wheelchair is being charged for a second month rental, how should this coded? E1050
31. What is the first level of HCPCS? CPT

32. What HCPCS codes are used for ambulance services? A0021-A0999
33. If a patient has repair of three wounds, what HCPCS modifier would be attached? A3
34. If a patient is admitted to the hospital and given 1500 cc of D5W to treat dehydration, how would this be coded? J7070X2
35. If the patient is given medication by IV and IM, will the same HCPCS code be used? Why or why not? NO, 2 DIFFERENT ROUTES OF ADMINISTRATION
36. When assigning HCPCS modifiers to fingers and toes, where does the counting begin? THUMB/TOE AND OUT FROM THERE
37. What are the anesthesia codes for a patient who had a lobectomy of the right lung due to small cell carcinoma which metastasized to the kidney and who was admitted to the hospital with severe difficulty breathing which was also complicated by pneumoniae pneumonia? C79.00, C34.90, J13, 00546
38. What physical status modifier would be applicable to a patient who is hospitalized for septicemia with shock? P4
39. What are the anesthesia codes for a patient who has an esophagectomy performed due to esophageal cancer that has metastasized to the liver and brain? C15.9, C79.31, C78.7, 00320
40. What are the anesthesia codes for removal of an infected dental molar from a 3-year-old which required general anesthesia? K04.4, 00170-23
41. What are the anesthesia codes for a 1-year-old child who had tubes placed in her ears for suppurative otitis media? H66.43, 00126
42. What are the codes for a 48-year-old patient who had a computed axial tomography of T1-T3 with contrast material for severe back pain and difficulty breathing? M54.9, R06.89, 72129
43. What are the codes for a 26-year-old patient who has gastroparesis and had a study for gastric emptying of the stomach? K31.84, 78264
44. What are the codes for a 66-year-old patient with ASHD who had angiography with noncardiac vascular flow imaging with cardiac stress test with treadmill with continuous monitoring and supervision by physician of the internal mammary artery? I25.10, 93015, 75756
45. What contrast materials are not coded as separate from the test? ORAL AND RECTAL
46. What are the codes for a 45-year-old patient who had imaging for carcinoma of the thyroid with urinary recovery which was found to be positive? C73, 78016
47. What are the codes for a 67-year-old patient who has tests for carbon dioxide, potassium, bilirubin, chloride, sodium, and glucose for a well check? V70.1, 80051, 82247, 82947
48. What are the codes for a patient who had training for the use of a TENS unit? 90901
49. What are the codes for a 52-year-old patient with ESRD who had monthly dialysis services with only 13 days of services this past month? N18.6 90970x13
50. What are the codes for a 43-year-old patient with complaints of severe abdominal pain who has an IVP with KUB study for possible kidney stones? R10.9, 74400
51. What are the codes for a 3-year-old patient who is seen today for her well-check and received oral polio and DTP whole cell IM with flu vaccine which were administered by the nurse? Z76.1, Z23, 90460, 90461, 99392, 90712, 90720
52. What are the codes for a 27-year-old patient seen in ICU by his PCP after having emergency CABG by a cardiologist due to ASHD? The patient is seen by the PCP from

10:30 am to 11:15 am and then from 1:40 pm to 2:20 pm and pulse oximetry is provided I25.10, 99291, 99292

53. What are the codes for 62-year-old patient who had an audiological screening of both ears due to tinnitus? H93.19, 92551
54. What are the codes for a 2-year-old who is seen today for a well check as part of continuing pediatric care with the office? Z00.129, 99392
55. What are the codes for a patient who was seen today for ORIF of his compound fracture of his right humerus in the emergency room. After this procedure, the patient is driving back to his hometown five hours away and won't be seen again by this physician? S42.309B, 23615
56. What are the codes for a patient who is seen for the first time today as a referral from his PCP for possible anemia due to extreme fatigue with the history being PF, exam EPF and moderate MDM? R53.83, 99201
57. What are the codes for a 32-year-old patient who receives 45 minutes of electrical stimulation and acupuncture to help relieve chronic neck and back pain? M54.9, M54.2, 97813, 97814X2
58. What are the codes for a 34-year-old patient who was treated today for sepsis due to MRSA with an antibiotic injection of Avelox? A41.01, 038.12, 96372, J2280
59. What are the codes for a 15-year-old patient who had three scratch allergy tests of which two are extracts and the other is drug which were negative? Z01.89, 95004X2
60. Define which of the following scenarios are unit/floor time, face-to-face or neither:
    a. Discussion with nurses on the patient's floor about schedules for staff. NEITHER
    b. Phone call to patient's parents from doctor's office. NEITHER
    c. Family consultation at nurse' station on patient's unit. FACE
    d. Review of patient's chart at nurse's station. UNIT/FLOOR TIME
    e. Review of research at doctor's office relative to patient's care. NEITHER

INTEGUMENTARY QUIZ 28

1) In the ICU, after prepping with ChloraPrep, we used some 0.25% Marcaine with epinephrine. The patient is on the ventilator. The lower piercings were used first where a post went through and through. The area was localized with some 1% Xylocaine. The lower left side was removed first. We grasped the ball, screwed off the external cap, and then brought it into the oral cavity and removed the entire post and the inside cap. We then in a like manner, removed the lower cap on the right side, screwing off the external cap and grasping it internally and then reducing it through the internal cavity. Then the patient had 2 areas of the left cheek and the right cheek where there was a diamond-like cap that was attached to a plate that was beneath. I had to make a small incision and first the left side was done. It was anesthetized, ChloraPrep was used and we grasped it. Made a small incision with #11 blade, removed the plate that was holding it beneath, and the incision was small enough that it did not need a suture on the left side. On the right side, a like procedure was carried out. There was a small incision made. It was large enough that we removed the plate. We had to use a 4-0 nylon suture. This controlled the bleeding. He tolerated all this well and the procedure was ended. M79.5, 10120, 20100-RT, 20100-LT

2) What are the codes for an 8-year-old patient who had suffered second and third degrees burns over both fronts of her legs four months ago which totaled 15% of TBSA with 7% third degree? She is seen today for STSG from her back to cover the burned area. T24.302S, L90.5, 15002, 15100, 15101X2, 15003X2

3) What are the codes for a 32-year-old patient who had 17 skin tags removed electrosurgically? L91.9, 11200, 11201

4) What are the codes for a 23-year-old patient who cut her right index finger which was 3 cm while preparing dinner which required 8 stitches in the emergency room? History and exam were problem focused. S61.210A, 99281, 12002-F6

5) What are the codes for a 62-year-old diabetic patient who was treated for an infected right toe requiring extensive debridement and wound repair with single layer suturing? L08.9, E11.9, 12041-RT

6) What are the codes for a 47-year-old patient who had 3.5 cc of collagen injected into her chin to reduce wrinkles? L98.8, 11951

7) What are the codes for a 42-year-old patient who presents with an infection from her previous CABG for ASHD and MI two weeks ago? She is found to have MRSA and the site is prepared for drainage with continued monitoring with the patient remaining in the hospital for further observation. History and exam were detailed. I25.10, B95.62, Z95.1, T81.4XXA, 99221

8) What are the codes for a 38-year-old female who had a mastectomy of both breasts which included removal of the axillary lymph nodes due to carcinoma of the breast with a

TRAM? C50.919, 19307-50, 19367-50

9) What are the codes when a pathologist finds malignancy from a needle core biopsy of the left breast of a 32-year-old woman? C50.919, 19100-LT

10) What are the codes for an 82-year-old nursing home patient who had excision of a sacral ulcer repaired with suturing and requiring an ostectomy? L98.429, 15933

11) What are the codes for a 49-year-old patient who was involved in a car accident and suffered extensive lacerations and broken collarbone? The patient had a BAC level of 1.0 as he has suffered for many years with alcoholism and went on a binge today. Lacerations were numerous including a 3.0 cm laceration of the right forearm which required layered closure, a 5.5 cm laceration of the right thigh which required retention sutures and ligation of arteries, 4.8 cm laceration of the chest which required simple closure but extensive debridement due to glass fragments, a 2.8 cm laceration of the right cheek which required layered closure, and a 3.0 cm laceration of the left thigh which required retention sutures. S51.811A, S71.111A, S21.119A, S01.411A, S71.112A, 810.00, , 12034, 13121, 12052

12) What are the codes for a pathologist when a 2.5 cm malignant lesion of the left arm was destroyed? No code, no pathology on destroyed lesion.

13) What are the codes for a 22-year-old patient who had 5 corns removed by paring? L84, 11057

14) What are the codes for a 58-year-old patient who had excision of basal cell carcinoma of the back (2.2 cm) which was repaired with a Z-plasty? C44.519, 14000

15) The patient was brought to the operative suite, prepped and draped in the usual manner. A time-out was accomplished. Preop antibiotics were given and SCDs applied. The patient morbidly obese. The left chest wall mass, which was about 3.5 cm was removed first. An elliptical incision was made. Bleeding controlled with electrocautery. Mass was removed. Subcutaneous tissue was closed with 3-0 Vicryl. The skin was closed with interrupted 3-0 Prolene. This appeared to be a large inclusion cyst. Right breast mass was then removed. A circumareolar incision made in the outer quadrant. This mass was removed. All bleeding was controlled. The mass will be submitted to pathology for review. Rule out carcinoma. The subcutaneous tissue was closed with 3-0 Vicryl after hemostasis had been accomplished and then skin was closed with interrupted 3-0 Prolene. Following this, we turned his head slightly, removed the right posterior neck mass. An elliptical incision was made. Bleeding controlled with electrocautery. Mass was removed and we closed with some interrupted 3-0 Prolene. Sterile dressing applied to each of these incisions. We used 0.25% Marcaine with epinephrine and each one of them sent to recovery room in satisfactory condition. N63, L72.3, 19120, 11404, 11420

16) What are the codes for a 44-year-old patient who is seen today for the first time with a history and exam that were expanded problem focused and who had a 3.2-cm mass of the

back which was infected and required drainage which was found to be a sebaceous cyst? L72.3, 10061, 99202-25

17) What are the codes for a 15-year-old patient who was seen in the emergency room due to complaints of severe abdominal pain and hemoptysis? The patient was found to have Staph food poisoning and discharged with prescriptions. The history was expanded problem focused and the exam was problem focused. A05.0, 99281

18) What are the codes for a pathologist who performs the pathological review of the two biopsies of specimens from Moh's surgery for a 4.2 cm lesion on the back of a 48-year-old man? L98.9, 88305x2

19) What are the codes for a 38-year-old female who had a suspicious lump in her left breast with fine needle aspiration being completed and specimen sent to pathology? N63, 10021-LT

20) What are the codes for a 17-year-old patient who is seen today for repair of burns sustained four months ago when hot water spilled on her? Her body had sustained second and third degree burns over 25% of her body (forearms and chest) with 13% of the burns being third degree. Repair at this time was a 50 sq. cm FTSG taken from her back and placed on the chest area which was 35 sq. cm in size. L90.5, T22.311S, T22.312S, T21.31XS, 15002, 15200, 15201

MUSCULOSKELETAL QUIZ 29

1) What are the codes for a 62-year-old patient who experienced blunt trauma to the left orbit with a hematoma on the forehead which resulted in neuropathy and blindness in the left eye. The patient was found to have an extensive blowout fracture of the left orbital floor which was treated with a periorbital open procedure. S02.3XXA, H46.9, S04.019A, S09.93XA, 21386-LT

2) What are the codes for a 23-year-old patient who had removal of screws in the right knee due to fracture repair 5 months ago? Z47.2, 20680-RT

3) What are the codes for a 15-year-old patient who received arthroscopy of the left knee. There was exploration of the knee in the suprapatellar and patellofemoral region, and a partial medial meniscectomy was completed to repair a tear. There was no evidence of remaining loose body or other abnormality. A posterior horn tear of the medial meniscus was debrided back to a stable margins. The chondromalacia of the patella were noted and chondroplasty was performed. S83.212A, M22.40, 29881-LT

4) What are the codes for a 17-year-old patient who was involved in a car accident and suffered skull fracture which required closed treatment of skull fracture in the emergency room with a history and exam that were both detailed? S02.91XA, 99284

5) What are the codes for a 42-year-old patient who had repair of an artificial fracture at a former pin site from a previous fracture of the right upper ulna which did not heal together properly and was repaired with external fixation? S52.001K, 20690

6) What are the codes for a 13-year-old patient who had removal of glass from a wound of the right forearm into the dermis and fascia? S51.821A, 20103

7) What are the codes for a 48-year-old patient who had repair of a bunion on the left foot with removal of the medial eminence with resection of part of the proximal phalanx and osteotomy with implantation of screw in addition to arthroplasty to repair the hammertoe of the second toe? M20.10, M20.40, 28298-LT

8) What are the codes for a 28-year-old patient who had received craniofacial reconstruction in the past and was now experiencing loosening of plate and screws. There were some irregularity in the temporal parietal bones. Old scar was excised and revised of both coronal sides. The plates, screws and wires were all removed from the area. Attention was directed to the craniofacial orbital region where some of the excess bone was reduced. L90.5, T85.618A, Z47.2, 13131, 20680, 21209

9) What are the codes for a 64-year-old patient who had a comminuted displaced distal fracture of the shaft of right radius and ulna which was repaired with ORIF? S52.251A, S52.351A, 25575

10) What are the codes for a 62-year-old patient who had resection of the base of the DIP of

the second toe on the left side with hemiphalengectomy and syndactylization due to Freiberg's? M92.62, 28280

11) What are the codes for the secondary procedure for a patient who had repair of a cranial deformity defect with a piece of titanium mesh as the primary procedure. Once this was complete, the secondary procedure was begun where a vertical incision was made transversely to the left side in order to allow exposure of the prominent right parietal bone with a contouring bur and reduced in size. Due to extensive tension on the wound repair, the old scar was removed. This was trimmed appropriately and hemostasis was achieved with electrocautery and closure with 2-0 Vicryl interrupted sutures and 3-0 nylon. Q75.9, L90.5, 213209, 13131

12) What are the codes for a 64-year-old patient with a history of insulin-dependent diabetes mellitus, coronary artery disease, chronic renal failure and heart failure who was initially admitted for congestive heart failure and nonhealing bilateral mid-foot ulcers treated for years with debridement and whirlpool. The patient was readmitted for acute diabetic right foot to be treated with incision and drainage of his right foot and first ray amputation but the infection had spread so right below-knee amputation was performed. 858.9, 250380, L97.429, L97.419, I25.9, I50.9, Z79.4, T79.8XXA, 27598-RT

13) What are the codes for a 71-year-old patient who has osteoarthritis of the left thumb which required fusion? M18.9, 26841

14) What are the codes for a 77-year-old patient who received some traction with some manipulation and reduction for intertrochanteric fracture of the left hip in addition to A 6-inch incision was made beginning at the tip of the greater trochanter and going distally along the lateral thigh. The fascia was incised in line with the incision, and the vastus lateralis muscle was split by sharp resection down to the underlying femur and a Bennett retractor placed. A guide wire was placed and a 90-mm compression hip screw was then placed over the guidewire. Next, the 135° angle, four-hole sideplate was slipped over the shaft of the screw and fixed to the femoral shaft. Four screws were then placed by drilling, measuring, and putting in four tap screws. S72.052A, 27244

15) What are the codes for a 32-year-old female who had a neoplasm removed from her left posterior shoulder in addition to a biopsy of the left axillary sentinel lymph node? C43.62, 38500

RESPIRATORY QUIZ 30

1) Insertion of a tube into the mouth and down into the trachea is known as what? tracheostomy

2) What are the codes for a 52-year-old patient with metastatic cancer of the pleura from breast cancer a year ago which was excised at that time and is being seen today for tube thoracostomy and chest tube insertion? C38.4, Z85.3, 32551

3) What are the codes for a 67-year-old patient who is seen today for pleural effusion secondary to small cell carcinoma of the upper left lung with tube thoracostomy including indwelling cathether? J91.0, C34.12, 32550-LT, 32551-LT

4) What are the codes for this 52-year-old patient who has a history of pulmonary nodule in the left lung? She was seen today for a CT of the Chest and Adrenals with oral and intravenous contrast. Today there is a 2-cm area of parenchymal density which has the appearance of interstitial changes without findings of significant nodule or mass. This finding can relate to scarring. There is no other nodule, mass, or effusion. No evidence of adenopathy in the mediastinum. The heart and great vessels are normal in appearance. No findings with the liver, spleen, kidneys, adrenals, or pancreas. Z12.2, 71260, 74262

5) What are the codes for a 14-year-old patient who had cauterization and packing of both sides of nose posteriorly to control expistaxis? R04.0, 30905-50

6) Excision of polyps is known as what? polypectomy

7) What are the codes for a 5-year-old patient who received a tracheobronchoscopy performed through an established tracheostomy incision when he swallowed part of a plastic toy and had stopped breathing at the scene? T17.390A, 31615

8) What are the codes for a 16-year-old who had an emergency left thoracostomy with ligation of the eighth intercostal artery and partial upper lobectomy with placement of arterial femoral catheter due to severe lacerations of the left artery and lung due to a car accident? S27.331A, S25.502A, 32480, 37616, 32551

9) What are the codes for a 3-year-old patient who had a computer-assisted bronchoscopy for biopsy of right lung which revealed upon physician's review that there were three coins. T17.898A, 31627, 31625

10) What are the codes for a 71-year-old patient who has a long history of lung disease due to being a lifelong smoker. History of hypertension. The patient also had COPD and asthma with bullous emphysema. A PET scan was reviewed by the physician and revealed that she has a 3.5-cm nodule in the upper left lobe which is malignant. A lobectomy was performed. I10, Z86.79, Z87.891, J43.8, J44.9, C34.10, 78811-26, 32480-LT

11) What are the codes for an 18-year-old patient who has trouble breathing due to airway obstruction. It was found that this is due to turbinate hypertrophy and deviated septum protruding into the left nasal airway for which a septoplasty and bilateral turbinectomy was performed. J34.3, Q67.4, 30130-50, 30520

12) What are the codes for a 38-year-old patient who presents with the complaint of SOB and dyspnea with wheezing that began approximately four hours ago and has worsened? She is seen in the emergency room today. Her medical history showed a history of asthma. The patient states that she had a cough for the past day but she denies any other problems. She denies any fever or chills. She denies any chest pain or palpitations. The patient had an asthma attack a month ago which required hospitalization and treatment. The patient has no other past surgical history. The patient does have HTN and hypercholesterolemia. The patient lives alone and she works at a local school. She has smoked for more than 20 years. Her father is deceased due to emphysema. ROS shows that the patient has no problems in any system including no abdominal pain, chest pain, or edema other than previously mentioned. Physical exam showed the patient to be tachypneic. She is well developed and well nourished with respiratory rate of 20 and blood pressure of 124/86. HEENT is normocephalic and atraumatic. Pupils equal and round, regular, reactive to light. Extraocular muscles intact. Nares and oropharynx negative. Neck is supple; no JVD, no lymphadenopathy, no carotid bruits, no thyromegaly. Lungs reveal bilateral wheeze diffusely. There are some decreased breath sounds bilaterally. No rhonchi. Cardiovascular: Regular rate and rhythm, without murmurs, gallops, or rubs. Normal S1 and S2. No S3, S4. Abdomen: Normal active bowel sounds, soft, nontender, nondistended. No hepatosplenomegaly. Extremities: No cyanosis, clubbing or edema. Today in the emergency room the patient received 4 nebulization treatments for her acute exacerbation of her asthma but continued to be hypoxic with room air oxygen saturation of 84%. She had some slight improvement in her wheeze with the nebulization treatments but without further improvement she was admitted to the hospital to be continued on Solu-Medrol 125 mg IV and supplemental O2. E78.0, I10, J44.1, 99285

13) What are the codes for this 41-year-old patient who had an esophagoscopy and microlaryngoscopy of the neck to determine if there was cancer secondary to lung cancer. The scope was advanced into the cervical esophagus which was found to be normal. It was noticed that there was tumor involving the anterior wall of the right portion of the neck extending approximately 1 cm below the pharyngeal epiglottic fold and into the hypopharyngeal wall of which a sample was obtained. The specimen was found to be malignant.C78.89, C34.90, 43202, 31510

14) What are the codes for a 2-year-old patient who had a tracheobronchoscopy to remove a toy that he swallowed. The scope was established through a tracheostomy incision. T17.398, 31615

CPT CARDIOVASCULAR QUIZ 31

1) What are the codes for a 49-year-old male with insulin-dependent diabetes mellitus has been admitted with diabetic ketoacidosis and not having peripheral vein access. Through a percutaneous puncture, the subclavian vein was located, and using the Seldinger technique, a triple-lumen catheter was inserted without difficulty. There was observed a good blood return from all three ports, and then the port was irrigated. One single stitch was used to secure the catheter in place. E11.69, 36561

2) What are the codes for a 61-year-old right-handed patient with history of hypertension, CKD, and schizophrenia with OCD symptoms who presents to the ER as having dysphasia and numbness/weakness on the right side that she noticed yesterday and has not resolved since. She explained that she had a similar incident a month before but it resolved. The patient's parents are both alive and well. She does not smoke or drink. Her ROS was negative for all other systems. Exam revealed temp of 98.7, blood pressure of 168/92. HEENT is clear. Lungs clear. Heart regular rate and rhythm. Abdomen shows surgical scar. Normal bowel sounds. Extremities show no clubbing, cyanosis or edema. She was alert and oriented times 3. She had difficulty with speech, mostly lingual sounds. No aphasic symptoms. Normal flow, normal rate and normal content. No breathlessness noted. Cranial nerves showed right fundi with sharp discs, pupils reactive 3 to 2 bilaterally, full extraocular movements and full visual fields. Corneal reflexes were present bilaterally. Decreased V1 through V3 pinprick on the face. Masticatory muscles were normal. Face was symmetric. Eye closure, puffed cheeks and smile were symmetric. Uvula and tongue were midline. Her gag was present bilaterally, left greater than right. Motor examination showed increased tone in the left arm. Strength was 4/4 in the right upper and lower extremities and 5/5 in the left upper and lower extremities. Reflexes were 2+ throughout with downgoing toes. Sensory examination showed decreased pinprick on the right side. The patient was given an EKG which revealed that the patient had experienced an MI previously and a CVA within the past several days. N18.9, I25.2, I12.9, I69.921, F20.9, 99285, 93000

3) Where are the two ways that electrodes can be placed for a pacemaker? EPICARDIAL OR TRANSVENOUS

4) What are the codes for a 49-year-old patient who has a history of ASHD. Left femoral artery was chosen for access because of recent cardiac catheterization from the right side. A diagnostic left coronary angiogram was performed which was advanced over a wire to the left coronary ostium. It revealed no change in the mid-LAD lesion. The wire was advanced across the lesion without difficulty, and initial PTCA was accomplished. Angiogram revealed less than 10% residual lesion, but in the left anterior oblique cranial view a nonocclusive dissection limited to the lesion was noted, therefore, stenting was performed. I25.10, 92980

5) What are the codes for an alcoholic 57-year-old patient who presents with compensated biliary cirrhosis and is suffering from recurrent variceal hemorrhage for which renal portal decompression with anastomosis was provided? K74.3, I85.01, 37140

6) What are the codes for a 58-year-old patient who had a triple coronary artery bypass with sequential left internal mammary artery anastomosis on the second diagonal of the left anterior descending, saphenous vein graft to the second obtuse marginal and the same to the posterior descending coronary artery due to ST elevated MI? I21.29, 33517, 33534

7) What is a PTCA? PERCUTANEOUS TRANSLUMINAL CORONARY ANGIOPLASTY

8) The improper connection of the great arteries is known as what? TRANSPOSITION

9) What are the codes for a 73-year-old patient with a history of aortic valve replacement and severe cardiomyopathy, chronic left bundle-branch block and diabetes who presents after having experience arrest early this morning characterized earlier by difficulty breathing and chest pain. The patient was cardioverted multiple times by EMTs and placed in ICU where he was seen several times from 8:00 am to 9:00 am, 11:30 to 12:45, and 4:15 pm to 5:30 pm but remained mostly unresponsive. Subsequent rhythm was sinus tachycardiac with a left bundle-branch block. He had a cardiac catheterization at the time of aortic valve replacement which showed normal coronary vessels three years ago. The patient does drink and smoke occasionally. His father died of a heart attack at age 75. ROS was unobtainable as the patient was not responsive. Exam showed blood pressure of 145/87, Pulse was 108 and respirations are 12 on ventilator. The patient is afebrile. HEENT show PERRLA. Neck is supple. Carotids have diminished upstroke without bruits. Lungs are clear. Anteriorly heart is tachycardiac . There is a prosthetic S2. The abdomen is soft and nontender without masses. Extremities have trace edema. Distal pulses are present. Neurologic exam: The patient is unresponsive. EKG shows sinus tachycardia with left bundle-branch block. Neurological and pulmonary evals are recommends. EKG should be repeated. Possible catheterization should be performed. I42.5, I44.7, I46.9, R00.0, E11.9, Z98.89, Z82.49, Z94.1, F17.200, 99291, 99292X5

10) What codes are used if a procedure is changed from a laparoscopic procedure to an open procedure? V64.41

11) What are the codes for a 49-year-old patient who had a permanent pacemaker implanted with leads placed into the right ventricle and right atrium due to bradycardia. A pocket was made in the left anterior chest wall into which the pulse generator was inserted. R00.1, 33208

12) What are the codes for a 12-month-old baby with ventricular septal defect who had patch closure? Q21.0, 33681

13) What are the codes for a 53-year-old male who was brought to the operating room and pulmonary artery catheter was inserted into the right internal jugular vein. The distal right saphenous vein was harvested from the medial malleolus to just above the knee. A midline sternotomy was performed and it was found that the ascending aorta was extremely calcified with diffuse atherosclerosis. Coronaries were marked for bypass,

including posterior descending artery and a posterolateral branch One liter of cardioplegia was given antegrade to arrest the heart. Bypasses were accomplished, first using the reverse saphenous vein in an end-to-side fashion to the PDA. The second bypass was to the posterolateral branch. A bolus of cold cardioplegia was given, and the patient was rewarmed. With the crossclamp still in place, a single aortotomy was made in the ascending aorta. The area was thickened and calcified, but had a decent lumen to allow suture of the proximal end of the PDA up to the ascending aorta. The remaining proximal anastomosis of the posterolateral branch was brought onto the hood of the PDA graft. The PDA was isolated with bulldog clamps. Venotomy was made, and the end-to-side anastomosis of the posterior left ventricle to the PDA was accomplished. The lungs were inflated. The patient was ventilated and weaned off bypass successfully without the aid of inotropic support. I70.0, 33511

14) What are the codes for a 55-year-old patient who had an acute MI with edema and received an intracorporeal left ventricular assist device as a bridge to cardiac transplantation several months ago. Now, after 100 days of support, the left ventricular assist device malfunctioned and the pump had to be replaced. Z45.09, 33982

15) What are the codes for a 47-year-old patient with renal failure requiring hemodialysis so an AV cannula was placed for access? N19, 36810

CPT DIGESTIVE QUIZ 32

1) The patient was brought to the operative suite, prepped and draped in the usual manner. A right paramedian incision was made basically just above the umbilicus. Bleeding controlled with electrocautery. The rectus muscle was split and the peritoneal cavity was entered. We used 0.25% Marcaine with epinephrine prior to making the incision. We had to lengthen it to get some exposure. I had problems finding the appendix, as the appendix with generalized peritonitis came off and was tethered into the retroperitoneal area. I asked Dr. Vaughan to assist for exposure. We were able to basically mobilize the right colon and then we dissected the appendix from the cecum but once we found it, it was coming out fairly high off of the cecum. We tied it twice, divided it, cauterized the tip, then dissected, used the LigaSure for the mesentery and dissected it off of the duodenum. All bleeding was controlled. We irrigated thoroughly with saline, made certain that the bowel was properly placed back into the abdomen. Omentum was placed over it. We used a sheet of Seprafilm over the cecum and the right colon and another one over the omentum. The sponge, instrument, and needle count was correct and then we closed with double looped Maxon for the fascia, subcutaneous tissue closed with 2-0 Vicryl and skin was closed with V-Loc. Steri-Strip was applied. Sterile dressing was applied. Sent to recovery room in satisfactory condition. Tolerated the procedure well. K35.2, 44140

2) What are the codes for a 54-year-old patient who had a Roux-en-Y reconstruction following a complete gastrectomy for stomach cancer? C16.2, 43621

3) What are the codes for a 57-year-old patient who had a diverting colostomy with Hartmann pouch with sepsis and excision and debridement of a stage 3 sacral decubitus ulcer with ostectomy which had become necrotic. L89.153, A41.9, 15933, 44143

4) What are the codes for a 62-year-old hypertensive patient who had a colostomy placed 9 days ago after resection of colonic carcinoma. Earlier today, he felt nauseated and stated that his colostomy stopped filling. He also had a sensation of "heartburn." He denies vomiting but has been nauseated. He denies diarrhea. He denies hematochezia, hematemesis, or melena. He denies abdominal pain or fever. Bowel obstruction was found and the colostomy had to be repaired. I10, K94.03, C18.9, K56.60, 44345

5) What are the codes for a 41-year-old patient who had an ERCP for identification and removal of gallstones?
K80.20, 432164

6) What are the codes for a 44-year-old patient in whom a videoendoscope was inserted under direct vision. The patient was found to have a meat bolus in the distal esophagus with diffuse inflammation causing compression. The bolus was displaced into the stomach. The stomach itself had an inflamed gastric mucosa as well as the first segment of the duodenum. Biopsies were obtained of the stomach and duodenum which were negative and esophageal dilatation which did not find anything. T18.110A, K20.9, K29.60, 43239

7) What are the codes for a 41-year-old patient who was complaining of a bulging mass in the right side of the abdomen which correlated with a ventral hernia of the right abdominal wall. At this point, plication of the rectus abdominis muscle was done and Marlex mesh was applied. K43.9, 49560, 49568

8) What are the codes for a 52-year-old patient who was placed in the supine position and the F2 focus of the MSL 5000 lithotriptor, shock wave lithotripsy was started at 17 kV and went up to 23, where a total of 3000 shocks were given to the stone with fragmentation of this left renal calculi. N2.0, 50590

9) The patient brought to the operative suite, prepped and draped in the usual manner. Timeout was accomplished. Preoperative antibiotics were given and SCDs applied. Low midline incision was made, bleeding controlled with electrocautery. Fascia divided and peritoneal cavity was entered. Bookwalter retractor was placed. We able to see the area where India ink had been injected in the sigmoid colon. We used the GIA proximally and distally, divided the mesentery using the ligature. One vessel was stick-tied with 3-0 silk. We then opened the specimen and there was no polyp in it, so we then opened the bowel proximally thinking that the polyp might be just above where we had resected and, indeed, we found the polyp on a very long stalk. Resected another portion of the colon, then used a pursestringer. Placed a pursestring proximally. Used the dilators. A 29 EEA was selected. We tied the pursestring and then brought the EEA in from below, made the anastomosis. We then tested it, and there were some air bubbles, and so we had to use 3-0 silk. There was a small rent in the anastomosis on the right lateral side. This was sutured. We then tested it again. Put the anastomosis under water and produced air from below using an Asepto syringe. There were no leaks. After making sure we had a good tight anastomosis, I also brought some surrounding fat over the area where we had reinforced and put a couple more silks anteriorly. Left a 19 Blake drain through a separate stab incision through the right side, sutured in place with a 2-0 Prolene. Then used 2 sheets of Seprafilm by the omentum over the small bowel. Had a correct sponge, instrument, and needle count. Closure was a double loop of Maxon along with some interrupted #1 Vicryl, subcutaneous tissue closed with 2-0 Vicryl, and skin was closed with V-Loc subcuticular. Steri-Strip applied. Sterile dressing applied. Sent to recovery room in satisfactory condition. Tolerated the procedure well. K63.5, 44140

10) What are the codes for a 78-year-old patient who has had profound microcytic, hyperchromic anemia, initially presenting with a hemoglobin of 6.5. A few weeks ago, she was transfused, discharged, and then returned with a hemoglobin of 6.4 with recurrent anginal pectoris and marked fatigue. She reports having black tarry stool immediately prior to admission. The scope was passed through the oropharynx into the stomach. The esophagus was well seen and was normal. There was a small hiatal hernia but no evidence of erosions in the gastric mucosa. The body of the stomach distended. The instrument was withdrawn into the stomach at this point. The enteroscope was then passed into the descending duodenum and down to the jejunum. The patient was given oral contrast to facilitate visualization of the small bowel. No abnormalities or neoplasia. D50.8, K92.1, K44.9, I20.9, 43235

CPT GENITOURINARY QUIZ 33

1) What are the codes for a 37-year-old ESRD patient who is seen for insertion of dialysis catheter. Attention was directed to the right neck and with direct puncture the right internal jugular vein was cannulated with a guidewire. Advanced over the guidewire were two-vessel dilators, then the Schon temporary dialysis catheter advanced. N18.6, 36800

2) What are the codes for this 41-year-old with urodynamically documented intrinsic sphincter deficiency. Attention was turned to the anterior vaginal wall. The sling material was then prepared with packing on either side of the dissection. A strip of cadaveric fascia was incised for its width and tacked at each of the corners. A series of four interrupted sutures of 2-0 PDS were then used to tack the sling at the UVJ and down the urethra to minimize the risk of the sling rolling under the urethra. The sling was under minimal tension under the urethra. Generous purchases of the cadaveric fascia were taken and tacked. N36. 42, 57288

3) What are the codes for a 38-year-old patient who had a percutaneous nephrostomy due to hydronephrosis with right ureteral obstruction? N13.30, N13.8, 52334

4) What are the codes for a 32-year-old patient who had a scar in the right upper quadrant, and through that same scar the abdominal cavity was entered. Upon entering the abdominal cavity, the gallbladder was evaluated and was noted to be full of stones and phlegm. The operative cholangiogram showed some stenotic area along the common bile duct and the hepatic duct with some dilatation, but there was no obstruction. At this point the gallbladder was removed. K80.20, K83.1, 47605

5) What are the codes for this 23-year-old patient who has volunteered to be a living, related kidney donor to her brother, who suffers from end-stage renal disease? Z52.4, 50320

6) What are the codes for a 42-year-old patient who had fulguration of cancerous tumors in the urethra? C68.0, 53220

7) What are the codes for a 42-year-old patient who had calculus of the right kidney which was removed with ESWL? N20.0, 50590

8) What are the codes for 35-year-old unmarried patient who has 7 children. After obtaining informed consent and also discussing with the patient the alternatives, including natural family planning, birth control pills, tubal ligation, barrier methods of birth control, and vasectomy; the patient chose to continue with a vasectomy. In the operating room, the left vas deferens was identified and isolated adjacent to the scrotal skin. A 2.5-cm segment of vas deferens was then excised between hemostats. The ends of the vasa were then cauterized with Bovie electrocautery. The distal end was suture-ligated and folded back upon itself with 3-0 chromic. The proximal end was suture-ligated and then, using a second suture of 2-0 chromic, ligated and folded back upon itself. Next, attention was

directed to the right side where the procedure was performed, done in identical mirror-image fashion. Z3.02, 55250

9) What are the codes for this 38-year-old man with carcinoma of the prostate who is seen today for lymphadenectomy which was done by mobilizing pelvic tissue on both sides. Frozen section revealed these to be negative. The posterior urethra was now incised and there was retropubic resection of the prostate off the rectum. A portion of this ejaculatory duct was removed with the seminal vesicles, and the bladder neck was mobilized against some mild traction of the Foley, sparing about a 1-cm section of prostatic urethra. This was everted with 3-0 chromic sutures on the seromuscular layer and anastomosed to the urethra using the Greenfield suture guide. C61, 55842

10) What are the codes for a 41-year-old patient who had repair of an inguinal hernia and hydrocelectomy on both sides as well as orchiopexy on the right for undescended testis? K40.20, Q53.9, 54640, 49505

11) What are the codes for a 28-year-old patient with excessive bleeding due to menorrhagia. The patient was then placed in Trendelenburg. Endocervical D&C was then done. A hysteroscope was placed through the cervix into the uterus. The uterine cavity was examined. There was a questionable polyp versus just a tear of the superficial endometrium noted anteriorly. The remainder of the cavity seemed normal, with normal ostia. Sharp curettage was done, and a small amount of tissue was obtained. The cervix was examined, and the hysteroscope was removed. There was no evidence of any abnormalities in the cervical canal. Specimens were submitted to pathology. N92.0, 58558

12) What are the codes for a 25-year-old patient who had TAH-BSO for uterine fibroids, endometriosis stage 4 and menometrorrhagia? N80.0, D25.9, N92.0, 58150

13) What are the codes for a 34-year-old patient who had surgery in which peritoneal biopsies were obtained scopically. Cul-de-sac biopsy and peritoneal omental biopsies were obtained. Uterosacral ligaments were clamped, cut, and ligated bilaterally. Uterine vessels were clamped, cut, and ligated bilaterally. Vessels in the broad ligament were clamped, cut, and ligated. There was visualization of uterine fibroids and the uterus and left ovary were then removed. D25.9 58542

14) What are the codes for a 23-year-old patient who had a LEEP procedure today due to abnormal PAP which showed cervical dysplasia? Z01.42, N87.9, 57460

15) What are the codes for a 23-year-old patient who progressed to delivery; however, there was shoulder dystocia. Epsiotomy was performed. Forceps were used but did not work but shortly after with additional push, the baby was delivered. The baby was 10 pounds 3 ounces. O66.0, Z37.0, O66.5, 59409

16) What are the codes for a 21-year-old patient who received a repeat low-abdominal Pfannenstiel incision from previous c-section due to obstructed labor. The rectus muscles

were divided in the midline by sharp dissection. The lower uterine segment was carefully incised with a scalpel and extended laterally. A living female infant was delivered from the vertex right occipitotransverse position. The head was noted to be wedged into the pelvis but was easily elevated with a hand. The baby was suctioned and cried immediately. There was marked bleeding coming from the laceration of the left uterine artery which was sutured. The first layer of uterine closure was with running-locking #1 chromic catgut suture. The second layer was with imbricating #1 chromic catgut suture. O34.21, O64.0XX0, Z37.0, 59514, 35221

17) What are the codes for a 31-year-old patient who is seen in ER this morning complaining of intense pelvic pain with vaginal bleeding. The patient is 8 weeks pregnant. She denies any dizziness or shoulder pain. The patient had a c-section previously and 2 normal vaginal births prior to that. She had one miscarriage. The patient smokes and does drink regularly and is diabetic. The patient's mother was also positive for diabetes and COPD with asthma. ROS negative for all systems other than previously stated. Exam revealed a well-developed, well-nourished female in no acute distress with stable vital signs and afebrile. HENT WNL. Neck is supple without masses. Lungs clear. Heart shows regular rate and rhythm without murmur or gallop.Bowel sounds are present. Pelvic shows normal external genitalia. Cervix shows some bleeding. Slightly tender to motion. Uterus: Tender. Ectopic pregnancy cannot be ruled out. Patient had an ultrasound which demonstrated ruptured tubal ectopic pregnancy which was removed laparoscopically. J44.9, E11.9, O00.1, 99283, 59150

18) What are the codes for this 42-year-old patient who has been having trouble sleeping. It Using the laryngeal mirror, the adenoid tissue was found to be very enlarged and totally obstructing the back of the nose which was excised and sent to pathology for diagnosis. Using the electrocautery, the hypertrophic right tonsil was amputated and sent to pathology for diagnosis. The left tonsil was then seen to have purulent material and also hypertrophic; therefore it was also excised. J35.3, 42821

19) What are the codes for a 45-year-old patient who had a total thyroidectomy with modified radical neck dissection on the right due to carcinoma metastatic to cervical lymph nodes? C73, 196.0, 60254-RT

20) What are the codes for a 39-year-old patient who noticed a large lump in the left side of their neck. The large left thyroid lobe was dissected from its loose attachments laterally. This was sent for pathologic examination and found to be carcinoma. It was elected to proceed with a total thyroidectomy. The superior parathyroid gland was found, dissected off the thyroid gland, and left intact. C73, 60240

CPT NERVOUS/SENSES QUIZ 34

1) What are the codes for a 44-year-old patient who had epidural blocks to treat herniated discs at L4-S1? M51.27, 62311

2) What are the codes for a 61-year-old patient who has left lower extremity footdrop and received an EMG which was abnormal and confirmed peroneal nerve dysfunction on the left side at the fibular head and does not seem to suggest a problem regarding the L5 nerve root. M21.372, 95860-LT

3) What are the codes for a 37-year-old patient with chronic low back pain which is sympathetic. I have suggested to the patient that we go ahead and perform a rhizotomy. A line was drawn to mark the sacral ala and the medial and superior aspects of each transverse process. There was radiofrequency facet denervation from L1-S1. A total of 10 lesioning denervation rhizotomies sites were performed. M54.5, 63190

4) What are the codes for a 69-year-old patient who had excision of intervertebral discs C4-6 with arthrodesis using an anterior approach for spondylosis and displacement with myelopathy? M47.12, 22554X2

5) What are the codes for a 33-year-old patient who had release of right carpal tunnel? G56.01, 64721-RT

6) What are the codes for a 22-year-old patient who had left frontal burr hole for placement of ventriculostomy due to brain swelling suffered after falling from a roof? G93.6, 61210

7) What are the codes for a 42-year-old patient who had decompression at the L4-S1 levels due to severe back pain. The fusion was done using the posterior lumbar interbody technique with BAK instrumentation. X-rays were taken throughout the procedures with fluoroscopy. There was an abundant quantity of bone from the laminectomy, so no bone graft was needed from elsewhere. This bone graft was packed into the cage at the distal end and then the cage was inserted. The proximal end of the cage was then packed with bone as well. The same technique was then done on the right-hand side and the same technique was done at the L5-S1 level, for a total of four cages. Because this was a two-level cage procedure, the pedicle screw instrumentation was used to augment the stabilization. M54.5, 63051-50

8) What are the codes for a patient whose right eye was prepared and draped in the usual sterile fashion. Conjunctival incisions were made nasally and temporally, and a 4-mm infusion cannula was sutured into the inferotemporal quadrant 4 mm posterior to the limbus using a 4-0 Vicryl suture. After cannula tip placement in the vitreous cavity had been verified, infusion was begun. Supranasal and superotemporal sclerotomies were performed, and the trocar and cannula system was introduced to correct primary open-angle glaucoma, severe stage. The vitrectomy was performed. The posterior vitreous was not detached. It was elevated from the posterior pole and trimmed back into the far periphery. We then selected a biopsy site inferiorly and cut out a 2 x 2-mm piece of retina

at 6 o'clock at the border of infected and noninfected retina. There was no significant bleeding. We then performed a fluid-gas exchange, flatting the retina through the biopsy site. Laser was placed around the biopsy for 360 degrees to demarcate the peripheral retinitis. We then filled the eye with silicone oil. The sclerotomies were sutured shut with 7-0 Vicryl, and the conjunctiva was closed with 6-0 plain. Sub-Tenon's Ancef and Decadron were injected. The patient tolerated the procedure well and was returned to the recovery room in stable condition. H40.00X3, 65850-RT

9) What are the codes for this 48-year-old patient whose right eye was prepped and draped for the procedure. Chalazion forceps were used to grasp the upper right eyelid. The pretarsal conjunctival surface of the chalazion was incised. The contents of the chalazion were curetted. H00.00, 67800-RT

10) What are the codes for a 68-year-old patient who was seen for pseudophakic bullous keratopathy of left eye. Blepharostat was inserted and sutured to the episclera. A 7.5-mm trephine was then used for the recipient until penetration occurred. Curved corneal scissors to the right and left were used to completely excise the recipient button. The pupil was enlarged and small amounts of capsule and cortical material were also excised. The donor corneal button was transferred to the operative field, where it was secured. The intraocular Healon was evacuated and replaced with balanced salt solution. The blepharostat was removed and subconjunctival injections of gentamicin, Ancef and Celestone were given and a drop of Betagan 0.5% was instilled. H18.12, Z96.1, 65755-LT

11) What are the codes for this 47-year-old patient who had a amyloid pterygium marked and subconjunctival injection of 1% lidocaine with epinephrine. The pterygium of the left eye was then resected. The head of the pterygium was dissected off the cornea. A conjunctival graft measuring 10 × 8 mm was harvested from the superior bulbar conjunctiva and replanted. H11.012, 65426-LT

12) What are the codes for this 63-year-old patient who had the excess skin of upper lid of both eyes crease demarcated to repair paralytic ptosis. Utilizing sharp dissection, the eyelid skin and orbicularis were removed. H02.433, 67901-50

13) What are the codes for a 42-year-old patient who had a MSICS and capsulotomy of the nucleus, due to diabetic cataracts. A phacoemulsification tip was introduced and a large bowl sculpted. The remaining nucleus was brought into the anterior chamber, and with the pulse mode and phacoemulsification with high vacuum, the remaining nucleus was prolapsed and removed without complication. A posterior chamber lens implant of the appropriate power was placed. E11.36, 66984

14) What are the codes for this 47-year-old patient who had strabismus surgery two years ago and is seen today for the same which was for correction of monocular A pattern esotropia of the left eye? H50.022, 67331-LT, 67312-LT

15) What are the codes for this 64-year-old patient who had repair of retinal detachment with

single break of the right eye by cryothermy and photocoagulation? H33.011, 67101

16) What are the codes for a 61-year-old patient who has been experiencing slow, decreasing vision in the right eye secondary to punctate cataract formation. A fornix-based conjunctival flap was formed with Westcott scissors. Clear-cornea paracentesis wound was made. A crescent blade was used to fashion a scleral tunnel through which the anterior chamber was entered and anterior capsulotomy performed with a capsulorrhexis technique. The nucleus was hydrodissected with balanced salt solution and emulsified with the phacoemulsification device. The remaining cortex was removed using irrigation and aspiration. Using a smooth lens forceps, we introduced the lens into the eye. H25.093, 66982-RT

17) What are the codes for this 8-year-old patient seen today for chronic suppurative otitis media of both ears. Using the Zeiss operating microscope, the left tympanic membrane was visualized. The canal was cleaned of cerumen. A radial incision was made in the anteroinferior quadrant. "Glue" was found behind this ear, and this was suctioned. A 0.40 Shepard tube was put into place. Cortisporin Otic suspension drops were instilled, and a cotton ball was placed at the meatus. The right tympanic membrane was then visualized using the same Zeiss operating microscope. The canal was cleaned of cerumen. Using the laryngeal mirror, the adenoid tissue was found to be moderately enlarged but was not removed. H66.3X3, 381.81, 69433-50, 69990

18) What are the codes for a 6-year-old patient who had bilateral myringotomy and tubes for chronic Eustachian tube dysfunction and recurrent acute serous otitis media? H69.83, H65.06, 69433-50

19) What are the codes for patient in whom a scope was used to visualize and inspect. There was a small retention cyst noted arising from the anterior medial wall of the left maxillary sinus which was filled full of a whitish glue-type material and inflamed, although it was nonpurulent and so an antrostomy was performed to remove it in addition to ethmoidectomy. J34.1, 31254, 31267

20) What are the codes for this 12-year-old patient who has continued to have problems with acute serous otitis media so an anterior inferior myringotomy was performed on the left tympanic membrane. An Armstrong tube was placed and ear drops following into the canal. With the use of an operating microscope, an anterior inferior myringotomy was performed on the right tympanic membrane, and through it no effusion was suctioned. An Armstrong tube was placed and ear drops following into the canal. H65.03, 69433-50, 69990

TEST 4 ANSWERS

1. What are the codes for this 8-year-old patient seen today for chronic suppurative otitis media of both ears. Using the Zeiss operating microscope, the left tympanic membrane was visualized. The canal was cleaned of cerumen. A radial incision was made in the anteroinferior quadrant. "Glue" was found behind this ear, and this was suctioned. A 0.40 Shepard tube was put into place. Cortisporin Otic suspension drops were instilled, and a cotton ball was placed at the meatus. The right tympanic membrane was then visualized using the same Zeiss operating microscope. The canal was cleaned of cerumen. Using the laryngeal mirror, the adenoid tissue was found to be moderately enlarged but was not removed. H66.3X3, 381.81, 69433-50, 69990
2. What are the codes for a 6-year-old patient who had bilateral myringotomy and tubes for chronic Eustachian tube dysfunction and recurrent acute serous otitis media? H69.83, H65.06, 69433-50
3. What are the codes for a patient whose right eye was prepared and draped in the usual sterile fashion. Conjunctival incisions were made nasally and temporally, and a 4-mm infusion cannula was sutured into the inferotemporal quadrant 4 mm posterior to the limbus using a 4-0 Vicryl suture. After cannula tip placement in the vitreous cavity had been verified, infusion was begun. Supranasal and superotemporal sclerotomies were performed, and the trocar and cannula system was introduced to correct primary open-angle glaucoma, severe stage. The vitrectomy was performed. The posterior vitreous was not detached. It was elevated from the posterior pole and trimmed back into the far periphery. We then selected a biopsy site inferiorly and cut out a 2 x 2-mm piece of retina at 6 o'clock at the border of infected and noninfected retina. There was no significant bleeding. We then performed a fluid-gas exchange, flatting the retina through the biopsy site. Laser was placed around the biopsy for 360 degrees to demarcate the peripheral retinitis. We then filled the eye with silicone oil. The sclerotomies were sutured shut with 7-0 Vicryl, and the conjunctiva was closed with 6-0 plain. Sub-Tenon's Ancef and Decadron were injected. The patient tolerated the procedure well and was returned to the recovery room in stable condition. H40.00X3, 65850-RT
4. An incision was made supertemporally to expose the right medial rectus muscle which was disinserted from the globe and reattached to the glob for treatment of esotropia. The right superior rectus muscle was then hooked to the muscle, disinserted and reattached to the globe. The left medial rectus muscle was then recessed in a similar manner. H50.011, 67312-RT, 67314-RT
5. What are the codes for a 68-year-old patient who was seen for pseudophakic bullous keratopathy of left eye. Blepharostat was inserted and sutured to the episclera. A 7.5-mm trephine was then used for the recipient until penetration occurred. Curved corneal scissors to the right and left were used to completely excise the recipient button. The pupil was enlarged and small amounts of capsule and cortical material were also excised. The donor corneal button was transferred to the operative field, where it was secured. The intraocular Healon was evacuated and replaced with balanced salt solution. The blepharostat was removed and subconjunctival injections of gentamicin, Ancef and Celestone were given and a drop of Betagan 0.5% was instilled. H18.12, Z96.1, 65755-LT

6. What are the codes for this 47-year-old patient who had a conjunctival pterygium marked and subconjunctival injection of 1% lidocaine with epinephrine. The pterygium was then resected. The head of the pterygium was dissected off the cornea. A conjunctival graft measuring 10 × 8 mm was harvested from the superior bulbar conjunctiva and replanted. H11.041, 65426
7. What are the codes for this 63-year-old patient who had the excess skin of upper lid of both eyes crease demarcated to repair paralytic ptosis. Utilizing sharp dissection, the eyelid skin and orbicularis were removed. H02.433, 67901-50
8. What are the codes for a 61-year-old patient who has been experiencing slow, decreasing vision in the right eye secondary to punctate cataract formation. A fornix-based conjunctival flap was formed with Westcott scissors. Clear-cornea paracentesis wound was made. A crescent blade was used to fashion a scleral tunnel through which the anterior chamber was entered and anterior capsulotomy performed with a capsulorrhexis technique. The nucleus was hydrodissected with balanced salt solution and emulsified with the phacoemulsification device. The remaining cortex was removed using irrigation and aspiration. Using a smooth lens forceps, we introduced the lens into the eye. H25.093, 66982-RT
9. What are the codes for a 61-year-old patient who has left lower extremity footdrop and received an EMG which was abnormal and confirmed peroneal nerve dysfunction on the left side at the fibular head and does not seem to suggest a problem regarding the L5 nerve root. 736.79, 95860-LT
10. What are the codes for a 37-year-old patient with chronic low back pain which is sympathetic. I have suggested to the patient that we go ahead and perform a rhizotomy. A line was drawn to mark the sacral ala and the medial and superior aspects of each transverse process. There was radiofrequency facet denervation from L1-S1. A total of 10 lesioning denervation rhizotomies sites were performed. M54.5, 63190
11. What are the codes for a 42-year-old patient who had decompression at the L4-S1 levels due to severe back pain. The fusion was done using the posterior lumbar interbody technique with BAK instrumentation. X-rays were taken throughout the procedures with fluoroscopy. There was an abundant quantity of bone from the laminectomy, so no bone graft was needed from elsewhere. This bone graft was packed into the cage at the distal end and then the cage was inserted. The proximal end of the cage was then packed with bone as well. The same technique was then done on the right-hand side and the same technique was done at the L5-S1 level, for a total of four cages. Because this was a two-level cage procedure, the pedicle screw instrumentation was used to augment the stabilization. M54.5, 63051-50
12. What are the codes for this 42-year-old patient who has been having trouble sleeping. It Using the laryngeal mirror, the adenoid tissue was found to be very enlarged and totally obstructing the back of the nose which was excised and sent to pathology for diagnosis. Using the electrocautery, the hypertrophic right tonsil was amputated and sent to pathology for diagnosis. The left tonsil was then seen to have purulent material and also hypertrophic; therefore it was also excised. J35.3, 42821
13. What are the codes for a 45-year-old patient who had a total thyroidectomy with modified radical neck dissection on the right due to carcinoma metastatic to cervical lymph nodes? C73, 196.0, 60254-RT
14. What are the codes for a 47-year-old patient with ESRD. The patient had no superficial

veins large enough on the distal forearm that would suffice for bypass and AV fistula creation. An incision was made in the antecubital fossa, dissection carried down to identify the brachial artery and the basilic vein . Second small incision was made on the volar aspect of the forearm distally and graft was sutured in the vein in end-to-side fashion with running 6-0 Prolene suture. Attention was directed to the brachial artery, vascular clamp was applied, arteriotomy made and a 4-mm end of the graft was sutured end-to-side to the artery. Attention was directed to the right neck and by direct puncture the right internal jugular vein was cannulated with a guidewire and two-vessel dilators advanced, then the temporary dialysis catheter advanced over the guidewire and superior cava. N18.6, 36819, 36825, 36558, 36147

15. What are the codes for a 23-year-old patient who progressed to delivery; however, there was shoulder dystocia. Epsiotomy was performed. Forceps were used but did not work but shortly after with additional push, the baby was delivered. The baby was 10 pounds 3 ounces. O66.0, Z37.0, O66.5, 59409
16. What are the codes for a 21-year-old patient who received a repeat low-abdominal Pfannenstiel incision from previous c-section due to obstructed labor. The rectus muscles were divided in the midline by sharp dissection. The lower uterine segment was carefully incised with a scalpel and extended laterally. A living female infant was delivered from the vertex right occipitotransverse position. The head was noted to be wedged into the pelvis but was easily elevated with a hand. The baby was suctioned and cried immediately. There was marked bleeding coming from the laceration of the left uterine artery which was sutured. The first layer of uterine closure was with running-locking #1 chromic catgut suture. The second layer was with imbricating #1 chromic catgut suture. O34.21, O64.0XX0, Z37.0, 59514, 35221
17. What are the codes for a 31-year-old patient who is seen in ER this morning complaining of intense pelvic pain with vaginal bleeding. The patient is 8 weeks pregnant. She denies any dizziness or shoulder pain. The patient had a c-section previously and 2 normal vaginal births prior to that. She had one miscarriage. The patient smokes and does drink regularly and is diabetic. The patient's mother was also positive for diabetes and COPD with asthma. ROS negative for all systems other than previously stated. Exam revealed a well-developed, well-nourished female in no acute distress with stable vital signs and afebrile. HENT WNL. Neck is supple without masses. Lungs clear. Heart shows regular rate and rhythm without murmur or gallop.Bowel sounds are present. Pelvic shows normal external genitalia. Cervix shows some bleeding. Slightly tender to motion. Uterus: Tender. Ectopic pregnancy cannot be ruled out. Patient had an ultrasound which demonstrated ruptured tubal ectopic pregnancy which was removed laparoscopically. J44.9, E11.9, O00.1, 99283, 59150
18. What are the codes for a 25-year-old patient who had cerclage due to cervical incompetence? N88.3, 57700
19. What are the codes for this 47-year-old patient who had an exploratory laparotomy. revealed a large left 15-cm ovarian mass in the right adnexa.. To facilitate dissection of the large left ovarian mass, we dissected the left ureter which was occluded and adherent to the mass. We were eventually able to completely perform extrafascial hysterectomy, and the uterus (filled with fibroids), large left adnexal mass, right ovarian endometrioma, and tubes were removed as a single specimen. N83.20, N80.1, D25.9, 58150

20. What are the codes for a 29-year-old patient who had scopic removal of a polyp with D&C on the vaginal wall due to postmenopausal bleeding with glandular dilatation and proliferative endometrium? N95.0, N84.2, 58558
21. What are the codes for a 27-year-old patient with ectopic pregnancy which required a salpingectomy on the left? O00.9, 59120-LT
22. What are the codes for a 31-year-old patient with incompetent cervix at 8 weeks which required a McDonald cerclage placement? O34.31, 59320
23. What are the codes for this 38-year-old man with carcinoma of the prostate who is seen today for lymphadenectomy which was done by mobilizing pelvic tissue on both sides. Frozen section revealed these to be negative. The posterior urethra was now incised and there was retropubic resection of the prostate off the rectum. A portion of this ejaculatory duct was removed with the seminal vesicles, and the bladder neck was mobilized against some mild traction of the Foley, sparing about a 1-cm section of prostatic urethra. This was everted with 3-0 chromic sutures on the seromuscular layer and anastomosed to the urethra using the Greenfield suture guide. C61, 55842
24. What are the codes for a 59-year-old who was found to have prostate cancer. Routine bilateral pelvic lymph node dissections were performed. The lymph node packets were sent for final histopathologic diagnosis. Retropubic dissection of the prostate was then performed rectopubically. C61, 55845
25. What are the codes for a 41-year-old patient who had repair of an inguinal hernia and hydrocelectomy on both sides as well as orchiopexy on the right for undescended testis? K40.20, Q53.10, 49505, 54640
26. What are the codes for a 48-year-old patient who had cystoscopy and ureteroscopy which revealed ureteral calculus in the left which was treated with lithotripsy and basket extraction with bilateral retrograde pyelograms? N20.1, 52353-LT
27. What are the codes for a 53-year-old male who has BPH and also has recurrent UTIs now. Today he had TURP and removal of prostatic chips which were occluding the bladder vault using a resectoscope. A 22-French Foley catheter 30-cc balloon was inserted. The balloon was inflated to 55 cc. The catheter was irrigated. The return was blood tinged. The catheter was connected to straight drainage. N40.1, N39.0, 52630
28. What are the codes for a 37-year-old ESRD patient who is seen for insertion of dialysis catheter. Attention was directed to the right neck and with direct puncture the right internal jugular vein was cannulated with a guidewire. Advanced over the guidewire were two-vessel dilators, then the Schon temporary dialysis catheter advanced. N18.6, 36800
29. Crushing of a stone in the bladder and washing out the fragments through a catheter is known as what? LITHOTRIPSY
30. What are the codes for this 41-year-old with urodynamically documented intrinsic sphincter deficiency. Attention was turned to the anterior vaginal wall. The sling material was then prepared with packing on either side of the dissection. A strip of cadaveric fascia was incised for its width and tacked at each of the corners. A series of four interrupted sutures of 2-0 PDS were then used to tack the sling at the UVJ and down the urethra to minimize the risk of the sling rolling under the urethra. The sling was under minimal tension under the urethra. Generous purchases of the cadaveric fascia were taken and tacked. The sling was well positioned but not under any tension from the urethra. The bladder was then inspected with a cystoscope. The urethra was normal. There was no evidence of any trauma to the urethra or bladder. The urine was clear. N36.4, 57288

31. What are the codes for this 78-year-old patient status post multiple colon resections for carcinoma. She has received radiation chemotherapy and was recently noted on CT scan to have bilateral hydronephrosis, right worse than left, and therefore for further evaluation underwent the above procedure. Findings were Retroperitoneal fibrosis. The cystoscope was introduced per urethra without any difficulty. Under vision it was placed into the bladder. There was no evidence of stone or tumor. Retrograde pyelogram was undertaken. Cystoscope was removed and the ureteroscope was inserted under direct vision and with hydrostatic dilatation it was advanced up to the point of obstruction where complete obstruction was visualized secondary to extrinsic compression likely from mild retroperitoneal fibrosis. A guidewire was inserted through the working port of the ureteroscope and advanced up the collecting system as confirmed under fluoroscopic control. Retrograde pyelogram demonstrated the guidewire to be in the renal collecting system. The ureteroscope was then removed and the cystoscope was reintroduced over the guidewire. A 6-French, 24-cm double-J stent was inserted over the guidewire and advanced up the collecting system as confirmed under fluoroscopic control. The string was cut from the stent and then the guidewire was removed. N13.30, N13.8, Z85.038, 52341, 52332, 74420
32. What are the codes for a 42-year-old patient who had calculus of the right kidney which was removed with ESWL? N20.0, 50590
33. What are the codes for a 45-year-old patient who was diagnosed with carcinoma of the bladder. Resectoscope was placed and cystopanendoscopy was performed. The urethra was within normal limits. There was a large fungating bladder carcinoma which was obviously necrotic. The tumor extended to the entire surface of the left lateral wall and was resected using the resectoscope. No other lesions were identified. A separate biopsy of the prostatic urethra was obtained. The chips were removed and the bladder was once again inspected and found to be free of evidence of injury, and the ureteral orifices were intact at the conclusion of the procedure. C67.2, 52240
34. The patient was brought to the operative suite, prepped and draped in the usual manner. A right paramedian incision was made basically just above the umbilicus. Bleeding controlled with electrocautery. The rectus muscle was split and the peritoneal cavity was entered. We used 0.25% Marcaine with epinephrine prior to making the incision. We had to lengthen it to get some exposure. I had problems finding the appendix, as the appendix came off and was tethered into the retroperitoneal area. I asked Dr. Vaughan to assist for exposure. We were able to basically mobilize the right colon and then we dissected it from the cecum but once we found it, it was coming out fairly high off of the cecum. We tied it twice, divided it, cauterized the tip, then dissected, used the LigaSure for the mesentery and dissected it off of the duodenum. All bleeding was controlled. We irrigated thoroughly with saline, made certain that the bowel was properly placed back into the abdomen. Omentum was placed over it. We used a sheet of Seprafilm over the cecum and the right colon and another one over the omentum. The sponge, instrument, and needle count was correct and then we closed with double looped Maxon for the fascia, subcutaneous tissue closed with 2-0 Vicryl and skin was closed with V-Loc. Steri-Strip was applied. Sterile dressing was applied. Sent to recovery room in satisfactory condition. Tolerated the procedure well. K35.80, 44140
35. What are the codes for a 54-year-old patient who had a Roux-en-Y reconstruction following a complete gastrectomy for stomach cancer? C16.9, 43621

36. What are the codes for a 57-year-old patient who had a diverting colostomy with Hartmann pouch with sepsis and excision and debridement of a sacral decubitus ulcer stage 3 with ostectomy which had become necrotic . L89.153, A41.9, 44143, 15933
37. What are the codes for a 41-year-old patient who was complaining of a bulging mass in the right side of the abdomen which correlated with a ventral hernia of the right abdominal wall. At this point, plication of the rectus abdominis muscle was done and Marlex mesh was applied. K43.9, 49560, 49568
38. What are the codes for a 52-year-old patient who was placed in the supine position and the F2 focus of the MSL 5000 lithotriptor, shock wave lithotripsy was started at 17 kV and went up to 23, where a total of 3000 shocks were given to the stone with fragmentation of this left renal calculi. N20.0, 50590
39. The patient brought to the operative suite, prepped and draped in the usual manner. Timeout was accomplished. Preoperative antibiotics were given and SCDs applied. Low midline incision was made, bleeding controlled with electrocautery. Fascia divided and peritoneal cavity was entered. Bookwalter retractor was placed. We able to see the area where India ink had been injected in the sigmoid colon. We used the GIA proximally and distally, divided the mesentery using the ligature. One vessel was stick-tied with 3-0 silk. We then opened the specimen and there was no polyp in it, so we then opened the bowel proximally thinking that the polyp might be just above where we had resected and, indeed, we found the polyp on a very long stalk. Resected another portion of the colon, then used a pursestringer. Placed a pursestring proximally. Used the dilators. A 29 EEA was selected. We tied the pursestring and then brought the EEA in from below, made the anastomosis. We then tested it, and there were some air bubbles, and so we had to use 3-0 silk. There was a small rent in the anastomosis on the right lateral side. This was sutured. We then tested it again. Put the anastomosis under water and produced air from below using an Asepto syringe. There were no leaks. After making sure we had a good tight anastomosis, I also brought some surrounding fat over the area where we had reinforced and put a couple more silks anteriorly. Left a 19 Blake drain through a separate stab incision through the right side, sutured in place with a 2-0 Prolene. Then used 2 sheets of Seprafilm by the omentum over the small bowel. Had a correct sponge, instrument, and needle count. Closure was a double loop of Maxon along with some interrupted #1 Vicryl, subcutaneous tissue closed with 2-0 Vicryl, and skin was closed with V-Loc subcuticular. Steri-Strip applied. Sterile dressing applied. Sent to recovery room in satisfactory condition. Tolerated the procedure well. D12.6, 44140
40. What are the codes for an 8-year-old patient who had suffered second and third degrees burns over both fronts of her legs four months ago which totaled 15% of TBSA with 7% third degree? She is seen today for STSG from her back to cover the burned area. T24.302S, L90.5, 15002, 15100, 15101X2, 15003X2
41. What is an I&D? INCISION AND DRAINAGE
42. What are the codes for a 32-year-old patient who had 17 skin tags removed electrosurgically? L91.9, 11200, 11201
43. What are the codes for a 38-year-old female who had a mastectomy of both breasts which included removal of the axillary lymph nodes due to carcinoma of the breast with a TRAM? C50.919, 19307-50, 19367-50
44. What are the codes when a pathologist finds malignancy from a needle core biopsy of the left breast of a 32-year-old woman? C50.919, 19100-LT

45. What are the codes for an 82-year-old nursing home patient who had excision of a sacral pressure ulcer stage 2 repaired with suturing and requiring an ostectomy? L89.152, 15933
46. What are the codes for a 49-year-old patient who was involved in a car accident and suffered extensive lacerations and broken collarbone? The patient had a BAC level of 1.0 as he has suffered for many years with alcoholism and went on a binge today. Lacerations were numerous including a 3.0 cm laceration of the right forearm which required layered closure, a 5.5 cm laceration of the right thigh which required retention sutures and ligation of arteries, 4.8 cm laceration of the chest which required simple closure but extensive debridement due to glass fragments, a 2.8 cm laceration of the right cheek which required layered closure, and a 3.0 cm laceration of the left thigh which required retention sutures. S51.811A, S71.111A, S21.119A, S01.411A, S71.112A, 810.00, , 12034, 13121, 12052
47. What are the codes for a 44-year-old patient who is seen today for the first time with a history and exam that were expanded problem focused and who had a 3.2-cm mass of the back which was infected and required drainage which was found to be a sebaceous cyst? L72.3, 10061, 99202-25
48. What are the codes for a 15-year-old patient who was seen in the emergency room due to complaints of severe abdominal pain and hemoptysis? The patient was found to have Staph food poisoning and discharged with prescriptions. The history was expanded problem focused and the exam was problem focused. A05.0, 99281
49. What are the codes for a pathologist who performs the pathological review of the two biopsies of specimens from Moh's surgery for a 4.2 cm lesion on the back of a 48-year-old man? L98.9, 88305X2
50. What are the codes for a 64-year-old patient with a history of insulin-dependent diabetes mellitus, coronary artery disease, chronic renal failure and heart failure who was initially admitted for congestive heart failure and nonhealing bilateral mid-foot ulcers treated for years with debridement and whirlpool. The patient was readmitted for acute diabetic right foot to be treated with incision and drainage of his right foot and first ray amputation but the infection had spread so right below-knee amputation was performed. 858.9, 250380, L97.429, L97.419, I25.9, I50.9, Z79.4, T79.8XXA, 27598-RT
51. What are the codes for a 67-year-old patient who is seen today for pleural effusion secondary to small cell carcinoma of the upper left lung with tube thoracostomy including indwelling cathether? J91.0, C34.12, 32550-LT, 32551-LT
52. What are the codes for this 52-year-old patient who has a history of pulmonary nodule in the left lung? She was seen today for a CT of the Chest and Adrenals with oral and intravenous contrast. Today there is a 2-cm area of parenchymal density which has the appearance of interstitial changes without findings of significant nodule or mass. This finding can relate to scarring. There is no other nodule, mass, or effusion. No evidence of adenopathy in the mediastinum. The heart and great vessels are normal in appearance. No findings with the liver, spleen, kidneys, adrenals, or pancreas. Z12.2, 71260, 74262
53. What are the codes for a 71-year-old patient who has a long history of lung disease due to being a lifelong smoker. History of hypertension. The patient also had COPD and asthma with bullous emphysema. A PET scan was reviewed by the physician and revealed that she has a 3.5-cm nodule in the upper left lobe which is malignant. A

lobectomy was performed. I10, Z86.79, Z87.891, J43.8, J44.9, C34.10, 78811-26, 32480-LT

54. What are the codes for an 18-year-old patient who has trouble breathing due to airway obstruction. It was found that this is due to turbinate hypertrophy and deviated septum protruding into the left nasal airway for which a septoplasty and bilateral turbinectomy was performed. J34.3, Q67.4, 30130-50, 30520
55. What are the codes for a 38-year-old patient who presents with the complaint of SOB and dyspnea with wheezing that began approximately four hours ago and has worsened? She is seen in the emergency room today. Her medical history showed a history of asthma. The patient states that she had a cough for the past day but she denies any other problems. She denies any fever or chills. She denies any chest pain or palpitations. The patient had an asthma attack a month ago which required hospitalization and treatment. The patient has no other past surgical history. The patient does have HTN and hypercholesterolemia. The patient lives alone and she works at a local school. She has smoked for more than 20 years. Her father is deceased due to emphysema. ROS shows that the patient has no problems in any system including no abdominal pain, chest pain, or edema other than previously mentioned. Physical exam showed the patient to be tachypneic. She is well developed and well nourished with respiratory rate of 20 and blood pressure of 124/86. HEENT is normocephalic and atraumatic. Pupils equal and round, regular, reactive to light. Extraocular muscles intact. Nares and oropharynx negative. Neck is supple; no JVD, no lymphadenopathy, no carotid bruits, no thyromegaly. Lungs reveal bilateral wheeze diffusely. There are some decreased breath sounds bilaterally. No rhonchi. Cardiovascular: Regular rate and rhythm, without murmurs, gallops, or rubs. Normal S1 and S2. No S3, S4. Abdomen: Normal active bowel sounds, soft, nontender, nondistended. No hepatosplenomegaly. Extremities: No cyanosis, clubbing or edema. Today in the emergency room the patient received 4 nebulization treatments for her acute exacerbation of her asthma but continued to be hypoxic with room air oxygen saturation of 84%. She had some slight improvement in her wheeze with the nebulization treatments but without further improvement she was admitted to the hospital to be continued on Solu-Medrol 125 mg IV and supplemental O2. E78.0, I10, J44.1, 99285
56. What are the codes for this 41-year-old patient who had an esophagoscopy and microlaryngoscopy of the neck to determine if there was cancer secondary to lung cancer. The scope was advanced into the cervical esophagus which was found to be normal. It was noticed that there was tumor involving the anterior wall of the right portion of the neck extending approximately 1 cm below the pharyngeal epiglottic fold and into the hypopharyngeal wall of which a sample was obtained. The specimen was found to be malignant.C78.89, C34.90, 43202, 31510
57. What are the codes for a 73-year-old patient with a history of aortic valve replacement and severe cardiomyopathy, chronic left bundle-branch block and diabetes who presents after having experience arrest early this morning characterized earlier by difficulty breathing and chest pain. The patient was cardioverted multiple times by EMTs and placed in ICU where he was seen several times from 8:00 am to 9:00 am, 11:30 to 12:45, and 4:15 pm to 5:30 pm but remained mostly unresponsive. Subsequent rhythm was sinus tachycardiac with a left bundle-branch block. He had a cardiac catheterization at the time of aortic valve replacement which showed normal coronary vessels three years ago. The patient does drink and smoke occasionally. His father died of a heart attack at age

75. ROS was unobtainable as the patient was not responsive. Exam showed blood pressure of 145/87, Pulse was 108 and respirations are 12 on ventilator. The patient is afebrile. HEENT show PERRLA. Neck is supple. Carotids have diminished upstroke without bruits. Lungs are clear. Anteriorly heart is tachycardiac . There is a prosthetic S2. The abdomen is soft and nontender without masses. Extremities have trace edema. Distal pulses are present. Neurologic exam: The patient is unresponsive. EKG shows sinus tachycardia with left bundle-branch block. Neurological and pulmonary evals are recommends. EKG should be repeated. Possible catheterization should be performed. I42.5, I44.7, I46.9, R00.0, E11.9, Z98.89, Z82.49, Z94.1, F17.200, 99291, 99292X5

58. What are the codes for a 49-year-old patient who had a permanent pacemaker implanted with leads placed into the right ventricle and right atrium due to bradycardia. A pocket was made in the left anterior chest wall into which the pulse generator was inserted. R00.1, 33208
59. What are the codes for a 55-year-old patient who had an acute MI with edema and received an intracorporeal left ventricular assist device as a bridge to cardiac transplantation several months ago. Now, after 100 days of support, the left ventricular assist device malfunctioned and the pump had to be replaced. Z45.09, 33982
60. What are the codes for a 47-year-old patient with renal failure requiring hemodialysis so an AV cannula was placed for access? N19, 36810

OTHER BOOKS BY DR. LYN OLSEN

AVAILABLE NOW AT AMAZON.COM

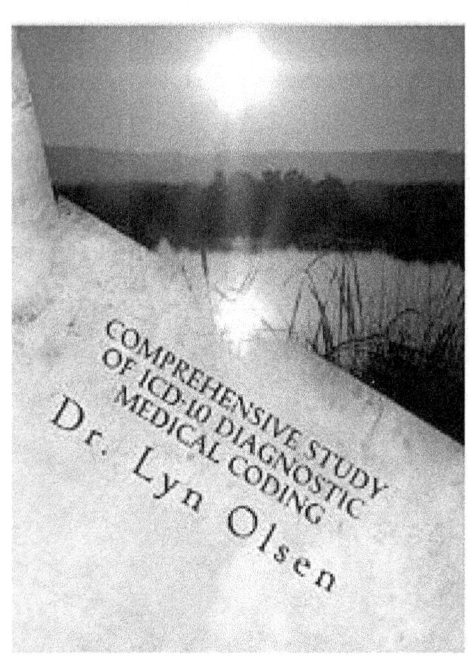

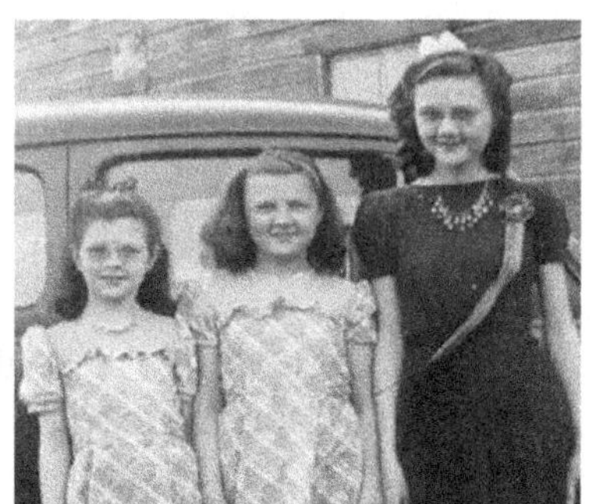

THE THREE SISTERS TRIED AND TRUE RECIPES OF BUTTE MONTANA

DR. LYN OLSEN

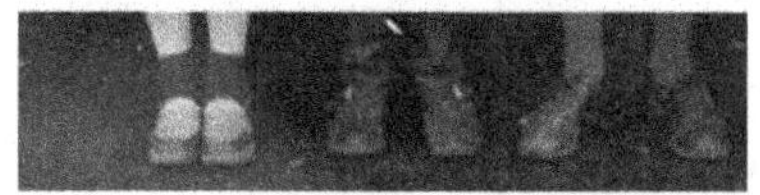

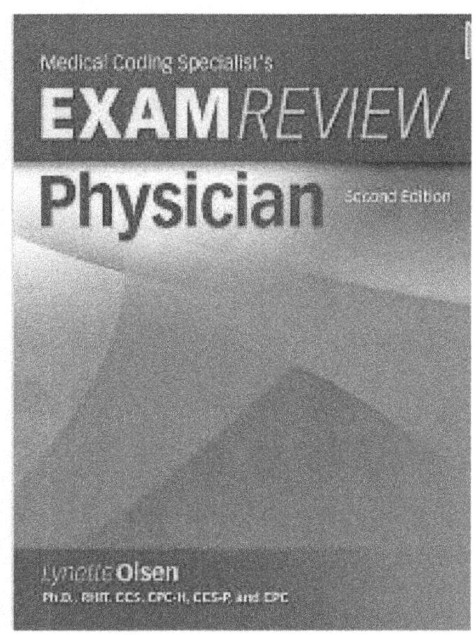

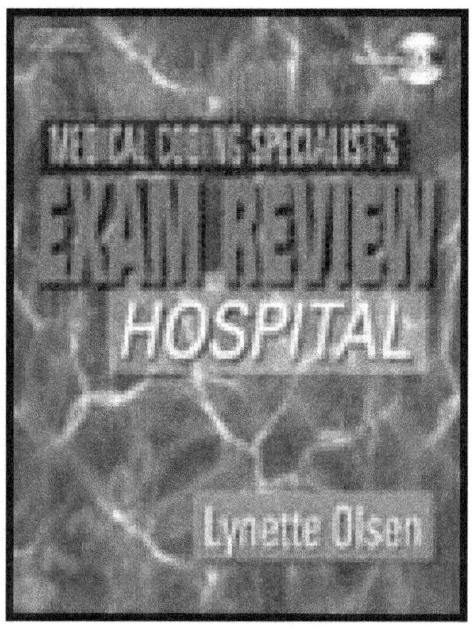

www.ingramcontent.com/pod-product-compliance
Lightning Source LLC
Chambersburg PA
CBHW082118210326
41599CB00031B/5806

* 9 7 8 0 6 9 2 5 7 3 2 8 0 *